Management of Urology

Series Editors
Sanchia S. Goonewardene, Norfolk and Norwich University Hospital
Norwich, UK
Raj Persad, North Bristol NHS Trust
BRISTOL, UK

This series addresses the need for an increase in the quantity of literature focused upon the effects of cancer in urology. Books within it will draw attention to the management of subtype specific urology cancer patients at each step of their pathway with suggestions on how care can potentially be improved. Therefore, it is of interest to a range of trainee and practicing physicians in a range of disciplines including urology oncology, specialist nurse and general practitioners.

Selcuk Sarikaya · Giorgio Ivan Russo
David Ralph
Editors

Andrology and Sexual Medicine

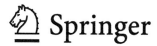 Springer

Editors
Selcuk Sarikaya
Department of Urology
Gulhane Research and Training Hospital
University of Health Sciences
Ankara, Turkey

Giorgio Ivan Russo
Department of Urology
University of Catania
Catania, Italy

David Ralph
Department of Urology
University College London Hospitals
London, UK

ISSN 2730-6372   ISSN 2730-6380   (electronic)
Management of Urology
ISBN 978-3-031-12048-0   ISBN 978-3-031-12049-7   (eBook)
https://doi.org/10.1007/978-3-031-12049-7

This Springer imprint is published by the registered company Springer Nature Switzerland AG
The registered company address is: Gewerbestrasse 11, 6330 Cham, Switzerland

Contents

Introduction, Epidemiology and Etiology of Sexual Dysfunctions in Men and Women

Joana Carvalho and Borja García-Gómez

Abstract

The epidemiology and etiology of male and female sexual dysfunctions should be addressed within a comprehensive biopsychosocial perspective. This perspective considers the interaction between the organic, psychological and cultural factors shaping human sexual response and functioning, allowing for more complete and tailored interventions. In this chapter, we will provide an overview of the epidemiology and etiology of male and female sexual dysfunctions, considering their position within a medical and a psychosocial framework, and further present evidence-based etiological and maintenance factors specific to men and women's sexual difficulties. We also discuss the interplay of the medical and psychosocial spaces and how both spaces can improve healthcare in the context of sexual dysfunctions. We stress current limitations in the field of epidemiology and etiology of sexual dysfunctions, such as the great gap in evidence regarding sexual and gender minorities, or the lack of a cultural frame regarding how epidemiology and etiology have been approached in sexual dysfunctions research.

Sexual Dysfunctions in the Biopsychosocial Context

Sexual dysfunctions in men and women are believed to be better approached by a biopsychosocial perspective. This perspective brings together the organic, psychological, and social components of sexuality, considering their interaction in the

J. Carvalho (✉)
Centro de Psicologia da Universidade do Porto, Faculdade de Psicologia e de Ciências da Educação da Universidade do Porto, Porto, Portugal

B. García-Gómez
Urology Department, Hospital Universitario 12 de Octubre and Hospital Universitario HM Montepríncipe, Madrid, Spain

© The Author(s), under exclusive license to Springer Nature Switzerland AG 2022
S. Sarikaya et al. (eds.), *Andrology and Sexual Medicine*, Management of Urology, https://doi.org/10.1007/978-3-031-12049-7_1

etiology, maintenance, and adaptation to sexual dysfunctions. The definition of sexual health established by the World Health Organization (WHO) has greatly contributed to the communication and partnership between different scientific areas. The concept of sexual health, defined as a state of physical, emotional, mental, and social well-being in the way individuals experience their sexuality, rather than the mere absence of physical illness or dysfunction [1], has promoted the dialog between medical and social sciences. This biopsychosocial perspective leads us to the understanding of the individuals in their context, which necessarily involves the consideration of background variables, including individuals' historical and even political scene, in the expression of sexual difficulties and their treatment. Currently, several scientific and professional organizations embrace this biopsychosocial dimension, which has echoed in the way we look at the etiology and/or maintenance of sexual dysfunctions. The etiological aspects are paramount in the way we design the therapeutic plan; an integrative view of the organic, psychological, and social aspects regarding the etiology of sexual dysfunctions will result in a more careful and refined analysis of the predisposition and maintenance mechanisms of sexual dysfunctions. Eventually, that will improve the definition of the therapeutic targets; therapeutic targets will be adjusted to individuals' context, and, therefore, treatments may have better chances of success.

In this chapter, we propose to present the epidemiology of male and female sexual dysfunctions, acknowledging that the evidence includes both clinical populations, i.e., those who received a formally recognized diagnosis, and data collected from the general/non-clinical population. In the last one, the concept of sexual difficulty, rather than sexual dysfunction, has empirical value and gives us a broader view of how individuals experience their sexuality. Additionally, the etiological aspects will be considered, not only from an organic and medical perspective but also from a psychosocial view. Specificities regarding sexual dysfunctions in men and women, as well as etiological aspects regarding particular sexual conditions, will be considered as well. In the end, we hope to present some remarks on the interplay role of the medical and psychosocial aspects in order to promote lines of action for clinical practice.

Epidemiology of Women's Sexual Dysfunctions

The estimated prevalence of female sexual dysfunction is quite high, with around 40% of women reporting one or more sexual complaints [2]. Evidence about sexual desire difficulties in Britain indicates that 34.2% of women report low sexual desire; the highest prevalence is found in the range between 55 and 64 years old [3]. In Canada, similar data show that 40% of women between 40 and 59 years old report low sexual desire [4]. If we consider data regarding the difficulty in spontaneous versus responsive sexual desire (data from Flanders), 19% of women report lack of spontaneous sexual desire, 14% report difficulties in responsive desire, and 9% report difficulties in both [5]. It is important to mention that 15% to 35% of women report a discrepancy between their sexual desire and their partner's sexual desire

[3], and the distress associated with this discrepancy is a variable of great clinical interest [6]. Complaints of low sexual desire are expected to be the most frequent sexual complaints in women, although in non-Western countries complaints associated with orgasm or arousal/lubrication difficulties are the most frequent [7]. Additionally, women with low sexual desire are nine times more likely to report sexual arousal problems [8]. Vaginal lubrication difficulties are seen in 8% to 28% of women [9, 10], although the associated distress rates are only 3.3% [10]. With regard to Persistent Genital Arousal Disorder (PGAD) its prevalence is unknown, although it is estimated that between 0.6% to 1% of women may suffer from this condition [11, 12]. The percentage of women reporting orgasm difficulties can range from 3% to 34% [13], although more recent data point that 3% to 10% of women in the European and North American context may suffer from those [14]. Surprisingly, only half of women seem to report distress associated with the inability to reach orgasm [15]. Data on genito-pelvic pain indicate that 10% to 28% of women of reproductive age have genital pain [16]. With regard to vaginismus, data are equally limited, suggesting that the prevalence may reach 6.2% [17], but may rise to 68% in non-Western and more conservative communities [18]. In fact, epidemiological data seem to be quite dependent on the cultural context. The "sexual regime" of each country or culture seems to play a fundamental role, with the prevalence of female sexual dysfunctions being higher in patriarchal systems [19].

In the epidemiological context of sexual dysfunctions in women, it is important to acknowledge that the evidence is quite dated and that the data vary depending on the different terminology that researchers use. It is equally important to recognize the role of the cultural context in the expression of sexual complaints as the evidence suggests that culture plays a role in the type and prevalence of reported symptoms, with differences between Western and non-Westerns cultures.

Epidemiology of Men's Sexual Dysfunctions

Data on the prevalence of male sexual dysfunctions reveal that erectile dysfunction is highly prevalent, increasing with age [20]. Prevalence rates have varied from 9.5% to 18% (findings from Australia, United Kingdom and U.S.A; [3, 21, 22]). Despite the prevalence can go up to 75% in men older than 70 years old [9], approximately 10% of men under the age of 40 may present erectile difficulties [22]. Indeed, data regarding men seeking first time help for erectile dysfunction showed that one out of four men were younger than 40 [23]. Incidence data point to 25.9 new cases per 1000 men in the U.S.A, naturally increasing along each decade of age [24]. In the Dutch context, the incidence rate (cases per 1000 person-year) was 99, ranging from 77 to 205 (age 50–59 and 70–78, respectively) [25]. Recent data on the prevalence of erectile difficulties is somehow surprising, as numbers are quite high, varying from 37.2% to 48.6% (Brazil and Italy, respectively) [26]. In obese, non-diabetic men, erectile difficulties are frequent as well—42.1% [27]. Prevalence rates of premature ejaculation strongly depend on the diversity of definitions and whether or not the condition was assigned by a trained clinician [28]. Still, rates ranging from 20% to 30% have been found [28], with specific rates of 2.3% to 3% regarding lifelong premature ejaculation, 3.9% to 4.8% regarding acquired premature ejaculation, 8.5% to 11% regarding variable premature ejaculation, and 5% to 7% regarding subjective premature ejaculation [29, 30]. Despite these numbers, and the overlapping between premature ejaculation and psychological comorbidities, men seem to seek little assistance [31]. As for delayed ejaculation, the prevalence rates seem to be little expressive, with only about 3% of men presenting the condition [32]. Yet, in U.S.A 8% to 20% of men reported difficulties achieving climax or ejaculation [33], but only 0.7% reported the same difficulty in Britain [34]. Older age may be associated with delayed ejaculation [32].

Despite sexual desire difficulties are often seen in the context of female sexuality, 3% to 28% of men reported low sexual desire [35, 36]. In young men (18–29 years), the prevalence can range from 6% to 19%, while in older men can go up to 27% (60–67 years) [33, 37, 38]. Data can be different if we consider solitary versus dyadic sexual desire (desire to engage in sexual behavior with one's self versus with a partner, respectively). Fourteen percent of men seem to report low dyadic sexual desire, and 68% report low solitary sexual desire [39]. The incidence rate was seen to be higher regarding solitary desire [40]. Looking at sexual fantasies, which are an important marker, absence of sexual fantasies is more prevalent in older men (20%) [41]. Sexual desire difficulties may be prevalent in gay men, with numbers ranging from 19% to 57% [42, 43].

Finally, is worth recognizing that the numbers here presented vary as a function of the assessment methodologies that were used by researchers. Also, the numbers may not be representative of the countries and cultures that receive little attention in sexuality research.

Medical Approach to the Etiology of Sexual Dysfunctions

Specific Etiological Factors in Women

Both in men and women, testosterone, or its biochemical metabolite 5α-DHT, modulates many physiological and biochemical pathways. Considering only its sexual implications, in adulthood, it determines sexual differentiation, contributes to maintain the functional state, and modulates the sexual behavior [44]. Although the underlying mechanisms are not completely understood, testosterone positively modulates sexual desire in women in the central nervous system, and it has a role, together with estradiol, in the increased blood flow to the vagina, labia, vulva and clitoris, and in the lubrication of the vagina during sexual arousal [45]. Similarly to men, androgen levels decline progressively with age in women, and with the decreased ovarian function and adrenal precursor steroids availability [46]. However, menopause seems to have no effect in this process, as long as the androgen levels found in women in their 70s are similar to those premenopausal. Different studies have failed to demonstrate a correlation between the presence of hypoactive sexual desire in women or its severity, and the levels of testosterone. In fact, when reaching levels of testosterone above those present in the premenopausal period, sexual desire may actually decrease, suggesting a bimodal effect [47].

In contrast, after menopause, an abrupt drop in circulating estrogens is observed. These changes lead to many changes in the physiology of women, including the deterioration of the vagina epithelia. It appears flattened, with an absence of papillae, and a lower proportion of cells containing glycogen, which leads to a decrease of Lactobacilli and an increase in the pH. Also, the collagen I/III ratio is lower, resulting in reduced tissue strength [48], so it is more susceptible to trauma and it can result in pain, ulceration or bleeding during or after sexual intercourse. This scenario can result in inflammation and further worsening of the atrophy [49].

Although some relation has been observed, there is no clear correlation between hormone levels and PGAD. This disorder has been related with a myriad of other conditions as bipolar disorder, anxiety, depression, overactive bladder, interstitial cystitis and pudendal neuralgia; but their pathophysiological mechanisms remain widely unknown [50].

Specific Etiological Factors in Men

In the last 30 years there has been an increasing interest in the study of the physio-pathology of sexual dysfunctions in both men and woman, but there is still a long way to go in some disorders. Erection is the result of a complex coordination of neural, vascular and hormonal mechanisms that work together to achieve and maintain rigidity during sexual intercourse [51]. When some of these mechanisms is disrupted, different types of ED are defined: vascular, neurological or hormonal, with a variable presence of psychological factors in almost all of them, that can ease or worsen the previous condition. Isolated psychogenic ED is a non-well defined entity, that usually affects younger patients, with rates of prevalence as high as 30% of those adults under 40 [52]. The relationship between vascular ED and cardiovascular disease (CVD) has been well established through the last 20 years, considering in fact ED as an independent risk factor for CVD, and to be present an average of 2–3 years before the onset of the first coronary event [53]. Therefore, comorbidities known to cause CVD, as smoking, diabetes, hypertension, dyslipidemia, overweight, or sedentary lifestyle, are mandatory to assess and investigate when a man complains about ED [54]. The high prevalence of these comorbidities in general population makes vasculogenic ED, by far, the most common subtype of ED [55]. Age is an independent risk factor for both ED and CVD [56]. Thereby, a recent study found a decrease in the peak systolic flow of the cavernosal arteries in a cohort of healthy male patients through the years, supporting the idea that even in men without comorbidities, ED will be more prevalent with age [57]. With respect to diabetes, two pathogenic pathways, neurologic and vascular, can be present, resulting in very high prevalence rates as high as 52.5% in this subgroup of patients [58]. The progressive obliteration of the arteries due to arteriosclerosis usually associated with a poor glucose control can be followed or preceded by a lesion of the distal branches of the pudendal nerve, making it difficult to transfer the erectogenic stimuli. This is the reason why this subgroup of patients is considered difficult to treat [59], and why neurogenic ED can be present in other disorders causing central or peripheral nerve damage, as multiple sclerosis, spinal cord injuries or chronic renal failure [60]. The most common cause of iatrogenic ED is after radical pelvic surgery, where nerve damage is supposed to have an important role and has been widely investigated in the literature. However, the reported incidence of ED after surgery shows an extremely variability, with figures ranging from 12% to 96%, due to methodological differences [61].

Late onset hypogonadism, also referred as age-associated testosterone deficiency syndrome or, more recently and correct, as "functional hypogonadism", is a biochemical and clinical syndrome characterized for the presence of a wide spectrum of clinical symptoms and low testosterone levels, which is related to age. In men, average levels of androgens decline constant and progressively through the years [62]. Focusing on sexual function, it is known that testosterone deficiency can cause low sexual desire, and also a decrease in morning erections and ED. So when a man complain of these conditions, it is mandatory to assess testosterone levels [63], especially in the elder population, given that androgen therapy could improve or solve these problems [64].

Despite the high prevalence of ejaculation disorders, as PE and DE, their biological pathophysiology has not been so widely investigated and has not been precisely established [65]. Acquired PE has been related to conditions as inflammation or infection of the prostate, abnormal hormonal levels (LH, prolactin and TSH), and low levels of serotonin, which, in some cases, could be successfully treated to improve the dysfunction [66]. In the case of lifelong PE, the most widely accepted hypothesis is that in men with low 5-hydroxytryptamine (5-HT) the hyposensitivity of the 5-HT_{2C}, or the hypersensitivity of the 5-HT_{1A} receptors that are located in the neuronal centers, can lead to a more rapid threshold for ejaculation, with lower stimulation [67]. This theory also explains that those men with a higher set point can better control the process, and that those with an abnormally high set point experience delayed, or even absent ejaculation with normal erection [68]. Several studies in the literature have used imaging techniques as magnetic resonance to investigate the functional and structural neural basis of PE, with findings as higher activation in the middle temporal gyrus; larger volume of the caudate nucleus; cortical, parietal, occipital and cingulate cortical thickening; altered structural connectivity of the fronto-cingulate-parietal control network; and lower activation of the left inferior frontal gyrus and left insula [65]. Although all of them try to better understand the condition, and to put some light in the darkness, there is still a need to put together these results and demonstrate the importance of these findings in daily clinical practice.

Psychosocial Approach to the Etiology of Sexual Dysfunctions

Over the last few decades, several models conceptualizing sexual dysfunctions have emerged. These models vary in the way they regard the role of different psychosocial factors in the etiology and/or maintenance of sexual dysfunctions. The precursor model of Masters and Johnson (the so-called linear model of sexual response) which was aimed at characterizing the physiological processes involved in arousal, plateau, orgasm, and resolution stages [69], gave little emphasis to the subjective and contextual processes involved in sexual response [70]. Nevertheless, the model proposed two core etiological factors regarding sexual dysfunctions: performance anxiety and *spectatoring*, i.e., spectator of oneself during sexual activity. The phenomenon of sexual performance anxiety appears to characterize individuals with sexual difficulties and emerges as a specific component of the broader concept of anxiety [71]. Therefore, while anxiety has the potential to increase the sexual response in men and women, increasing their erectile response and vaginal lubrication, more specific components such as the anticipation of failure or poor sexual performance are associated with clinical conditions of sexual dysfunction [72]. In the clinical context, is it important for the health professional to define the weight of this etiological variable, as well as the sources that promote it, e.g., cultural standards? partner pressure? Regarding the role of anxiety and its triggers, Barlow proposes a more elaborate model with greater empirical value, mostly focused on male sexual dysfunction, and in particular, on erectile dysfunction [73]. From a series of studies focusing on physiological variables (namely, erectile response) but also psychological or subjective measures, it became clear that what most differentiated men with and without erectile dysfunction, more than their erectile response, was the fact that men with dysfunction respond with more negative affect through sexual stimulation, a feeling of loss of control, preoccupation with performance or the negative consequences of sexual performance, and an underestimation of their erectile response [74]. The man with sexual dysfunction ends up focusing on non-erotic cues, with implications for his adaptive response. Basson, who were more aligned with the domain of female sexuality, proposed an alternative model, considering relationship aspects, namely, emotional intimacy [75]. Emotional intimacy is seen as a driving source of sexual response, especially in terms of sexual arousal and desire. Although a basic condition is necessary—be it organic or psychological—that guarantees the ability to process sexual stimuli, there is an important relational purpose for the understanding of sexual (dys)function [76].

Another interesting model is that of the sexual scripts of Gagnon and Simon [77]. Sexual scripts emerge from more general scripts, i.e., social scripts, and result from a social learning process that defines what is correct and expected at a given time, in a given society. These scripts incorporate a sociocultural, interpersonal, and individual dimension that guides individuals in how they should live their sexuality and build their sexual interactions [78]. These sexual scripts will thus guide individuals in what they should and should not do sexually, how, and with whom. According to this model, it is expected that individuals with sexual dysfunctions present more rigid, conventional, or routine sexual scripts, which contribute to the maintenance of their symptoms [79]. A contextual look would therefore be essential for understanding the etiology and maintenance factors of sexual dysfunctions. More recently, and in articulation with a cognitive-behavioral clinical intervention proposal, Nobre suggested the cognitive-emotional model according to which a series of cognitive structures, of information processing, are at the core of erroneous interpretations of negative sexual events (e.g., sexual failure). These cognitive structures promote a vicious cycle that feeds dysfunctional thoughts in the sexual context as well as emotional states that are not compatible with the capacity to perform sexually [80, 81]. Data collected over several years and in independent investigations allowed researchers to characterize different sexual difficulties, in men and women, with and without heterosexual preferences, pointing potential etiological and maintenance factors of sexual dysfunctions [82]. Examples of these factors are lack of erotic thoughts, preoccupation with erections during sexual activity, the anticipation of failed sexual performance, thoughts of sexual abuse, or preoccupation with body image [82]. Finally, and because we will not cover all models of a psychosocial nature, we highlight the Dual Control Model of sexual response. This model postulates that the sexual response results from the balance between relatively independent mechanisms of sexual arousal and inhibition [83, 84]. In this regard, it is interesting to analyze the factorial structure of the model, as it resulted in an excitation mechanism and two inhibition mechanisms [85, 86]. The latter refers to the predisposition to sexual inhibition due to the fear of sexual performance failure, and inhibition due to the fear of the negative consequences associated with the sex (e.g., STD, unwanted pregnancy). It is interesting to see that sexual inhibition due to fear of sexual performance failure echoes other models (Barlow model, Nobre and Pinto-Gouveia model), supporting the role of learned cultural standards about sexual performance—often, unrealistic standards—, in male and female sexual functioning. Empirical evidence on the Dual Control Model suggests that sexual inhibition, especially the fear of sexual performance failure, is a vulnerability factor for sexual dysfunction in men and women [87, 88].

Furthermore, there is a consensus to improve the focus on the individuals' proximal relationship context. Accordingly, it is paramount that the focus is on the dyad or partners and not on the individual carrying the symptom or the sexual complaint. What sometimes causes the complaint is not the sexual symptoms themselves, but the fact that there is a discrepancy in the sexual response between the elements of the couple, or the fact that one of the elements has unrealistic and very high expectations regarding the sexual functioning of the other. This contextual and relationship view becomes an asset in understanding the etiological and maintenance variables of sexual complaints.

Specific Etiological Factors in Women

In addition to the models presented, a series of studies have made it possible to assess psychosocial etiological factors specific to each sexual dysfunction or difficulty. For example, in women's sexual desire difficulties, the quality of the relationship seems to be a determining factor, to the point that satisfaction with the partner in one specific day, promotes sexual activity the next day [89]. Relationship duration seems to play a negative role [90], while conservative sexual beliefs and medical aspects have an indirect effect, influencing female sexual desire through lack of erotic thoughts and perception of sexual failure [91]. Insecure and anxious attachment styles, i.e., dysfunctional relationship styles, characterized the expression of sexual desire in women [92]. Thoughts of sexual abuse were also associated with lower sexual desire [93]. Additionally, communication in the relational context has also a central role, being a key target in therapy [94]. On the other hand, cultural aspects can be important etiological mechanisms of sexual desire difficulties in women. These include social narratives favoring female passivity and responsiveness [95], poor sex education, overload of professional and parental tasks, or even demanding and unrealistic standards of female attractiveness [96]. Likewise, and considering patterns of sexual arousal, while sexually explicit stimuli (stimuli with a focus on genital interaction) seem to induce greater genital activation, subjective sexual arousal in women is prompted by stimuli that suggest a relational context [97, 98]. In fact, relational satisfaction seems to be associated with fewer arousal difficulties [99]. In addition, women with PGAD reported more dysfunctional sexual beliefs (sexual conservatism or sexual desire regarded as a sin), as well as thoughts of sexual abuse and lack of affection during sexual activity [100]; likewise, the quality of the dyadic relationship was associated with the levels of distress [101].

With regard to orgasm difficulties, the data suggest that a history of sexual victimization may play an etiological role, particularly in women who experienced physical sensations and orgasm during abuse [102]. Similar to desire difficulties, the presence of thoughts of sexual failure and lack of erotic thoughts during sexual activity predicted orgasm difficulties in women [103]. Women with genito-pelvic pain also reported a higher probability of sexual and physical abuse [104, 105], which places this problem in a relational and interpersonal context. Anxiety factors such as catastrophizing thoughts and hypervigilance towards pain also triggered the perception of genito-pelvic pain [106].

Specific Etiological Factors in Men

Regarding male sexual dysfunctions, there is also evidence about vulnerability factors specific to each clinical condition. Cases of erectile dysfunction are often accompanied by depressive and anxiety symptoms, resulting in a context of psychological distress [107]. Lower erectile capacity is also associated with situational events where psychological distress arises in response to a critical event [108]. On the other hand, the perception of intimacy has been shown to be a protective factor in erectile dysfunction [109]. Additionally, much has been written about the importance of cognitive factors in erectile dysfunction. High expectations of sexual performance coupled with dysfunctional processing styles of sexual information result in a sense of loss of control, guilt for poor sexual performance, and cognitive distraction during sexual activity, contributing to the maintenance of erectile difficulties [82]. In the context of non-heterosexual relationships, sexual minority associated distress seems to be linked with erectile difficulties in men who have sex with men [110]. All these factors are relevant in the design of biopsychosocial interventions for erectile dysfunction. Although the evidence is more limited, cases of premature ejaculation seem to be characterized by a style of internalization, in which the man attributes to himself the responsibility for his dysfunctional sexual response, blaming himself and monitoring the partner for confirmation signs of his poor sexual performance [111]. These men have a more preoccupied personality style and are less motivated to look for new sensations, fearing novelty [112]. Delayed ejaculation cases also appear to be characterized by an anxiety profile, lack of confidence, in which a pattern of negative self-talk interferes with reaching climax even with a good erectile response [113]. Regarding the difficulties of sexual desire in men, although the literature is also insufficient, the data suggest that some psychosocial determinants such as duration of the relationship, professional stress, little confidence in achieving an erection, higher education and more demanding careers, or even the desire to having children or having young children are associated with lower sexual desire in men [39, 114–116]. The combination of cognitive and emotional aspects proved to be an important predictor of desire difficulties, with a special emphasis on concerns with erectile capacity and the lack of erotic thoughts during sexual intercourse [117].

Combining the Medical and Psychosocial Factors Toward a Comprehensive Approach to Sexual Dysfunction

The biopsychosocial view of sexual dysfunctions promotes a more comprehensive analysis of the etiological and maintenance factors of sexual difficulties, focusing on the interaction between etiological aspects and looking for better forms of intervention, as well as more adjusted ways to address the specificities of each individual or partner(s). Therefore, it is a vision that makes it possible to overcome the reductionist dichotomy of organic versus psychological, improving assessment and intervention practices, and stimulating the articulation between the different scientific and professional domains [118]. The different fields are not incompatible; on the contrary, they make it possible to maximize interventions. In this regard, some scientific and professional societies have promoted this vision, resulting in proposals for the integrative assessment and intervention in sexual problems. Indeed, existing integrative approaches have shown promising results [119]. In order to further explore the link between the organic and the psychosocial, important networks, including the European Sexual Medicine Network, have invested in this approach as a way to ensure greater interdisciplinary and, therefore, better services in the field of human sexuality [120]. This biopsychosocial approach to the etiological aspects of sexual dysfunctions needs further empirical work, especially if we consider that the etiological factors of a psychosocial order are permeable to the cultural, historical, and even political context, and those are in constant change. It is, therefore, essential to follow this evolutionary process for a better understanding of the etiology and maintenance factors of sexual dysfunctions.

Final Remarks

This section intended to present evidence on the epidemiology and etiological factors associated with sexual dysfunction in men and women. It is important to highlight methodological limitations. Among them, we highlight the reduced information about the etiological aspects and prevalence in sexual and gender minorities. This limitation clearly excludes the possibility of a rigorous analysis of the etiological aspects or the specific needs of these populations, resulting in a less effective and less socially fair intervention approach. Furthermore, and although this chapter has focused on the context of sexual dysfunctions, the tendency to look at other equally relevant constructs such as issues of sexual pleasure or sexual well-being is also worthy of attention. Indeed, the gap between men and women in access to sexual pleasure requires an analysis of the factors that promote this gap and the respective consideration by professionals and clinicians in the area of sexuality [121]. The same is true for the concept of sexual distress. It has emerged as a more comprehensive view of sexual dysfunction, referring to the negative emotional response resulting from the sexual functioning of individuals, and being a fundamental criterion for the diagnosis of sexual dysfunction [122, 123]. In fact, the prevalence of sexual dysfunctions is lower when this criterion is considered [124]; the application of cutoff points (e.g., IIEF or FSFI) to understand the prevalence and etiology of sexual dysfunctions is insufficient as it assumes the presence versus absence of dysfunction as a fundamental criterion, rather than the actual impact of the symptomatology on the life of individuals [125]. Finally, we consider that some evidence about the psychosocial etiological factors is dated. Available data may fail to reflect the transformative character of the biopsychosocial vision.

References

1. World Health Organization. Sexual health. https://www.who.int/health-topics/sexual-health#tab=tab_2. Accessed December, 6, 2021.
2. McCool-Myers M, Theurich M, Zuelke A, Knuettel H, Apfelbacher C. Predictors of female sexual dysfunction: a systematic review and qualitative analysis through gender inequality paradigms. BMC Womens Health. 2018;8(1):108.
3. Mitchell KR, Mercer CH, Ploubidis GB, Jones KG, Datta J, Field N, Copas AJ, Tanton C, Erens B, Sonnenberg P, Clifton S, Macdowall W, Phelps A, Johnson AM, Wellings K. Sexual function in Britain: findings from the third National Survey of Sexual Attitudes and Lifestyles (Natsal-3). Lancet. 2013;382(9907):1817–29.
4. Quinn-Nilas C, Milhausen RR, McKay A, Holzapfel S. Prevalence and predictors of sexual problems among midlife Canadian adults: results from a National Survey. J Sex Med. 2018;15(6):873–9.
5. Hendrickx L, Gijs L, Enzlin P. Prevalence rates of sexual difficulties and associated distress in heterosexual men and women: results from an Internet survey in Flanders. J Sex Res. 2014;51(1):1–12.
6. Marieke D, Joana C, Giovanni C, Erika L, Patricia P, Yacov R, Aleksandar Š. Sexual desire discrepancy: a position statement of the European Society for Sexual Medicine. Sex Med. 2020;8(2):121–31. https://doi.org/10.1016/j.esxm.2020.02.008.

7. Atallah S, Johnson-Agbakwu C, Rosenbaum T, Abdo C, Byers ES, Graham C, Nobre P, Wylie K, Brotto L. Ethical and sociocultural aspects of sexual function and dysfunction in both sexes. J Sex Med. 2016;13(4):591–606.

8. Graham CA, Boynton PM, Gould K. Women's sexual desire: challenging narratives of "dysfunction". Eur Psychol. 2017;22(1):27–38.

9. Lewis RW, Fugl-Meyer KS, Corona G, Hayes RD, Laumann EO, Moreira ED Jr, Rellini AH, Segraves T. Definitions/epidemiology/risk factors for sexual dysfunction. J Sex Med. 2010;7(4 Pt 2):1598–607.

10. Shifren JL, Monz BU, Russo PA, Segreti A, Johannes CB. Sexual problems and distress in United States women: prevalence and correlates. Obstet Gynecol. 2008;112(5):970–8.

11. Jackowich R, Pukall C. Prevalence of persistent genital arousal disorder criteria in a sample of Canadian undergraduate students. J Sex Med. 2017;14(6):e369.

12. Garvey LJ, West C, Latch N, Leiblum S, Goldmeier D. Report of spontaneous and persistent genital arousal in women attending a sexual health clinic. Int J STD AIDS. 2009;20(8):519–21.

13. Graham CA. The DSM diagnostic criteria for female orgasmic disorder. Arch Sex Behav. 2010;39(2):256–70.

14. Carpenter KM, Williams K, Worly B. Treating women's orgasmic difficulties. In: Peterson Z, editor. The Wiley handbook of sex therapy. Hoboken: Wiley-Blackwell; 2017. Chapter 5.

15. Laan E, Rellini AH, Barnes T, International Society for Sexual Medicine. Standard operating procedures for female orgasmic disorder: consensus of the International Society for Sexual Medicine. J Sex Med. 2013;10(1):74–82.

16. Pukall CF, Goldstein AT, Bergeron S, Foster D, Stein A, Kellogg-Spadt S, Bachmann G. Vulvodynia: definition, prevalence, impact, and pathophysiological factors. J Sex Med. 2016;13(3):291–304.

17. Oberg K, Sjögren Fugl-Meyer K. On Swedish women's distressing sexual dysfunctions: some concomitant conditions and life satisfaction. J Sex Med. 2005;2(2):169–80.

18. Amidu N, Owiredu WK, Woode E, Addai-Mensah O, Quaye L, Alhassan A, Tagoe EA. Incidence of sexual dysfunction: a prospective survey in Ghanaian females. Reprod Biol Endocrinol. 2010;8:106.

19. Hall KSK, Graham CA. The privilege of pleasure: sex therapy in global cultural context. In: Hall KSK, Binik YM, editors. Principles and practice of sex therapy. New York: Guilford; 2020. Chapter 11.

20. Lewis RW, Fugl-Meyer KS, Bosch R, Fugl-Meyer AR, Laumann EO, Lizza E, Martin-Morales A. Epidemiology/risk factors of sexual dysfunction. J Sex Med. 2004;1(1):35–9.

21. Richters J, Grulich AE, de Visser RO, Smith AM, Rissel CE. Sex in Australia: sexual difficulties in a representative sample of adults. Aust N Z J Public Health. 2003;27(2):164–70.

22. Selvin E, Burnett AL, Platz EA. Prevalence and risk factors for erectile dysfunction in the US. Am J Med. 2007;120(2):151–7.

23. Capogrosso P, Colicchia M, Ventimiglia E, Castagna G, Clementi MC, Suardi N, Castiglione F, Briganti A, Cantiello F, Damiano R, Montorsi F, Salonia A. One patient out of four with newly diagnosed erectile dysfunction is a young man—worrisome picture from the everyday clinical practice. J Sex Med. 2013;10(7):1833–41.

24. Johannes CB, Araujo AB, Feldman HA, Derby CA, Kleinman KP, McKinlay JB. Incidence of erectile dysfunction in men 40 to 69 years old: longitudinal results from the Massachusetts male aging study. J Urol. 2000;163(2):460–3.

25. Schouten BW, Bosch JL, Bernsen RM, Blanker MH, Thomas S, Bohnen AM. Incidence rates of erectile dysfunction in the Dutch general population. Effects of definition, clinical relevance and duration of follow-up in the Krimpen Study. Int J Impot Res. 2005;17(1):58–62.

26. Goldstein I, Goren A, Li VW, Tang WY, Hassan TA. Epidemiology update of erectile dysfunction in eight countries with high burden. Sex Med Rev. 2020;8(1):48–58.

27. Molina-Vega M, Asenjo-Plaza M, Banderas-Donaire MJ, Hernández-Ollero MD, Rodríguez-Moreno S, Álvarez-Millán JJ, Cabezas-Sanchez P, Cardona-Díaz F, Alcaide-Torres J, Garrido-Sánchez L, Castellano-Castillo D, Tinahones FJ, Fernández-García JC. Prevalence

of and risk factors for erectile dysfunction in young nondiabetic obese men: results from a regional study. Asian J Androl. 2020;22(4):372–8.

28. Althof SE. Treatment of premature ejaculation. In: Hall KSK, Binik YM, editors. Principles and practice of sex therapy. New York: Guilford; 2020. Chapter 6.

29. Serefoglu EC, Yaman O, Cayan S, Asci R, Orhan I, Usta MF, Ekmekcioglu O, Kendirci M, Semerci B, Kadioglu A. Prevalence of the complaint of ejaculating prematurely and the four premature ejaculation syndromes: results from the Turkish Society of Andrology Sexual Health Survey. J Sex Med. 2011;8(2):540–8.

30. Gao J, Zhang X, Su P, Liu J, Xia L, Yang J, Shi K, Tang D, Hao Z, Zhou J, Liang C. Prevalence and factors associated with the complaint of premature ejaculation and the four premature ejaculation syndromes: a large observational study in China. J Sex Med. 2013;10(7):1874–81.

31. Porst H, Montorsi F, Rosen RC, Gaynor L, Grupe S, Alexander J. The Premature Ejaculation Prevalence and Attitudes (PEPA) survey: prevalence, comorbidities, and professional help-seeking. Eur Urol. 2007;51(3):816–23. discussion 824

32. Perelman MA, Rowland DL. Retarded ejaculation. World J Urol. 2006;24(6):645–52.

33. Laumann EO, Paik A, Rosen RC. Sexual dysfunction in the United States: prevalence and predictors. JAMA. 1999;281(6):537–44.

34. Mercer CH, Fenton KA, Johnson AM, Copas AJ, Macdowall W, Erens B, Wellings K. Who reports sexual function problems? Empirical evidence from Britain's 2000 National Survey of Sexual Attitudes and Lifestyles. Sex Transm Infect. 2005;81(5):394–9.

35. Fugl-Meyer AR, Fugl-Meyer KS. Sexual disabilities, problems and satisfaction in 18–74 year old Swedes. Scand J Sex. 1999;3:79–105.

36. Laumann E, Nicolosi A, Glasser D, et al. Sexual problems among women and men aged 40–80 y: prevalence and correlates identified in the Global Study of Sexual Attitudes and Behaviors. Int J Impot Res. 2005;17:39–57.

37. Najman JM, Dunne MP, Boyle FM, Cook MD, Purdie DM. Sexual dysfunction in the Australian population. Aust Fam Physician. 2003;32(11):951–4.

38. Traeen B, Stigum H. Sexual problems in 18-67-year-old Norwegians. Scand J Public Health. 2010;38(5):445–56.

39. Martin S, Atlantis E, Wilson D, Lange K, Haren MT, Taylor A, Wittert G, Members of the Florey Adelaide Male Ageing Study. Clinical and biopsychosocial determinants of sexual dysfunction in middle-aged and older Australian men. J Sex Med. 2012;9(8):2093–103.

40. Martin S, Haren M, Taylor A, Middleton S, Wittert G, FAMAS. Cohort profile: the Florey Adelaide Male Ageing Study (FAMAS). Int J Epidemiol. 2007;36(2):302–6.

41. Corona G, Isidori AM, Aversa A, Burnett AL, Maggi M. Endocrinologic control of men's sexual desire and arousal/erection. J Sex Med. 2016;13(3):317–37.

42. Hirshfield S, Chiasson MA, Wagmiller RL Jr, Remien RH, Humberstone M, Scheinmann R, Grov C. Sexual dysfunction in an Internet sample of U.S. men who have sex with men. J Sex Med. 2010;7(9):3104–14.

43. Peixoto MM, Nobre P. Prevalence of sexual problems and associated distress among lesbian and heterosexual women. J Sex Marital Ther. 2015;41(4):427–39.

44. Parish SJ, Simon JA, Davis SR, Giraldi A, Goldstein I, Goldstein SW, et al. International Society for the Study of Women's Sexual Health Clinical Practice Guideline for the use of systemic testosterone for hypoactive sexual desire disorder in women. J Women's Health. 2021;30(4):474–91.

45. Cappelletti M, Wallen K. Increasing women's sexual desire: the comparative effectiveness of estrogens and androgens. Horm Behav. 2016;78:178–93.

46. Burger HG, Dudley EC, Cui J, Dennerstein L, Hopper JL. A prospective longitudinal study of serum testosterone, dehydroepiandrosterone sulfate, and sex hormone-binding globulin levels through the menopause transition. J Clin Endocrinol Metab. 2000;85(8):2832–8.

47. Krapf JM, Simon JA. A sex-specific dose-response curve for testosterone: could excessive testosterone limit sexual interaction in women? Menopause. 2017;24(4):462–70.

48. Miller EA, Beasley DE, Dunn RR, Archie EA. Lactobacilli dominance and vaginal pH: why is the human vaginal microbiome unique? Front Microbiol. 2016;7:1936.

49. Alvisi S, Gava G, Orsili I, Giacomelli G, Baldassarre M, Seracchioli R, et al. Vaginal health in menopausal women. Medicina (Mex). 2019;55(10):615.

50. Pease ER, Ziegelmann M, Vencill JA, Kok SN, Collins CS, Betcher HK. Persistent genital arousal disorder (PGAD): a clinical review and case series in support of multidisciplinary management. Sex Med Rev. 2022;10(1):53–70.

51. Irwin GM. Erectile dysfunction. Prim Care. 2019;46(2):249–55.

52. Nguyen HMT, Gabrielson AT, Hellstrom WJG. Erectile dysfunction in young men—a review of the prevalence and risk factors. Sex Med Rev. 2017;5(4):508–20.

53. Montorsi P, Ravagnani PM, Galli S, Rotatori F, Veglia F, Briganti A, et al. Association between erectile dysfunction and coronary artery disease. Role of coronary clinical presentation and extent of coronary vessels involvement: the COBRA trial. Eur Heart J. 2006;27(22):2632–9.

54. Burnett AL, Nehra A, Breau RH, Culkin DJ, Faraday MM, Hakim LS, et al. Erectile dysfunction: AUA guideline. J Urol. 2018;200(3):633–41.

55. Yafi FA, Jenkins L, Albersen M, Corona G, Isidori AM, Goldfarb S, et al. Erectile dysfunction. Nat Rev Dis Primers. 2016;2:16003.

56. Miner M, Parish SJ, Billups KL, Paulos M, Sigman M, Blaha MJ. Erectile dysfunction and subclinical cardiovascular disease. Sex Med Rev. 2019;7(3):455–63.

57. Pathak RA, Broderick GA. Color Doppler duplex ultrasound parameters in men without organic erectile dysfunction. Urology. 2020;135:66–70.

58. Kouidrat Y, Pizzol D, Cosco T, Thompson T, Carnaghi M, Bertoldo A, et al. High prevalence of erectile dysfunction in diabetes: a systematic review and meta-analysis of 145 studies. Diabet Med. 2017;34(9):1185–92.

59. Gandhi J, Dagur G, Warren K, Smith NL, Sheynkin YR, Zumbo A, et al. The role of diabetes mellitus in sexual and reproductive health: an overview of pathogenesis, evaluation, and management. Curr Diabetes Rev. 2017;13(6):573–81.

60. Thomas C, Konstantinidis C. Neurogenic erectile dysfunction. Where do we stand? Med Basel Switz. 2021;8(1):3.

61. Emanu JC, Avildsen IK, Nelson CJ. Erectile dysfunction after radical prostatectomy: prevalence, medical treatments, and psychosocial interventions. Curr Opin Support Palliat Care. 2016;10(1):102–7.

62. Wang C, Nieschlag E, Swerdloff R, Behre HM, Hellstrom WJ, Gooren LJ, et al. Investigation, treatment and monitoring of late-onset hypogonadism in males: ISA, ISSAM, EAU, EAA and ASA recommendations. Eur J Endocrinol. 2008;159(5):507–14.

63. Corona G, Goulis DG, Huhtaniemi I, Zitzmann M, Toppari J, Forti G, et al. European Academy of Andrology (EAA) guidelines on investigation, treatment and monitoring of functional hypogonadism in males: endorsing organization: European Society of Endocrinology. Andrology. 2020;8(5):970–87.

64. Taniguchi H, Shimada S, Kinoshita H. Testosterone therapy for late-onset hypogonadism improves erectile function: a systematic review and meta-analysis. Urol Int. 2021;2:1–14.

65. Lu J, Chen Q, Li D, Zhang W, Xing S, Wang J, et al. Reconfiguration of dynamic functional connectivity states in patients with lifelong premature ejaculation. Front Neurosci. 2021;15:721236.

66. Crowdis M, Nazir S. Premature ejaculation. In: StatPearls. Treasure Island, FL: StatPearls Publishing; 2021. https://www.ncbi.nlm.nih.gov/books/NBK546701/.

67. Saitz TR, Serefoglu EC. Advances in understanding and treating premature ejaculation. Nat Rev Urol. 2015;12(11):629–40.

68. Giuliano F, Clement P. Neuroanatomy and physiology of ejaculation. Annu Rev Sex Res. 2005;16:190–216.

69. Masters WH, Johnson VE. Human sexual response. Boston: Little Brown; 1966.

70. Rosen CR, Beck JG. Patterns of sexual arousal: psychophysiological processes and clinical applications. New York: Guilford; 1988.

71. Masters WH, Johnson VE. Human sexual inadequacy. Boston: Little Brown; 1970.

72. Kane L, Dawson S, Shaughnessy K, Reissing ED, Ouimet AJ, Ashbaugh AR. A review of experimental research on anxiety and sexual arousal: implications for the treatment of sexual dysfunction using cognitive behavioral therapy. J Exp Psychopathol. 2019;10(2):1–24.

73. Barlow DH. Causes of sexual dysfunction: the role of anxiety and cognitive interference. J Consult Clin Psychol. 1986;54(2):140–8.

74. Abrahamson DJ, Barlow DH, Abrahamson LS. Differential effects of performance demand and distraction on sexually functional and dysfunctional males. J Abnorm Psychol. 1989;98(3):241–7.

75. Basson R. The female sexual response: a different model. J Sex Marital Ther. 2000;26(1):51–65.

76. Basson R. Human sex-response cycles. J Sex Marital Ther. 2001;27(1):33–43.

77. Gagnon JH, Simon W. Sexual conduct: the social sources of human sexuality. Chicago: Aldine; 1973.

78. Gagnon JH, Simon W. The sexual scripting of oral genital contacts. Arch Sex Behav. 1987;16(1):1–25.

79. Gagnon JH, Rosen RC, Leiblum SR. Cognitive and social aspects of sexual dysfunction: sexual scripts in sex therapy. J Sex Marital Ther. 1982;8(1):44–56.

80. Nobre PJ. Treating men's erectile problems. In: Peterson Z, editor. The Wiley-Blackwell handbook of sex therapy. Hoboken, NJ: Wiley-Blackwell; 2017. Chapter 4.

81. Nobre PJ. Treatments for sexual dysfunctions. In: Hoffman S, editor. Clinical psychology: a global perspective. Hoboken, NJ: Wiley-Blackwell; 2017. Chapter 14.

82. Tavares IM, Moura CV, Nobre PJ. The role of cognitive processing factors in sexual function and dysfunction in women and men: a systematic review. Sex Med Rev. 2020;8:403–30.

83. Bancroft J, Janssen E. The dual control model of male sexual response: a theoretical approach to centrally mediated erectile dysfunction. Neurosci Biobehav Rev. 2000;24(5):571–9.

84. Janssen E, Bancroft J. The dual control model: the role of sexual inhibition and excitation in sexual arousal and behavior. In: Janssen E, editor. The psychophysiology of sex. Bloomington: Indiana University Press; 2007. Chapter 10.

85. Janssen E, Vorst H, Finn P, Bancroft J. The Sexual Inhibition (SIS) and Sexual Excitation (SES) Scales: I. Measuring sexual inhibition and excitation proneness in men. J Sex Res. 2002;39(2):114–26.

86. Carpenter D, Janssen E, Graham C, Vorst H, Wicherts J. Women's scores on the sexual inhibition/sexual excitation scales (SIS/SES): gender similarities and differences. J Sex Res. 2008;45(1):36–48.

87. Bancroft J, Graham CA, Janssen E, Sanders SA. The dual control model: current status and future directions. J Sex Res. 2009;46(2-3):121–42.

88. Sanders SA, Graham CA, Milhausen RR. Predicting sexual problems in women: the relevance of sexual excitation and sexual inhibition. Arch Sex Behav. 2008;37(2):241–51.

89. Dewitte M, Mayer A. Exploring the link between daily relationship quality, sexual desire, and sexual activity in couples. Arch Sex Behav. 2018;47(6):1675–86.

90. Mark KP, Leistner CE, Garcia JR. Impact of contraceptive type on sexual desire of women and of men partnered to contraceptive users. J Sex Med. 2016;13(9):1359–68.

91. Carvalho J, Nobre P. Sexual desire in women: an integrative approach regarding psychological, medical, and relationship dimensions. J Sex Med. 2010;7(5):1807–15.

92. Attaky A, Kok G, Dewitte M. Attachment orientation moderates the sexual and relational implications of sexual desire discrepancies. J Sex Marital Ther. 2022;48(4):343–62.

93. Carvalho J, Nobre P. Predictors of women's sexual desire: the role of psychopathology, cognitive-emotional determinants, relationship dimensions, and medical factors. J Sex Med. 2010;7(2 Pt 2):928–37.

94. Brotto LA, Velten J. Sexual interest/arousal disorder in women. In: Hall KSK, Binik YM, editors. Principles and practice of sex therapy. New York: Guilford; 2020. Chapter 1.

95. Boul L, Hallam-Jones R, Wylie KR. Sexual pleasure and motivation. J Sex Marital Ther. 2009;35(1):25–39.

96. Tiefer L, Hall M, Tavris C. Beyond dysfunction: a new view of women's sexual problems. J Sex Marital Ther. 2002;28(Suppl 1):225–32.

97. Laan E, Everaerd W, van Bellen G, Hanewald G. Women's sexual and emotional responses to male- and female-produced erotica. Arch Sex Behav. 1994;23(2):153–69.

98. Carvalho J, Gomes AQ, Laja P, Oliveira C, Vilarinho S, Janssen E, Nobre P. Gender differences in sexual arousal and affective responses to erotica: the effects of type of film and fantasy instructions. Arch Sex Behav. 2013;42(6):1011–9.

99. Jiann BP, Su CC, Yu CC, Wu TT, Huang JK. Risk factors for individual domains of female sexual function. J Sex Med. 2009;6(12):3364–75.

100. Carvalho J, Veríssimo A, Nobre PJ. Cognitive and emotional determinants characterizing women with persistent genital arousal disorder. J Sex Med. 2013;10(6):1549–58.

101. Carvalho J, Veríssimo A, Nobre PJ. Psychological factors predicting the distress to female persistent genital arousal symptoms. J Sex Marital Ther. 2015;41(1):11–24.

102. Buehler S. What every mental health professional needs to know about sex. New York: Springer; 2017.

103. Tavares IM, Laan ETM, Nobre PJ. Cognitive-affective dimensions of female orgasm: the role of automatic thoughts and affect during sexual activity. J Sex Med. 2017;14(6):818–28.

104. Khandker M, Brady SS, Stewart EG, Harlow BL. Is chronic stress during childhood associated with adult-onset vulvodynia? J Womens Health (Larchmt). 2014;23(8):649–56.

105. Landry T, Bergeron S. Biopsychosocial factors associated with dyspareunia in a community sample of adolescent girls. Arch Sex Behav. 2011;40(5):877–89.

106. Bergeron S, Corsini-Munt S, Aerts L, et al. Female sexual pain disorders: a review of the literature on etiology and treatment. Curr Sex Health Rep. 2015;7:159–69.

107. Li K, Liang S, Shi Y, Zhou Y, Xie L, Feng J, Chen Z, Li Q, Gan Z. The relationships of dehydroepiandrosterone sulfate, erectile function and general psychological health. Sex Med. 2021;9(4):100386.

108. Carvalho J, Campos P, Carrito M, Moura C, Quinta-Gomes A, Tavares I, Nobre P. The relationship between COVID-19 confinement, psychological adjustment, and sexual functioning, in a sample of Portuguese men and women. J Sex Med. 2021;18(7):1191–7.

109. Sivaratnam L, Selimin DS, Abd Ghani SR, Nawi HM, Nawi AM. Behavior-related erectile dysfunction: a systematic review and meta-analysis. J Sex Med. 2021;18(1):121–43.

110. Parent MC, Wille L. Heterosexual self-presentation, identity management, and sexual functioning among men who have sex with men. Arch Sex Behav. 2021;50(7):3155–62.

111. Giuri S, Caselli G, Manfredi C, Rebecchi D, Granata A, Ruggiero GM, Veronese G. Cognitive attentional syndrome and metacognitive beliefs in male sexual dysfunction: an exploratory study. Am J Mens Health. 2017;11(3):592–9.

112. Gao P, Gao J, Wang Y, Peng D, Zhang Y, Li H, Zhu T, Zhang W, Dai Y, Jiang H, Zhang X. Temperament-character traits and attitudes toward premature ejaculation in 4 types of premature ejaculation. J Sex Med. 2021;18(1):72–82.

113. Perelman MA. Delayed ejaculation. In: Hall KSK, Binik YM, editors. Principles and practice of sex therapy. New York: Guilford; 2020. Chapter 7.

114. Carvalheira A, Traeen B, Štulhofer A. Correlates of men's sexual interest: a cross-cultural study. J Sex Med. 2014;11(1):154–64.

115. Nimbi FM, Tripodi F, Rossi R, Simonelli C. Expanding the analysis of psychosocial factors of sexual desire in men. J Sex Med. 2018;15(2):230–44.

116. Durette R, Marrs C, Gray PB. Fathers faring poorly: results of an Internet-based survey of fathers of young children. Am J Mens Health. 2011;5(5):395–401.

117. Carvalho J, Nobre P. Biopsychosocial determinants of men's sexual desire: testing an integrative model. J Sex Med. 2011;8(3):754–63.

118. Kalogeropoulos D, Larouche J. An integrative biopsychosocial approach to the conceptualization and treatment of erectile disorder. In: Hall KSK, Binik YM, editors. Principles and practice of sex therapy. New York: Guilford; 2020. Chapter 4.

119. Brotto L, Atallah S, Johnson-Agbakwu C, Rosenbaum T, Abdo C, Byers ES, Graham C, Nobre P, Wylie K. Psychological and interpersonal dimensions of sexual function and dysfunction. J Sex Med. 2016;13(4):538–71.

120. European Sexual Medicine Network. Memorandum of understanding for the implementation of the cost action European Sexual Medicine Network. Brussels: European Sexual Medicine Network; 2018.
121. de Oliveira L, Carvalho J. Women's sexual health during the pandemic of COVID-19: declines in sexual function and sexual pleasure. Curr Sex Health Rep. 2021;3:1–13.
122. Stephenson KR, Meston CM. Differentiating components of sexual well-being in women: are sexual satisfaction and sexual distress independent constructs? J Sex Med. 2010;7(7):2458–68.
123. Pescatori ES, Giammusso B, Piubello G, Gentile V, Farina FP. Journey into the realm of requests for help presented to sexual medicine specialists: introducing male sexual distress. J Sex Med. 2007;4(3):762–70.
124. Hayes RD, Dennerstein L, Bennett CM, Fairley CK. What is the "true" prevalence of female sexual dysfunctions and does the way we assess these conditions have an impact? J Sex Med. 2008;5(4):777–87.
125. Santos-Iglesias P, Mohamed B, Walker LM. A systematic review of sexual distress measures. J Sex Med. 2018;15(5):625–44.

Diagnosis of Male Sexual Dysfunction

2

Alexander Bjørneboe Nolsøe, Emil Durukan,
Christian Fuglesang S. Jensen, and Mikkel Fode

Abstract

Sexual behavior is influenced by biology, psychology, interpersonal relationships, and culture. The investigation and diagnosis of sexual dysfunctions require an exploratory and holistic approach where the health professional includes the whole patient together with their interactions with others (Levine, J Sex Med 4:853–54, 2007; Lipshultz et al., Management of sexual dysfunction in men and women: An interdisciplinary approach, 2016). In this chapter, we describe the essential concepts in diagnosing male sexual dysfunctions. We demonstrate the basics in history-taking presenting general principles in the communication process and present the central components in the physical examination.

Setting the Scene

Investigating a patient's sexual problems might take place in a wide variety of settings whether it be long-term sexual therapy or a doctor's consultation in a hospital outpatient clinic. It is therefore important to create a comfortable setting shielded from external disturbances so the patient feels safe and has the fundamental sense of time and respect [1]. Also, make room for a possible partner since the partner can play an active role in the treatment process. For example, men with erectile dysfunction (ED), who are treated with pro-erection medication, may not always return to a completely fulfilled and satisfying sexual relationship. The partner's role is the best predictor of maintaining pleasurable sexual experiences [2].

A. B. Nolsøe · E. Durukan · C. F. S. Jensen · M. Fode (✉)
Department of Urology, Copenhagen University Hospital, Herlev and Gentofte Hospital, Copenhagen, Denmark

Department of Clinical Medicine, University of Copenhagen, Copenhagen, Denmark

S. Sarikaya et al. (eds.), *Andrology and Sexual Medicine*, Management of Urology,
https://doi.org/10.1007/978-3-031-12049-7_2

Clearly emphasize confidentiality for example by directly expressing that the communication between the patient and health professional is confidential and protected. It may be particularly relevant with younger patients [3].

Sexual health can greatly impact the overall quality of life and is one of the most intimate and vulnerable aspects of human life. Accordingly, health professionals must maintain a supportive and non-judgmental attitude and be aware of social or cultural biases that one might have when investigating sexual problems. Be open and receptive to the patient's own experiences, wants, and needs both vocally and nonverbally. Managing sexual problems is a collaborative effort that embraces the patient's perspectives, thoughts, feelings, expectations, and values and in addition, includes cultural and ethnic facets, as well as religious views [4].

Sexual History Taking

For most individuals, sexuality is a highly private matter, and patients may find it difficult to seek treatment or disclose sexual concerns. It is important to address such concerns especially during consultations for conditions or treatments that might affect sexual health. The health care professional can ease the interview by using open, inviting, generalizing, and appreciative questions such as:

- We ask about sexual health because we experience that patients going through the same condition as you have felt changes in their intimate and sexual lives. Is it alright for me to ask questions about your sexual life?
- In your current situation, I can imagine that it may affect your sexual life. What is your experience?

By openly addressing sexual matters, health professionals demonstrate acknowledgment of the importance of sexuality in the patient's life and their willingness to discuss it professionally. Actively state that problems and thoughts related to topics such as sex life and relationships are normal and is a routine aspect of health care [5].

In sexual medicine, people who do not identify with the gender they were assigned at birth may seek professional help due to a sexual problem relating to their gender identity. Examples include patients expressing reflections or doubts regarding gender identity both during sex and out of a sexual context and/or if the patient considers or undergoes gender-affirming surgery. Gender identity is subjective and as a health professional, you can only listen to and observe the patient's self-perception and experiences. The patient may understand gender in various ways. Some trans people and nonbinary people are satisfied and pleased with their bodies, while others experience discomfort [6]. The patient's sex and gender identity can be relevant information to access during a consultation in several situations. Ask about the patient's sex and gender identity when clinically relevant while simultaneously assuring the professional reason for doing so. For example, when assessing the risk of developing cancer in the reproductive system. As each patient is unique, a health professional should never make assumptions about sexual orientation or behavior before conducting a full sexual history [7].

Sexual history taking is usually overlooked or rushed, yet it is a crucial part of therapy. The health professional should strive towards taking a full history for a thorough understanding of the patient's issues. However, the sexual history can never be complete because the information given varies depending on the specialty of the health professional, the issue, and the patient's motivation to talk about the problem [8]. By being aware of the general structure of the dialogue, you limit the likelihood of any areas being neglected. First, align expectations to the consultation at the very beginning and establish an agenda when taking the sexual history. What are the patient's viewpoints and expectations, and what do you expect you can accomplish in the time frame? Then, let the patient describe the current problem in their own words and explore the issue with questions like:

- How big is the problem for you?
- How has it evolved?
- How long has it been going on?
- How much does it affect the patient and partner?
- What else happened in the patient's life around this time?

Simultaneously, special attention should be paid to the biological and psychosocial factors when interviewing the patient. A comprehensive bio-psychosocial evaluation is essential for a successful diagnostic process. Mental or relational problems may cause physical symptoms, while physical problems can have psychological implications. Even if the problem mainly is psychological, the physical examination may alleviate fear or anxiety of an underlying disease. Note the patient's demeanor and speech during the consultation as it can be indicative of anxiety or depression.

A systematic history taking that covers all relevant elements of the patients' lives reduces the risk of overlooking important factors and it usually reveals that biological and psychosocial issues are inextricably intertwined. The bio-psychosocial evaluation may reveal underlying comorbid medical issues and can help distinguish between possible organic and psychogenic causes in the etiology of a patient's sexual dysfunction [9].

The Bio-Psychosocial Approach

To fully and openly understand and treat a patient's sexual problem, information regarding the following four domains of the patient's life should be collected. Unlike a medical examination, a therapeutic evaluation is less transparent and needs the healthcare professional to explore various facets of a patient's life to understand the root of the problem. This includes individual, relational, familial, and sociocultural aspects [10, 11]. However, depending on the scenario, the healthcare professional should weigh the various factors or leave them out entirely. For example, there is a strong and clear correlation between ED following prostatectomy, and a comprehensive familial history taking in this situation would be irrelevant. Likewise, an extensive physical examination of a younger person with a primary mental condition may lead to an unnecessary sense of morbidity.

When diagnosing and evaluating a patient's sexual problem, it is important to recognize during the interview whether the problem exceeds the health professional's abilities. In such cases, the patient needs to be referred for the appropriate help [9].

Individual

The diagnosis process begins with gathering general information about the patient. Secondly, the biological and psychological background is explored including a full medical history, current medication, chronic, and recent medical conditions. Information about previous surgeries should be included especially in relation to the pelvic area. It is important to note if the patient is using herbal or other natural substances to enhance their performance and overall sexual satisfaction. Psychological well-being should then be explored with a focus on sexuality and their current relationship [12].

Relational

Identify the current state of the relationship and how the patient and their partner interact with each other not only in relation to sexuality but also in relation to other problems other than sexual issues for example conflict management and communication styles. Establish an overview of the commitment level and if there are any incongruent levels of sexual desire. Most often, sexual issues affect a relationship, and a relationship affects a couple's sex life [12, 13].

Family History

To establish a thorough foundation of information for the later therapeutic process, it is important to investigate the patient's familial history. This includes information about sex education, sexual attitudes, and any history of trauma, abuse, or sexual health problems [12].

Sociocultural Context

Explore the patient's culture, religion, and other significant experiences growing up. The patient's socio-cultural background can affect their sexual attitudes, practices, and behavior. Ask the patient if any earlier experiences have had an impact on them as an adult [12].

Physical Examination

As with the medical history taking it is crucial to create a comfortable environment for the physical examination. It is often deeply private and for some a great cause of psychological discomfort, shame, and embarrassment. Therefore, informing the patient of what is going to happen during the physical exam and aligning expectations prior to the actual exam is necessary.

The Role of the Physical Examination

The extent of the examination should reflect the tentative diagnosis derived from the patient's sexual- and medical history. Even though the physical examination may not directly identify the specific etiology or cause of sexual dysfunction [14], the physical findings can help confirm or deny any tentative diagnoses and differentiate between differential diagnoses. In addition, the physical examination can provide valuable information of any underlying conditions that may be linked to the patient's sexual problem.

In fact, men with sexual dysfunction have a high prevalence of comorbidities such as diabetes, metabolic syndrome, lower urinary tract symptoms (LUTS) hypertension, dyslipidemia, and cardiovascular disease (CVD) [15–18], which all require treatment if they are not already being treated. As an example, ED is strongly linked to CVD and often precedes CVD by a couple of years opening a window for early preventive treatment that could reduce any future and potentially fatal cardiovascular events [18].

It also seems that there is a higher prevalence of sexual comorbidities in patients with sexual dysfunction, that is when a man with one sexual dysfunction such as premature ejaculation is also suffering from ED, although the etiology of this is not known [19]. A general physical assessment should therefore almost always be conducted, whereas more specific testing should only be performed if indicated by specific findings from the medical history or physical examination.

Finally, the physical examination can help provide information on medical history that the patient may have not thought of during the initial history taking. This could be a patient who complains about ED, about not being able to attain a sufficient erection but is not able to elaborate further when inquired. The physical examination may reveal phimosis that is so tight it results in insufficient tumescence leading to ED.

General Health Assessment

The physical examination should start with a general health assessment. This should include height, weight, BMI or waist circumference, blood pressure, and heart rate. Together with the patient's medical history, this will indicate the need for risk stratification for CVD. There are many risk prediction tools available [20] and they are easily accessible at https://u-prevent.com/. Healthcare workers evaluating patients with ED should always assess this risk and refer the patient to his general practitioner or a cardiologist when relevant.

Next, the general physical attributes should be assessed including secondary sexual characteristics such as deepening of the voice, bodily and facial hair, muscle mass, and fat distribution. Lack of bodily and facial hair, gynecomastia, and female fat distribution can be signs of hypogonadism and would require further lab-testing to confirm and distinguish between primary-, secondary-, or adult-onset hypogonadism.

A general abdominal examination will reveal any possible hernias or any signs of previous abdominal/pelvic surgery that the patient may have omitted in their medical history.

The neurological state of the perineal region and lower limbs can sometimes be relevant for evaluation. If neurological deficiencies are suspected, then a more thorough evaluation should be conducted including testing of the perianal reflex involving nerves that arise from the S2-S4 segment. The reflex is elicited by stroking the skin around the anus which results in a contraction of the anal sphincter. Another test is the bulbocarvernosus reflex that tests the nerves arising from the S3-S4-segment. Here the glans of the penis is squeezed causing the anal sphincter to contract.

Genital Exam

As with the general assessment, a genital exam should always be conducted to a variable extent at some point in men with sexual dysfunction.

Initially evaluating the degree of pubic hair growth, penis, and testes size using the Tanner scale [21].

Examine the penis for any abnormalities starting with visual examination and moving on to palpation. If beginning distally, start by noting any edema or reddening of the foreskin on uncircumcised patients as seen in balanitis. Observe any ulcers or nodules and then progress to retract the foreskin to check for phimosis and frenulum breve, stop if it becomes too painful/tight. Alternatively, ask the patient to do it themselves. Then check the glans for ulcers, scars, nodules or chancre, rashes or any signs of infection or visible discharge, and different meatus placements. In hypospadias the orifice is located on the ventral surface of the shaft, most often distally on the ventral side of the glans then midshaft and proximal [22]. Most will have had surgery performed as a child but not all and it may be the cause of embarrassment leading to sexual dysfunction.

The best view of the meatus to check for discharge is achieved by gently compressing the glans distally which opens the meatus. It is also worth noting any foul odor as this could imply an infection.

Go on to check the shaft and base of the penis for reddening, edema, and if relevant, different urethral meatus placements.

Some patients will present with edema of the shaft/base of the penis which can have different etiologies ranging from infections to more rare causes as reactive inflammations due to self-administered filler injections with unapproved foreign materials or ointment application arising from a desire for more girth or length [23].

Thoroughly palpate the entire penis for any induration, abnormalities, or pain, one way to do this is by squeezing the penis between the thumb and two first fingers. Check for plaques consistent with Peyronie's disease. If the medical history indicates Peyronie's disease it may be helpful with an injection of a vasoactive substance to see the degree of the problem. Alternatively, the patient may bring a photo of his penis in the erect state. For patients that have sexual dysfunction due to concern over a small penis that may be inclined to go for penile augmentation surgery, measurements should be obtained as maximum stretched length and width by grasping the glans and pulling the penis to full stretch at 90 degrees from the plane of the body [24]. Stretched penile length is close to the length of the erect penis.

When examining the testicles, start by having the patient standing facing you and assess the size of the scrotum, look for any swelling or reddening of the skin, edema, and check for any visible varicocele. If the scrotum seems very small remember that if it is cold or the patient is nervous the cremasteric reflex may have retracted the testicles. An enlarged scrotum can be due to anything from hydrocele to a tumor or epididymitis. It is important to palpate thoroughly and if possible, use an ultrasound probe. In the case of epididymitis, it might be relevant as well to check for potential STDs, especially in the younger patient group.

Palpate the testes, epididymis, and spermatic cord, and check for any signs of varicoceles which is a dilatation of the pampiniform plexus, most commonly found on the left side. Examine the size and consistency, check for nodules and any pain that is more than the discomfort of the examination. The size of the testes can be measured by a Prader orchidometer or in a specialty setting by ultrasound with the latter being more precise [25]. Small testes are not necessarily a sign of an underlying disease, however, they are more often found in some medical conditions and it might be relevant to test for chromosomal abnormality (karyotype) and hormone levels. Nodules and/or irregular surfaces of the testes should be examined by ultrasound and possibly bloodwork incl LDH, AFP and HCG. If the testes are retracted it may be of help to have the patient sit down on the exam table to relax and make sure to have warm hands. It may also be due to an undescended testis. Approximately 80% of undescended testes are still palpable in the inguinal canal [26] and whether or not it is palpable influences the surgical approach, so make sure to palpate sufficiently and see if it is possible to bring the testes back down to the scrotum, however, in the majority of cases cryptorchidism is diagnosed during a routine check of infants.

The final part of the physical exam is a digital rectal exam to assess the prostate, however, it should only be performed if there is a relevant medical history or physical findings to support it. Here the size and consistency of the prostate is evaluated and related to possible symptoms such as LUTS. In fact, LUTS and ED share pathophysiological mechanisms and LUTS may even precede ED. Therefore, patients with LUTS should always have a rectal exam performed and be asked about ED [17, 27]. The prostate should be evaluated for any pain which could signify an infection, and irregularities or nodules as prostate cancer is the second most common cancer in men. It is especially important to assess in men that are to receive testosterone replacement, as abnormalities can be present even in men with a normal PSA level.

Laboratory Tests and Specialized Tests

There are many laboratory tests and/or specialized functional tests that may be relevant depending on the tentative diagnosis one wants to confirm or deny. For example, if underlying diabetes or cardiovascular disease is suspected one should initially perform a test for Haemoglobin A1c and Lipid Profile. If the medical history or physical findings hints at endocrine involvement one should initially test Testosterone and related pituitary hormones, LH and FSH. Symptoms of hypogonadism are unspecific but include decreased libido, infertility, ED, while physical findings include small testes a high pitched voice and little to no hair growth or in especially older men, loss of muscles mass, abnormal breast growth or female fat distribution.

One of the most commonly used specialized diagnostic tests when treating male sexual dysfunction is the ultrasound examination. It is relevant especially when a testes examination requires further investigation due to abnormal findings or size. It may also be used to assess Peyronie's plaques and with induction of an erection and use of color doppler the penile flow can be assessed. This test should be used with caution as there is patient discomfort and a risk of priapism with penile injections, while the clinical implications of the test are limited.

Nocturnal penile tumescence and rigidity testing may be used to differentiate between primary organic and primary psychogenic ED but are rarely indicated in clinical practice [14].

Summary

Sexual medicine involves biological, psychological, interpersonal relationships, and cultural factors. When setting the scene and investigating sexual dysfunctions, ensure confidentiality, take your time, and remember to involve the whole patient and include the factors above when relevant. The physical examination does not only help us distinguish between tentative diagnosis, but it can also uncover underlying issues that the patient may not be aware of and which may require further treatment as in the case of CVD.

References

1. Tomlinson J. ABC of sexual health: taking a sexual history. BMJ. 1998;317:1573–6.
2. Metz ME, McCarthy BW. The "good-enough sex" model for couple sexual satisfaction. Sex Relatsh Ther. 2007;22:351–62.
3. Thomas N, Murray E, Rogstad KE. Confidentiality is essential if young people are to access sexual health services. Int J STD AIDS. 2006;17:525–9.

4. Hertlein KM, Weeks GR, Sendak SK. A clinician's guide to systemic sex therapy. New York: Routledge; 2009.
5. French P. BASHH 2006 National Guidelines—consultations requiring sexual history-taking. Int J STD AIDS. 2007;18:17–22.
6. Glynn TR, Gamarel KE, Kahler CW, Operario D, Iwamoto M, Nemoto T. The role of gender affirmation in psychological well-being among transgender women. Psychol Sex Orientat Gend Divers. 2016;3:336.
7. Sadovsky R, Nusbaum M. Sexual health inquiry and support is a primary care priority. J Sex Med. 2006;3:3–11.
8. Levine SB. The first principle of clinical sexuality. J Sex Med. 2007;4:853–4.
9. Hatzichristou D, Rosen RC, Broderick G, et al. Clinical evaluation and management strategy for sexual dysfunction in men and women. J Sex Med. 2004;1:49–57.
10. Seshadri G, Knudson-Martin C. How couples manage interracial and intercultural differences: implications for clinical practice. J Marital Fam Ther. 2013;39:43–58.
11. Kedde H, Van De Wiel H, Schultz WW, Vanwesenbeeck I, Bender J. Sexual health problems and associated help-seeking behavior of people with physical disabilities and chronic diseases. J Sex Marital Ther. 2012;38:63–78.
12. Wylie K, Rudolph E, Boffard C. Sexual History Taking. In P.S. Kirana, F. Tripodi, Y. Reisman, H. Porst (Eds.), The EFS and ESSM syllabus of clinical sexology—ESSM. 2013. p. 400–401.
13. Crowe M. Couple relationship problems and sexual dysfunctions: therapeutic guidelines. Adv Psychiatr Treat. 2012;18(2):154–9. https://doi.org/10.1192/apt.bp.109.007443.
14. Hatzichristou D, Rosen RC, Derogatis LR, Low WY, Meuleman EJH, Sadovsky R, Symonds T. Recommendations for the clinical evaluation of men and women with sexual dysfunction. J Sex Med. 2010;7:337–48.
15. Burke JP, Jacobson DJ, McGree ME, Nehra A, Roberts RO, Girman CJ, Lieber MM, Jacobsen SJ. Diabetes and sexual dysfunction: results from the olmsted county study of urinary symptoms and health status among men. J Urol. 2007;177:1438–42.
16. Corona G, Mannucci E, Schulman C, Petrone L, Mansani R, Cilotti A, Balercia G, Chiarini V, Forti G, Maggi M. Psychobiologic correlates of the metabolic syndrome and associated sexual dysfunction. Eur Urol. 2006;50:595–604.
17. Martin SA, Atlantis E, Lange K, Taylor AW, O'Loughlin P, Wittert GA. Predictors of sexual dysfunction incidence and remission in men. J Sex Med. 2014;11:1136–47.
18. Gandaglia G, Briganti A, Jackson G, Kloner RA, Montorsi F, Montorsi P, Vlachopoulos C. A systematic review of the association between erectile dysfunction and cardiovascular disease. Eur Urol. 2014;65:968–78.
19. Rowland DL, Oosterhouse LB, Kneusel JA, Hevesi K. Comorbidities among sexual problems in men: results from an internet convenience sample. Sex Med. 2021;9:100416.
20. Rossello X, Dorresteijn JA, Janssen A, Lambrinou E, Scherrenberg M, Bonnefoy-Cudraz E, Cobain M, Piepoli MF, Visseren FL, Dendale P. Risk prediction tools in cardiovascular disease prevention: A report from the ESC Prevention of CVD Programme led by the European Association of Preventive Cardiology (EAPC) in collaboration with the Acute Cardiovascular Care Association (ACCA) and the As. Eur Hear J Acute Cardiovasc Care. 2020;9:522–32.
21. Marshall WA, Tanner JM. Variations in the pattern of pubertal changes in boys. Arch Dis Child. 1970;45:13.
22. van der Horst HJR, de Wall LL. Hypospadias, all there is to know. Eur J Pediatr. 2017;176:435–41.
23. Ahmed U, Freeman A, Kirkham A, Ralph DJ, Minhas S, Muneer A. Self injection of foreign materials into the penis. Ann R Coll Surg Engl. 2017;99:e78.
24. Wessells H, Lue TF, Mcaninch JW. Penile length in the flaccid and erect states: guidelines for penile augmentation. J Urol. 1996;156:995–7.
25. Sønksen J, Ohl DA, Giwercman A, Biering-Sørensen F, Skakkebaek NE, Kristensen JK. Effect of repeated ejaculation on semen quality in spinal cord injured men. J Urol. 1999;161:1163–5.

26. Radmayr C, Dogan HS, Hoebeke P, Kocvara R, Nijman R, Stein R, Undre S, Tekgul S. Management of undescended testes: European Association of Urology/European Society for Paediatric Urology Guidelines. J Pediatr Urol. 2016;12(6):335–43. https://doi.org/10.1016/j.jpurol.2016.07.014.
27. McVary KT. Erectile dysfunction and lower urinary tract symptoms secondary to BPH. Eur Urol. 2005;47:838–45.

Erectile Dysfunction: From Diagnosis to Treatment

3

Selcuk Sarikaya

Abstract

Erectile dysfunction (ED) is inability to achieve and maintain erection for satisfactory sexual intercourse persistently. ED can be classified according to the etiological factors as organic, psychogenic and mixed. Endothelial dysfunction takes important role in the pathophysiologic mechanism of vascular ED as well as cardiovascular diseases so that they share similar risk factors. The diagnosis and evaluation of ED start with a comprehensive medical, psychosocial and sexual history. International Index of Erectile Function (IIEF-5, IIEF-15) and Sexual Health Inventory for Men (SHIM) can be used for the evaluation. Physical examination includes detailed urogenital examination, examination for neurologic system, cardiovascular system, endocrin system and general examination. Basic laboratory tests (biochemical tests including blood glucose, lipid profile, creatinine, blood urea nitrogen, electrolytes and hormonal profile including testosterone, Follicle-Stimulating Hormone (FSH), Luteinizing Hormone (LH), Prolactin (PRL), catecholamine, Thyroid-Stimulating Hormone (TSH), thyroid hormones) are used for both diagnosis and assessing the severity of ED. Specific diagnostic tests (psychologic evaluation, nocturnal penile tumescence, color duplex doppler ultrasonography, injection test, arteriography, cavernosometry, cavernosography, electromyography, pudendal nerve evoked potential, biopsy etc.) would be also necessary. Treatment of erectile dysfunction basically depends on the etiologic factors. Treatment options are lifestyle modifications, oral phosphodiesterase type 5 inhibitors (PDE5i), vacuum erection devices (VED), extracorporeal shock wave therapy (ESWT), stem cell therapy (SCT) and platelet-rich plasma injection (PRP), intracavernosal injections (ICI), intrauretral agents, penile prosthesis implantation (PPI), vascular surgery and other options.

S. Sarikaya (✉)
Department of Urology, Gulhane Research and Training Hospital, University of Health Sciences, Ankara, Turkey

© The Author(s), under exclusive license to Springer Nature Switzerland AG 2022
S. Sarikaya et al. (eds.), *Andrology and Sexual Medicine*, Management of Urology, https://doi.org/10.1007/978-3-031-12049-7_3

29

Introduction, Etiology and Epidemiology

Erectile dysfunction (ED) is inability to achieve and maintain erection for satisfactory sexual intercourse persistently [1]. ED is the most common sexual disorder among men [2]. ED may affect the psychological condition as well as social life that is directly in relation with quality of life (QoL) [1]. Several epidemiologic studies have been conducted in order to reveal the prevalence of ED. Epidemiological data pointed the ED prevalence between 16–25% [3]. The studies have shown 52% rates among men between 40–70 years and increasing with age [4]. ED is associated with several comorbidities as diabetes mellitus (DM), cardiovascular pathologies, metabolic syndrome and depression [5]. The most important associations were found with age and depression at initial admission for ED [6]. ED can be classified according to the etiological factors as organic, iatrogenic, psychogenic and mixed [1, 7] (Table 3.1). Organic etiologies include vascular, neurogenic, anatomic and endocrine factors [2]. Psychogenic ED is generally seen at younger ages especially under the age of 40 [3]. Over the age of 50, psychogenic ED is between 10–45% [3]. Psychogenic reasons are depression, anxiety and traumatic experiences that directly affect the self-confidence [3]. Studies have shown the bidirectional relationship between ED and depression [8]. Pharmacologic agents for cardiovascular diseases (thiazide diuretics and beta blockers) have negative effects on erectile functions [1]. Pelvic and urogenital surgical procedures including radical prostatectomy may cause erectile dysfunction and penile rehabilitation would be needed in the postoperative period [9]. Analysis of the patients during the post-prostatectomy period showed that one-third of impotent patients did not try treatment options for erectile dysfunction in postoperative period and there were moderate to severe problems for these patients regarding this pathologic condition [10]. Studies show similar pathophysiologic mechanisms that are associated with ED and lower urinary tract symptoms (LUTS). This strong correlation must be considered for both diagnosis and treatment of these pathologies [11].

Table 3.1 Etiologic factors

Organic	Iatrogenic	Psychogenic
Vascular [1, 2]	Pharmacotherapeutic agents [1] (Antihypertensives, Antidepressants, Chemotherapeutics, Anticholinergics, Benzodiazepines)	Depression [3, 6]
Neurogenic [1]	Alcohol [1]	Performance anxiety [3]
Endocrinologic [1]	Tobacco [1]	Traumatic experiences [3]
Primary disorders [1]	Recreational drugs [1]	Lack of self-confidence [3]
	Pelvic & Colorectal surgery [9]	Relationship conflicts [1]
	Radical prostatectomy [9]	

Penile Anatomy

The corpora cavernosa are located dorsolaterally and they are surrounded by thick fibrous tunica albuginea [12]. Corpora cavernosa include multiple smooth muscles and sinusoids that allow penile extension [12]. Corpus spongiosum is single and ventrally located that is surrounded by thinner layer of tunica albuginea and it surrounds urethra [12]. Tunica albuginea is a dense and fibroelastic layer that surrounds corpora cavernosa and corpus spongiosum [13]. Superficial to the tunical layer, there is Buck's fascia and the three corpora are surrounded by Buck's fascia [12, 13]. The bulbospongiosus and ischiocavernosus muscles are located superiorly to the Buck's fascia [13]. More superficially, there is areolar dartos or Colles' fascia [13]. Internal pudendal artery which provides main arterial blood supply of penis continues as penile artery and it gives bulbar artery branch that gives arterial supply to the proximal part [12]. Internal pudendal arteries continue as penile arteries after passing the urogenital diaphragm [13]. Penile artery divides into dorsal and cavernosal arteries and cavernosal artery provides arterial blood supply to the corpora cavernosa with hellicine arteries and also supplies sinusoids with arterioles [12]. Besides the cavernosal arteries, penile arteries give dorsal, bulbar and urethral arterial branches [13]. The main veins are superficial and deep dorsal veins of the penis. Emissary veins drain into deep dorsal vein [12]. The glans penis drains through the superficial dorsal vein and it drains into the left saphenous vein [13]. Spongiosal, circumflex and cavernosal veins also take role in venous drainage [12]. Corpus spongiosum drains via urethral and circumflex veins that join with deep dorsal vein [13].

Physiology of Erection

Hypothalamus is stimulated with several neurotransmitters during the sexual activity and dopamine takes an important erectogenic role in this process [14]. Erectile tissues, specifically cavernous smooth muscles and arterial, arteriolar walls play key role in the process [15]. Erection would be both psychogenically-mediated and tactile-mediated [14]. Cavernous nerve activation would result in Nitric Oxide release by the Nitric Oxide Synthase (NOS) enzyme and it activates Guanylate Cyclase (GC) which results in breakdown of guanosine triphosphate into 3'5'-cyclic guanosine monophosphate (cGMP) [14]. Starting with the sexual stimulus, smooth muscle relaxation starts, blood flow increases with arterial dilation, blood is trapped in the expanded sinusoidal structures, venous outflow decrease with the compression on venous structures, intracavernous pressure increases and finally an additional pressure increase is seen with ischiocavernosus muscle contraction as it results with rigid erection [15]. With the phophodiesterase subtype 5, cGMP and cAMP (cyclic adenosine monophosphate) are hydrolyzed and these lead to vasodilation and smooth muscle relaxation [14].

Pathophysiology of Erectile Dysfunction

Endothelial dysfunction takes important role in the pathophysiologic mechanism of vascular ED as well as cardiovascular diseases so that they share similar risk factors [16]. Erectile tissue defects due to several comorbidities and risk factors would result in erectile dysfunction [14]. Arteriogenic ED mainly depends on structural changes (oxygen tension decrease in corpus cavernosum), vasoconstruction (enhanced myogenic tone and increased resistance in vascular structures) and endothelium impairments [17]. Cavernosal (venogenic) ED mainly depends on veno-occlusive dysfunction due to the presence of large venous structures and degenerative or traumatic changes (peyronie's disease, diabetes, penile fracture) [17].

Diagnosis

There are several diagnostic tools that can be used in the diagnosis of erectile dysfunction (Table 3.2).

Medical and Sexual History

The diagnosis and evaluation of ED start with a comprehensive medical, psychosocial and sexual history [14]. Diagnosis is basically depends on patient complaints, diagnostic tests and partner reports [7]. Signs and symptoms of possible etiologic factors must be assessed in detail [14].

Table 3.2 Diagnostic approaches

Medical and Sexual History [7, 14]	Comprehensive Medical, Psychosocial and Sexual history
Questionnaires and Diagnostic Tools [1, 16]	International Index of Erectile Function (IIEF-5, IIEF-15), Sexual Health Inventory for Men (SHIM), Beck Depression Inventory
Physical examination [1]	Urogenital examination, Examination for Neurologic system, Cardiovascular system, Endocrin system and General examination.
Laboratory Tests [1, 16]	Blood glucose, Lipid profile, Creatinine, Blood Urea Nitrogen (BUN), Electrolytes and Hormonal Profile (Testosterone, Follicle-Stimulating Hormone (FSH), Luteinizing Hormone (LH), Prolactin (PRL), Catecholamine, Thyroid-Stimulating Hormone (TSH), Thyroid Hormones
Specific Diagnostic Tests [1, 16]	Psychologic Evaluation, Nocturnal Penile Tumescence, Color Duplex Doppler Ultrasonography, Injection test, Arteriography, Cavernosometry, Cavernosography, Electromyography, Pudendal Nerve Evoked Potential, Biopsy

Questionnaires and Diagnostic Tools

International Index of Erectile Function (IIEF-5, IIEF-15) and Sexual Health Inventory for Men (SHIM) can be used for the evaluation [1, 16]. Beck Depression Inventory is used for depressive patients [1]. These questionnaires give detailed information about the presence and the severity of sexual dysfunction.

Physical Examination

Physical examination includes detailed urogenital examination, examination for neurologic system, cardiovascular system, endocrin system and general examination [1]. Primary disorders, sex characteristics, and deformities would be observed. Physical examination would reveal primary disorders such as Peyronie's disease (PD), malignant urogenital tumors, prostatic pathologies and also hypogonadism signs and symptoms [1].

Basic Laboratory Tests

Basic laboratory tests (biochemical tests including blood glucose, lipid profile, creatinine, blood urea nitrogen, electrolytes and hormonal profile including testosterone, Follicle-Stimulating Hormone (FSH), Luteinizing Hormone (LH), Prolactin (PRL), catecholamine, Thyroid-Stimulating Hormone (TSH), thyroid hormones) are used for both diagnosis and assessing the severity of ED [16]. Fasting blood glucose, lipids and HbA1c must be assessed if they have not been assessed during the previous 1 year period and total testosterone must be assessed in early morning hours [1].

Specific Diagnostic Tests

Specific diagnostic tests (psychologic evaluation, nocturnal penile tumescence, color duplex doppler ultrasonography, injection test, arteriography, cavernosometry, cavernosography, electromyography, pudendal nerve evoked potential, biopsy etc.) would be also necessary for selected patients [16]. Nocturnal penile tumescence and rigidity (NPTR) test can reveal erectile episodes, tumescence and rigidity and nocturnal erection durations [1]. Intracavernous injection test gives information about the vascular status and color duplex doppler ultrasonography reveals haemodynamic condition of penis [1].

Treatment

Lots of treatment approaches have been reported in the literature and also they are effective treatment approaches for erectile dysfunction (Table 3.3).

Initial Approach, Lifestyle Modification and Psychological Therapy

Treatment of erectile dysfunction basically depends on the etiologic factors. Lifestyle changes including weight loss, physical exercises, dietary changes, quit smoking and reducing alcohol must be considered in the first line of treatment and prevention [18]. Detailed evaluation of the patients can lead the appropriate treatment option. Curable causes must be considered and treated first. Patients with psychogenic ED need psychological evaluation and they would receive psychosexual therapy. As the bidirectional relationship between ED and depression has been revealed, it is very important to treat depression for getting improvement in sexual functions [8]. The choice of antidepressants is also important because they can directly affect the sexual response [8]. Selective serotonin reuptake inhibitors (SSRI) increase the serotonin levels and this may result in inhibition of sexual function [8]. Most of the patients can be treated with treatment options that are not cause-specific [1]. Specific treatment options are applied for psychogenic ED, post-traumatic arteriogenic subtype and hormonal reasons such as hypogonadism [1].

Table 3.3 Treatment options

Lifestyle modifications [18]	Weight loss, Physical exercises, Dietary changes, Smoking cessation and reducing Alcohol
Oral phosphodiesterase type 5 inhibitors (PDE5i) [18–20]	Sildenafil, Tadalafil, Vardenafil and Avanafil
Vacuum erection devices (VED) [18, 21]	Negative Pressure results with Erection
Extracorporeal shock wave therapy (ESWT) [22–26]	900 shocks at 0.09 mJ/mm^2 energy to right and left corpora cavernosa and the crura/total number of 3600 shocks per session are applied at four sessions
Stem cell therapy (SCT) and Platelet-rich plasma injection (PRP) [27–29]	Intracavernosal stem cell injection therapy, Platelet-Rich Plasma (PRP) injection
Intracavernosal injections (ICI) [1, 30, 31]	Diagnosis and Treatment. Alprostadil (PGE1 - Caverject, Edex/Viridal), Bimix: Papaverine: 7.5–45 mg + Phentolamine: 0.25–1.5 mg and Trimix: Papaverine: 8–16 mg + Phentolamine: 0.2–0.4 mg + Alprostadil: 10–20 µg
Intrauretral agents [1, 18]	Alprostadil (PGE1) - with permeation enhancer (200 and 300 µg)/specific formulation (125–1000 µg)-MUSE
Penile prosthesis implantation (PPI) [1, 32]	Non-inflatable (Malleable) and Inflatable
Vascular surgery [1, 33]	Penile revascularisation
Other options [34–36]	Mirabegron, Intracavernous injection of onabotilinum toxin-A, Acupuncture

Oral Phosphodiesterase Type 5 Inhibitors (PDE5i)

Oral treatment options include phosphodiesterase type 5 (PDE5) inhibitors. PDE5 specifically target cyclic Guanylate Monophosphate (cGMP) that is generated by guanylyl cyclase and mediated by nitric oxide (NO) [19]. Oral PDE5 inhibitors include sildenafil, tadalafil, vardenafil and avanafil [18]. PDE5 inhibitors provide vasodilatation by blocking the breakdown of cGMP. Patients with low testosterone levels and low sexual desire, erectile dysfunction can receive testosterone therapy in addition to PDE5 inhibitors. Studies showed the beneficial effect of testosterone therapy with PDE5 inhibitors for the patients that did not have effective treatment response to PDE5 inhibits alone and did not have a contraindication for testosterone therapy [20].

Vacuum Erection Devices (VED)

Vacuum erection devices (VED) are important options for the patients with DM and arteriogenic ED [21]. It is also an alternative treatment option for the patients who denied oral therapeutic agents [21]. VED generates negative pressure that collects blood in cavernosal structures and results with erection [18].

Extracorporeal Shock Wave Therapy (ESWT)

Studies have shown the positive effects of extracorporeal shock wave therapy (ESWT) in organic ED [22]. 900 shocks at 0.09 mJ/mm^2 energy were applied to right and left corpora cavernosa and the crura of the penile shaft and total number of 3600 shocks per session are applied at four sessions [23]. Successful outcomes were reported for 80% of the patients and the average 9 points increase in IIEF scores were observed in patients [23]. Low-intensity extracorporeal shock wave therapy (LI-ESWT) is effective and safe method for rehabilitation of penile traumas and deviations [24]. LI-ESWT also improves the response to PDE5 inhibitors among the patients that are difficult to treat [25]. Studies also showed the efficacy of ESWT in improvement of erectile functions for younger patients with mild vasculogenic ED [26].

Stem Cell Therapy (SCT) and Platelet-Rich Plasma Injection (PRP)

Stem cell treatment is an important option with safety and efficacy [27]. Intracavernosal stem cell injection therapy is an alternative method for the patients that have resistant ED to conventional drugs and the patients with DM [28]. This therapy has been found to improve sexual function as well as ultrasonography parameters of patients with DM [28]. Platelet-rich plasma (PRP) injection would be performed for the patients with ED and this treatment remains promising, however recommendation cannot be made as a standard treatment option because additional evidence and literature-based outcomes are needed [29].

Intracavernosal Injections (ICI)

Intracavernosal injections are both used for diagnosis and treatment in erectile dysfunction [30]. Doppler ultrasonography after injections is an important diagnostic tool [30]. According to the guideline recommendations peak systolic velocity (PSV) of >30 cm/s, end-diastolic velocity (EDV) of <3 cm/s and resistive index (RI) of >0.8 are considered as normal [30]. EDV >5 cm/s and RI <0.75 are defined as venous leakage and some authors define PSV between 25–35 cm/s, EDV between 5–7 cm/s as grey zone [30]. Intracavernous vasoactive drug injection is an alternative medical therapy for ED. Intracavernous injection of prostaglandin E1 is an effective treatment option that improves rigidity and the duration of erection [31]. Alprostadil (Caverject, Edex/Viridal) was the first option approved for ED (5–40 µg) [1]. Combination of agents would be also preferred. (Bimix: Papaverine: 7.5–45 mg + Phentolamine: 0.25–1.5 mg and Trimix: Papaverine: 8–16 mg + Phentolamine: 0.2–0.4 mg + Alprostadil: 10–20 µg).

Intrauretral Agents

Alprostadil as an exogenous form of prostaglandin E1 (PGE1) could be used as intraurethral treatment option [18]. It allows erection by diffusion into corpus cavernosum or via collateral vessels and acts via increase of cyclic Adenosin Monophosphate (cAMP) in smooth muscles [18]. The first option is used with permeation enhancer that allows alprostadil absorption (200 and 300 µg) [1]. The second way is intraurethral insertion of specific formulation (125–1000 µg) with medicated pellet (MUSE) [1].

Penile Prosthesis Implantation (PPI)

Penile prosthesis implantation (PPI) is mainly offered for the patients over 40 years that do not respond to oral and intracavernous treatment options or reject these treatments [32]. Penile prostheses are basically divided into two groups as non-inflatable (malleable) and inflatable prostheses [32]. Two main surgical approaches are penoscrotal and infrapubic [1]. Malleable prostheses were found to be associated with less complication rates as the outcomes of the studies in this field [32]. Main perioperative complications are urethral perforation, cavernosal crossover, crural perforation and main postoperative complications are infection, hematoma, bending during the sexual intercourse, lower urinary tract symptoms, breakage, concord deformity and mechanical failure [32].

Vascular Surgery

Some of the patients that are resistant to oral treatment are diagnosed as cavernous leakage (CVL) [33]. Studies showed improvement in erectile functions and successful intercourse with embolisation and open surgery for these patients [33]. This option would be preferred for the patients at younger ages and patients that did not prefer penile prosthesis implantation [33]. Penile revascularisation has 60–70% long-term success rates [1].

Other Options

Studies showed the efficacy of Mirabegron for improvement of sexual function that is associated with lower urinary tract symptoms [34].

Intracavernous injection of onabotilinum toxin-A was pointed as an effective alternative for refractory ED [35].

Acupuncture can be considered as adjunctive treatment option for especially psychogenic ED [36].

References

1. Salonia A, Bettocchi C, Boeri L, Capogrosso P, Carvalho J, Cilesiz NC, et al. European Association of Urology Guidelines on Sexual and Reproductive Health-2021 update: male sexual dysfunction. Eur Urol. 2021;80(3):333–57. https://doi.org/10.1016/j.eururo.2021.06.007.
2. Ravikanth R. Diagnostic categorization of erectile dysfunction using duplex color doppler ultrasonography and significance of phentolamine redosing in abolishing false diagnosis of venous leak impotence: a single center experience. Indian J Radiol Imaging. 2020;30(3):344–53. https://doi.org/10.4103/ijri.IJRI_419_19.
3. Celik O, Ipekci T, Akarken I, Ekin G, Koksal T. To evaluate the etiology of erectile dysfunction: what should we know currently? Arch Ital Urol Androl. 2014;86(3):197–201. https://doi.org/10.4081/aiua.2014.3.197.
4. Rodler S, von Buren J, Buchner A, Stief C, Elkhanova K, Wulfing C, et al. Epidemiology and treatment barriers of patients with erectile dysfunction using an online prescription platform: a cross-sectional study. Sex Med. 2020;8(3):370–7. https://doi.org/10.1016/j.esxm.2020.04.001.
5. Panken EJ, Fantus RJ, Chang C, Kashanian JA, Helfand BT, Brannigan RE, et al. Epidemiology and diagnosis of erectile dysfunction by urologists versus non-urologists in the united states: an analysis of the National Ambulatory Medical Care Survey. Urology. 2021;147:167–71. https://doi.org/10.1016/j.urology.2020.09.016.
6. Korenman SG. Epidemiology of erectile dysfunction. Endocrine. 2004;23(2–3):87–91. https://doi.org/10.1385/ENDO:23:2-3:087.
7. Caskurlu T, Tasci AI, Resim S, Sahinkanat T, Ergenekon E. The etiology of erectile dysfunction and contributing factors in different age groups in Turkey. Int J Urol. 2004;11(7):525–9. https://doi.org/10.1111/j.1442-2042.2004.00837.x.
8. Perelman MA. Erectile dysfunction and depression: screening and treatment. Urol Clin North Am. 2011;38(2):125–39. https://doi.org/10.1016/j.ucl.2011.03.004.
9. Seo YE, Kim SD, Kim TH, Sung GT. The efficacy and safety of tadalafil 5 mg once daily in the treatment of erectile dysfunction after robot-assisted laparoscopic radical prostatectomy: 1-year follow-up. Korean J Urol. 2014;55(2):112–9. https://doi.org/10.4111/kju.2014.55.2.112.

10. Baunacke M, Schmidt ML, Groeben C, Borkowetz A, Thomas C, Koch R, et al. Treatment of post-prostatectomy urinary incontinence and erectile dysfunction: there is insufficient utilisation of care in German cancer survivors. World J Urol. 2021;39(8):2929–36. https://doi.org/10.1007/s00345-020-03526-z.

11. Kirby M, Chapple C, Jackson G, Eardley I, Edwards D, Hackett G, et al. Erectile dysfunction and lower urinary tract symptoms: a consensus on the importance of co-diagnosis. Int J Clin Pract. 2013;67(7):606–18. https://doi.org/10.1111/ijcp.12176.

12. Halls J, Bydawell G, Patel U. Erectile dysfunction: the role of penile doppler ultrasound in diagnosis. Abdom Imaging. 2009;34(6):712–25. https://doi.org/10.1007/s00261-008-9463-x.

13. Dwyer ME, Salgado CJ, Lightner DJ. Normal penile, scrotal, and perineal anatomy with reconstructive considerations. Semin Plast Surg. 2011;25(3):179–88. https://doi.org/10.1055/s-0031-1281487.

14. Albersen M, Mwamukonda KB, Shindel AW, Lue TF. Evaluation and treatment of erectile dysfunction. Med Clin North Am. 2011;95(1):201–12. https://doi.org/10.1016/j.mcna.2010.08.016.

15. El-Sakka AI, Lue TF. Physiology of penile erection. ScientificWorldJournal. 2004;4(Suppl 1):128–34. https://doi.org/10.1100/tsw.2004.58.

16. Ma M, Yu B, Qin F, Yuan J. Current approaches to the diagnosis of vascular erectile dysfunction. Transl Androl Urol. 2020;9(2):709–21. https://doi.org/10.21037/tau.2020.03.10.

17. Dean RC, Lue TF. Physiology of penile erection and pathophysiology of erectile dysfunction. Urol Clin North Am. 2005;32(4):379–95., v. https://doi.org/10.1016/j.ucl.2005.08.007.

18. Karakus S, Burnett AL. The medical and surgical treatment of erectile dysfunction: a review and update. Can J Urol. 2020;27(S3):28–35.

19. Ahmed WS, Geethakumari AM, Biswas KH. Phosphodiesterase 5 (PDE5): structure-function regulation and therapeutic applications of inhibitors. Biomed Pharmacother. 2021;134:111128. https://doi.org/10.1016/j.biopha.2020.111128.

20. Alhathal N, Elshal AM, Carrier S. Synergetic effect of testosterone and phophodiesterase-5 inhibitors in hypogonadal men with erectile dysfunction: a systematic review. Can Urol Assoc J. 2012;6(4):269–74. https://doi.org/10.5489/cuaj.11291.

21. Pajovic B, Dimitrovski A, Fatic N, Malidzan M, Vukovic M. Vacuum erection device in treatment of organic erectile dysfunction and penile vascular differences between patients with DM type I and DM type II. Aging Male. 2017;20(1):49–53. https://doi.org/10.1080/13685538.2016.1230601.

22. Porst H. Review of the current status of low intensity extracorporeal Shockwave Therapy (Li-ESWT) in erectile dysfunction (ED), Peyronie's disease (PD), and sexual rehabilitation after radical prostatectomy with special focus on technical aspects of the different marketed ESWT devices including personal experiences in 350 patients. Sex Med Rev. 2021;9(1):93–122. https://doi.org/10.1016/j.sxmr.2020.01.006.

23. Stone L. Sexual dysfunction: shock treatment for erectile dysfunction. Nat Rev Urol. 2015;12(2):62. https://doi.org/10.1038/nrurol.2014.354.

24. Stoykov B, Kolev N, Dunev V, Genov P. Low-intensity extracorporeal shockwave therapy in the treatment of erectile dysfunction after penile trauma. Urol Case Rep. 2020;30:101133. https://doi.org/10.1016/j.eucr.2020.101133.

25. Vena W, Vaccalluzzo L, SLA V, Morenghi E, D'Agostino C, Perri A, et al. Low-intensity shockwave treatment (liswt) improves penile rigidity in eugonadal subjects with erectile dysfunction: a pilot study. Minerva Endocrinol (Torino). 2021; https://doi.org/10.23736/S2724-6507.21.03686-1.

26. Ortac M, Ozmez A, Cilesiz NC, Demirelli E, Kadioglu A. The impact of extracorporeal shock wave therapy for the treatment of young patients with vasculogenic mild erectile dysfunction: a prospective randomized single-blind, sham controlled study. Andrology. 2021;9(5):1571–8. https://doi.org/10.1111/andr.13007.

27. Protogerou V, Chrysikos D, Karampelias V, Spanidis Y, Sara EB, Troupis T. Erectile dysfunction treatment using stem cells: a review. Medicines (Basel). 2021;8(1):2. https://doi.org/10.3390/medicines8010002.

28. Mirzaei M, Bagherinasabsarab M, Pakmanesh H, Mohammadi R, Teimourian M, Jahani Y, et al. The effect of intracavernosal injection of stem cell in the treatment of erectile dysfunction in diabetic patients: a randomized single-blinded clinical trial. Urol J. 2021;18(6):675–81. https://doi.org/10.22037/uj.v18i.6503.

29. Alkandari MH, Touma N, Carrier S. Platelet-rich plasma injections for erectile dysfunction and Peyronie's disease: a systematic review of evidence. Sex Med Rev. 2022;10(2):341–52. https://doi.org/10.1016/j.sxmr.2020.12.004.

30. Jakubczyk T. Intracavernosal injections in the diagnosis and treatment of PDE-5 resistant erectile dysfunction. Cent European J Urol. 2013;66(2):215–6. https://doi.org/10.5173/ceju.2013.02.art26.

31. Bassiem MA, Ismail IY, Salem TA, El-Sakka AI. Effect of intracavernosal injection of prostaglandin E1 on duration and rigidity of erection in patients with vasculogenic erectile dysfunction: is it dose dependent? Urology. 2021;148:173–8. https://doi.org/10.1016/j.urology.2020.09.030.

32. Kisa E, Keskin MZ, Yucel C, Ucar M, Yalbuzdag O, Ilbey YO. Comparison of penile prosthesis types' complications: a retrospective analysis of single center. Arch Ital Urol Androl. 2020;92(4) https://doi.org/10.4081/aiua.2020.4.386.

33. Allaire E, Sussman H, Zugail AS, Hauet P, Floresco J, Virag R. Erectile dysfunction resistant to medical treatment caused by cavernovenous leakage: an innovative surgical approach combining pre-operative work up, embolisation, and open surgery. Eur J Vasc Endovasc Surg. 2021;61(3):510–7. https://doi.org/10.1016/j.ejvs.2020.08.048.

34. Elbaz R, El-Assmy A, Zahran MH, Hashem A, Shokeir AA. Mirabegron for treatment of erectile dysfunction concomitant with lower urinary tract symptoms in patients with benign prostatic obstruction: a randomized controlled trial. Int J Urol. 2022;29(5):390–6. https://doi.org/10.1111/iju.14792.

35. El-Shaer W, Ghanem H, Diab T, Abo-Taleb A, Kandeel W. Intra-cavernous injection of BOTOX((R)) (50 and 100 Units) for treatment of vasculogenic erectile dysfunction: randomized controlled trial. Andrology. 2021;9(4):1166–75. https://doi.org/10.1111/andr.13010.

36. Lai BY, Cao HJ, Yang GY, Jia LY, Grant S, Fei YT, et al. Acupuncture for treatment of erectile dysfunction: a systematic review and meta-analysis. World J Mens Health. 2019;37(3):322–38. https://doi.org/10.5534/wjmh.180090.

Ejaculation and Orgasmic Disorders

4

Emre Altintas (iD) and Murat Gül (iD)

Abstract

Ejaculation is a complex physiological event in which multiple factors play a role. It requires a properly functioning central and peripheral nervous system and the absence of any anatomical and functional pathology. Pathologies occurring in any or more of these parameters cause ejaculation disorder. Ejaculation disorders are examined in a wide range, including premature ejaculation, delayed ejaculation, retrograde ejaculation, painful ejaculation, haemospermia, and anejaculation.

Although orgasm is often a term used instead of ejaculation, it is a different physiological state and is a sense of pleasure that manifests itself with various body changes. Although orgasmic disorders are not as common as erectile dysfunction or premature ejaculation in clinical practice, they can cause serious sexual problems in men. Orgasmic disorders are mainly examined under anorgasmia and postorgasmic illness syndrome. While anorgasmia is primarily evaluated together with delayed ejaculation disease, postorgasmic illness syndrome is a different orgasmic disorder.

Ejaculation Disorders

Men's sexual cycle consists of four phases: desire, erection, ejaculation (orgasm), and resolution. Although orgasm and ejaculation are utilised in the same manner, they are complex and physiologically different events [1]. Ejaculation, which marks the culmination of sexual intercourse, has two phases involving neurological and hormonal pathways [2, 3]. In the emission phase, phasic contractions release

E. Altintas · M. Gül (✉)
Department of Urology, Selcuk University School of Medicine, Konya, Turkey

© The Author(s), under exclusive license to Springer Nature
Switzerland AG 2022
S. Sarikaya et al. (eds.), *Andrology and Sexual Medicine*, Management of Urology,
https://doi.org/10.1007/978-3-031-12049-7_4

41

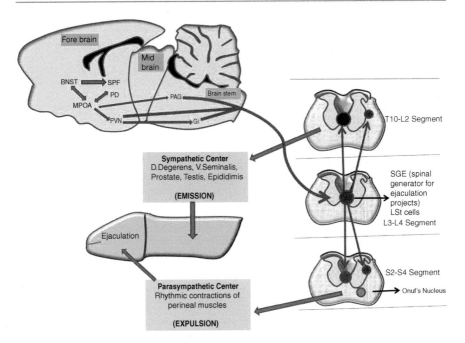

Fig. 4.1 Schematic view of the brain and spinal network of ejaculation. BNTS bed nucleus of the stria terminalis posteromedial, Gi gigantocellular, MPOA medial preoptic area, PAG periaqueductal grey, PD posterodorsal preoptic, PVN hypothalamic paraventricular, SPF subparafascicular parvicellular

seminal fluids from the testicles and accessory sex glands to the posterior urethra. The contraction of the pelvic-perineal striated muscles then triggers the expulsion phase.

Sensory receptors, afferent pathways, efferent pathways, spinal motor centers, and cerebral sensory and motor centers work together to generate the ejaculation reflex. They are supported by neurochemical pathways populated by neurotransmitters, primarily dopamine and serotonin, followed by oxytocin, acetylcholine, norepinephrine, GABA, and nitric oxide [4]. Pathological conditions related to the ejaculation reflex can result in various ejaculation disorders (Fig. 4.1).

Premature Ejaculation

Definition

Though premature ejaculation (PE) is one of the most common sexual dysfunctions found in men [5], there is no consensus on its definition [6]. Men and their sexual partners have different perceptions on average ejaculation time, which generates uncertainty and makes arriving at a standard definition difficult [7].

Although many definitions exist, some standout—in particular, those offered by the International Society of Sexual Medicine (ISMM), International Statistical

Table 4.1 Definition of PE according to different international communities

ICD (11th revision, 2018)	Male early ejaculation is characterized by ejaculation that occurs prior to or within a very short duration of the initiation of vaginal penetration or other relevant sexual stimulation, with no or little perceived control over ejaculation. The pattern of early ejaculation has occurred episodically or persistently over a period at least several months, and is associated with clinically significant distress [8]	
DSM-5 (APA, 2013)	Persistent or recurrent pattern of ejaculation occurring during partnered sexual activity within approximately 1 min following vaginal penetration and before the individual wishes it.	
	•	This symptom must have been present for at least 6 months and must be experienced on almost all or all (approximately 75–100%) occasions of sexual activity,
	•	This symptom must cause clinically significant distress in the individual,
	•	This sexual dysfunction is not better explained by a nonsexual mental disorder or as a result of severe relationship distress or other important stressors and is not attributable to the effects of a substance/medication or another medical disorder [9]
ISSM	PE (lifelong and acquired) is a male sexual dysfunction characterised by the following:	
	•	ejaculation that always or nearly always occurs prior to or within about 1 min of vaginal penetration (lifelong PE) or a clinically significant and bothersome reduction in latency time, often to about 3 min or less (acquired PE);
	•	inability to delay ejaculation on all or nearly all vaginal penetrations;
	•	negative personal consequences, such as distress, bother, frustration, and/or the avoidance of sexual intimacy [10]

ISMM International Society of Sexual Medicine, *ICD* International Statistical Classification of Disease, *DSM* Diagnostic and Statistical Manual of Mental Disorders

Classification of Disease (ICD), and Diagnostic and Statistical Manual of Mental Disorders (DSM). The various definitions are given in Table 4.1.

The EAU Guidelines accepted ISSM's definition as the first evidence-based definition [10]. Unlike previous definitions, ISSM's definition includes the time criterion. Again, the DSM-5 added the time criterion to their definition and divided PE into three: mild PE (30–60 s after coitus), moderate PE (15–30 s after coitus), and severe PE (coitus lasting less than 15 s).

In addition to the previous definitions, two more definitions of PE have been proposed [11]:

Variable PE: Inconsistent and irregular premature ejaculation, which is considered a normal variation in sexual performance.

Subjective PE: Subjectively rapid ejaculation during intercourse, with the ejaculation latent time within normal limits (sometimes even longer). It is recommended not to consider this condition a disease or symptom.

Epidemiology

The validity and standardisation problem in identifying PE has made it difficult to evaluate its prevalence studies [12, 13]. Especially since the previous epidemiological studies were not observational, the biggest and most common problem was the lack of a universally accepted definition while conducting surveys [13]. Moreover, during face-to-face interviews, they could not clearly express this problem due to the social stamping of men with PE [14].

In a large-scale study conducted in England in 1998, 14% of the patients stated that they had PE in the last 3 months and 31% at some point in their lives [15]. Since the mean age of the patients was 51, the incidence of erectile dysfunction (ED) was also higher. In a study conducted by the National Health and Social Life Survey (NHSLS), which included 1410 men (19–59 years), the participants were asked whether they "ejaculated too quickly in the past one year" [14]. They could answer yes or no. The prevalence of PE for ages 18–29 was 30%; 30–39, 32%; 40–49, 28%; and 50–59, 55%. The overall prevalence was high, at 31%, probably due to the close-ended question (yes/no).

An internet-based survey (PEPA), where the prevalence of PE for men over 24 was 22.7%, concluded that PE did not change according to age [16]. Moreover, the prevalence was 24% in the USA, 20.3% in Germany, and 20% in Italy. In a study conducted in Turkey, the prevalence of lifetime PE was 2.3%, acquired PE 3.9%, variable PE 8.5%, and subjective PE 5.1% [17]. Men with lifetime PE do not seek treatment as much as those with acquired PE, this may lead to incomplete prevalence data. This may also apply to other PE subtypes and it may make it difficult to determine PE's true measure of incidence [17]. The approximately 5% prevalence of acquired PE and lifetime PE in the general population is consistent with the epidemiological data, according to which approximately 5% of the population has an ejaculation time of less than 2 min [7].

Pathophysiology, Aetiology, and Risk Factors

PE's pathophysiology is not clearly known, with studies finding the involvement of more than one factor [7]. PE's main aetiological factors were traditionally thought to be psychological and sexual experience-related factors [18, 19], but recent studies have found that somatic and neurobiological factors may also play a role [20]. In particular, the definition of different types of PE has made it more important to investigate the aetiological factors [21, 22].

Lifelong PE, according to Waldinger's neurobiological-genetic theory [23], is related to the serotoninergic central nervous system mechanisms that regulate the ejaculation reflex through the lumbar spinothalamic cells [24]. These mechanisms can also be explained by the hypertonic state of sexual behaviour. In addition, dopaminergic, oxytocinergic, genetic, and epigenetic factors were found to contribute to lifelong PE [24]. Acquired PE may occur due to psychological problems (sexual performance anxiety, psychological relationship problems, female sexual dysfunctions, and so on) and/or some comorbid conditions (such as ED, prostatitis, and hyperthyroidism) [25–27]. Finally, subjective PE has been suggested to have roots in cultural or psychological reasons [6].

While PE was found to be not affected by marriage and marital status, it was found to be related to lower educational levels [14, 28]. In addition, the prevalence of PE was observed to be higher in black, Hispanic, and Islamic societies [12, 29]. PE's aetiological factors are presented in Table 4.2.

Table 4.2 Premature Ejaculation Etiological Factors [30]

Psychological factors	Biological factors	
Relationship problems	Endocrinopathies	Diabetes, Hyperthyroidism
Performance anxiety	Neurological Pathologies	MS, Peripheral Neuropathy
Early sexual experiences	Urological Pathologies	ED, Prostatitis
Body dysmorphic disorders	Genetic	5-HTLPR gene polymorphism
	5-hydroxytryptamine receptor dysfunction:	5-HT2C receptor hyposensitivity and/or 5-HT1A receptor hypersensitivity
	Drug-induced	Amphetamine, cocaine, and dopaminergic drugs
	Other pathologies	İncreased Penile sensitivity, Chronic Renal Disease

5-HTLPR serotonin-transporter-linked promoter region, *5-HT2C* 5-hydroxytryptamine 2C, *5-HT1A* 5-hydroxytryptamine 1A, *MS* multiple sclerosis, *ED* erectile dysfunction

Table 4.3 Classification of premature ejaculation [30]

	Lifelong PE	Acquired PE	Variable PE	Subjective PE
IELT	<60–90 s	<90–180 s	3–8 min (Normal)	3–30 min (Normal or long)
Symptoms	Continuous	New-onset	Inconsistent	Subjective perception of PE despite normal ejaculation
Etiology	Genetic and Neurobiological	Medical and/or psychological	Normal variation	Psychological
Prevalence	Low (2.3%)	Low (3.9%)	High (8.5%)	High (5.1%)

Classification

There is still little consensus on the definition and classification of PE). Currently, it is accepted that PE is a broad term that includes many concepts. Previously, PE was divided into two, namely, lifelong and acquired PE. A subsequent study has shown that men with normal intravaginal ejaculation latency time (IELT) can use medication to delay ejaculation [31]. As a result, "subjective PE" and "variable PE" types of PE were defined [32]. Thus, four different subtypes of PE are documented in the literature (Table 4.3).

Lifelong PE: From the first sexual intercourse, ejaculation occurs in a very short time in almost every relationship and every woman. Ejaculation can occur intraportal, anteportal, or during foreplay. Anteportal ejaculation is considered the most severe form of PE.

Acquired PE: It is the condition of PE that develops later in individuals who have normal ejaculation at a certain period of their life. Most of these patients have an organic/psychological pathology that causes this condition.

Subjective PE: It is the condition of complaining of PE despite normal (3–20 min) or prolonged ejaculation times. Although it is not an organic pathology, there is a

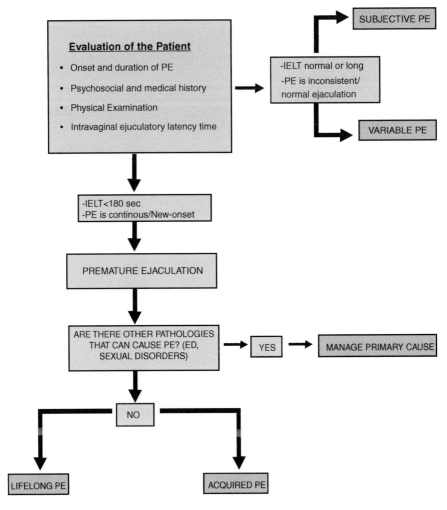

Fig. 4.2 Evaluation of PE [34]

misconception of ejaculation time. On the other hand, the late orgasm of the partner can also cause this situation.

Variable PE: These patients occasionally complain of PE. This is considered a normal variation of sexual performance.

Diagnosis

The diagnosis of PE is based on the patient's medical and sexual history [7]. After the general medical history of the patients, psychosocial evaluation is also recommended. The use of laboratory tests in routine evaluation is not recommended. However, if the clinical picture is accompanied by conditions such as ED or loss of libido, hormonal tests such as serum testosterone, prolactin, and thyroid-stimulating hormone (TSH) may be requested [33] (Fig. 4.2).

Table 4.4 Suggested and optional questions for the diagnosis of PE [7]

Recommended questions for diagnosis	What is the time between penetration and ejaculation (cumming)?
	Can you delay ejaculation?
	Do you feel bothered, annoyed, and/or frustrated by your premature ejaculation?
Optional questions:	When did you first experience premature ejaculation?
Differentiate lifelong and acquired PE	Have you experienced premature ejaculation since your first sexual experience on every/almost every attempt and with every partner?
Optional questions:	Is your erection hard enough to penetrate?
Assess erectile function	Do you have difficulty in maintaining your erection until you ejaculate during intercourse?
	Do you ever rush intercourse to prevent loss of your erection?
Optional questions:	How upset is your partner with your premature ejaculation?
Assess relationship impact	Does your partner avoid sexual intercourse?
	Is your premature ejaculation affecting your overall relationship?
Optional question: Previous treatment	Have you received any treatment for your premature ejaculation previously?
Optional questions:	Do you avoid sexual intercourse because of embarrassment?
Impact on quality of life	Do you feel anxious, depressed, or embarrassed because of your premature ejaculation?

History

Patients presenting with PE may be shy about explaining their complaints [35]. Therefore, they usually expect the doctor to ask their complaints [36]. For diagnosis, first of all, the time elapsed between the beginning of sexual intercourse and ejaculation, whether the patient can delay ejaculation and whether he feels sad or angry due to PE should be questioned. It should also be asked whether PE occurs after each sexual experience from the first sexual intercourse. This is important in distinguishing between lifelong and acquired PE.

ED can be seen together with PE. In most patients with ED, secondary PE may develop due to the anxiety experienced in maintaining an erection [37]. On the other hand, some patients may complain of ED even though the primary problem is PE (not aware of the expected loss of erection after ejaculation) [38]. Table 4.4 lists the questions that should be asked to patients complaining of PE (suggested and optional questions) [7].

Physical Examination

Routine physical examination is not mandatory for patients presenting with lifelong and acquired PE. However, some patients can rely on a physical examination. Especially in acquired PE, physical examination can be performed to distinguish comorbidities (urinary tract and reproductive system infections, Peyronie's disease, endocrine dysfunctions, etc.) and risk factors.

Stopwatch Assessment of Ejaculatory Latency (IELT)

IELT is an objective criterion in diagnosis, but it is not sufficient in itself to define PE [39]. Although the measurement of IELT with a stopwatch is used in experimental and clinical studies, it is not routinely recommended [7]. It is not used in the routine because it tends to be intrusive and may disrupt sexual pleasure [17]. In a few studies, it was determined that the self-reported ejaculation time of the patient or his partner was similar to IELT. Therefore, the self-estimated IELT has been reported to be sufficient in routine clinical practice [40, 41].

PE Assessment Questionnaires

To standardize the diagnosis of PE, validated questionnaires can also be used in clinical practice [42]. Only five comprehensive (with psychometric tests and validation) questionnaires have been developed to evaluate lifelong and acquired PE in the literature [43–47]. Among these, two questionnaires can distinguish between those with and without PE, namely, Premature Ejaculation Diagnostic Tool (PEDT) and Arabic Index Premature Ejaculation (AIPE) (Table 4.5).

PEDT: The premature ejaculation diagnostic tool (PEDT) consists of a five-question questionnaire. A total score of >11 indicates a diagnosis of PE, and a score of 9–10 shows a possible diagnosis of PE. A score of <8 shows a low probability of PE. Although PEDT is widely used, a low correlation has been reported for the diagnosis of PE [48].

AIPE: AIPE is a questionnaire consisting of seven questions. PE severity is classified as severe (score: 7–13), moderate (score: 14–19), mild-moderate (score: 20–25), and mild (score: 26–30).

PEP or AIPE is preferred to evaluate lifetime or acquired PE subtypes, especially in monitoring response to treatment. Although these questionnaires are helpful for us in the clinic, the importance of sexual history is crucial. Although questionnaires facilitate the methodology of drug studies related to PE, more cross-cultural validation is needed [41].

Table 4.5 PE questionnaires assessing lifelong and acquired subtypes

Name	Content	Advantages	Limitations
Premature Ejaculation Diagnostic Tool (PEDT)	Assesses control	Screening questionnaire with cut off Scores	
	Frequency	Brief and easy to administer	
	Minimal stimulation		
	Distress		
	İnterpersonal difficulty		
Arabic Premature Ejaculation Index (AIPE)	Sexual desire	Assesses outcome	Lacks norms and diagnostic cutoffs
	Hard erections for sufficient intercourse	Relatively brief and easy to administer	
	Time to ejaculation	Evaluates the subjective and clinically relevant domains	
	Control		
	Satisfaction of the patient and partner		
	Anxiety or depression		

Psychiatric Evaluation

Psychiatric evaluation of the patient is essential in the diagnosis of PE. The patient should be seen both with his partner and alone. In addition, confidentiality should be observed during the interview. When questioning the relationship of the patients with their partners, one should not be judgmental and directive. While taking a sexual history, generalizing and normalizing may relieve the patient and improve the examination process. The patient's anxiety for PE and problems between partners can be understood by psychiatric evaluation, and thus the patient is referred to psychiatric treatment.

Treatment

Identifying the subtype of PE is the essential step before starting treatment. Along with the treatment, it is necessary to understand the expectations of the patient. While pharmacotherapy is the first-line treatment in lifelong PE, treating the underlying cause (ED, prostatitis, anxiety, hyperthyroidism, etc.) in acquired PE should be the first target [7]. Men with lifelong PE are effectively treated with selective serotonin reuptake inhibitors (SSRIs) or local anesthetic gels/creams in daily practice. However, the psychosexual problems of the patient and his partner should also be paid attention [7]. SSRIs and topical anesthetics can be used if there is no underlying pathology in acquired PE [7]. Patients with variable PE usually do not seek treatment because they sometimes ejaculate prematurely. These patients can be educated about their sporadic PE and may benefit from psychosexual counseling [20, 49]. The treatment of men with subjective PE with SSRI is controversial because they have normal IELT values [49]. These patients should be offered psychotherapy, behavioral sex therapy, and couple therapy [49].

Psychological Approach

Although limited, some studies have addressed the psychological factors underlying PE. Possible risk factors in PE include anxiety, early sexual experiences, low frequency of sexual intercourse, and relationship problems [34, 50–52]. Among these, it is still a controversial issue whether anxiety is the cause or the result of PE [53]. Men with PE anticipate failure, have trouble loosening their bodies when sexually aroused, and become overly focused on their partner's body and reactions [54]. In addition, these men blame themselves for their dysfunctional sexual response (not related to PE) and may ignore it even if they have a positive sexual experience [55]. On the other hand, performance anxiety increases in men after each PE [38]. Afterwards, the dissatisfaction of the spouses increases, and PE starts to negatively affect the quality of life (QoL) of the couplE. This eventually leads couples to seek treatment options for PE [55]. Psychosexual interventions (individually or with a partner) aim to teach techniques for controlling ejaculation, gaining confidence in sexual performance, reducing anxiety, and solving problems between couples [56].

Behavioral Strategies

Behavioral strategies have been proposed based on the hypothesis that men with PE cannot delay their increased sense of arousal and control their inevitable ejaculation

[18]. Behavioral treatments include stop-start, squeeze, pelvic floor exercises, and precoital masturbation.

Semens suggested that an abnormally rapid ejaculation reflex causes PE [57]. Based on this, he stated that the stop-start technique acts by changing the neuromuscular reflex mechanism of ejaculation [57]. In this technique, the penis is stimulated by the partner until the feeling of ejaculation is felt. When the feeling of ejaculation emerges, the man stops his partner. He waits until the feeling of ejaculation is gone, and then the intercourse is continued. In the squeeze technique, when the man feels the urge to ejaculate, his partner squeezes the frenulum of the penis for a few seconds. Once the feeling of ejaculation disappears, PE is delayed. In the literature, a 62% success rate was reported for the stop-start technique [58], 64% of ejaculation control was reported for the squeeze technique [59]. However, it has been reported that only one-third of the patients continued their ejaculation control in the third year [60].

Pelvic floor muscle (PFM) exercises may also help delay ejaculation. In Kegel exercises the patient is advised to stop the urine while urinating or squeeze the rectal area to hold the stool. It is recommended to perform these exercises at least three times a day and ten times at a time [61]. Another method is masturbation 1–2 h before sexual intercourse. This method is used primarily by young men. Desensitization occurs in the penis, and ejaculation is delayed after the refractory period [62]. Yet another method is to prohibit coitus for a certain period. Thus, performance anxiety can be reduced by enabling the patient and his partner to focus on areas of sexual intercourse other than coitus [63]. Regular physical exercise was also shown to relieve the symptoms of PE. In a study, PE was not detected in any of those who did regular physical activity. In addition, a significant difference was found between PEDT scores and IELT in the group that exercised regularly compared to the group with a sedentary lifestyle [64].

In behavioral therapies, it is aimed to increase the awareness of men with respect to sexual sensations, reduce anxiety, and focus on sexual intercourse. There are no controlled and randomized studies supporting the effectiveness of behavioral treatments. However, these treatments have been observed to provide specific improvement in the short term. Current guidelines recommend using behavioral therapies in conjunction with pharmacological treatment in the treatment of PE [65].

Pharmacological Treatment

Due to the complex pathophysiology of PE, many treatment alternatives have been proposed. While pharmacotherapy is prominent in lifelong PE, primary pathology should be treated first in PE due to secondary causes (prostatitis, ED, urinary tract infection) [66–68]. In the treatment of PE, long-acting SSRI, clomipramine, short-acting SSRI (dapoxetine), topical anesthetics, tramadol, and phosphodiesterase type 5 inhibitors (PDE5i) are used [7]. None of the drugs used in the treatment of PE have Food and Drug Administration (FDA) approval. Of these, only Dapoxetine and prilocaine-lidocaine topical aerosol spray obtained European Medical Agency (EMA) approval for the treatment of PE. Other drugs are used off-label. Medicolegal problems should be kept in mind in off-label use.

On-Demand Treatment Options
Topical Anesthetics
In patients with PE, the response threshold to penile sensory stimulation occurs at lower levels. The sensory point in the glans penis and penile shaft can be measured with a biothesiometer. The sensory response to penile stimulation was found lower in patients with PE than in normal individuals by biothesiometer (95% confidence limit of perception threshold on the glans penis 0.053–0.062 vs. 0.194–0.259 μ, respectively, $p < 0.001$) [69]. On the other hand, abnormalities in some reflexes (such as the bulbocavernosus reflex response) can affect penile hypersensitivity, leading to PE [70]. Based on this, topical anesthetics have been started to be used to treat PE. Prilocaine–lidocaine-containing cream (EMLA) was given 30 min before sexual intercourse, and approximately 85% of the patients stated that ejaculation control was better [71]. In addition, it was observed that IELT in EMLA use patients was between 5 and 20 min [71]. In another randomized controlled study, an increase in IELT value of approximately five times was observed in men given EMLA compared to the placebo group [72]. Aerosol sprays have been observed to be effective in the treatment of PE, and the use of aerosol sprays containing prilocaine (50 mg/mL)-lidocaine (150 mg/mL) in the treatment of PE has been approved by the EMA. In a phase II study, it was determined that the use of prilocaine-lidocaine mixture aerosol spray in the treatment of PE increased the IELT value by 2.4 times compared to placebo [73]. In another study, a new prilocaine-lidocaine aerosol spray (PSD502) was compared with a placebo in the treatment of lifelong PE. In the group given PSD502, the duration of IELT increased significantly more than the placebo (0.56–2.60 vs. 0.53–0.80 min) [74]. Side effects of topical anesthetics were reported as penile irritation, vaginal numbness, and penile numbness [72–74]. Although most patients on topical anesthetics for the treatment of PE are satisfied, they discontinue topical anesthetics after a certain period. Data on the long-term use of these drugs are limited [75].

On-Demand Dapoxetine Treatment
Dapoxetine, the first drug approved by the EMA for the treatment of PE, is a short-acting SSRI. Pharmacokinetic studies have shown that dapoxetine is rapidly eliminated from plasma (T_{max} 1.3 h), and 95% clearance is achieved within 24 h [76, 77]. Owing to these, on-demand dapoxetine has been accepted in the treatment of PE. In a phase III study in which 1162 men with PE were included, it was observed that the IELTs of those who used 30 and 60 mg of dapoxetine 1–3 h before intercourse increased significantly compared to the placebo group. The mean IELT value increased in all groups compared to baseline levels (placebo group from 0.9 to 1.9 min, Dapoxetine 30 mg group from 0.9 to 3.2 min, Dapoxetine 60 mg group from 0.9 to 3.5 min). This increase was statistically significant in the dapoxetine 30 and 60 mg groups compared to placebo ($p < 0.001$) [78]. Again, a few clinical studies observed that the use of dapoxetine increased IELT by an average of 3.6–4.5 times [48, 79]. In addition, these studies reported decreased performance anxiety and increased satisfaction [48, 78, 79]. It is known that a significant portion of men with PE complain of ED [37]. It was observed that IELT increased 3.5 times after 3 months of dapoxetine treatment (30 or 60 mg) in patients using PDE5i for ED [80].

The most common side effects related to dapoxetine (seen in 30%) were nausea, headache, diarrhea, and dizziness. Although side effects associated are not common, they are dose-dependent. The drug withdrawal rate is 10% for those using 60 mg of dapoxetine, while around 4% for those using 30 mg dapoxetine [81]. For this reason, the treatment should be started with 30 mg dapoxetine first and if there is no adequate response after using at least 6 times, the dose should be increased to 60 mg [7]. If the treatment is well tolerated but has no response, 60 mg can be started. A multicenter observational study reported that dapoxetine has a safer side effect profile with respect to mood, neurocognitive, urogenital, and sexual function than other SSRIs [82]. Therefore, patients should be informed about potential side effects before using dapoxetine. Contrary to long-acting SSRIs, no suicide attempt or drug discontinuation syndrome is observed with dapoxetine use [83]. No drug interactions have been reported with dapoxetine to date. In a study on the use of combined dapoxetine/sildenafil (Dapoxil® TB) in patients with concomitant PE and ED, significant increases were observed in both IELT and IIEF scores [84]. Therefore, its use is also effective and safe in patients receiving PDE5i therapy [85].

Off-Label Treatments
Daily Treatment of SSRIs and Clomipramine
Ejaculation is a process controlled by the spinal ejaculation center in which both the brain and the peripheral nerves take part. Serotonin receptors are specifically involved in the ejaculation process. 5-HT1A receptor stimulation facilitates ejaculation, whereas 5-HT1B and 5-HT2C receptors activation delay ejaculation [86]. Figure 4.3 shows the mechanism of action of the receptors and the delaying effect of ejaculation [87].

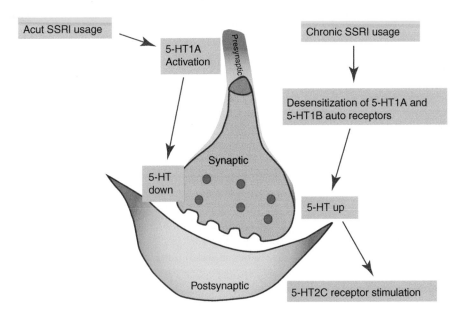

Fig. 4.3 Mechanism of action of serotonin receptors on ejaculation

SSRIs used in the treatment of PE are paroxetine (20–40 mg daily), clomipramine (12.5–50 mg), sertraline (25.50 and 100 mg daily), fluoxetine (10–60 mg), and citalopram (20–60 mg daily) [88–91]. SSRIs should be started at the lowest dose, and dose adjustments should be made over time. Although a delay in ejaculation occurs a few days after SSRI intake, 1–3 weeks should pass for maximum effect. This activity mostly continues, but in some cases, the activity may decrease after 6 months due to tachyphylaxis [92]. SSRIs can be used before sexual intercourse (3–6 h before) instead of daily. In previous studies conducted, the use of SSRIs before intercourse provides less delay in ejaculation than daily use [7, 92].

In a randomized controlled study investigating the efficacy of different types of SSRIs on PE, paroxetine was observed as the most potent SSRI that delays ejaculation. The increase in mean IELT was 110 s in the SSRI group versus 20 s in the placebo group [93]. According to the increase in IELT, paroxetine was followed by fluoxetine, sertraline respectively ($p < 0.001$, $p < 0.001$, and $p = 0.0017$, respectively). While the fluvoxamine group increased the IELT value by an average of 40 s, an increase of 20 s was observed in the placebo group, and there was no statistically significant difference ($p = 0.38$) [93]. In a meta-analysis, it was observed that paroxetine, sertraline, fluoxetine, clomipramine increased IELT statistically significantly compared to placebo ($p < 0.001$). Mean IELT increase rates were 783% in paroxetine, 360% in clomipramine, 313% in sertraline, 295% in fluoxetine, and 47% in placebo [94]. In a recent Cochrane Database systematic review, including 8254 patients, demonstrated that those who used SSRIs showed improvement in symptoms, satisfaction with sexual intercourse, and control over the perception of ejaculation compared to the placebo group [95]. In addition, the mean rate of increase in mean IELT was 4.85-fold for citalopram, 1.52 for duloxetine, 2.46 for fluoxetine, 0.59 for fluvoxamine, 6.51 for paroxetine, and 2.55 for sertraline ($p < 0.001$) [95]. In a meta-analysis involving 710 patients, it was observed that clomipramine increased IELT on average 1.47-fold over placebo ($p < 0.001$) [96]. Clomipramine may be recommended in cases where SSRIs are ineffective or cannot be tolerated.

Although the benefits of SSRIs on PE patients were clearly shown, none of the currently available SSRIs has been approved by the FDA and EMA for the treatment of PE. For this reason, care should be taken, especially with respect to side effects and off-label use. Side effects such as fatigue, drowsiness, nausea, dry mouth, sweating, gaining weight, or diarrhea can be seen in the use of SSRIs. While these side effects are more common at the beginning of the treatment, they decrease over time [92]. Besides, some sexual problems such as decreased libido, ED, and anejaculation can also be seen [7]. Long-term side effects include bleeding, priapism, restless genital syndrome, and infertility as a result of impaired sperm motility [49, 97]. Rarely, neurocognitive side effects (extreme irritability, hypomania) can be seen. Therefore, SSRIs should not be given to patients with major depression or bipolar disorder. A meta-analysis reported that the use of SSRIs in young people with depression and anxiety disorders caused a slight increase in suicidal thoughts and attempts [98]. If depressive disorders accompany PE in young patients, caution should be taken in the use of SSRIs.

PDE5Is

Although the therapeutic mechanism of PDE5Is on PE is not clearly understood, PDE5Is are thought to delay ejaculation both centrally and peripherally [99]. PDE5s cross the blood-brain barrier increase cGMP and NO activity in the medial preoptic area. As a result of this effect, the sympathetic tone fired from the central nervous system decreases and eventually delayed ejaculation [100]. On the other hand, PDE5Is help delay ejaculation by providing relaxation of organs (vas deferens, seminal vesicle, prostate, urethra, etc.) involved in the emission phase of ejaculation from the peripheral route via cGMP/NO [101].

A randomized placebo-controlled study evaluated the use of sildenafil in men with PE. Although there was no significant increase in IELT, sildenafil use was associated with increased sexual satisfaction, decreased anxiety, and reduces refractory period [102]. In a meta-analysis published in 2020, including 471 patients, a significant increase in IELT was observed. It was observed that the IELT value increased by an average of 2.6 times in those using PDE5Is, and the sexual satisfaction scale score increased by an average of 2.04 times compared to those using the placebo ($p < 0.00001$ and $p = 0.002$, respectively) [103]. In some studies, it was observed that the combined use of PDE5Is and SSRIs increased the mean IELT more than the use of SSRIs and PD5Is alone [104, 105]. The rate of increase in IELT was 94% in the SSRI group alone, 61% in the PDE5Is group alone, and 145% in the combination therapy group [104]. In the other study, two groups of patients who received dapoxetine alone and mirodenafil together with dapoxetine were given 12 weeks of treatment. The increase in the mean IELT value after the treatment was statistically significantly higher in the group receiving combination therapy (3.6 min in the dapoxetine group, 6.1 min in the combination group, $p = 0.026$) [105]. Although PDE5Is are considered first-line therapy for ED, a meta-analysis supports the use of PDE5Is in patients with PE [99]. The 2021 European Association of Urology (EAU) guidelines "strongly" recommend the use of sildenafil for PE (without ED), either alone or as part of combination therapies [65]. The American Urological Association (AUA) [106] and the International Society for Sexual Medicine (ISSM) do not recommend the use of PDE5 alone in patients with PE [7]. The most reported adverse events related to PDE5 use were flushing, headache, fatigue, and indigestion [107, 108].

On-Demand Tramadol Treatment

Tramadol is a centrally acting analgesic and an opioid receptor agonist. It also differs from other opioids due to its norepinephrine and serotonin reuptake inhibitor effect [109]. After oral ingestion, it reaches its maximum concentration in plasma at approximately 2 h, and its half-life is approximately 5–7 h [110]. The first study showing the efficacy of tramadol on PE was published in 2006 [111]. Men with untreated PE with an IELT value below 2 min were given 50 mg of tramadol per day. After 8 weeks of treatment, the mean IELT time increased from 19 to 243 s in the tramadol group, while it increased from 21 to 34 s in the placebo group ($p < 0.001$) [111]. A randomized placebo-controlled study evaluated patients with lifetime PE with an IELT value of less than 2 min. A 2.5-fold increase in IELT was observed in those receiving tramadol 82 mg, and a 2.4-fold increase in those receiving tramadol 62 mg [112]. In another study, it was found that tramadol (25–89 mg) taken 2 h before sexual intercourse increased IELT by an average of 2.77 times [113]. A meta-analysis published in 2021 stated that tramadol is an effective drug in the treatment of PE (although the available evidence is low or moderate) [114]. Side effects such as nausea, vomiting, dizziness, constipation, drowsiness, and dry mouth can be seen due to tramadol use [111]. In addition, serotonergic syndrome with symptoms such as tachycardia, agitation, and hyperthermia may be observed when tramadol is used alone or in combination with SSRIs [115, 116]. Considering the risk of addiction and side effects associated with opioids, tramadol may be used with caution as third-line therapy in cases where SSRI and clomipramine have been ineffective [65].

Emerging Treatment Options for PE
Oral Pharmacological Agents

DA-8031
DA-8031 is a potent SSRI. A few preclinical and phase I studies have been published so far on DA-803 [117–119]. A phase II study is still in progress [120]. DA-8031 showed high selectivity and specificity for 5-HT receptors while having a low affinity with other receptors [117, 118]. In a phase I randomized study, DA-8031 was divided into seven different groups according to the dose, and 70 healthy subjects were included [121]. In this study, doses ranging from 20 to 80 mg were within the safe range. QTc prolongation was observed in 75% of those who used 120 mg of DA-8031. All adverse events were mild or moderate in proportion to the dose [121]. Nausea and headache due to orthostatic hypotension were the most common side effects. More clinical studies are needed to use DA-8031 in the treatment of PE with its pharmacokinetic properties and safety.

On-Demand Clomipramine
A few studies have been conducted in recent years on the use of on-demand clomipramine in the treatment of PE. In a phase II study, those who received clomipramine 15 and 30 mg were compared with the placebo group [122]. Those taking clomipramine had significantly increased IELT values compared to the placebo group. After treatment, mean IELT values increased 3.24 ± 3.42 in the 15 mg group, 2.89 ± 1.98 in the 30 mg group, and 1.75 ± 0.84 in the placebo group ($p = 0.0115$). Gastrointestinal and psychiatric side effects were more common in the groups receiving, especially those taking 30 mg clomipramine (adverse effects 32.35% in the 15 mg clomipramine group, 57.57% in the 30 mg clomipramine group, 11.76% in the placebo group) [122]. Another study compared those taking 15 mg of clomipramine with those taking a placebo. The mean fold increase in IELT after 12 weeks of treatment was significantly higher in the 15 mg clomipramine group compared to placebo (mean ± SD 4.40 ± 5.29 vs. 2.68 ± 2.03, $p < 0.05$) [123]. Although the efficacy of 15 mg clomipramine has been demonstrated in these studies, its use is limited as patients are not included according to the PE criteria based on the latest definitions.

GSK958108

There are two studies on GSK958108, a 5-HT1A receptor antagonist. The results of the phase I study have been published previously [124, 125]. In this study, the GSK958108 3 and 7 mg groups were compared with the placebo group, and 35 men with PE were included. IELT increased by 16% in the 3 mg group compared to the placebo group and increased by approximately 56% in the 7 mg group [126]. The most frequently reported adverse events were somnolence, headache, and tinnitus. Although the results are promising, phase II and phase III studies are needed to confirm its efficacy.

Modafinil

Modafinil((2-[(diphenylmethyl)sulfinyl] acetamide)) is a wake-promoting enhancing drug used in the treatment of narcolepsy [127]. Although its pharmacokinetic properties are not fully known, it may delay ejaculation by activating serotoninergic activity while inhibiting dopaminergic activity via D2 receptors. In the first study conducted on rats, it was observed that modafinil caused a delay in ejaculation compared to placebo [128]. In a case report in 2016, 100 mg modafinil was given to a man with lifetime PE for 2 weeks. It was observed that the patient's IELT value increased to 15 min after the treatment [129]. In a later study, 55 patients with lifetime PE received 100 mg of d-modafinil [130]. After 1 month of treatment, the IELT and PEP of the patients were evaluated. Patients reported a modest increase in IELT (24.82 ± 16.10 vs. 49.82 ± 31.46 s, $p = 0.0001$), greater satisfaction with sexual intercourse (0.98 ± 0.78 vs. 1.40 ± 0.85, $p = 0.0001$), and an anxiety reduction [130]. The most common side effect (10.9%) was insomnia. Although modafinil was shown beneficial in the treatment of PE, more clinical studies are needed for its efficacy and safety.

Alpha (α) Blockers

α-1 blockers can cause abnormal ejaculation by providing relaxation in the prostate, seminal vesicles, vas deferens, and urethra, which are involved in the emission phase of ejaculation [131]. In a study, the effects of different α-1 adrenoreceptor antagonists on IELT were compared [132]. Silodosin 4 mg was observed as the most effective α-1 adrenoreceptor antagonist with an eightfold increase in IELT. There were also significant changes in the PEP and QoL index reported by patients in this study. In a randomized controlled trial (RCT) that gave silodosin or placebo to patients with PE dissatisfied with dapoxetine, silodosin significantly improved IELT [133]. In line with these data, on-demand silodosin is more effective in treating PE than other α-1 adrenoreceptor antagonists. The most important side effect of silodosin is decreased ejaculation volume, a serious problem for some patients. In a prospective study conducted in 2017, the impact of naftopidil and silodosin on 26 patients with PE was investigated [134]. The increase in IELT was higher in the silodosin group than in the naftopidil group (median IELT; naftopidil group 4.1 ± 2.8 min, silodosin group 7.6 ± 5.1 min, $p < 0.001$), but the decrease in semen volume was significantly higher in the silodosin group [134]. For this reason, patients who will be started on silodosin should be informed about decreased ejaculation before the treatment.

Oxytocin Receptor Antagonist

The effect of oxytocin on male sexual health is not clear. It has been suggested in previous studies that oxytocin receptor antagonists delay ejaculation by desensitizing the 5HT1-A receptor [135, 136]. GSK557296, an oxytocin receptor antagonist, was given to rats intracerebroventricularly (i.c.v.), intrathecally (i.t.), and intravenously [137]. It was observed that i.c.v. and i.t. administration of GSK557296 to the T12-L1 interval delayed ejaculation [137]. Following promising results shown in animal studies, epelsiban (GSK557296), an oxytocin antagonist, given 50–150 mg, was compared with placebo [138]. However, there was no significant difference in IELT durations in the placebo and epelsiban groups in this study. This was attributed to the fact that epelsiban could not pass into the central nervous system. IX-01 (cligosiban), another oxytocin receptor antagonist, was used due to its both central and peripheral effects. Wayman et al. demonstrated the effect of cligosiban in inhibiting ejaculation in rodents [139]. Two phase II studies (PEPIX, PEDRIX) have been recently performed on cligosiban [140, 141]. In the PEPIX study, after 4 weeks of treatment, the mean increase in IELT was 61 s for cligosiban versus 16.4 s for placebo ($p = 0.0086$) [140]. In the PEDRIX study, no statistical difference in IELT values (geometric change) was observed between different doses of cligosiban (400, 800, and 1200 mg) and placebo [141]. The side effect and safety profile of cligosiban were acceptable when compared to placebo. In light of these data, more evidence is needed for oxytocin receptor antagonists to be used routinely in the treatment of PE.

Penile Nerve Resection and Pudendal Neuromodulation

Some studies in the literature have suggested selective resection of penile dorsal nerves (SRDN) in the treatment of PE. In an RCT of 101 patients with PE, 40 patients underwent penile SRDN, while 61 patients were designated as the control group (circumcision only) [142]. In the SRDN group, the mean IELT value increased significantly compared to the pre-procedure (1.1 ± 0.9 vs. 3.8 ± 3.1 min, $p < 0.01$). In the control group, there was no significant difference in the mean IELT before and after the procedure (0.2 ± 0.7 vs. 1.5 ± 1.1 min, $p > 0.05$) [142]. In another study, cryoablation of the dorsal penile nerve was performed under computed tomography guidance in 24 patients with PE [143]. While the baseline mean IELT was 54.7 ± 7.8 s, the mean IELT was 82.5 ± 87.8 s ($p < 0.0001$) at 3 months after the procedure, and 140.9 ± 83.6 s ($p < 0.001$) at 1 year [143]. In an RCT performed in China, 46 patients with excess foreskin and 96 patients with PE were compared for the number of dorsal penile nerve branches. Dorsal nerve branches were found to be more and thicker in patients with PE. It was also observed that SRDN increased the average IELT value more (257.7 ± 205.7 vs. 49.3 ± 26.1 s, $p = 0.02$) [144]. The EAU, AUA, and ISSM guidelines do not recommend this form of treatment.

Glans Penis Hyaluronic Acid Injection

In hyaluronic acid (HA) injection, it is aimed to decrease the access of stimuli to tactile receptors by increasing the volume of the glans penis. Thereupon, a few studies have been published on HA in the treatment of PE [145, 146]. In an RCT in

2019, 30 patients with PE infused with HA and saline into the glans penis were evaluated [147]. IELT values of the patients were recorded 1 week, 1 month, 3 months, 6 months, and 9 months after the procedures, and the AIPE scores were noted. After 1 month, the mean IELT increased significantly in the HA group compared to the saline group (two-way repeated ANOVA, $p = 0.001$). In addition, the AIPE scores increased significantly in the HA group compared to the pre-procedure ($p = 0.002$). Although the mean IELT values in the HA group decreased over time, they were higher than the baseline level at the end of the ninth month (median IELT values; baseline, 1 week, 1 month, 6 months and 9 months after - 34, 44.5, 120.85 and 45 s, respectively) [147]. Although side effects such as pain at the injection site and ecchymosis were noted, no severe side effects were observed. Due to insufficient studies on HA, it is not routinely used in the treatment of PE today.

Botulinum Toxin-A Injection

Botulinum toxin inhibits the release of acetylcholine from presynaptic receptors [148, 149]. In a study on rats, botulinum toxin was injected into the bulbospongiosus muscle, and its effect on ejaculation was investigated. A significant delay in ejaculation times was observed in rats injected with botulinum toxin without changing their sexual habits [150]. Following animal studies, a randomized phase II study was conducted involving 59 patients with PE. In the study, bilateral botulinum injections (minimum 5 units–maximum 100 units) were applied to the bulbospongiosus muscles. After botulinum injection at different doses, the mean IELT value increased statistically at each dose compared to placebo [120]. Later, in a study conducted in China, patients with primary PE were divided into two groups. While botulinum injection was applied to the bulbospongiosus muscle in one group, the saline infusion was used in the other group [151]. After 1 month, the IELT values and PEP score were significantly found higher in the botulinum group. Although botulinum toxin-A has been observed to increase IELT in some studies, this treatment should be considered experimental and should not be recommended for patients with PE. Further phase III and IV studies are needed for the efficacy and safety of botulinum in the treatment of PE.

Neuromuscular Electrical Stimulation

Pelvic floor muscles (PFMs), especially bulbospongiosus and ischiocavernosus, take part in the expulsion phase of the ejaculation process [152]. In one study, PFM rehabilitation was applied to 40 patients with lifelong PE. After 3 months of treatment, the mean IELT of the patients was found to be statistically significantly higher than the baseline values (31.7 ± 14.8 vs. 146.2 ± 38.3 s, $p < 0.0001$). The authors also stated that PFM rehabilitation is more cost-effective than other common treatment modalities (SSRIs, PED5Is and topical anesthetics) [153]. The same investigators conducted an RCT study involving 40 patients with PE to compare on-demand dapoxetine (30 or 60 mg) and PFM rehabilitation. After 12 weeks of treatment, there was a significant increase in mean IELT values from baseline in both groups ($p < 0.0001$). However, the mean IELT value increased more in the dapoxetine group (199.14 ± 37.26) than in the PFM rehabilitation group (126.2 ± 37.2 s) ($p < 0.001$)

[154]. In 2017, transcutaneous electrical stimulation (TES) applied to the perineal region was suggested in the treatment of PE [155]. The aim was to prevent the rhythmic movements of the bulbospongiosus and ischiocavernosus muscles by causing them to contract with continuous stimuli [155]. Later, in a study conducted with TES, patients were divided into two groups (active vs. sham). In the active TES treatment group, the mean masturbation ejaculatory latency time (MELT) prolonged significantly than the sham treatment, corresponding to an approximately fourfold increase in MELT (311.4 ± 237.14 vs. 124.6 ± 107.02 s, $p = 0.0009$) [156].

Transcutaneous Posterior Tibial Nerve Stimulation

Transcutaneous posterior tibial nerve stimulation (TPTNS) is a frequently used method in pelvic floor physiotherapy. The rationale behind the electrostimulation therapy is based on the complex sensorimotor function of the posterior-tibial nerve stemming from T4-S3 roots. Therefore TPTNS has been suggested that ejaculation may affect the emission (via the sympathetic system) and expulsion (via parasympathetic - somatic ejaculation system) phases. In a phase II study, 11 patients with PE were treated with TPTNS three times a week for 3 months. After treatment, the mean IELT value increased three times in six patients compared to baseline ($p = 0.037$) [157]. In a study conducted in 2020, 60 patients were divided into two groups (30 patients in the TPTNS group, 30 patients in the placebo group) and treated once a week for 12 weeks. Compared to the mean IELT values (seconds) at baseline, post-treatment mean IELT values increased significantly in both groups (Placebo group increased from 37.9 ± 11.81 to 42.5 ± 11.64, $p = 0.030$ and treatment group increased from 40.4 ± 13.21 to 51.25 ± 10.5, $p < 0.001$). However, there was no significant difference in mean post-treatment IELT values between groups ($p = 0.532$) [158]. Although preliminary results of TPTNS treatment appear good, randomized studies with larger samples are needed.

Future Treatment

Studies are conducted on some plant extracts (Satureja montana, Rhodiola rosea, Tribulus terrestris) in the treatment of PE [159–161]. Studies on the neurobiology of PE examine the.

antagonism of PIEZO2 proteins, a brain-derived neurotrophic factor [162, 163]. In conclusion, there are still uncertainties regarding the definition, pathophysiology, and treatment of PE. Therefore, studies are continuing especially for the treatment of PE.

Delayed Ejaculation

Definition

Delayed ejaculation (DE) is a rare ejaculation disorder. DE can be used synonymously with anejaculation or anorgasmia. DE can create significant problems for both the man and his partner. Definitions of DE according to various international disciplines are given in Table 4.6.

Table 4.6 Definition of DE according to different international communities

DSM-V	Almost all or all of the co-sexual activity (75–100%); marked delay or absence of ejaculation
	Continuing for at least 6 months
	A condition in which these symptoms cause significant distress to the individual
	(Sexual dysfunction; should not result from severe relationship distress, stress factors, or substance/drug use)
SMSNA	Inability to ejaculate despite good erection and adequate stimulation
ISSM	It is the state of delayed ejaculation even though a man has a full erection due to good stimulation

DSM-V Diagnostic and Statistical Manual of Mental Disorders, *SMSNA* Sexual Medicine Society of North America, *ISSM* International Society of Sexual Medicine

Epidemiology

The prevalence of DE is uncertain due to the lack of epidemiological studies. In some studies in the literature, the prevalence of DE varies between 3% and 11% [164–166]. It is stated that the prevalence of DE is related to age and the prevalence increases in advanced ages [167]. According to subtypes, 25% of cases with DE were primary, and 75% were acquired [165].

Pathophysiology, Etiology, and Risk Factors

The exact pathophysiology of especially primer DE is not fully elucidated. Pathologies in the emission and expulsion phases of ejaculation or the central and peripheral nervous systems may cause DE. An underlying cause is usually detected in men with secondary PE.

Drugs and psychological and organic pathologies are involved in the etiology of DE [168, 169]. Some psychological theories are thought to cause DE [170]. These theories are inadequate penile or mental stimulation, masturbation habits, sexual desire disorders, or having a psychic conflict [165, 171–173]. Especially psychic conflicts fear that ejaculation may harm the partner may arise from anger, fear of having children, or strict religious rules [170]. Some men with DE may have idiosyncratic masturbation [172]. This masturbation situation occurs at the speed, pressure, and intensity determined by the person himself. It is tough to repeat this situation in sexual intercourse with a partner. In addition, the person may feel a decrease in sexual stimulation due to the difference between the fantasy experienced during masturbation and sexual intercourse, which may result in [165]. Sexual performance anxiety may also contribute to DE. This may be due to a lack of confidence in satisfying their partner sexually [170]. In addition, this state of anxiety can distract the man's attention from stimuli that increase arousal [174]. Other etiological factors that can cause DE are listed in Table 4.7.

Classification

DE can be primary (present since the person has been sexually active) or acquired. On the other hand, it can be seen globally (with all sexual stimulations and all partners) or situational (only with certain sexual stimuli or partners).

Table 4.7 Etiological causes of delayed ejaculation and anejaculation

Organic	*Congenital* [175]: Mullerian duct cyst, Prune Belly Syndrome, Imperforate Anus
	Anatomic [176]: TUR-P, Ejaculatory duct obstruction, Circumcision
	Neurogenic causes [177–179]: Diabetic autonomic neuropathy, MS, Spinal cord injury, Radical prostatectomy, Para-aortic lymphadenectomy
	Infectıve/Inflammation[180]: Urethritis, Genitourinary tuberculosis, prostatitis
	Endocrine: [25, 26] Hypogonadism, Hypothyroidism, Prolactin disorders
Pharmacological [181, 182]	Alpha-adrenergic blockers, Antiandrogens, Ganglion blockers, SSRI, Alcohol, Antihypertensives (thiazide diuretics)
Psychogenic	Relationship distress, cute psychological distress, Psychosexual skill deficit, Masturbation style

TUR-P transurethral resection of prostate, *MS* multiple sclerosis, *SSRI* selective serotonin reuptake inhibitors

Diagnosis

In evaluating patients with DE, assessing all phases of the male sexual cycle (sexual desire, arousal, orgasm, resolution) is necessary. A detailed history (medical and sexual) should be collected, and a physical examination should be performed. The primary/acquired and global/situational distinction of DE should be made. In the patient's medical history, the drugs used, comorbidities, psychological status, cultural and family structure, and sexual orientation should be questioned. Frequency and type of sexual intercourse and IELT should be asked in the sexual history. In addition, the relationship between the patient and his partner other than sexuality should be questioned. Negative situations such as disappointment, avoidance of sexuality, and performance anxiety should be asked. To complete the psychological evaluation, a sex therapist can evaluate the patient [34]. The bilateral testicles should be examined in detail in the physical examination, and the presence of the epididymis and vas deferens should be checked. Prostate size, anal sphincter tone, or bulbocavernosus reflex can also be evaluated by digital rectal examination (DRM). Total testosterone levels should be measured in all patients. If necessary, other hormonal tests and imaging tests may be requested (Fig. 4.4).

Treatment

Although the basic principle in treatment is aimed at the etiological cause, a multidisciplinary approach is recommended. It has been shown that psychotherapy, especially together with medical treatment, increases the effectiveness of treatment [168].

Pharmacotherapy

There is no drug treatment approved for indication in the treatment of DE, but there are drugs in clinical use (Table 4.8.)

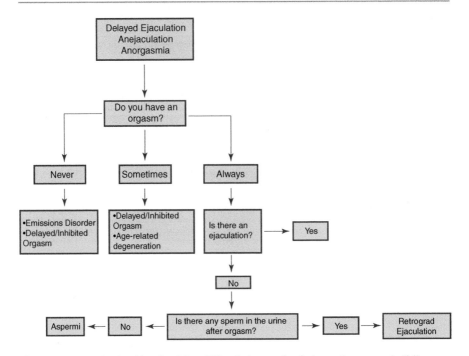

Fig. 4.4 Diagnostic algorithm for delayed Ejaculation, anejaculation and anorgasmia [34]

Table 4.8 The mechanism of action, dosage and side effect profile of drugs used in the treatment of DE

Drugs	Effect mechanism	Usage dose	Side effects
Cyproheptadine [183, 184]	5-HT and H1 receptor antagonist	Before intercourse 4–12 mg p.o.	Nausea, dizziness, urinary retention, rash, itching
Amantadine [185, 186]	– Central dopamine agonist,	5–6 h before intercourse	Nausea, dizziness, depression, hallucination, hypotension
	– Stimulating effect on sexual reflexes and ejaculation	100–400 mg p.o.	
Cabergoline [187, 188]	– Dopamine-2 receptor agonist	twice a week	Dizziness, drowsiness, anxiety, abdominal pain, hot flush
	– Erection and orgasm enhancing effect (in studies in Parkinson's patients)	0.25–2 mg p.o.	
Oxytocin [189, 190]	– Peptide hormone (increases ejaculation frequency and sexual desire)	– 10 min before intercourse, 24 IU intranasal	Nausea, vomiting, headache
	– Effective in orgasm and ejaculation processes	– 10–20 min before intercourse, 24 IU sublingual	

Table 4.8 (continued)

Drugs	Effect mechanism	Usage dose	Side effects
Bupropion [191, 192]	– Dopamine-norepinephrine reuptake inhibitor	2–3 times a day	Palpitations, frequent urination, blurred vision
	– It is an the most effective drug in the treatment of DE caused by SSRIs	75 mg p.o.	
Buspirone [193]	5-HT1A receptor agonist	2 times a day	Dizziness, nausea, fatigue, blurred vision
		5–15 mg p.o.	
Yohimbine [194]	Herbal alkaloid with alpha-2 antagonist effect	3 times a day	Nervousness, tremor, hyperglycemia, urinary retention
		5.4 mg p.o.	
Betanechol [195]	Long-acting muscarinic receptor agonist	1–2 h before intercourse 20 mg p.o.	Abdominal pain, nausea, miosis, diarrhea
Apomorphine [196]	Dopamine receptor agonist	20 min before intercourse,	Dyskinesia, rhinorrhea, hallucination, anxiety
	Effective in sexual and ejaculation dysfunctions in patients with Parkinson's	0.5–1.5 mg intranasal	

Penile Vibrator Stimulation

In the treatment of penile vibrator stimulation (PVS), it is aimed to induce ejaculation due to stimulation of the afferent nerves. In a previous study, frenulum vibration stimulation was given to patients with DE at regular intervals for 3–6 months, and a success rate of 72% was reported [197]. In another study, it was observed that PVS treatment together with medical treatment increased the success in DE [198]. Despite these results, studies with a high level of evidence are required to use PVS effectively.

Psychotherapy

Concurrent psychotherapy with medical treatment in patients with DE increases the effectiveness of treatment and detects other underlying psychopathologies [168]. Reducing anxiety, masturbation exercises, and increasing genital stimulation are methods used in psychotherapy to treat DE [34]. In addition, the management of the patient's relationship with his partner provides benefits in the treatment [165].

Anejaculation

Definition

Anejaculation (AE) is the complete absence of both antegrade and retrograde ejaculation (RE) despite adequate stimulation of the penis. It occurs as a result of the failure of semen emission [199].

Epidemiology

Since the difference between DE and AE is not clearly defined, epidemiological studies are insufficient, and the prevalence of AE is unknown.

Pathophysiology, Etiology, and Risk Factor

The etiology of AE is similar mainly to DE and RE. The most common etiologic causes in patients presenting with AE are retroperitoneal lymph node dissection (RPLND) and spinal cord traumas [200]. Postoperative AE may develop in men undergoing RPLND (especially when nerve-sparing cannot be performed) for testicular tumor treatment. After nerve-sparing RPLND, over 80% ejaculation can be preserved [201]. A 15% reduction in the ejaculate or AE has been reported in patients receiving radiotherapy to the abdominal area for testicular cancer [202]. AE can also be seen frequently in patients who have undergone radical prostatectomy, abdominoperineal resections for rectal cancer, and medulla spinalis surgery [200]. Spinal cord injury causes significant ejaculatory dysfunction [179]. Ejaculation problems can be seen in more than 95% of upper motor neuron damage patients. Various ejaculation problems (such as RE, AE, and DE) are seen in 1/3 of patients with diabetes mellitus [178]. In cases that obstruct the ejaculatory ducts for various reasons (such as congenital Mullerian duct cysts, prostatitis, and urogenital tuberculosis) AE can be seen.

Classification

AE is divided into two, namely, orgasmic and anorgasmic. Anorgasmic AE is usually evaluated as DE and treated similarly.

Diagnosis

A detailed anamnesis should be taken in the evaluation of patients with AE. A situational/global distinction of AE and an orgasmic/anorgasmic distinction should be made. Underlying etiological causes should be investigated, and neurological examination should be performed when necessary, in addition to genital examination. If RE is suspected, urine analysis should be performed after ejaculation. Prostate midline cysts can be palpated by DRM. Imaging may be performed if obstruction of the ejaculatory ducts is suspected (transrectal ultrasound (TRUS) or pelvic magnetic resonance imaging (MRI) (Fig. 4.4).

Treatment

The treatment of AE in which no cause has been determined is performed similarly to the treatment of DE. Alpha agonists can be given in the treatment of patients with orgasmic AE. In a previous study, ejaculation (antegrade or retrograde) was achieved in more than 50% of patients treated with midodrine [203]. PVS is the preferred method, especially in T10 or higher spinal cord injury cases. PVS acts on the ejaculation reflex by stimulating the frenulum with vibration [204]. With this method, ejaculation is achieved in 81% of patients [205]. Since PVS may cause autonomic dysreflexia in lesions above T6, pre-procedure administration of 10–30 mg of nifedipine makes the procedure safe [206]. In cases where PVS fails, electro-ejaculation with a rectal probe can be applied to obtain sperm [207]. With the rectal probe, ejaculation is stimulated by a direct effect on the seminal vesicles and vas deferens nerves. The procedure is performed under general anesthesia, and the bladder should be emptied before the procedure. With this technique, ejaculation is achieved in more than 90% of patients [208]. Ejaculation can also be retrograde. Apart from these methods, surgical methods of obtaining sperm can be used according to the couple's wish for a child.

Painful Ejaculation

Definition
Painful ejaculation is a condition that can range from mild discomfort to severe pain during or after the patient's ejaculation. Painful ejaculation is also called disejaculation, dysorgasmia, or orgasmalgia [209]. Pain may be felt in the penis, scrotum, and perineum. The duration of the pain can vary from a few seconds to a few days.

Epidemiology
Painful ejaculation is a symptom that patients do not often report. It can be an isolated symptom or seen together with lower urinary system symptoms. In 2003, 12,815 men aged 50–80 years were surveyed about lower urinary tract symptoms., It was found that 6.7% of the participants complained of painful ejaculation [210]. In a study involving 2000 sexually active men, 25.9% reported discomfort during ejaculation. In epidemiological studies, it is stated that painful ejaculation is seen at rates ranging from 1.9% to 12% [209, 211].

Pathophysiology, Etiology, and Risk Factors
Painful ejaculation may be idiopathic or may be due to multiple causes. Common causes include infectious diseases of the urinary system such as orchitis, epididymitis, prostatitis, and urethritis [212]. Patients with BPH were observed to have more painful ejaculation symptoms than the normal population (without BPH) [213]. Again, after radical prostatectomy, painful orgasm was found in 9–33% of patients [2, 214]. It may cause painful ejaculation in cases of ejaculatory duct obstruction (such as seminal vesicle stones, midline prostate cysts, and seminal vesiculitis) [215, 216]. Painful ejaculation can be seen due to ejaculatory duct obstruction in Zinner syndrome [217]. Painful ejaculation can also be seen in chronic pelvic pain syndrome and after pelvic radiation, vasectomy surgery, inflammation in the vas deferens due to the use of mesh in inguinal hernia repair, and mercury toxicity [218–220]. Painful ejaculation has been reported from time to time using antidepressant drugs (such as imipramine, clomipramine, amoxapine, fluoxetine, and venlafaxine) [221].

Diagnosis
Detailed history and physical examination are essential in the diagnosis of painful ejaculation. The urogenital system should be evaluated in detail in the physical

examination, and a DRM should be performed for the prostate. Depending on the underlying cause, laboratory tests (such as prostate-specific antigen (PSA), urinalysis, and urine culture) may be requested. TRUS and pelvic MRI may be ordered for pathologies that may cause possible ejaculatory duct obstruction. Cystoscopy can be performed in cases with suspected urethral stricture [209].

Treatment

In treating painful ejaculation, the treatment is planned according to the primary cause. If the painful ejaculation develops due to infectious-inflammatory reasons, antibiotics and anti-inflammatory drugs are given together. Painful ejaculation due to radical prostatectomy or BPH is treated with alpha-blockers. Behavioral treatments, pelvic floor exercises, and drugs such as opioids can be given in cases where an underlying cause cannot be determined [222, 223].

Surgical methods can be used for seminal vesicle-related pain (such as transurethral seminal vesiculoscopy and ejaculatory duct resection). In cases of pain (due to possible fibrosis) after inguinal hernia repair, the surrounding of the vas deferens and the ilioinguinal nerve can be dissected [224].

Retrograde Ejaculation

Definition

RE is the condition in which the semen goes retrogradely into the bladder instead of being ejected from the penile urethra. As a result, partial or complete antegrade ejaculation does not occur. In RE, the sensation of orgasm may be reduced or normal [2].

Epidemiology

As the incidence of RE varies in different patient populations, it is difficult to determine the true incidence. RE occurs due to resections starting from the bladder neck and extending to the verumontanum, especially during prostate resection. While 53–75% of RE is seen in patients who underwent transurethral resection of the prostate, it is seen at a rate of 5–45% in patients who underwent transurethral prostate incision [225, 226]. After the newly introduced holmium laser prostate enucleation method, RE is seen at a rate of 54–75% [176]. In a study conducted with infertile couples, the incidence of RE was between 0.3% and 2% among male-induced infertility causes [227]. In a prospective study conducted on patients with diabetes, 34.6% of the patients showed RE [228]. A detailed list of etiological factors causing RE is given in Table 4.9.

Pathophysiology, Etiology, and Risk Factors

The ejaculation reflex consists of the synchronous operation of the emission, expulsion, and orgasm phases. The emission phase is when the sympathetic nervous system is responsible (T10-L2), and the spermatozoa merge with the seminal fluid and pass into the posterior urethra. In the expulsion phase, adrenoreceptors in the

Table 4.9 Etiology of retrograde ejaculation

Neurogenic	Spinal cor injury
	Multiple sclerosis
	Autonomic neuropathy
	Parkinson's disease
	Diabetes Mellitus
	Retroperitoneal lymphadenectomy, sympathectomy
	Cauda equina lesions
Urethral	Urethral stricture
	Ectopic ureterocele
	Urethral valves or verumontaneum hyperplasia
Pharmacological	Antihypertensives, thiazide diuretics
	Alfa-1-adrenoceptor antagonist
	Antipsychotics
Endocrine	Hypogonadism
	Hyperprolactinaemia
	Hypothyroidism
Bladder neck incompetence	Congenital defects/dysfunction of hemitrigone
	Bladder neck resection
	Prostatectomy

bladder neck are stimulated by sympathetic nerves, and the bladder neck is closed, preventing the passage of semen into the retrograde bladder. Then, PFMs contract, and expulsion occurs through the pudendal plexus (S2–S4) and parasympathetic nervous system. During the orgasm phase, increased pressure in the posterior urethra and contraction of the accessory glands stimulate sensory receptors in the verumontanum. As a result, an orgasm response occurs through the central nervous system [1]. In RE, the emission phase continues physiologically, but the bladder neck tone required for the initiation of the ejection phase cannot be achieved. As a result, the semen cannot be expelled from the urethra and is directed toward the bladder [229].

Diagnosis

In the diagnosis of RE, anamnesis, history, physical examination, and laboratory tests are evaluated together. Men with RE often complain of reduced semen or no semen at all. Orgasm may be normal or decreased. Patients usually state that they have cloudy urine after ejaculation. Some patients apply with the complaint of infertility (primary or secondary) [34]. Physical examination is usually normal in men with RE. However, the bilateral testes, epididymis, and vas deferens should be examined in detail. In addition, DRM should be performed except for young men. In prostate size consistency, the anal tone should be checked with DRM.

The reference range of semen volume according to the World Health Organization is 1.4–1.7 mL. The absence of ejaculate is defined as "aspermia," whereas an ejaculate below 1.4 mL is defined as "hypospermia" [230]. In these two cases, RE or ejaculatory duct obstruction should be considered [34].

The definitive diagnosis of RE is made by the first urinalysis after masturbation or postcoital intercourse. The presence of spermatozoa in the first urine sample suggests RE. On the other hand, the presence of azoospermia/oligospermia in semen analysis, low viscosity, low fructose, and pH values suggest ejaculatory duct obstruction. In some studies, 10–15 spermatozoa in the postcoital first urine sample at 400× magnification are considered sufficient for the diagnosis of RE, whereas in other studies, more than one million spermatozoa in the urine sample are considered correct for the diagnosis of RE [231].

Treatment

Pharmacological Treatment
Drug therapy is the primary treatment for RE. The most commonly used drugs are sympathomimetic agents [232]. Sympathomimetics increase noradrenaline secretion, activate adrenergic receptors (alpha and beta), and provide antegrade ejaculation as a result of closing the bladder neck. Synephrine, pseudoephedrine, ephedrine, and phenylpropanolamine are commonly used sympathomimetic drugs [233]. In a previous review, the success rate of sympathomimetic drugs in providing antegrade ejaculation was 28% [234]. The most common side effects are dryness of the mucosal membranes and hypertension [235]. Most of the studies showing the efficacy of sympathomimetics in treating RE have small samples and generally consist of case reports [236]. Today's most common sympathomimetic use is 60–120 mg orally administered pseudoephedrine 1–2 h before sexual intercourse [237]. Imipramine is a tricyclic antidepressant and has both alpha-adrenergic and anticholinergic effects. It has been reported that imipramine (25 and 50 mg) provides antegrade ejaculation in patients with type 2 diabetes and patients undergoing RPLND for testicular tumors [238, 239]. In a study conducted in Japan, it was reported that amoxapine, a second-generation tricyclic antidepressant, is also beneficial in the treatment of RE [240]. Sympathomimetic drugs with imipramine or brompheniramine combination of anticholinergic drugs, increases the success of RE treatment [234].

Surgical Treatment
Abram performed bladder neck reconstruction in two patients who developed RE after surgery, and antegrade ejaculation was provided [241]. Bladder neck reconstruction, which was later used in urinary incontinence, was performed in five patients with RE. Antegrade ejaculation was achieved in four of these patients [242]. It was observed that ejaculation returned to normal in a case with RE, who was injected with collagen into the bladder neck [243]. Although surgical procedures have been tried to treat RE, studies with large case series are not available. Therefore, there is no accepted surgical treatment for RE.

Approach to Infertility
Although RE causes many problems in patients, the most important problem of patients who want to have children is infertility. Apart from routine sperm retrieval methods, there are several different sperm retrieval methods for managing infertility in patients with RE.

Centrifugation and Resuspension
Patients with RE are primarily given a few recommendations for dilution of urine. Giving sodium bicarbonate or increasing fluid intake is some of these suggestions. As a result, a better environment is provided for the sperm. Then, a urine sample is collected from the patient after orgasm. Urine can be collected spontaneously after voiding or by catheter. The collected urine sample is centrifuged and suspended in heterogeneous liquids such as bovine albumin and human serum albumin. The obtained sperm can then be used in assisted reproductive techniques. In a systematic review, a pregnancy rate of 15% was reported as a result of this method [234].

Hotchkiss (or Modified Hotchkiss) Method
In this method, the bladder is first emptied with a catheter, and washed with ringer lactate. A small amount of ringer lactate is then introduced into the bladder. After this procedure, the patient is asked to ejaculate. After ejaculation, the contents of the bladder are removed by a catheter or spontaneous voiding. Subsequently, spermatozoa are used in assisted reproductive techniques [244]. Modified techniques were defined by changing the suspension fluids used in this technique. In studies conducted with the Hotchkiss method, a pregnancy rate of 24% was achieved [234].

Ejaculation on a Full Bladder
There are only a few studies on this method [245, 246]. The patient is encouraged to ejaculate with a full bladder in this method. After ejaculation, the semen is placed in Baker's tampon. This ingredient is then used in assisted reproductive techniques. In a previous study, which included five patients in total, pregnancy was reported in three patients [234].

Hemospermia

Definition
Hemospermia is the presence of blood in the ejaculate. Although it mainly occurs due to benign causes, it should be kept in mind that serious pathologies can cause hemospermia [65, 247].

Epidemiology
Hemospermia can be seen in all age groups. In previous studies, hemospermia was found at a rate of 1–1.5% among urological pathologies [247, 248]. In a study conducted on patients presenting with hemospermia, the risk of genitourinary malignancy was found to be approximately 3.5% [249]. In another study in which 26,600 men were screened for prostate cancer, prostate cancer was diagnosed in 19 (13.7%) out of 139 men who reported hemospermia [250]. In a study in which the patients presented with hemospermia were included, the rate of urinary tract infection was high in patients younger than 40 years old, whereas the rate of stone disease and malignancy was high in the group over 40 years old. In addition, no underlying pathology was detected in 81% of the patients [247].

Table 4.10 Possible causes of hemospermia

Category	Causes
Congenital	Seminal vesicle (SV) or ejaculatory duct cysts
Inflammatory	Urethritis, prostatitis, epididymitis, tuberculosis, CMV, HIV, Schistosomiasis, hydatid, condyloma of urethra and meatus, urinary tract infections
Obstruction	Prostatic, SV and ejaculatory duct calculi, post-inflammatory, seminal vesicle diverticula/cyst, urethral stricture, utricle cyst, BPH
Tumors	Prostate, bladder, SV, urethra, testis, epididymis, melanoma
Vascular	Prostatic varices, prostatic telangiectasia, haemangioma, posterior urethral veins, excessive sex or masturbation
Trauma/ iatrogenic	Perineum, testis, instrumentation, post-haemorrhoid injection, prostate biopsy, vaso-venous fistula
Systemic	Hypertension, haemophilia, purpura, scurvy, bleeding disorders, chronic liver disease, renovascular disease, leukaemia, lymphoma, cirrhosis, amyloidosis

Pathophysiology, Etiology, and Risk Factors

Multiple factors can cause hemospermia. These factors can be categorized as congenital, inflammatory, obstruction, trauma, malignancy, and systemic causes. Detailed possible causes of hemospermia are given in Table 4.10.

Diagnosis

Clinical history should be collected in detail in the evaluation of hemospermia. Both symptom-specific and systemic evaluations should be performed. First of all, a distinction should be made between hemospermia and pseudohemospermia. Pseudohemospermia develops during coitus due to vaginal bleeding or secondary to hematuria. To distinguish this, the patient empties into the condom, and the absence of blood in the semen makes the diagnosis of pseudohemospermia [251]. Rarely, in cases where malignant melanoma invades the genitourinary system, melanospermia may occur, and the diagnosis is made by demonstrating melanoma in the semen [252].

It has been reported that some sexually transmitted microorganisms cause hemospermia (herpes simplex virus, *Chlamydia trachomatis*, *Enterococcus faecalis*, *Ureaplasma urealyticum*, and cytomegalovirus) [253]. Travel history should also be questioned, especially where schistosomiasis and tuberculosis are endemic [253]. Although causal links have not been proven yet, many systemic conditions are associated with hemospermia. Hemospermia may be seen in patients with uncontrolled hypertension [254]. Blood in the ejaculate may be seen in bleeding diatheses such as hemophilia and Von Willebrand's disease [255]. Similarly, severe liver diseases in which coagulation factors are insufficiently synthesized may accompany hemospermia [256]. Detailed physical examination is important in patients with hemospermia. Abdominal examination should be done for mass or organomegaly. The perineal and genital examination should be done in detail. The urethral meatus should be examined for the presence of trauma, condylomas, and mass pathologies. The testicular examination is important because hemospermia can be seen in testicular tumors. In addition, a detailed examination of the testis and epididymis can help reveal inflammatory pathologies such as tuberculosis. Possible prostate pathologies can be detected by rectal examination. Especially in elderly patients, the detection of hardness or nodule along with hemospermia in the rectal examination may be a sign of prostate cancer [257].

Although there is no consensus with respect to the first tests to be requested in the diagnosis, urinalysis should be requested in addition to the urine culture. Semen analysis should be performed in cases with suspected tuberculosis or schistosomiasis. Urine, blood, and necessary samples should be collected for sexually transmitted diseases [258]. PSA should be checked for patients over the age of 40. If a systemic disease is present, whole blood, liver function tests, and coagulation parameters should be checked. If further investigation is required, the patient's risk factors should be decided [250]. TRUS or MRI can be used to evaluate pathologies such as stone or tumor in the prostate, seminal vesicle, vas deferens, or ejaculatory ducts. TRUS is primarily preferred for imaging. If pathology is detected during TRUS, it also provides the possibility of biopsy simultaneously [259]. The use of MRI has been increasing recently. In addition to structural pathologies, MRI shows prostatic middle or paramedian cysts in detail and is useful in making surgical decisions [260].

In persistent or unresponsive hemospermia, the lower urinary tract may need to be evaluated with cystoscopy. With the advancement of technology, the ejaculatory duct and seminal vesicles can be directly visualized through optics. In a previous study, 106 patients with recurrent hemospermia were evaluated by TRUS and seminal vesiculoscopy, and 87% of the patients were diagnosed with these methods. The diagnostic rate of seminal vesiculoscopy was found to be higher than that of TRUS [261].

In a study published in 2021, 283 patients were grouped according to the Charlson Comorbidity Index and EAU guidelines [262]. According to the EAU guidelines, approximately 90% of patients were high-risk for hemospermia. However, there was no significant difference between the low risk and high-risk groups, except for hypertension and PSA value. A new hemospermia risk model was created using all of the data. As a result of the study, it was seen that the EAU hemospermia risk classification may be insufficient and that the hemospermia cases that are not high-risk but can go away spontaneously are considered high-risk. Therefore, the authors stated that a new risk classification would be more accurate in cases with hemospermia [262].

Treatment

The main goal of treatment is to exclude serious pathologies such as prostate or bladder cancer and to treat other underlying causes. With respect to treatment management, patients are classified as low or high-risk [263, 264]. The conservative approach is the primary treatment in patients with low risk. Symptomatic treatment can be given to these patients when necessary [265]. Detailed examinations should be performed in the high-risk patient group, and necessary treatment should be planned. The management algorithm for hemospermia is given in Fig. 4.5 [263, 264, 266].

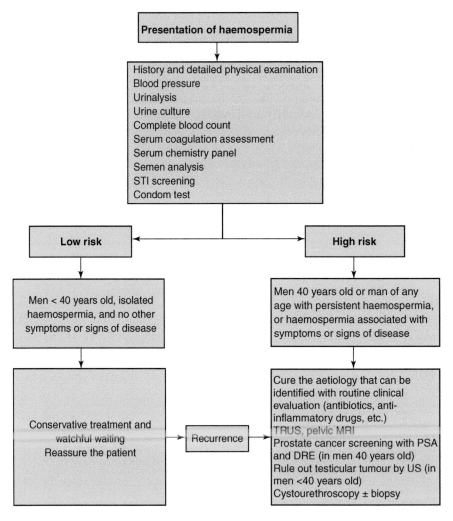

Fig. 4.5 Management algorithm for haemospermia [249, 263, 264, 266]

Appropriate antibiotic therapy is given in cases of infection (urogenital infection or sexually transmitted infections). When a vascular pathology is detected, seminal vesicle and prostate cysts can be aspirated transurethrally while fulgarization is performed [248]. Resection can be performed in ejaculatory duct obstruction [267]. In cases of hemospermia due to systemic diseases, the primary target in treatment is the underlying pathology [264]. In a previous study conducted on 60 patients with idiopathic hemospermia, finasteride was found to be more successful than a placebo [268].

Orgasmic Disorders

Orgasm is a neurobiological process involving a complex series of events and the neurophysiological mechanism of orgasm has not been demonstrated [269]. Orgasm occurs due to the collective work of the spinal cord ejaculation center, central nervous system, parasympathetic-sympathetic pathways, pelvic nerves, and muscles [270–272]. As a result of examining the centers in the brain with PET in the presence of sexual stimuli, the most intense activity during orgasm was detected in the ventral tegmental region of the mesencephalon [273]. Apart from this region, many areas of the brain are associated with orgasm (such as lateral putamen, subparafascicular nucleus, cerebellum, Brodmann areas 18, 21, and 23).

In men, orgasm and ejaculation are often simultaneous. However, in some cases, ejaculation may not be accompanied by orgasm. Orgasmic disturbances are not as common as ED and PE. The absence of orgasm is often associated with DE, and etiological factors, clinical presentation, and treatment approaches are similar. Therefore, orgasmic disorders should be evaluated together with DE.

Anorgasmia

Definition
Anorgasmia is the absence of the sensation of orgasm. It appears as a situation independent of whether there is ejaculation or not.

Epidemiology
Since anorgasmia is a rare condition, it is difficult to determine the true prevalence. It mostly co-occurs with DE, and the prevalence of DE is around 3% in studies in the literature [166, 274, 275]. According to DSM-5, it has been reported that only 25% of men reach orgasm during all sexual intercourse [9]. In addition, men over the age of 80 have twice as many orgasm-related complaints as men under 60 [9]. A few studies have reported the prevalence of primary anorgasmia to be 1.5 per 1000 and the prevalence of secondary anorgasmia to be 2–4 per 1000 [276, 277].

Pathophysiology, Etiology and Risk Factors
Since anorgasmia is often seen with DE and is considered a symptom of DE, risk factors are considered the same as DE. Anorgasmia usually develops secondary to antipsychotic, antidepressant, or anticonvulsant drugs used in psychiatric disorders [278]. In addition, such as anxiety, fear, obesity, drug use, testosterone deficiency and hypothyroidism may cause anorgasmia [198, 279]. As a result of peculiar masturbation techniques (idiosyncratic masturbation) of some men, penile sensitivity decreases. To increase this diminishing feeling, they increase the strength of masturbation and as a result, a vicious cycle begins. During sexual intercourse with the

partner, it is difficult to reach orgasm and, penile stimulation decreases. In this case, hyperstimulation occurs and anorgasmia may develop [34, 165].

Spinal cord trauma and surgical procedures (such as radical prostatectomy) that cause penile hypoesthesia or penile sensory loss, which increases with aging, may cause anorgasmia [198, 280].

Classification
Primary anorgasmia: Anorgasmia that continues continuously from the first sexual intercourse.

Secondary anorgasmia: It is the state of having an orgasm in the previous sexual intercourse but not having an orgasm in the following sexual intercourse [281].

Diagnosis
First of all, taking a good medical and psychosexual history is essential for diagnosis. Drug use (especially psychiatric drugs such as SSRIs) should be questioned. Comorbid conditions that may cause loss of penile sensation, such as DM, should be revealed. In cases where penile sensory loss is suspected, biothesiometry and pudendal somatosensory evoked potentials (SSEP) may be useful for diagnosis. Endocrine pathologies (hypothyroidism, hyperprolactinemia, testosterone deficiency) should be questioned. Laboratory tests may be requested in cases where endocrinopathy is suspected. If the patient masturbates, the frequency and type of masturbation should be asked. Relationship status and satisfaction, problems with his partner, external stress factors are psychologically important. It should be questioned when anorgasmia begins. Thus, the distinction between primary and secondary anorgasmia can be clarified.

Treatment

Psychosexual Counseling
If there is no organic pathology causing anorgasmia, psychotherapy with the partner may be beneficial. Psychotherapy techniques such as masturbation training, changes in arousal methods, reducing sexual anxiety, and increasing genital stimulation can be used [170, 186].

Pharmacotherapy
Buspirone (150 mg/day) has been tried and found beneficial in men with life-long anorgasmia reported [282]. Cyproheptadine, an antihistamine that increases brain serotonin levels,- has been used in some studies to treat anorgasmia [184, 191]. Again, amantadine was tried in anorgasmia (100–200 mg 5–6 h before sexual intercourse) caused by SSRIs and observed to stimulate ejaculation [283]. In a study with yohimbine, an alpha-2 adrenergic receptor blocker, where 29 patients were included due to infertility or orgasmic dysfunction, approximately half of the patients reached orgasm after using yohimbine [194]. In a case report on oxytocin, intranasal oxytocin in anorgasmic man has been proven to be successful [190].

To date, there is no FDA-approved drug for anorgasmia. The effects of these drugs have been tested on a small number of patients. Large-batch cohort studies are needed for pharmacotherapy in anorgasmia.

Other Treatment Methods

Cabergoline is effective in treating both ED and sexual dysfunction in hyperprolactinemia [187]. It has been observed that the replacement of testosterone increases orgasm in cases of testosterone deficiency [284]. When these treatment methods fail, penile vibrator stimulation, electro-ejaculation or (m)TESE may be preferred to obtain sperm in patients with anorgasmia [198].

If there is no organic pathology causing anorgasmia, psychotherapy with the partner may be beneficial. Psychotherapy techniques such as masturbation training, changes in arousal methods, reducing sexual anxiety, and increasing genital stimulation can be used [170, 186].

Postorgasmic Illness Syndrome (POIS)

Post-orgasmic illness syndrome (POIS) is characterized by extreme tiredness, weakness, fever or sweating, mood disturbances, incoherent speech, memory disorders, nasal congestion, and itchy eyes, which develop during orgasm or within a few hours after orgasm. It was first described in 2002 by Waldinger et al. [285]. Although POIS is a scarce condition, it seriously affects the quality of life. Due to its rarity, little is known about the etiology and epidemiology.

Symptoms occur in almost all ejaculation episodes. These symptoms disappear spontaneously in an average of 2–7 days. In a study of 45 men with POIS, it was observed that 87% of the patients had onset of POIS symptoms within 30 min after ejaculation [286]. Waldinger et al. stated that there was an atopic structure in 58% of the cases and the skin pick test performed with the men's own semen were positive in 88%. Therefore, type 1 hypersensitivity reaction was postulated as the reason of POIS [287]. Changes similar to opioid withdrawal in the brain and irregularities in cytokine and chemokine response have also been suggested in the etiology [288].

Although there is no definitive treatment for POIS, SSRIs, antihistamines, and benzodiazepines are used in the treatment. Waldinger et al. reported that they treated two patients with POIS by subcutaneous injection of autologous semen (prolonged hyposensitization). In the study, it was reported that the treatment success decreased over time [287].

References

1. Clement P, Giuliano F. Physiology and pharmacology of ejaculation. Basic Clin Pharmacol Toxicol. 2016;119(Suppl 3):18–25.
2. Althof SE, McMahon CG. Contemporary management of disorders of male orgasm and ejaculation. Urology. 2016;93:9–21.

3. Giuliano F, Clement P. Neuroanatomy and physiology of ejaculation. Annu Rev Sex Res. 2005;16:190–216.
4. McMahon CG, et al. Disorders of orgasm and ejaculation in men. J Sex Med. 2004;1(1):58–65.
5. Rosen RC. Prevalence and risk factors of sexual dysfunction in men and women. Curr Psychiatry Rep. 2000;2(3):189–95.
6. Parnham A, Serefoglu EC. Classification and definition of premature ejaculation. Transl Androl Urol. 2016;5(4):416–23.
7. Althof SE, et al. An update of the International Society of Sexual Medicine's Guidelines for the diagnosis and treatment of premature ejaculation (PE). Sex Med. 2014;2(2):60–90.
8. World Health Organization. International Classification of Diseases 11th Revision for Mortality and MorbidityStatistics (ICD- 11-MMS): the global standard for diagnostic health information. Geneva: WHO; 2018.
9. American Psychiatric Association. Diagnostic and statistical manual of mental disorders (DSM-V). 5th ed. Arlington, VA: American Psychiatric Association; 2013.
10. Serefoglu EC, et al. An evidence-based unified definition of lifelong and acquired premature ejaculation: report of the second International Society for Sexual Medicine Ad Hoc Committee for the Definition of Premature Ejaculation. J Sex Med. 2014;11(6):1423–41.
11. Waldinger MD, Schweitzer DH. Changing paradigms from a historical DSM-III and DSM-IV view toward an evidence-based definition of premature ejaculation. Part II—proposals for DSM-V and ICD-11. J Sex Med. 2006;3(4):693–705.
12. Carson C, Gunn K. Premature ejaculation: definition and prevalence. Int J Impot Res. 2006;18(Suppl 1):S5–13.
13. Waldinger MD. The neurobiological approach to premature ejaculation. J Urol. 2002;168(6):2359–67.
14. Laumann EO, Paik A, Rosen RC. Sexual dysfunction in the United States: prevalence and predictors. JAMA. 1999;281(6):537–44.
15. Dunn KM, Croft PR, Hackett GI. Sexual problems: a study of the prevalence and need for health care in the general population. Fam Pract. 1998;15(6):519–24.
16. Porst H, et al. The Premature Ejaculation Prevalence and Attitudes (PEPA) survey: prevalence, comorbidities, and professional help-seeking. Eur Urol. 2007;51(3):816–23; discussion 824
17. Serefoglu EC, et al. Prevalence of the complaint of ejaculating prematurely and the four premature ejaculation syndromes: results from the Turkish Society of Andrology Sexual Health Survey. J Sex Med. 2011;8(2):540–8.
18. Masters W, Johnson V. Human sexual inadequacy. Boston: Little, Brown; 1970.
19. Schapiro B. Premature ejaculation: a review of 1130 cases. J Urol. 1943;50(9):374.
20. Waldinger MD. The pathophysiology of lifelong premature ejaculation. Transl Androl Urol. 2016;5(4):424–33.
21. McMahon CG, et al. An evidence-based definition of lifelong premature ejaculation: report of the International Society for Sexual Medicine (ISSM) ad hoc committee for the definition of premature ejaculation. J Sex Med. 2008;5(7):1590–606.
22. Waldinger MD. Recent advances in the classification, neurobiology and treatment of premature ejaculation. Adv Psychosom Med. 2008;29:50–69.
23. Waldinger MD, et al. Premature ejaculation and serotonergic antidepressants-induced delayed ejaculation: the involvement of the serotonergic system. Behav Brain Res. 1998;92(2):111–8.
24. Gao J, et al. Prevalence and factors associated with the complaint of premature ejaculation and the four premature ejaculation syndromes: a large observational study in China. J Sex Med. 2013;10(7):1874–81.
25. Carani C, et al. Multicenter study on the prevalence of sexual symptoms in male hypo- and hyperthyroid patients. J Clin Endocrinol Metab. 2005;90(12):6472–9.
26. Corona G, et al. Psycho-biological correlates of rapid ejaculation in patients attending an andrologic unit for sexual dysfunctions. Eur Urol. 2004;46(5):615–22.
27. McMahon CG, et al. The pathophysiology of acquired premature ejaculation. Transl Androl Urol. 2016;5(4):434–49.

28. Verze P, et al. Premature ejaculation among italian men: prevalence and clinical correlates from an observational, non-interventional, cross-sectional, epidemiological study (IPER). Sex Med. 2018;6(3):193–202.
29. Richardson D, Goldmeier D. Premature ejaculation—does country of origin tell us anything about etiology? J Sex Med. 2005;2(4):508–12.
30. El-Hamd MA, Saleh R, Majzoub A. Premature ejaculation: an update on definition and pathophysiology. Asian J Androl. 2019;21(5):425–32.
31. Waldinger MD, McIntosh J, Schweitzer DH. A five-nation survey to assess the distribution of the intravaginal ejaculatory latency time among the general male population. J Sex Med. 2009;6(10):2888–95.
32. Waldinger MD. Premature ejaculation: different pathophysiologies and etiologies determine its treatment. J Sex Marital Ther. 2008;34(1):1–13.
33. Shabsigh R. Diagnosing premature ejaculation: a review. J Sex Med. 2006;3(Suppl 4):318–23.
34. Rowland D, et al. Disorders of orgasm and ejaculation in men. J Sex Med. 2010;7(4 Pt 2):1668–86.
35. Schein M, et al. The frequency of sexual problems among family practice patients. Fam Pract Res J. 1988;7(3):122–34.
36. Humphery S, Nazareth I. GPs' views on their management of sexual dysfunction. Fam Pract. 2001;18(5):516–8.
37. Corona G, et al. Interplay between premature ejaculation and erectile dysfunction: a systematic review and meta-analysis. J Sex Med. 2015;12(12):2291–300.
38. Althof SE. Prevalence, characteristics and implications of premature ejaculation/rapid ejaculation. J Urol. 2006;175(3 Pt 1):842–8.
39. Giuliano F, et al. Premature ejaculation: results from a five-country European observational study. Eur Urol. 2008;53(5):1048–57.
40. Althof SE. Evidence based assessment of rapid ejaculation. Int J Impot Res. 1998;10(Suppl 2):S74–6; discussion S77–9
41. Rosen RC, et al. Correlates to the clinical diagnosis of premature ejaculation: results from a large observational study of men and their partners. J Urol. 2007;177(3):1059–64; discussion 1064
42. Corona G, Jannini EA, Maggi M. Inventories for male and female sexual dysfunctions. Int J Impot Res. 2006;18(3):236–50.
43. Althof S, et al. Development and validation of a new questionnaire to assess sexual satisfaction, control, and distress associated with premature ejaculation. J Sex Med. 2006;3(3):465–75.
44. Arafa M, Shamloul R. Development and evaluation of the Arabic Index of Premature Ejaculation (AIPE). J Sex Med. 2007;4(6):1750–6.
45. Patrick DL, et al. The premature ejaculation profile: validation of self-reported outcome measures for research and practice. BJU Int. 2009;103(3):358–64.
46. Symonds T, et al. Further evidence of the reliability and validity of the premature ejaculation diagnostic tool. Int J Impot Res. 2007;19(5):521–5.
47. Yuan YM, et al. Sexual function of premature ejaculation patients assayed with Chinese Index of Premature Ejaculation. Asian J Androl. 2004;6(2):121–6.
48. McMahon C, et al. Treatment of premature ejaculation in the Asia-Pacific region: results from a phase III double-blind, parallel-group study of dapoxetine. J Sex Med. 2010;7(1 Pt 1):256–68.
49. Waldinger MD. Pharmacotherapy for premature ejaculation. Expert Opin Pharmacother. 2015;16(17):2615–24.
50. Rosen RC, Althof S. Impact of premature ejaculation: the psychological, quality of life, and sexual relationship consequences. J Sex Med. 2008;5(6):1296–307.
51. Rowland DL, et al. The psychological burden of premature ejaculation. J Urol. 2007;177(3):1065–70.
52. Giuri S, et al. Cognitive attentional syndrome and metacognitive beliefs in male sexual dysfunction: an exploratory study. Am J Mens Health. 2017;11(3):592–9.

53. Kempeneers P, et al. Sexual cognitions, trait anxiety, sexual anxiety, and distress in men with different subtypes of premature ejaculation and in their partners. J Sex Marital Ther. 2018;44(4):319–32.
54. Metz ME, Pryor JL. Premature ejaculation: a psychophysiological approach for assessment and management. J Sex Marital Ther. 2000;26(4):293–320.
55. Rowland DL, Dabbs CR, Medina MC. Sex differences in attributions to positive and negative sexual scenarios in men and women with and without sexual problems: reconsidering stereotypes. Arch Sex Behav. 2019;48(3):855–66.
56. Althof SE. Psychosexual therapy for premature ejaculation. Transl Androl Urol. 2016;5(4):475–81.
57. Semans JH. Premature ejaculation: a new approach. South Med J. 1956;49(4):353–8.
58. Kilmann PR, et al. Perspectives of sex therapy outcome: a survey of AASECT providers. J Sex Marital Ther. 1986;12(2):116–38.
59. Hawton K, Catalan J. Prognostic factors in sex therapy. Behav Res Ther. 1986;24(4):377–85.
60. Hawton K, et al. Long-term outcome of sex therapy. Behav Res Ther. 1986;24(6):665–75.
61. La Pera G, Nicastro A. A new treatment for premature ejaculation: the rehabilitation of the pelvic floor. J Sex Marital Ther. 1996;22(1):22–6.
62. Ma GC, et al. Regular penis-root masturbation, a novel behavioral therapy in the treatment of primary premature ejaculation. Asian J Androl. 2019;21(6):631–4.
63. Öztürk MO, Uluşahin A. Ruh Sağlığı ve Bozuklukları. Istanbul: Nobel Tıp Kitabevleri; 2014.
64. Yildiz Y, Kilinc MF, Doluoglu OG. Is there any association between regular physical activity and ejaculation time? Urol J. 2018;15(5):285–9.
65. Salonia A, et al. European Association of Urology guidelines on sexual and reproductive health—2021 update: male sexual dysfunction. Eur Urol. 2021;80(3):333–57.
66. Lue TF, et al. Summary of the recommendations on sexual dysfunctions in men. J Sex Med. 2004;1(1):6–23.
67. Chierigo F, et al. Lower urinary tract symptoms and depressive symptoms among patients presenting for distressing early ejaculation. Int J Impot Res. 2020;32(2):207–12.
68. Qin Z, et al. Safety and efficacy characteristics of oral drugs in patients with premature ejaculation: a Bayesian network meta-analysis of randomized controlled trials. Int J Impot Res. 2019;31(5):356–68.
69. Xin ZC, et al. Penile sensitivity in patients with primary premature ejaculation. J Urol. 1996;156(3):979–81.
70. Wyllie MG, Hellstrom WJ. The link between penile hypersensitivity and premature ejaculation. BJU Int. 2011;107(3):452–7.
71. Berkovitch M, Keresteci AG, Koren G. Efficacy of prilocaine-lidocaine cream in the treatment of premature ejaculation. J Urol. 1995;154(4):1360–1.
72. Busato W, Galindo CC. Topical anaesthetic use for treating premature ejaculation: a double-blind, randomized, placebo-controlled study. BJU Int. 2004;93(7):1018–21.
73. Dinsmore WW, et al. Topical eutectic mixture for premature ejaculation (TEMPE): a novel aerosol-delivery form of lidocaine-prilocaine for treating premature ejaculation. BJU Int. 2007;99(2):369–75.
74. Dinsmore WW, Wyllie MG. PSD502 improves ejaculatory latency, control and sexual satisfaction when applied topically 5 min before intercourse in men with premature ejaculation: results of a phase III, multicentre, double-blind, placebo-controlled study. BJU Int. 2009;103(7):940–9.
75. Martyn-St James M, et al. Topical anaesthetics for premature ejaculation: a systematic review and meta-analysis. Sex Health. 2016;13(2):114–23.
76. Dresser MJ, et al. Pharmacokinetics of dapoxetine, a new treatment for premature ejaculation: impact of age and effects of a high-fat meal. J Clin Pharmacol. 2006;46(9):1023–9.
77. Andersson KE, Mulhall JP, Wyllie MG. Pharmacokinetic and pharmacodynamic features of dapoxetine, a novel drug for 'on-demand' treatment of premature ejaculation. BJU Int. 2006;97(2):311–5.

78. Buvat J, et al. Dapoxetine for the treatment of premature ejaculation: results from a randomized, double-blind, placebo-controlled phase 3 trial in 22 countries. Eur Urol. 2009;55(4):957–67.
79. Kaufman JM, et al. Treatment benefit of dapoxetine for premature ejaculation: results from a placebo-controlled phase III trial. BJU Int. 2009;103(5):651–8.
80. McMahon CG, et al. Efficacy and safety of dapoxetine in men with premature ejaculation and concomitant erectile dysfunction treated with a phosphodiesterase type 5 inhibitor: randomized, placebo-controlled, phase III study. J Sex Med. 2013;10(9):2312–25.
81. McMahon CG, et al. Efficacy and safety of dapoxetine for the treatment of premature ejaculation: integrated analysis of results from five phase 3 trials. J Sex Med. 2011;8(2):524–39.
82. Verze P, et al. Comparison of treatment emergent adverse events in men with premature ejaculation treated with dapoxetine and alternate oral treatments: results from a large multinational observational trial. J Sex Med. 2016;13(2):194–9.
83. Levine S, Casey R, Mudumbi R, Hashmonay R. Evaluation of withdrawal effects with dapoxetine in the treatment od premature ejaculation [abstract no. 82]. J Sex Med. 2007;4(Suppl. 1):91.
84. Tuken M, Culha MG, Serefoglu EC. Efficacy and safety of dapoxetine/sildenafil combination tablets in the treatment of men with premature ejaculation and concomitant erectile dysfunction-DAP-SPEED Study. Int J Impot Res. 2019;31(2):92–6.
85. Porst H, et al. Baseline characteristics and treatment outcomes for men with acquired or lifelong premature ejaculation with mild or no erectile dysfunction: integrated analyses of two phase 3 dapoxetine trials. J Sex Med. 2010;7(6):2231–42.
86. Giuliano F. 5-Hydroxytryptamine in premature ejaculation: opportunities for therapeutic intervention. Trends Neurosci. 2007;30(2):79–84.
87. Olivier B, van Oorschot R, Waldinger MD. Serotonin, serotonergic receptors, selective serotonin reuptake inhibitors and sexual behaviour. Int Clin Psychopharmacol. 1998;13(Suppl 6):S9–14.
88. Atmaca M, et al. The efficacy of citalopram in the treatment of premature ejaculation: a placebo-controlled study. Int J Impot Res. 2002;14(6):502–5.
89. McMahon CG. Treatment of premature ejaculation with sertraline hydrochloride: a single-blind placebo controlled crossover study. J Urol. 1998;159(6):1935–8.
90. Waldinger MD, Hengeveld MW, Zwinderman AH. Paroxetine treatment of premature ejaculation: a double-blind, randomized, placebo-controlled study. Am J Psychiatry. 1994;151(9):1377–9.
91. Kara H, et al. The efficacy of fluoxetine in the treatment of premature ejaculation: a double-blind placebo controlled study. J Urol. 1996;156(5):1631–2.
92. Waldinger MD. Premature ejaculation: definition and drug treatment. Drugs. 2007;67(4):547–68.
93. Waldinger MD, et al. Effect of SSRI antidepressants on ejaculation: a double-blind, randomized, placebo-controlled study with fluoxetine, fluvoxamine, paroxetine, and sertraline. J Clin Psychopharmacol. 1998;18(4):274–81.
94. Waldinger MD, et al. Relevance of methodological design for the interpretation of efficacy of drug treatment of premature ejaculation: a systematic review and meta-analysis. Int J Impot Res. 2004;16(4):369–81.
95. Sathianathen NJ, et al. Selective serotonin re-uptake inhibitors for premature ejaculation in adult men. Cochrane Database Syst Rev. 2021;3(3):CD012799.
96. Wu PC, et al. Tolerability and optimal therapeutic dosage of clomipramine for premature ejaculation: a systematic review and meta-analysis. Sex Med. 2021;9(1):100283.
97. Waldinger MD, et al. Stronger evidence for small fiber sensory neuropathy in restless genital syndrome: two case reports in males. J Sex Med. 2011;8(1):325–30.
98. Stone M, et al. Risk of suicidality in clinical trials of antidepressants in adults: analysis of proprietary data submitted to US Food and Drug Administration. BMJ. 2009;339:b2880.

99. Asimakopoulos AD, et al. Does current scientific and clinical evidence support the use of phosphodiesterase type 5 inhibitors for the treatment of premature ejaculation? A systematic review and meta-analysis. J Sex Med. 2012;9(9):2404–16.

100. Pfaus JG. Neurobiology of sexual behavior. Curr Opin Neurobiol. 1999;9(6):751–8.

101. Chen J, et al. The role of phosphodiesterase type 5 inhibitors in the management of premature ejaculation: a critical analysis of basic science and clinical data. Eur Urol. 2007;52(5):1331–9.

102. Krishnappa P, et al. Sildenafil/Viagra in the treatment of premature ejaculation. Int J Impot Res. 2019;31(2):65–70.

103. Zhang X, et al. Phosphodiesterase-5 inhibitors for premature ejaculation: systematic review and meta-analysis of placebo-controlled trials. Am J Mens Health. 2020;14(3):1557988320916406.

104. Polat EC, et al. Combination therapy with selective serotonin reuptake inhibitors and phosphodiesterase-5 inhibitors in the treatment of premature ejaculation. Andrologia. 2015;47(5):487–92.

105. Lee WK, et al. Comparison between on-demand dosing of dapoxetine alone and dapoxetine plus mirodenafil in patients with lifelong premature ejaculation: prospective, randomized, double-blind, placebo-controlled, multicenter study. J Sex Med. 2013;10(11):2832–41.

106. Shindel AW, et al. Disorders of ejaculation: an AUA/SMSNA guideline. J Urol. 2022;207(3):504–12.

107. Aversa A, et al. Effects of vardenafil administration on intravaginal ejaculatory latency time in men with lifelong premature ejaculation. Int J Impot Res. 2009;21(4):221–7.

108. McMahon CG, et al. Efficacy of sildenafil citrate (Viagra) in men with premature ejaculation. J Sex Med. 2005;2(3):368–75.

109. Raffa RB, et al. Opioid and nonopioid components independently contribute to the mechanism of action of tramadol, an 'atypical' opioid analgesic. J Pharmacol Exp Ther. 1992;260(1):275–85.

110. Lee CR, McTavish D, Sorkin EM. Tramadol. A preliminary review of its pharmacodynamic and pharmacokinetic properties, and therapeutic potential in acute and chronic pain states. Drugs. 1993;46(2):313–40.

111. Safarinejad MR, Hosseini SY. Safety and efficacy of tramadol in the treatment of premature ejaculation: a double-blind, placebo-controlled, fixed-dose, randomized study. J Clin Psychopharmacol. 2006;26(1):27–31.

112. Bar-Or D, et al. A randomized double-blind, placebo-controlled multicenter study to evaluate the efficacy and safety of two doses of the tramadol orally disintegrating tablet for the treatment of premature ejaculation within less than 2 minutes. Eur Urol. 2012;61(4):736–43.

113. Martyn-St James M, et al. Tramadol for premature ejaculation: a systematic review and meta-analysis. BMC Urol. 2015;15:6.

114. Sharma AP, et al. Safety and efficacy of "on-demand" tramadol in patients with premature ejaculation: an updated meta-analysis. Int Braz J Urol. 2021;47(5):921–34.

115. Mittino D, Mula M, Monaco F. Serotonin syndrome associated with tramadol-sertraline coadministration. Clin Neuropharmacol. 2004;27(3):150–1.

116. Takeshita J, Litzinger MH. Serotonin syndrome associated with tramadol. Prim Care Companion J Clin Psychiatry. 2009;11(5):273.

117. Jeon HJ, et al. Candidate molecule for premature ejaculation, DA-8031: in vivo and in vitro characterization of DA-8031. Urology. 2011;77(4):1006.e17–21.

118. Kang KK, et al. Ejaculatory responses are inhibited by a new chemical entity, DA-8031, in preclinical rodent models of ejaculation. Urology. 2013;81(4):920.e13–920.e8.

119. Kang KK, et al. Effect of DA-8031, a novel oral compound for premature ejaculation, on male rat sexual behavior. Int J Urol. 2014;21(3):325–9.

120. Clinical trial to evaluate the efficacy and safety of DA-8031 in male patients with premature ejaculation. 2013. https://clinicaltrials.gov/ct2/show/NCT01798667

121. Shin D, et al. Pharmacokinetics and tolerability of DA-8031, a novel selective serotonin reuptake inhibitor for premature ejaculation in healthy male subjects. Drug Des Devel Ther. 2017;11:713–23.

122. Kim SW, et al. Tolerability and adequate therapeutic dosage of oral clomipramine for the treatment of premature ejaculation: a randomized, double-blind, placebo-controlled, fixed-dose, parallel-grouped clinical study. Int J Impot Res. 2018;30(2):65–70.
123. Choi JB, et al. Efficacy and safety of on demand clomipramine for the treatment of premature ejaculation: a multicenter, randomized, double-blind, phase III clinical trial. J Urol. 2019;201(1):147–52.
124. FITH Study with GSK958108. 2008. https://ClinicalTrials.gov/show/NCT00664365
125. Proof of mechanism in ELT. 2009. https://ClinicalTrials.gov/show/NCT00861484
126. Migliorini F, et al. A double-blind, placebo-controlled parallel group study to evaluate the effect of a single oral dose of 5-HT1A Antagonist GSK958108 on ejaculation latency time in male patients suffering from premature ejaculation. J Sex Med. 2021;18(1):63–71.
127. Lyons TJ, French J. Modafinil: the unique properties of a new stimulant. Aviat Space Environ Med. 1991;62(5):432–5.
128. Marson L, Yu G, Farber NM. The effects of oral administration of d-modafinil on male rat ejaculatory behavior. J Sex Med. 2010;7(1 Pt 1):70–8.
129. Serefoglu EC. On-demand d-modafinil may be an effective treatment option for lifelong premature ejaculation: a case report. Andrologia. 2016;48(1):121–2.
130. Tuken M, Kiremit MC, Serefoglu EC. On-demand modafinil improves ejaculation time and patient-reported outcomes in men with lifelong premature ejaculation. Urology. 2016;94:139–42.
131. Kawabe K, Yoshida M, Homma Y. Silodosin, a new alpha1A-adrenoceptor-selective antagonist for treating benign prostatic hyperplasia: results of a phase III randomized, placebo-controlled, double-blind study in Japanese men. BJU Int. 2006;98(5):1019–24.
132. Akin Y, et al. Comparison of alpha blockers in treatment of premature ejaculation: a pilot clinical trial. Iran Red Crescent Med J. 2013;15(10):e13805.
133. Bhat GS, Shastry A. Effectiveness of 'on demand' silodosin in the treatment of premature ejaculation in patients dissatisfied with dapoxetine: a randomized control study. Cent European J Urol. 2016;69(3):280–4.
134. Sato Y, et al. Silodosin versus naftopidil in the treatment of premature ejaculation: a prospective multicenter trial. Int J Urol. 2017;24(8):626–31.
135. de Jong TR, et al. Oxytocin involvement in SSRI-induced delayed ejaculation: a review of animal studies. J Sex Med. 2007;4(1):14–28.
136. Stoneham MD, et al. Oxytocin and sexual behaviour in the male rat and rabbit. J Endocrinol. 1985;107(1):97–106.
137. Clément P, et al. Inhibition of ejaculation by the non-peptide oxytocin receptor antagonist GSK557296: a multi-level site of action. Br J Pharmacol. 2013;169(7):1477–85.
138. Shinghal R, et al. Safety and efficacy of epelsiban in the treatment of men with premature ejaculation: a randomized, double-blind, placebo-controlled, fixed-dose study. J Sex Med. 2013;10(10):2506–17.
139. Wayman C, et al. Cligosiban, a novel brain-penetrant, selective oxytocin receptor antagonist, inhibits ejaculatory physiology in rodents. J Sex Med. 2018;15(12):1698–706.
140. McMahon C, et al. The oxytocin antagonist cligosiban prolongs intravaginal ejaculatory latency and improves patient-reported outcomes in men with lifelong premature ejaculation: results of a randomized, double-blind, placebo-controlled proof-of-concept trial (PEPIX). J Sex Med. 2019;16(8):1178–87.
141. Althof S, et al. The oxytocin antagonist cligosiban fails to prolong intravaginal ejaculatory latency in men with lifelong premature ejaculation: results of a randomized, double-blind, placebo-controlled phase IIb trial (PEDRIX). J Sex Med. 2019;16(8):1188–98.
142. Zhang GX, et al. Selective resection of dorsal nerves of penis for premature ejaculation. Int J Androl. 2012;35(6):873–9.
143. David Prologo J, et al. Percutaneous CT-guided cryoablation of the dorsal penile nerve for treatment of symptomatic premature ejaculation. J Vasc Interv Radiol. 2013;24(2):214–9.
144. Liu Q, et al. Anatomic basis and clinical effect of selective dorsal neurectomy for patients with lifelong premature ejaculation: a randomized controlled trial. J Sex Med. 2019;16(4):522–30.

145. Kim JJ, et al. Effects of glans penis augmentation using hyaluronic acid gel for premature ejaculation. Int J Impot Res. 2004;16(6):547–51.
146. Kwak TI, et al. Long-term effects of glans penis augmentation using injectable hyaluronic acid gel for premature ejaculation. Int J Impot Res. 2008;20(4):425–8.
147. Alahwany A, et al. Hyaluronic acid injection in glans penis for treatment of premature ejaculation: a randomized controlled cross-over study. Int J Impot Res. 2019;31(5):348–55.
148. Jankovic J. Botulinum toxin in clinical practice. J Neuro Neurosurg Psychiatry. 2004;75:951–7.
149. Jost WH, Naumann M. Botulinum toxin in neuro-urological disorders. Mov Disord. 2004;19(Suppl 8):S142–5.
150. Serefoglu EC, et al. Effect of botulinum-A toxin injection into bulbospongiosus muscle on ejaculation latency in male rats. J Sex Med. 2014;11(7):1657–63.
151. Li ZT, et al. Injection of botulinum-A toxin into bulbospongiosus muscle for primary premature ejaculation: a preliminary clinical study. Zhonghua Nan Ke Xue. 2018;24(8):713–8.
152. Pischedda A, et al. Pelvic floor and sexual male dysfunction. Arch Ital Urol Androl. 2013;85(1):1–7.
153. Pastore AL, et al. Pelvic floor muscle rehabilitation for patients with lifelong premature ejaculation: a novel therapeutic approach. Ther Adv Urol. 2014;6(3):83–8.
154. Pastore AL, et al. A prospective randomized study to compare pelvic floor rehabilitation and dapoxetine for treatment of lifelong premature ejaculation. Int J Androl. 2012;35(4):528–33.
155. Gruenwald I, et al. Transcutaneous neuromuscular electrical stimulation may be beneficial in the treatment of premature ejaculation. Med Hypotheses. 2017;109:181–3.
156. Shechter A, et al. Transcutaneous functional electrical stimulation-a novel therapy for premature ejaculation: results of a proof of concept study. Int J Impot Res. 2020;32(4):440–5.
157. Uribe OL, et al. Transcutaneous electric nerve stimulation to treat patients with premature ejaculation: phase II clinical trial. Int J Impot Res. 2020;32(4):434–9.
158. Aydos MM, Nas I, Önen E. The impact of transcutaneous posterior tibial nerve stimulation in patients with premature ejaculation. Eur Res J. 2020;6(5):457–63.
159. Zavatti M, et al. Experimental study on Satureja montana as a treatment for premature ejaculation. J Ethnopharmacol. 2011;133(2):629–33.
160. Cai T, et al. Rhodiola rosea, folic acid, zinc and biotin (EndEP®) is able to improve ejaculatory control in patients affected by lifelong premature ejaculation: results from a phase I-II study. Exp Ther Med. 2016;12(4):2083–7.
161. Sansalone S, et al. A combination of tryptophan, satureja montana, tribulus terrestris, phyllanthus emblica extracts is able to improve sexual quality of life in patient with premature ejaculation. Arch Ital Urol Androl. 2016;88(3):171–6.
162. Chen Z, et al. Significance of piezo-type mechanosensitive ion channel component 2 in premature ejaculation: an animal study. Andrology. 2020;8(5):1347–59.
163. Huang Y, et al. Expression of brain-derived neurotrophic factor in rapid ejaculator rats: a further study. Andrologia. 2021;53(8):e14134.
164. Kinsey AC, Pomeroy WR, Martin CE. Sexual behavior in the human male. 1948. Am J Public Health. 2003;93(6):894–8.
165. Perelman MA, Rowland DL. Retarded ejaculation. World J Urol. 2006;24(6):645–52.
166. Rowland DL, Keeney C, Slob AK. Sexual response in men with inhibited or retarded ejaculation. Int J Impot Res. 2004;16(3):270–4.
167. Lindau ST, et al. A study of sexuality and health among older adults in the United States. N Engl J Med. 2007;357(8):762–74.
168. Shin DH, Spitz A. The evaluation and treatment of delayed ejaculation. Sex Med Rev. 2014;2(3–4):121–33.
169. Abdel-Hamid IA, Ali OI. Delayed ejaculation: pathophysiology, diagnosis, and treatment. World J Mens Health. 2018;36(1):22–40.
170. Althof SE. Psychological interventions for delayed ejaculation/orgasm. Int J Impot Res. 2012;24(4):131–6.
171. Bancroft J. Human sexuality and its problem. Edinburgh: Churchill Living-stone; 2008.

172. Perelman MA. 1254: idiosyncratic masturbation patterns: a key unexplored variable in the treatment of retarded ejaculation by the practicing urologist. J Urol. 2005;173(4, Suppl):340.
173. Apfelbaum B. Retarded ejaculation: a much-misunderstood syndrome. In: Leiblum SR, Rosen RC, editors. Principles and practice of sex therapy: update for the 1990s. New York: Guilford; 1989. p. 168–206.
174. Brotto L, et al. Psychological and interpersonal dimensions of sexual function and dysfunction. J Sex Med. 2016;13(4):538–71.
175. Holt B, Pryor JP, Hendry WF. Male infertility after surgery for imperforate anus. J Pediatr Surg. 1995;30(12):1677–9.
176. Marra G, et al. Systematic review of lower urinary tract symptoms/benign prostatic hyperplasia surgical treatments on men's ejaculatory function: time for a bespoke approach? Int J Urol. 2016;23(1):22–35.
177. Minderhoud JM, et al. Sexual disturbances arising from multiple sclerosis. Acta Neurol Scand. 1984;70(4):299–306.
178. Dunsmuir WD, Holmes SA. The aetiology and management of erectile, ejaculatory, and fertility problems in men with diabetes mellitus. Diabet Med. 1996;13(8):700–8.
179. Hess MJ, Hough S. Impact of spinal cord injury on sexuality: broad-based clinical practice intervention and practical application. J Spinal Cord Med. 2012;35(4):211–8.
180. Kul'chavenia EV, et al. Ejaculatory disorders in some regions of the Russian Federation. Urologiia. 2010;3:49–52.
181. Montejo AL, et al. Incidence of sexual dysfunction associated with antidepressant agents: a prospective multicenter study of 1022 outpatients. Spanish Working Group for the Study of Psychotropic-Related Sexual Dysfunction. J Clin Psychiatry. 2001;62(Suppl 3):10–21.
182. IsHak WW. Textbook of clinical sexual medicine. Cham: Springer International Publishing AG; 2017.
183. Keller Ashton A, Hamer R, Rosen RC. Serotonin reuptake inhibitor-induced sexual dysfunction and its treatment: a large-scale retrospective study of 596 psychiatric outpatients. J Sex Marital Ther. 1997;23(3):165–75.
184. McCormick S, Olin J, Brotman AW. Reversal of fluoxetine-induced anorgasmia by cyproheptadine in two patients. J Clin Psychiatry. 1990;51(9):383–4.
185. Balon R. Intermittent amantadine for fluoxetine-induced anorgasmia. J Sex Marital Ther. 1996;22(4):290–2.
186. McMahon CG, et al. Standard operating procedures in the disorders of orgasm and ejaculation. J Sex Med. 2013;10(1):204–29.
187. Krüger TH, et al. Effects of acute prolactin manipulation on sexual drive and function in males. J Endocrinol. 2003;179(3):357–65.
188. Wittstock M, Benecke R, Dressler D. Cabergoline can increase penile erections and libido. Neurology. 2002;58(5):831.
189. Burri A, et al. The acute effects of intranasal oxytocin administration on endocrine and sexual function in males. Psychoneuroendocrinology. 2008;33(5):591–600.
190. IsHak WW, Berman DS, Peters A. Male anorgasmia treated with oxytocin. J Sex Med. 2008;5(4):1022–4.
191. Ashton AK, Rosen RC. Bupropion as an antidote for serotonin reuptake inhibitor-induced sexual dysfunction. J Clin Psychiatry. 1998;59(3):112–5.
192. Labbate LA, et al. Bupropion treatment of serotonin reuptake antidepressant-associated sexual dysfunction. Ann Clin Psychiatry. 1997;9(4):241–5.
193. Landén M, et al. Effect of buspirone on sexual dysfunction in depressed patients treated with selective serotonin reuptake inhibitors. J Clin Psychopharmacol. 1999;19(3):268–71.
194. Adeniyi AA, et al. Yohimbine in the treatment of orgasmic dysfunction. Asian J Androl. 2007;9(3):403–7.
195. Segraves RT. Reversal by bethanechol of imipramine-induced ejaculatory dysfunction. Am J Psychiatry. 1987;144(9):1243–4.
196. Bronner G, Vodušek DB. Management of sexual dysfunction in Parkinson's disease. Ther Adv Neurol Disord. 2011;4(6):375–83.

197. Nelson CJ, et al. Assessment of penile vibratory stimulation as a management strategy in men with secondary retarded orgasm. Urology. 2007;69(3):552–5; discussion 555–6
198. Jenkins LC, Mulhall JP. Delayed orgasm and anorgasmia. Fertil Steril. 2015;104(5):1082–8.
199. Geboes K, Steeno O, De Moor P. Primary anejaculation: diagnosis and therapy. Fertil Steril. 1975;26(10):1018–20.
200. Kamischke A, Nieschlag E. Update on medical treatment of ejaculatory disorders. Int J Androl. 2002;25(6):333–44.
201. van Basten JP, et al. Sexual functioning after multimodality treatment for disseminated non-seminomatous testicular germ cell tumor. J Urol. 1997;158(4):1411–6.
202. Jonker-Pool G, et al. Sexual functioning after treatment for testicular cancer: comparison of treatment modalities. Cancer. 1997;80(3):454–64.
203. Safarinejad MR. Midodrine for the treatment of organic anejaculation but not spinal cord injury: a prospective randomized placebo-controlled double-blind clinical study. Int J Impot Res. 2009;21(4):213–20.
204. Brindley GS. Reflex ejaculation under vibratory stimulation in paraplegic men. Paraplegia. 1981;19(5):299–302.
205. Ohl DA, Menge AC, Sønksen J. Penile vibratory stimulation in spinal cord injured men: optimized vibration parameters and prognostic factors. Arch Phys Med Rehabil. 1996;77(9):903–5.
206. Courtois F, et al. Sexual function and autonomic dysreflexia in men with spinal cord injuries: how should we treat? Spinal Cord. 2012;50(12):869–77.
207. Schatte EC, et al. Treatment of infertility due to anejaculation in the male with electroejaculation and intracytoplasmic sperm injection. J Urol. 2000;163(6):1717–20.
208. Ohl DA, et al. Electroejaculation and assisted reproductive technologies in the treatment of anejaculatory infertility. Fertil Steril. 2001;76(6):1249–55.
209. Ilie CP, Mischianu DL, Pemberton RJ. Painful ejaculation. BJU Int. 2007;99(6):1335–9.
210. Rosen R, et al. Lower urinary tract symptoms and male sexual dysfunction: the multinational survey of the aging male (MSAM-7). Eur Urol. 2003;44(6):637–49.
211. Matsushita K, Tal R, Mulhall JP. The evolution of orgasmic pain (dysorgasmia) following radical prostatectomy. J Sex Med. 2012;9(5):1454–8.
212. Wagenlehner FM, et al. National Institutes of Health Chronic Prostatitis Symptom Index (NIH-CPSI) symptom evaluation in multinational cohorts of patients with chronic prostatitis/chronic pelvic pain syndrome. Eur Urol. 2013;63(5):953–9.
213. Litwin MS, et al. The National Institutes of Health chronic prostatitis symptom index: development and validation of a new outcome measure. Chronic Prostatitis Collaborative Research Network. J Urol. 1999;162(2):369–75.
214. Barnas J, et al. The utility of tamsulosin in the management of orgasm-associated pain: a pilot analysis. Eur Urol. 2005;47(3):361–5; discussion 365
215. Lira FTN, et al. Management of ejaculatory duct obstruction by seminal vesiculoscopy: case report and literature review. JBRA Assist Reprod. 2020;24(3):382–6.
216. Zaidi S, et al. Etiology, diagnosis, and management of seminal vesicle stones. Curr Urol. 2019;12(3):113–20.
217. Sundar R, Sundar G. Zinner syndrome: an uncommon cause of painful ejaculation. BMJ Case Rep. 2015;2015:bcr2014207618.
218. Shoskes DA, et al. Impact of post-ejaculatory pain in men with category III chronic prostatitis/chronic pelvic pain syndrome. J Urol. 2004;172(2):542–7.
219. Calisir A, et al. Pain during sexual activity and ejaculation following hernia repair: a retrospective comparison of transabdominal preperitoneal versus Lichtenstein repair. Andrologia. 2021;53(2):e13947.
220. Senthilkumaran S, et al. Painful ejaculation. Something fishy. Saudi Med J. 2010;31(4):451–2.
221. Kraus MB, et al. Painful ejaculation with cyclobenzaprine: a case report and literature review. Sex Med. 2015;3(4):343–5.
222. Cornel EB, et al. The effect of biofeedback physical therapy in men with Chronic Pelvic Pain Syndrome Type III. Eur Urol. 2005;47(5):607–11.

223. Jordi P, et al. Management of ejaculation pain with topiramate: a case report. Clin J Pain. 2004;20(5):368–9.
224. Butler JD, Hershman MJ, Leach A. Painful ejaculation after inguinal hernia repair. J R Soc Med. 1998;91(8):432–3.
225. Edwards L, Powell C. An objective comparison of transurethral resection and bladder neck incision in the treatment of prostatic hypertrophy. J Urol. 1982;128(2):325–7.
226. Rassweiler J, et al. Complications of transurethral resection of the prostate (TURP)—incidence, management, and prevention. Eur Urol. 2006;50(5):969–79; discussion 980
227. Yavetz H, et al. Retrograde ejaculation. Hum Reprod. 1994;9(3):381–6.
228. Fedder J, et al. Retrograde ejaculation and sexual dysfunction in men with diabetes mellitus: a prospective, controlled study. Andrology. 2013;1(4):602–6.
229. Publishing HH. Retrograde ejaculation. 2022. https://www.drugs.com/health-guide/retrograde-ejaculation.html
230. Cooper TG, et al. World Health Organization reference values for human semen characteristics. Hum Reprod Update. 2010;16(3):231–45.
231. McMahon C. Disoerders of male orgasm and ejaculation. In: Wein AJ, Kavoussi LR, Partin AW, et al., editors. Campbell-Walsh urology. Philadelphia: Elsevier; 2016. p. 692–708.
232. Kedia K, Markland C. The effect of pharmacological agents on ejaculation. J Urol. 1975;114(4):569–73.
233. Proctor KG, Howards SS. The effect of sympathomimetic drugs on post-lymphadenectomy aspermia. J Urol. 1983;129(4):837–8.
234. Jefferys A, Siassakos D, Wardle P. The management of retrograde ejaculation: a systematic review and update. Fertil Steril. 2012;97(2):306–12.
235. Kamischke A, Nieschlag E. Treatment of retrograde ejaculation and anejaculation. Hum Reprod Update. 1999;5(5):448–74.
236. Mehta A, Sigman M. Management of the dry ejaculate: a systematic review of aspermia and retrograde ejaculation. Fertil Steril. 2015;104(5):1074–81.
237. Colpi G, et al. EAU guidelines on ejaculatory dysfunction. Eur Urol. 2004;46(5):555–8.
238. Arafa M, El Tabie O. Medical treatment of retrograde ejaculation in diabetic patients: a hope for spontaneous pregnancy. J Sex Med. 2008;5(1):194–8.
239. Ochsenkühn R, Kamischke A, Nieschlag E. Imipramine for successful treatment of retrograde ejaculation caused by retroperitoneal surgery. Int J Androl. 1999;22(3):173–7.
240. Koga M, Hirai T, Kiuti H, et al. Experience of two cases where tricyclic antidepressant amoxapine seemed to be useful for dry ejaculation. Jpn J Sex Med. 2003;18:170.
241. Abrahams JI, et al. The surgical correction of retrograde ejaculation. J Urol. 1975;114(6):888–90.
242. Middleton RG, Urry RL. The Young-Dees operation for the correction of retrograde ejaculation. J Urol. 1986;136(6):1208–9.
243. Reynolds JC, et al. Bladder neck collagen injection restores antegrade ejaculation after bladder neck surgery. J Urol. 1998;159(4):1303.
244. Hotchkiss RS, Pinto AB, Kleegman S. Artificial insemination with semen recovered from the bladder. Fertil Steril. 1954;6(1):37–42.
245. Crich JP, Jequier AM. Infertility in men with retrograde ejaculation: the action of urine on sperm motility, and a simple method for achieving antegrade ejaculation. Fertil Steril. 1978;30(5):572–6.
246. Templeton A, Mortimer D. Successful circumvention of retrograde ejaculation in an infertile diabetic man. Case report. Br J Obstet Gynaecol. 1982;89(12):1064–5.
247. Ng YH, Seeley JP, Smith G. Haematospermia as a presenting symptom: outcomes of investigation in 300 men. Surgeon. 2013;11(1):35–8.
248. Mulhall JP, Albertsen PC. Hemospermia: diagnosis and management. Urology. 1995;46(4):463–7.
249. Ahmad I, Krishna NS. Hemospermia. J Urol. 2007;177(5):1613–8.
250. Han M, et al. Association of hemospermia with prostate cancer. J Urol. 2004;172(6 Pt 1):2189–92.

251. Akhter W, Khan F, Chinegwundoh F. Should every patient with hematospermia be investigated? A critical review. Cent European J Urol. 2013;66(1):79–82.
252. Smith GW, Griffith DP, Pranke DW. Melanospermia: an unusual presentation of malignant melanoma. J Urol. 1973;110(3):314–6.
253. Pal DK. Haemospermia: an Indian experience. Trop Dr. 2006;36(1):61–2.
254. Close CF, Yeo WW, Ramsay LE. The association between haemospermia and severe hypertension. Postgrad Med J. 1991;67(784):157–8.
255. Lemesh RA. Case report: recurrent hematuria and hematospermia due to prostatic telangiectasia in classic von Willebrand's disease. Am J Med Sci. 1993;306(1):35–6.
256. Marshall VF, Fuller NL. Hemospermia. J Urol. 1983;129(2):377–8.
257. Papp G, Molnar J. Causes and differentialdiagnosis of hematospermia. Andrologia. 1981;13(5):474–8.
258. Bamberger E, et al. Detection of sexually transmitted pathogens in patients with hematospermia. Isr Med Assoc J. 2005;7(4):224–7.
259. Raviv G, Laufer M, Miki H. Hematospermia—the added value of transrectal ultrasound to clinical evaluation: is transrectal ultrasound necessary for evaluation of hematospermia? Clin Imaging. 2013;37(5):913–6.
260. Furuya S, et al. Magnetic resonance imaging is accurate to detect bleeding in the seminal vesicles in patients with hemospermia. Urology. 2008;72(4):838–42.
261. Xing C, et al. Prospective trial comparing transrectal ultrasonography and transurethral seminal vesiculoscopy for persistent hematospermia. Int J Urol. 2012;19(5):437–42.
262. Pozzi E, et al. Haemospermia in the real-life setting: a new high-risk stratification. Sci Rep. 2022; https://doi.org/10.21203/rs.3.rs-1028335/v1.
263. Mittal PK, et al. Hematospermia evaluation at MR imaging. Radiographics. 2016;36(5):1373–89.
264. Suh Y, et al. Etiologic classification, evaluation, and management of hematospermia. Transl Androl Urol. 2017;6(5):959–72.
265. Kumar P, Kapoor S, Nargund V. Haematospermia—a systematic review. Ann R Coll Surg Engl. 2006;88(4):339–42.
266. Hosseinzadeh K, et al. ACR Appropriateness Criteria® Hematospermia. J Am Coll Radiol. 2017;14(5s):S154–s159.
267. Fuse H, et al. Transurethral incision for hematospermia caused by ejaculatory duct obstruction. Arch Androl. 2003;49(6):433–8.
268. Kang DI, Chung JI. Current status of 5α-reductase inhibitors in prostate disease management. Korean J Urol. 2013;54(4):213–9.
269. Mulhall J. Premature ejaculation. In: Wein AJ, editor. Campell-Walsh urology. 10th ed. Philadelphia: Elsevier Saunders; 2011. p. 770–9.
270. Waldinger MD, Olivier B. Animal models of premature and retarded ejaculation. World J Urol. 2005;23(2):115–8.
271. Hellstrom WJ. Current and future pharmacotherapies of premature ejaculation. J Sex Med. 2006;3(Suppl 4):332–41.
272. Young B, Coolen L, McKenna K. Neural regulation of ejaculation. J Sex Med. 2009;6(Suppl 3):229–33.
273. Holstege G, et al. Brain activation during human male ejaculation. J Neurosci. 2003;23(27):9185–93.
274. Perelman MA. Patient highlights. Delayed ejaculation. J Sex Med. 2013;10(4):1189–90.
275. Chen J. The pathophysiology of delayed ejaculation. Transl Androl Urol. 2016;5(4):549–62.
276. Nathan SG. The epidemiology of the DSM-III psychosexual dysfunctions. J Sex Marital Ther. 1986;12(4):267–81.
277. Waldinger MD, Schweitzer DH. Retarded ejaculation in men: an overview of psychological and neurobiological insights. World J Urol. 2005;23(2):76–81.
278. Calabrò RS, et al. Anorgasmia during pregabalin add-on therapy for partial seizures. Epileptic Disord. 2013;15(3):358–61.

279. Jannini EA, Simonelli C, Lenzi A. Disorders of ejaculation. J Endocrinol Investig. 2002;25(11):1006–19.
280. Johnson RD, Murray FT. Reduced sensitivity of penile mechanoreceptors in aging rats with sexual dysfunction. Brain Res Bull. 1992;28(1):61–4.
281. Di Sante S, et al. Epidemiology of delayed ejaculation. Transl Androl Urol. 2016;5(4):541–8.
282. Abdel-Hamid IA, Saleh E-S. Primary lifelong delayed ejaculation: characteristics and response to bupropion. J Sex Med. 2011;8(6):1772–9.
283. Balogh S, Hendricks SE, Kang J. Treatment of fluoxetine-induced anorgasmia with amantadine. J Clin Psychiatry. 1992;53(6):212–3.
284. Corona G, et al. Testosterone supplementation and sexual function: a meta-analysis study. J Sex Med. 2014;11(6):1577–92.
285. Waldinger MD, Schweitzer DH. Postorgasmic illness syndrome: two cases. J Sex Marital Ther. 2002;28(3):251–5.
286. Waldinger MD, et al. Postorgasmic illness syndrome (POIS) in 45 Dutch caucasian males: clinical characteristics and evidence for an immunogenic pathogenesis (part 1). J Sex Med. 2011;8(4):1164–70.
287. Waldinger MD, Meinardi MM, Schweitzer DH. Hyposensitization therapy with autologous semen in two Dutch caucasian males: beneficial effects in postorgasmic illness syndrome (POIS; part 2). J Sex Med. 2011;8(4):1171–6.
288. Reinert AE, Simon JA. "Did you climax or are you just laughing at me?" Rare phenomena associated with orgasm. Sex Med Rev. 2017;5(3):275–81.

Andrologic Emergencies

5

Esaù Fernández-Pascual, Celeste Manfredi,
Davide Arcaniolo, and Juan Ignacio Martínez-Salamanca

Abstract

Andrological emergencies are conditions that require rapid medical or surgical intervention. Although some may be more frequent, such as testicular torsion, which requires emergent intervention to preserve gonad function, most of them have a much lower incidence. Some urgent pathologies are managed with conservative medical treatment, such as penile contusions or Mondor's disease, while others require minor surgical interventions that usually resolve the problem, such as ischemic priapism or paraphimosis, though occasionally major surgery may be required. Penile fracture is a closed trauma that requires surgical intervention to avoid subsequent sequelae. On the other hand, all penetrating injuries require urgent surgery, and some cases even require complex interventions such as partial or total amputation of the penis. Fournier's gangrene is a necrotic infection of the genitalia of maximum severity, which requires intensive management with early surgery if survival of the patient is to be achieved. The aim of this chapter is to provide a basic guide to the diagnosis and treatment of the most common andrological emergencies.

E. Fernández-Pascual
Department of Urology, Hospital Universitario La Paz, Madrid, Spain

LYX Institute of Urology, Universidad Francisco de Vitoria, Madrid, Spain

C. Manfredi · D. Arcaniolo
Department of Woman, Child and General and Specialized Surgery, Urology Unit, University of Campania "Luigi Vanvitelli", Naples, Italy

J. I. Martínez-Salamanca (✉)
LYX Institute of Urology, Universidad Francisco de Vitoria, Madrid, Spain

Department of Urology, Hospital Universitario Puerta del Hierro Majadahonda, Madrid, Spain

S. Sarikaya et al. (eds.), *Andrology and Sexual Medicine*, Management of Urology,
https://doi.org/10.1007/978-3-031-12049-7_5

Introduction

An emergency is defined as a sudden serious and dangerous event or situation that needs immediate action to deal with it. Time is the essential element to consider in an emergency condition. Identifying and treating the patient "in time" can mark the line between good and bad functional outcomes, and consequently between a satisfied and dissatisfied patient [1].

Andrology, like any other specialty, is characterized by possible emergency conditions that require rapid medical or surgical intervention. The main andrological emergencies include testicular torsion, ischemic priapism, paraphimosis, Fournier's gangrene, penile Mondor's disease, and genital trauma of which the most typical expression is the penile fracture. Vascular compromise appears as a pivotal pathophysiological factor in most andrological emergencies; more specifically, an impairment of both the venous and arterial components may be at the basis of emergency andrological conditions [2]. Since the area affected by andrological diseases is the genital one by definition, sexual function is the main domain that can be affected if an emergency is not properly managed, with a consequent negative impact on the patient's sexual quality of life [3].

Ischemic Priapism

Definition and Epidemiology

Ischemic (low-flow or veno-occlusive) priapism is a persistent painful erection that lasts for more than four hours characterized by absent or reduced intracavernous arterial inflow. More specifically, it can be considered a compartment syndrome, marked by increased pressure within the corpora cavernosa closed space and consequent impairment of circulation [4]. Emergency management is required to minimize irreversible complications, such as smooth muscle necrosis, corporal fibrosis and the development of permanent erectile dysfunction (ED) [5]. However, emergency department visits for priapism are relatively uncommon with a national incidence of 5.34 per 100,000 male subjects per year esteemed in the USA, being the ischemic priapism the most frequent subtype affecting the population (95%). Priapism can occur in any age group, however, a bimodal distribution of incidence was described, with a peak between 5 and 10 years in children and between 20 to 50 years in adults [1, 6, 7].

Etiology

Ischemic priapism is frequently idiopathic [1]; however, several potential etiological factors were recognized. Sickle cell disease (SCD) is the most frequent etiology of ischemic priapism in childhood (63% of cases), being the primary cause in 23% of adults [8]. Second-generation antipsychotics accounted for the largest percentage of drug-induced ischemic priapism cases (33%) [9]. Risk of priapism is <1% after intracavernous injection of prostaglandin E1 (PGE1) [10]. Phosphodiesterase type 5 inhibitors (PDE5Is) was associated with some cases of ischemic priapism (2.9% of drug-induced forms); however, most patients had additional risk factors, therefore it is unclear whether PDE5Is are actually an independent risk factor [4, 11]. Infrequently, ischemic priapism can due to neoplastic processes, more often arising from bladder or prostate. Several neurogenic, infective/toxin-mediated, and metabolic disorders can also rarely cause ischemic priapism [4, 12].

Diagnosis

The main condition that should be considered in the differential diagnosis with ischemic priapism is non-ischemic (high-flow or arterial) priapism (<5% of all cases). It is generally caused by a blunt perineal or penile trauma, which leads to the formation of a fistula between the artery and the lacunar spaces of the sinusoidal tissue. Non-ischemic priapism is not an emergency because the corpora cavernosa do not contain ischemic blood [13].

Medical history with physical examination, penile blood gas analysis, and penile doppler ultrasound (PDU) are the cornerstones for a correct diagnosis [14]. The main risk factors (e.g., hematological disorders, penile or perineal trauma, drugs intake) and the duration of erection should be investigated whenever priapism is suspected. Collecting information on pre-event erectile function can also be useful for medico-legal purposes [4]. Patients with ischemic priapism had a fully rigid and painful erection (Fig. 5.1), on the contrary, a not fully rigid and painless erection characterize the non-ischemic priapism [8, 13]. During an event of ischemic priapism there are time-dependent metabolic alterations within the corpora cavernosa progressively leading to hypoxia, hypercapnia and acidosis. The penile blood gas analysis shows a dark red blood, $pO_2 < 30$ mmHg, $pCO_2 > 60$ mmHg, and $pH < 7.25$. In non-ischemic cases there is not ischemic blood in the corpora cavernosa, therefore a bright red blood with arterial gas values ($pO_2 > 90$ mmHg, $pCO_2 < 40$ mmHg, and pH 7.4) can be found [4, 15]. If ischemic priapism occurs, PDU classically reveals minimal blood flow in the cavernosal arteries and low peak systolic velocity (PSV). However, there is no specific cut-off for PSV and in some cases it can be even high. Increased resistance index (RI) of the cavernosal arteries, thrombosis of the corpora cavernosa, and flow in the superficial penile veins are other possible data that can be recorded. In subjects with non-ischemic priapism the fistula appears as a characteristic color blush and turbulent high-velocity flow, besides, normal to high blood velocities are recorded in the cavernosal arteries [4, 16]. A blood count with white blood cell differential and a coagulation profile should be performed to evaluate any hematological abnormalities. Penile magnetic resonance imaging (MRI) can be useful in selected patients with ischemic priapism (i.e., refractoriness to non-surgical treatment and onset from 24–48 h) to investigate the presence of penile fibrosis/necrosis, in order to decide if an immediate penile prosthesis implantation should be considered [14].

Fig. 5.1 Patient with ischemic priapism

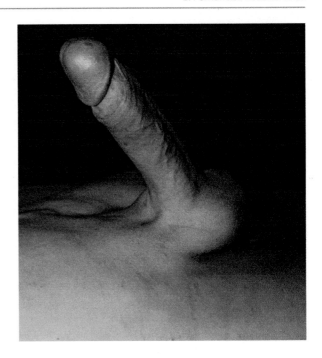

Treatment

The duration of ischemic priapism represents the most significant predictor for the development of ED. Indeed, interventions beyond 48–72 h of onset may help to relieve the erection and pain, but have little benefit in preventing long-term ED [17]. For this reason, management of ischemic priapism should start as early as possible (within 4–6 h from the onset) and follow a stepwise approach [14].

Auxiliary Strategies

Several first-line conservative treatments have been proposed including exercise, ejaculation, ice packs, cold baths, and cold-water enemas; however, the evidence for a benefit with these measures is very limited [4]. Anesthesia cannot relieve ischemic pain, but cutaneous anesthesia can reasonably facilitate subsequent treatments. Dorsal penile nerve block, circumferential penile block, and subcutaneous local penile shaft block are possible viable anesthesia techniques [14]. Cavernosal irrigation with 0.9% saline solution can be practiced with corporal blood aspiration and intracavernous injections, but data supporting better outcomes by combining irrigation are limited [18].

Corporal Blood Aspiration

Corporal blood aspiration is the first step in the management of ischemic priapism. It aims to drain the stagnant blood from the corpora cavernosa in order to relieve the compartment syndrome-like condition [14]. It can be performed with a 16–18 G angiocatheter or butterfly needle inserted into the glans or the lateral aspect of the proximal penile shaft. Aspiration should be continued until bright red (oxygenated) blood is aspirated and has up to a 30% chance of resolving the ischemic priapism [18].

Intracavernous Injection of Sympathomimetic Drugs

If priapism persists despite corporal blood aspiration, intracavernous injection of sympathomimetic drugs is indicated. However, this is the first step in the management of ischemic priapism secondary to intracavernous injections of vasoactive agents (e.g., PGE1) [14]. Phenylephrine is currently the drug of choice, due to its high selectivity for the α-1-adrenergic receptor. It is diluted in 0.9% saline solution to a concentration of 100–500 µg/mL. Usually, 200 µg are injected into the corpora cavernosa every 3–5 min until detumescence, maintaining a maximum dosage of 1 mg in 1 h [14, 19]. During the administration and for 60 min afterwards (every 15 min) blood pressure, pulse and cardiac rhythm should be monitored due to its potential cardiovascular adverse effects. Phenylephrine is contraindicated in patients with a history of cerebro-vascular disease and significant hypertension [4, 14, 19].

Penile Shunt Surgery

If priapism persists despite corporal blood aspiration and intracavernous injection of sympathomimetic drugs, these steps should be repeated several times (i.e., at least 1 h) before considering penile shunt surgery [14]. Penile shunt surgery aims to create a communication between the corpora cavernosa (incision through the tunica albuginea) and the glans, the corpus spongiosum or a vein, allowing ischemic blood drainage. Several penile shunt surgical techniques have been described over the years (e.g., Winter's procedure, Ebbehoj's technique, T-shunt, Al-Ghorab's procedure, Burnett's technique, Quackles's technique, Grayhack's procedure) [20]. Distal shunts are less invasive and associated with lower rate of ED, therefore, they are generally performed before considering proximal shunts. Tunneling can be combined with distal shunt if necessary [14]. Penile shunt surgery can be the cause of iatrogenic non-ischemic priapism, leading to a conversion of ischemic to non-ischemic priapism. Peri-procedural anticoagulation may decrease the priapism recurrence [21].

Penile Prosthesis Implantation

Immediate penile prosthesis implantation should be considered when ischemic priapism has lasted for more than 48 h (delayed presentation) or when all other interventions have failed (refractory case) [14]. Early implantation is associated with less difficulty and lower complications rate compared to late placement, because over time severe fibrosis of the corpora cavernosa develops. Besides, early implantation offers the opportunity to maintain penile size and prevent penile curvature due to corporal fibrosis. The optimal time for implantation is within the first 3 weeks from the onset [17, 22]. However, if a shunt has been performed the penile prosthesis insertion should be delayed (i.e., 2–4 weeks) to reduce the risk of infection and erosion [4, 14]. A malleable prosthesis might be reasonably preferable to minimize the complications, although limited evidence on the topic is available. If the patient wishes, it can be replaced later with an inflatable prosthesis that can allow the upsizing of the implant cylinders and more natural erections [14, 22].

Penile Mondor's Disease

Definition and Epidemiology

Mondor's disease is a thrombophlebitis of the superficial veins which can occur in various body regions. It manifests as a palpable cord-like induration on the body surface, localized under the skin. Henri Mondor was the first to describe the disease involving the chest in 1939. It was later discovered that it could also arise in other body regions such as abdominal wall, groin, axilla, and penis [23]. More specifically, penile Mondor's disease (PMD) is a thrombophlebitis of the superficial dorsal vein of the penis. However, some atypical cases with circumflex veins involvement have been described [24]. PMD is a rare condition, although its incidence is probably underestimated. Until 2014, only 53 cases of PMD were reported in the literature, affecting sexually active men of any age [25].

Etiology

Mondor's disease can be classified in primary (idiopathic) and secondary (due to an underlying disease). Secondary form can be caused by different conditions such as vasculitis, hypercoagulative states, and malignancies. Local triggers have also been associated with the onset of disease, including trauma and iatrogenic insults. The pathophysiology of PMD fits the Virchow's triad. In fact, vessel-wall damage (e.g., vigorous sexual activity, vacuum erection device, penile trauma, excessive masturbation), blood stasis (e.g., prolonged erection, prolonged sitting position, bladder overdistension), and hypercoagulation (e.g., urogenital infection, prostate biopsy, hematological diseases) seem to be the main risk factors that can lead to this condition [25, 26].

Diagnosis

An accurate history and physical examination are the essential steps for the diagnosis of PMD. The classic clinical manifestation is a palpable cord-like induration on the dorsal/dorsolateral aspect of the penis (Fig. 5.2). Some atypical cases with induration on the ventral aspect have been recorded [24]. Inflammatory skin changes such as erythema and edema can be associated. There is usually pain, typically exacerbated during erection. However, asymptomatic cases characterized only by cord-like induration have been described [25]. As previously reported, PMD can be preceded by an history of intense sexual activity or various types of penile trauma. Recurrent episodes have been described in literature [25, 26].

Fig. 5.2 Patient with penile Mondor's disease

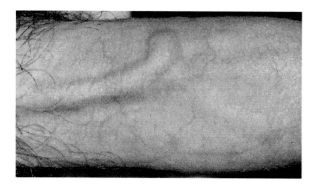

Patients should undergo laboratory tests to investigate any hypercoagulative states. In PMD, screening for main sexually transmitted diseases should also be considered. PDU is a useful imaging examination that reveals a non-compressible tubular structure and lack of flow signal. MRI can also be used as a diagnostic tool. A biopsy should be considered only when the lesion is highly suspected of malignancy or vasculitis, or when the lesion does not resolve within the expected time [26].

Important differential diagnoses are with Peyronie's disease (PD) sclerosing lymphangitis. PD is also associated with a hardened area of the penis and penile pain; however, its peculiar clinical (e.g., penile curvature) and instrumental (e.g., plaque of the albuginea on ultrasound) characteristics generally allow the distinction between the two diseases. Sclerosing lymphangitis is characterized by thickened and dilated lymphatic vessels that can be easily differentiated from PMD with PDU [27].

Treatment

PMD is typically a benign self-limiting (4–8 weeks) condition, however, sudden penile pain can lead to emergency department visit. There is no standard treatment or guideline recommendations. A limitation of sexual activity appears reasonable. Non-steroidal anti-inflammatory drugs (NSAIDs) can be prescribed to relieve pain. Anticoagulants are an option contemplated by the literature. In rare cases refractory to medical treatments (i.e., persistence of the symptomatology and absence of permeabilization of the vein after 6 weeks), thrombectomy or resection of the dorsal vein can be considered [25, 26].

Paraphimosis

Definition and Epidemiology

Paraphimosis or painful swelling of the distal foreskin is a common urologic emergency in which the foreskin, once retracted over the glans penis, cannot return to its normal position. There is a strangulation of the glans by a constricting band which is progressively worsened by oedema. Paraphimosis is considered an emergency. It is important to differentiate from the concept of phimosis which is a condition in which the contracted foreskin cannot be retracted behind the glans of the penis [28].

Etiology

Paraphimosis commonly occurs iatrogenically in uncircumcised males, whether due to genital manipulation or exploration, attempted grooming, balanitis, or placement of a urinary catheter. In very young boys paraphimosis is often seen after the foreskin has been traumatically reduced during an examination or sometimes due to excessive parental zeal for hygiene [29].

The constricting ring of skin, retracted behind the glans of the penis, causes venous and lymphatic congestion leading to oedema and enlargement of the glans, which makes the condition worse. As this condition progresses, arterial occlusion and necrosis of the glans can occur after some hours or days. Therefore, paraphimosis must be urgently reduced [30].

Diagnosis

The patient usually complains of swelling and pain of the glans penis. There is an enlargement and congestion of the glans and preputial mucosa, and a tight constrictive ring or band that prevents easy manual retraction of the foreskin over the glans without difficulty. Diagnosis is clinical by direct visualisation, as well as by the inability to easily reduce the retracted foreskin manually.

Treatment

A large proportion of paraphimoses are mild and uncomplicated and can be reduced without the need for local anaesthesia, sedation or oedema-reducing manoeuvres.

Although removal of Foley catheter may aid in the reduction of paraphimosis, most of the time, it is not necessary to successfully resolve the problem.

Non-surgical Reduction of Paraphimosis

Non-surgical reduction is possible with or without compression methods, using osmotic agents or puncture-aspiration techniques.

1. Methods for reduction of penile oedema

    Often, a simple manual compression of the glans during several minutes sufficiently reduces the oedema to be able to reverse the foreskin.

Alternatively, another good technique to reduce oedema is to apply a compressive elastic bandage over the swollen part of the penis for 10–20 min [31].

There are osmotic methods, in which substances with a high concentration of solutes are applied to the skin surface of the oedematous tissue. A thick layer of sugar is applied over the entire circumference of the penis and foreskin and wrapped with a gauze pad. Once the reduction of the oedema, the presence of wrinkles in the mucosa and the humidity of the sugar have been checked, the penis is washed, and the reversal manoeuvre is carried out [32]. A 20% mannitol solution has also been used as an osmotic agent [33].

Reduction of oedema by direct injection of hyaluronidase has been successfully described in children and infants. By increasing the diffusion of fluid trapped within the tissue planes of the foreskin, swelling and oedema are reduced [34].

Ice applied to oedematous areas have also been described although many authors advise against its use as it may further compromise arterial inflow to the possibly ischaemic portion of the penis.

2. Penile block

If the paraphimosis is long-standing, severe or extremely painful, a penile block is recommended for the comfort of the patient and the physician. The plan is to infiltrate the right and left penile nerve as proximal to the base of the penis as possible. A 27-gauge needle is used to create a puncture in the skin at 2 o'clock and 10 o'clock. The needle is then inserted into the centre of each dimple perpendicularly up to 0.5 cm deep, or until resistance is lost suggesting that the tip is in Buck's fascia.

3. Reversion manoeuver

Place both index fingers on the dorsal edge of the penis, behind the retracted foreskin, and both thumbs on the tip of the glans penis. Apply even and continuous pressure on the glans with the thumbs, while pulling the ring with the index and middle fingers over the glans. A little lubricant may help in this procedure, although excessive lubricant may take the skin too slippery for effective grasping.

After successful manual reduction, the foreskin should be carefully cleaned. Topical antibiotics should be applied if skin abrasions or tears are present. Patients should avoid any activity that contributes to paraphimosis or retracting the foreskin.

Surgical Reduction of Paraphimosis

When manual reduction methods are not sufficient, the problem must be solved by a surgical approach. Once adequate sterility has been prepared and a penile block has been made, two haemostatic forceps are applied to the skin of the ring at 12 o'clock. A 2 cm longitudinal cut is made, allowing the glans to be surpassed and the skin to be turned back. Subsequently, this incision is not reapproximated, but the edges are sutured back on themselves to prevent recurrence.

Although rare, ischaemia leading to necrosis and gangrene of the glans and distal urethra may occur. When such a serious eventuality occurs, debridement of the necrotic tissue with or without the need for glansectomy or even partial penectomy is usually necessary. Cases managed conservatively with apparent good results have been published in the literature.

Once the emergency is solved, circumcision or dorsal slit are recommended due to the risk of recurrence and associated complications [35].

Blunt Penile Trauma

Penile Fracture

Definition and Epidemiology

Penile fracture consists of injury of the tunica albuginea with associated tearing of the corpus cavernosum. Its incidence is low, although probably under-diagnosed due to lack of patient attendance at the hospital and is estimated at 1 case per 175,000 hospital admissions [36].

Etiology

It usually occurs during vigorous sexual intercourse, when the erect penis strikes the perineum or pubis and bends. The sudden increase in intracavernosal pressure is greater than the tensile strength of the albuginea, which, together with the thinning of the albuginea during erection, results in rupture. This mecanism has been called "faux pas de coit", "Texas trauma" and "bent nail syndrome" [37]. In Asian countries, the practice of taghaandan, based on bending the erect penis vigorously during masturbation to achieve rapid detumescence, makes it more frequent. It has also been described in a large number of situations: turning in bed, falling down while the penis is erect, etc. It usually affects the proximal third, dorsally or laterally, and is rarely bilateral [38]. Associated urethral injury occurs in 20–38% of cases, with a lower incidence in Asia and the Middle East due to the different mechanism of production [37, 39].

Diagnosis

The clinical presentation is very typical: popping sound, pain, sudden detumescence, contralateral deviation and sheath haematoma (Fig. 5.3).

The extent of the haematoma will depend on the involvement of Buck's fascia. If it is not affected, the haematoma remains contained between the skin and the tunica, causing an "aubergine" appearance. If ruptured, the haematoma may extend to the scrotum, perineum and suprapubic area, showing a "butterfly wing" appearance. Occasionally cases have been described where pain has not been present. The fracture line is sometimes palpable [40].

In case of urethral involvement, urethrorrhagia, haematuria or urinary retention are often associated, although it can be silent.

Ultrasonography is the best technique to assess penile trauma although it requires a high degree of skills (Fig. 5.4). In good hands, it allows delineation of the anatomical structures and extent of the haematoma and study of the penile vascularisation using Doppler [41, 42].

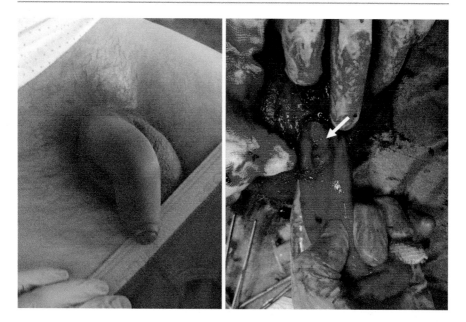

Fig. 5.3 Patient with penile fracture without urethral involvement. The tunica albuginea injury could be seen (arrow)

Fig. 5.4 Penile ultrasound showing a continuity solution in the tunica albuginea of a patient with penile fracture

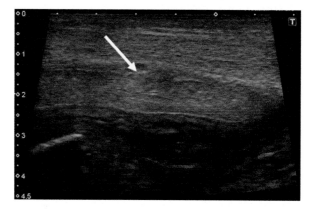

Other more invasive techniques such as cavernosography are not recommended, as they have a high false negative rate (15%) when the rupture is small or a clot prevents bleeding. It is also frequently associated with complications (infection, allergic reactions, fibrosis) [39].

Magnetic resonance imaging (MRI) is the technique with the highest diagnostic capacity, but its limited availability and high cost mean that it is rarely used and only in patients with atypical clinical and examination findings [43].

The differential diagnosis should be made with rupture of the dorsal penile artery or vein, Mondor's disease or rupture of the suspensory ligament.

Treatment

The published literature confirms that the recommended approach is immediate surgical intervention to evacuate the haematoma and close the tunica albuginea defect with 2/0 suture; avoiding excessive debridement or deep body vascular ligation [38, 44]. There is no agreement on the use of absorbable or non-absorbable suture. Although different approaches have been proposed, the circular incision with circumcision is the most commonly used. In case of urethral rupture, a thin, absorbable suture is placed over the urethral catheter, usually without the need for grafts, termino-terminally after spatulation of the urethral ends. Given that the urethral lesion usually coincides in location with the albuginea lesion of the corpus cavernosum, it is advisable to make a subdartos flap between the corpus cavernosum and the spongiosum to avoid fistulas. The catheter should be kept in place for 7–10 days, although it is not necessary if no urethral lesion has been detected [45].

The long-term sequelae of penile fracture are mainly fibrosis, penile curvature and erectile dysfunction, often varying depending on the type of treatment and timing of treatment. Many studies suggest that immediate surgical treatment achieves better long-term results than conservative treatment. In some series, the rate of sequelae is almost twice as high in patients managed conservatively [46], while delaying intervention increases the risk of sequelae fivefold in some comparative studies [47]. The success rate is around 90% if surgery is performed early [48].

Strangulation Injuries of the Penis

Definition and Epidemiology

Strangulation of the penis is a rare emergency complication. It can be caused by a variety of materials (condoms, metal rings, hair, etc.) forming a ring around the phallus, initially interrupting venous and lymphatic return, resulting in severe penile oedema. Subsequently, if compression is maintained, mechanical lesions will appear in varying degrees: skin ulcers, urethral fistula or loss of sensation. If arterial involvement is added, the constriction will cause ischaemic necrosis and tissue gangrene within a few hours.

In children, it usually occurs accidentally or as a means of avoiding nocturnal enuresis, although sexual abuse must be considered. In adults, it usually occurs during the development of sexual activity when rings are used to prolong erection but may also be associated with psychiatric disorders.

Diagnosis

Bhat et al. developed a classification of these lesions (Table 5.1) and noted that although non-metallic objects are easier to remove, they tend to produce more significant injuries as they are thinner and sharper [49].

The diagnosis is visual, but the assessment of lesions on the glans, skin and urethra cannot be determined until the object is removed (Fig. 5.5). In patients with loss of sensation or colour changes distal to the constriction, the outcome is usually

Table 5.1 Bhat classification of strangulation injuries

Bhat classification of strangulation injuries	
Grade 1	Oedema of distal penis. No evidence of skin ulceration or urethral injury.
Grade 2	Injury to skin and constriction of corpus spongiosum but no evidence of urethral injury. Distal penile oedema with decreased penile sensation.
Grade 3	Injury to skin and urethra but no urethral fistula. Loss of distal penile sensation.
Grade 4	Complete division of corpus spongiosum leading to urethral fistula and constriction of corpus cavernosum with loss of distal penile sensation.
Grade 5	Gangrene, necrosis or complete amputation of distal penis.

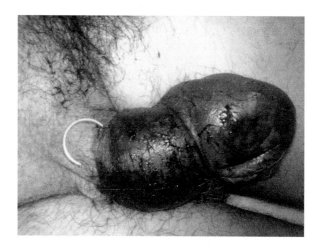

Fig. 5.5 Patient with penile strangulation due to metallic ring

satisfactory. Irreversible ischaemia is rare. Urinary fistulae are diagnosed with retrograde urethrography or methylene blue. Fluorescein can be used to delineate devitalised tissue for proper debridement. Doppler ultrasound can help diagnose vascular lesions, thrombosis and absence of flow, and some authors believe it should be used routinely.

Treatment

There is no single approach to removal of the constrictive object, and each case may require a different approach. We should base our treatment on the shape, material and size of the object, the time of evolution, the degree according to Bhat's classification, the availability of equipment and personnel skilled in its use, and the patient's ability to cooperate. Occasionally suprapubic drainage may be required for bladder emptying [50, 51].

The need for local anaesthesia/sedation should be based on the need for patient feedback that we require, especially to prevent iatrogenic thermal injury caused by industrial cutting instruments.

Removal with lubrication and traction should be attempted initially. Various mechanisms can be used to reduce distal penile oedema (explained in the Paraphimosis section). If the material is soft (hair, rubber, strings, etc.) it can be cut.

If this is not possible, the string method can be used. Wrap a thin piece of thread or dental floss tightly around the immediate distal circumference of the penis. Slip the end of the thread under the ring, pull it taut, and start unwinding it in the same direction to slowly pry off the object. It may be necessary to drain blood retained in the corpora cavernosa or the glans penis with a needle as the ring is advanced towards the distal part of the penis [52, 53].

When this is not achieved by the above techniques, metal cutting tools such as orthopaedic, dental or neurosurgical drills, or industrial equipment if available and available to trained personnel, are used, protecting the penis from heat, sparks, swarf etc. Tongue depressors, dressings, ribbed probes, laryngoscope blades or similar material may be used for this purpose. The use of ice is useful to avoid thermal injury [54, 55]. Finally, surgical techniques of skin denudation down to Buck's fascia can be used, with skin grafts or myocutaneous flaps for glans reconstruction.

When no pulse is found by Doppler, the use of heparin may be useful, as skin necrosis may not be visible until several hours after resolution of the strangulation [50].

Blunt Penile Contusion

Penile contusion frequently occurs in violent confrontations, high-risk sports, traffic accidents or falls from a straddle, with the penis in a flaccid state. A haematoma of the sheath or between Buck's and Colles' fasciae occurs, usually without rupture of the albuginea or classic symptoms, which rules out the need for surgical intervention. Treatment will consist of local cold, anti-inflammatory drugs, elevation of the penis and relative rest [44].

Although rare, cavernous haematomas may occur due to blunt trauma or crushing of the penile base against the pelvic bones, and are usually bilateral. A complication is high-flow priapism that occurs due to injury to the intracavernosal arteries, which in most cases resolves spontaneously. Penile Doppler ultrasound is the technique of choice, cavernous blood gas values do not reveal hypoxia or acidosis. Occasionally immediate invasive interventions such as embolisation or surgery may be necessary [45].

Penetrating Penile Trauma

Penetrating Wounds

Definition and Epidemiology

Penetrating penile injuries are infrequent, usually related to road traffic accidents, fights (domestic violence), accidents at work due to machinery, risky sports, complications during circumcision or self-mutilation.

Diagnosis

These are bleeding lesions, which require evaluation in a general context, as they may be accompanied by more complex lesions in other organs in up to 83% of cases [56]. The presence of urethral bleeding, difficulty urinating or swelling of the penis during urination requires urethral injury to be ruled out by retrograde urethrography, although its absence does not exclude it. Urethral injury can be found in up to 22% of gunshot wounds [57]. Therefore, in this type of aggression, where severity depends largely on the calibre and velocity of the projectile, retrograde urethrography should be considered even in the absence of any of the signs described above, and computed tomography should be performed to rule out injuries to neighbouring organs [58].

Treatment

The principles of treatment include: immediate examination, copious lavage and control of bleeding, removal of foreign bodies, correct antibiotic and tetanus prophylaxis and surgical closure. In case of urethral involvement, the use of a suprapubic diversion is recommended to avoid infection and to facilitate diagnosis and follow-up. Urethral repair is usually deferred in most cases, following the usual principles of urethroplasty. In the case of penile urethral injuries, there is controversy about management as some large series report urethral strictures in up to 78% if the repair is deferred, compared to 12.5% if the repair is primary [59, 60]. Most patients recover erection within 1–6 weeks.

The mechanism of injury is important in the therapeutic approach:

- Burns should be covered. If thermal, 1% argentic sulphadiazine cream is appropriate. Chemical burns should be irrigated with saline. Electrical burns require a watchful waiting attitude at first, as it is not possible to delineate the area requiring debridement until 12–24 h. Glans burns tend to heal with better cosmetic results by second intention [60, 61].
- Zip wounds are more frequent in children or intoxicated adults. Multiple manoeuvres have been described to achieve release, depending on the mechanism of skin entrapment [62]. The situation that is least frequent is when the moving part of the zip has gone beyond the place where the skin is trapped between the teeth of the zip. This situation is the easiest to resolve: cutting the zip from underneath and opening the teeth. The most frequent situation is that the movable part of the zip is the part that traps the foreskin. In this case, an attempt to unzip is made under local anaesthesia and with lubricant. If this is not possible, the movable part of the zip is cut into two pieces with a bone cutter [63]. Occasionally it is necessary to perform elliptical excisions or circumcision [64].
- Bite genital involvement is rare and is more common in children. The morbidity of the lesions caused is determined by the severity of the initial wound and the time until medical attention. In children, early consultation results in better outcomes. In contrast, human bites are usually referred later [39, 65] Basic treatment includes copious lavage, debridement, immediate primary closure in most

cases and broad-spectrum antibiotic therapy [44]. Subsequently, depending on the type of sequelae, reconstructive surgery will be performed as necessary.

- Pasterurella multocida infections are common (20–50% of dog bites and 70% of cat bites). It usually causes early cellulitis and, only rarely in patients with comorbidities (liver cirrhosis, glucocorticoids, alcoholism), late septic disease. They respond to beta-lactams together with beta-lactamase inhibitors, although fluoroquinolones, cotrimoxazole and chloramphenicol are possible alternatives. In human bites, empirical treatment should cover S. aureus, E. corrodens, Haemophilus and anaerobes [66]. The duration of antibiotic treatment/prophylaxis should be individualised and should last 10–14 days [67, 68]. The possibility of rabies infection should be considered and vaccination administered if deemed necessary. Appropriate tetanus vaccination is mandatory.

Penile Amputation

Definition and Epidemiology

Penile amputation is a rare emergency condition. In the paediatric population the most common aetiology is in relation to assault or as a complication following circumcision outside the health care setting. In adults, amputation is usually a self-inflicted injury, as a consequence of psychotic disorders in the context of intoxication (Klingsor syndrome), or in relation to religious or sexual identity issues [69].

Treatment

The treatment of penile amputation has three possibilities: reimplantation, suturing and closure of the wound (in case of non-complete amputation) or reconstruction of the penis.

Phallic reinsertion or reimplantation is the technique that obtains the best results from a functional point of view, especially when performed with vascular and nerve microsurgery of the dorsal neurovascular bundle. Urethral and corpus cavernosum suturing does not require microsurgery. Thus, the results are often surprisingly good, with 20% incidence of urethral strictures, 10% incidence of urethral fistula, 55% incidence of skin loss and 21% incidence of erectile dysfunction. Reanastomosis of the cavernous arteries is not recommended as their dissection may cause fibrosis and such anastomosis has a high likelihood of thrombosis given its calibre. Furthermore, it has not been proven to improve sexual function [60]. If microsurgical repair is not possible, macroscopic repair can be performed, although a loss of sensation is expected in 80–100% of patients [70]. After repair, a suprapubic cystostomy should be maintained until complete wound healing.

For reimplantation it must be possible to obtain the amputated penis, its correct preservation in saline and cold ischaemia (with double sterile bag technique, avoiding direct contact with ice) and stabilisation of the patient from a psychiatric and haemodynamic point of view. Reimplantation is successful after up to 16 h of cold ischaemia or 6 h of warm ischaemia. If this procedure is not possible, the usual steps of partial or total penile amputation should be completed, with suturing of the corpora cavernosa, spatulating the urethra to create a neomeatum. Another option, once the emergency has been resolved, is phalloplasty, which should be performed by experienced teams due to its high complication rate [39, 71].

Testicular Torsion

The presence of acute testicular pain or swelling is often defined as "acute scrotum" and can recognize many different etiologies. Acute scrotal pain should always be considered as an emergency condition and should be promptly faced [72]. It can derive from scrotal structures or referred from other sources. In Table 5.2 possible causes of acute testicular pain and the possible differential diagnosis to take into consideration are listed [73, 74]. Among them, the most common are torsion of the spermatic cord, epididymo-orchitis and torsion of the testicular appendages. The most important objective in these patients is to rule out testicular torsion, which should be quickly diagnosed and treated in order to avoid possible severe complications.

Torsion of the spermatic cord can be defined as the interruption of arterial blood flow in the testicle due to the twisting of the artery and associated structures. If not treated timely, it can determine infarction, necrosis and an irreversible ischemic injury of the affected testicle. Severity of testicular damage depends on grade and duration of the torsion [75]. It is considered the most common cause of acute scrotal pain and swelling in boys from birth until to 18 years of age. There are two peaks in the distribution of the age of onset, with the first one in the neonatal period and the second one around puberty. The estimated annual incidence is 3.8 per 100,000 males younger than 18 years [76] and it accounts for about 10% to 15% of acute scrotal disease in children [77]. Usually left testis is more commonly affected than the right (with a 6:4 ratio), probably due to the different length of spermatic cord that is greater on the left. In prenatal or neonatal age, a reduced fixation of the tissues to one another or retarded delivery of testes could be possible risk factors of torsion [78]. In young boys and adults, an abnormal anchorage of tunica vaginalis to the testicle results in increased mobility of the testicle within the tunica, facilitating possible cord torsion. Moreover, cold weather can be a risk factor for torsion as it facilitates cremasteric contraction. From the physiopatological point of view, during torsion the first event is the interruption of venous supply to testicle, leading to

Table 5.2 Differential diagnosis for acute testicular pain

Disease	
Testicular torsion	Adductor tendinitis
Torsion of appendages	Neoplasia
Acute epididymitis	Fournier's gangrene
Hydrocele/Varicocele	Dermatological lesions
Hernia	Trauma
Hematocele	Spermatocele
Cyst of epididymis	Vasculitis (Henoch-Schönlein purpura)
Idiopathic scrotal oedema	Idiopathic fat necrosis

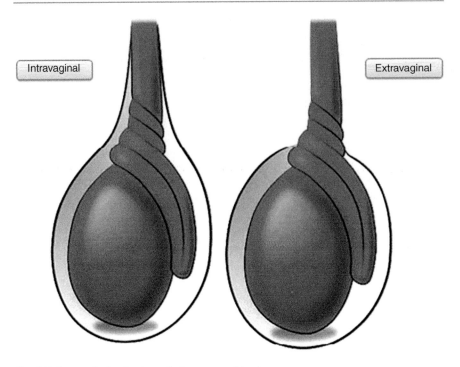

Fig. 5.6 Intravaginal and extravaginal sperm cord torsion

edema and swelling than arterial obstruction occurs determining subsequent ischemia and necrosis [79].

Depending on anatomical features, testicular torsion can be classified as either
intravaginal or as extravaginal (Fig. 5.6).

Intravaginal Torsion

It is considered the most common type of testicular torsion. The twisting of spermatic cords occurs into the tunica vaginalis. Intravaginal torsion probably due to an
abnormal fixation of the gubernaculum, epididymis, and testis, that determines for
the testicle an increased freedom to swing and rotate within the tunica [80]. This
anatomic relationship, in which the testicle has a transverse lie, is defined as the
"bell-clapper deformity" that is considered a risk factor for torsion. The *primum
movens* for the torsion is usually a sudden contraction of the cremaster muscle that
determines an initial rotation of the testis. This contortion is caused by the spiral
configuration of the muscle's insertion onto the cord, twisting it in such a way that
each testis' anterior surface rotates toward the midline.

Extravaginal Torsion

Extravaginal spermatic cord torsion is typical of prenatal and neonatal age. The lack
of fixation of the gubernaculum testis and testicular tunica to the scrotal wall leads
to torsion of testis, spermatic cord, and tunica vaginalis all together. Cryptorchidism
is considered the most important risk factor for this type of torsion [81].

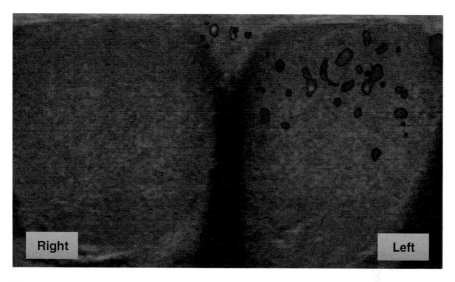

Fig. 5.7 Right sperm cord torsion (absence of blood flow compared to left testicle at color doppler ultrasound in transverse view)

Clinical Presentation and Diagnosis

The typical presentation of testicular torsion is described as an abrupt testicular pain, usually occurred during night that can awake patient from sleep. The venous outflow obstruction determines the rapid onset of swelling. Less frequently its onset is gradual with mild pain. Most times boys refer history of previous episodes of severe, self-limiting scrotal pain and swelling. Pain can be associated with nausea and vomiting and ipsilateral lower abdomen pain [80]. Intensity and frequency of pain can be useful for differential diagnosis. If the patient has mild pain that has increased over few days, the most probable diagnosis is a torsion of the testicular appendage. In case of intermittent acute pain, which completely resolves, it is probably due to an intermittent testicular torsion [82]. Usually, in case of sperm cord torsion, the pain is aggravating by walking.

Physical examination must start with the normal testicle that should be in the correct vertical position. Next, the spermatic cord of the affected testis is palpated. In case of torsion, it is painful and swollen. Then the position of the affected testis in the scrotal sac is checked [80].

Pain at the lower pole of the testis is more likely to signify torsion than pain at the upper pole of the testis. Hydrocele and scrotal oedema can be associated in some cases. The cremasteric reflex should be checked as in spermatic cord torsion it is usually absent [83].

In patients with signs and symptoms suggestive of testicular torsion imaging studies are not mandatory and they should undergo immediate surgical exploration in order to avoid further delay [84]. The most commonly used imaging modality is Doppler ultrasonography is the most commonly used imaging technique. It presents a high sensitivity (88.9%) and specificity (98.8%) with a very low rate of false negative (< 1%) [84]. Absence of blood flow in the testicle is consistent with the diagnosis of sperm cord torsion (Fig. 5.7). Even if the color doppler is not conclusive, in presence of a clinical examination strongly indicative for torsion, patients should undergo surgical intervention [85]. Emergency scrotal scintigraphy with radionuclide and MRI could be an alternative for diagnosis [86].

Treatment

Surgical treatment does not change between intravaginal and extravaginal torsion and consists of scrotal exploration. It is generally accepted that the testicle can be totally rescued after ≤6 h of torsion, but the probability decreases as time goes by, reaching the 50% at 12 h, until it becomes almost nil after 24 h [87, 88]. After the resolution of the sperm cord torsion, the affected testis should be enveloped in a warm gauze in order to check the possible return of the normal flow. If during this maneuver testis returns to its standard color and consistency, an orchidopexy can be performed; if not, orchiectomy should be performed. The presence of a necrotic testis always requires orchiectomy [89]. Usually, contralateral orchidopexy is performed especially in intravaginal torsion as the bell-clapper deformity is considered a bilateral defect in most cases, even if this approach is not universally accepted [90].

Manual detorsion could be attempted only if surgery is not delayed. The testicle is twisted from the medial to the lateral side (like opening a book) and sometimes more than one rotation is needed [91].

Fournier's Gangrene

Epidemiology and Risk Factors

Fournier's gangrene is a potential life-threatening disease defined as a progressive necrotizing fasciitis due to a synergistic polymicrobial infection of the perineum, peri-anal region, and/or external genitalia. The infection determines an obliterative endarteritis of subcutaneous vessels leading to gangrene and necrosis of the overlying tissue and skin [92, 93]. Incidence of Fournier's Gangrene is estimated in about 1.6 cases per 100,000 and increases with age with a peak between 60–70 years old and a M to F ratio of 10:1 [93]. Even if it can be considered a rare disease the mortality rate is high, ranging from 3% up to 88% [94].

Usually, Fournier's Gangrene derives from an infection of urinary tract, genitalia, anorectal area and skin, through which bacteria reaches the subcutaneous tissues. Fournier's Gangrene typically recognizes a polymicrobic etiology [94]. The synergistic action of aerobic and anaerobic bacteria can be considered as responsible of thrombosis and tissue necrosis. Local thrombosis determines ischemia and decrease in tissue oxygenation that yield spreading of the infection, leading to necrotising fasciitis [95]. E. coli is the most commonly pathogen detected (48%), followed by Enterococcus fecalis (28%). Microbiological agents responsible of the gangrene are listed in Table 5.3. Only in 10% of patients an etiological factor cannot be identified [96].

Main risk factors for Fournier's Gangrene development are diabetes mellitus, obesity, malignancies and chemotherapy, HIV infection, state of malnutrition,

Table 5.3 Etiological agents in Fournier's Gangrene

Gram-positive Aerobes
Corynebacterium spp.
Staphylococcus aureus
Streptococcus Beta-hemolytic
Streptococcus faecalis
Staphylococcus epidermidis
Gram-negative Aerobes
Escherichia coli
Enterococcus Faecalis
Proteus mirabilis
Pseudomonas aeruginosa
Klebsiella pneumoniae
Pseudomonas pyocyanea
Morganella morganii
Acinetobacter bauminii
Anaerobes
Bacteroides fragilis
Clostridium perfringens
Clostridium welchii
Citrobacter freundii
Fusobacterium
Mycobacteria
Mycobacterium tuberculosis
Yeasts
Candida albicans
Candida glabrata

history of alcohol abuse, genitourinary infections or trauma, liver and renal diseases and poor personal hygiene. Among these, diabetes mellitus is the most common predisposing factor (> 70% of all patients). All these conditions have impairment of host immunity and microcirculation as common denominator [97, 98].

Clinical Presentation and Diagnosis

Sign and symptoms of Fournier's Gangrene should be recognized promptly (Fig. 5.8). Even if it has a sudden onset, some prodromal symptoms like fever, asthenia, nausea and vomiting, tachycardia, perineal, perianal and/or scrotal pain, itching, edema and/or erythema of tissue surface can be present few days (2–7) before the gangrene manifestation [99, 100]. When present, subcutaneous crepitus due to tissue emphysema is considered to be pathognomonic for anaerobic bacteria involvement [95]. Typically, the gangrenous area spreads to adjacent tissues with a speed of 2/3 cm per hour, and this is why early diagnosis is so crucial for patients' survival. Potential life-threatening complication of FG are coagulopathy, cerebro-vascular accidents, septic shock and subsequent multiple organ failure [101]. Diagnostic criteria for Fournier's Gangrene are listed in Table 5.4.

Fig. 5.8 Fournier's
Gangrene

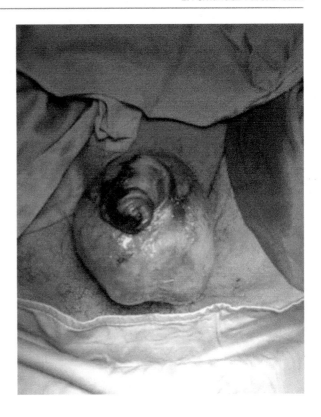

Table 5.4 Diagnostic criteria for Fournier's Gangrene

Infection of soft tissues that involves perineum, genitalia (usually scrotum) or anal region
Finding of air in subcutaneous tissue at clinical or radiological examination
Presence of necrotic tissues at surgical intervention and histological diagnosis of necrotizing fasciitis

Laboratory tests in Fournier's Gangrene are usually aspecific. Anemia, leukocytosis and thrombocytopenia can be found in these patients. In more advanced stages, hyponatremia, hypokalemia, hypocalcemia can be detected. Blood culture are positive only in about 20% of patients [102]. Imaging with X-ray of the abdomen, in order to recognize the presence of air in subcutaneous tissues, and CT or MRI, that are useful for defining extension of the gangrene could be useful as diagnostic tools [103]. MRI is considered the gold standard for planning surgical intervention [104].

Some prognostic tools have been proposed for clinical practice in order to predict outcomes of Fournier's Gangrene (Table 5.5).

Treatment
Treatment of Fournier's Gangrene is multimodal and involves intensive care, antibiotic therapy and surgery. Supportive cares should be given for anemia, hypotension

Table 5.5 Prognostic indexes for Fournier's Gangrene

Fournier's Gangrene Severity Index (FGSI) [101]	The score is calculated including patients' vital signs and metabolic parameters. It has been estimated that score > 9 have a 75% probability of death and an index score ≤ 9 is associated with 78% survival
Laboratory Risk Indicator for Necrotizing Fasciitis (LRINEC) [105]	this score stratifies patients into three different risk class for necrotising Soft-Tissue Infection (low, moderate or high risk) according to blood parameters (C-reactive proteins, WBC, Haemoglobin, Serum sodium, Serum creatinine, Plasma glucose)
Affected area calculation/ Extension of the necrosis [106]	It has been estimated that an affected area of less than 3% have a low risk of progression while if the area is above 5% the risk raises

Table 5.6 Recommended empiric treatment for Fournier's Gangrene (from [108])

Drugs	Dosage
Piperacillin-tazobactam plus Vancomycin	4.5 g every 6–8 h IV
	15 mg/kg every 12 h
Imipenem-cilastatin	1 g every 6–8 h IV
Meropenem	1 g every 8 h IV
Ertapenem	1 g once daily
Gentamicin	5 mg/kg daily
Cefotaxime plus metronidazole or clindamycin	2 g every 6 h IV
	500 mg every 6 h IV
	600–900 mg every 8 h IV
Cefotaxime plus fosfomycin plus metronidazole	2 g every 6 h IV
	5 g every 8 h IV
	500 mg every 6 h IV

and electrolytic impairment before patient undergoes surgery [107]. Immediate empiric parenteral antibiotic treatment should be started covering all probable causative organisms and then it should be corrected according to culture results. In fact, timing of antibiotic therapy is crucial for positive outcome. The recommended empiric antibiotic therapies are according to European Association of Urology Guidelines are showed in Table 5.6 [108].

Surgical debridement is the milestone of Fournier's Gangrene treatment and plays a crucial role in reducing mortality in FG patients (Fig. 5.9) [109]. The aim of surgery is to remove all the infected tissues. Debridement should be extended until the affected fascia is no longer easily dissociable from deep fascia and muscle. In many cases a subsequent delayed reconstructive surgery with skin flap or grafts is needed. If surgery is performed in the first 12–24 h the outcomes are significantly better than delayed surgery [110].

As hypoxia is one of the most important pathogenetic mechanisms of necrotizing infection, some authors reported a possible beneficial effect of Hyperbaric oxygen

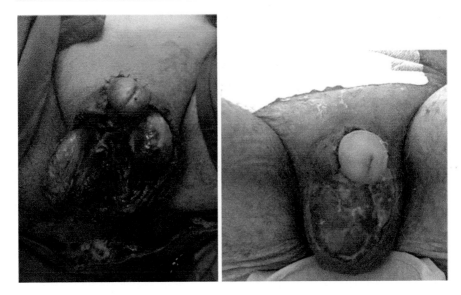

Fig. 5.9 Surgical debridement and reconstruction of the previous showed Fournier's Gangrene

therapy on Fournier's Gangrene [111]. Nevertheless, to date, no specific recommendation can be given on hyperbaric oxygen therapy [108].

References

1. Morgans A, et al. What is a health emergency? The difference in definition and understanding between patients and health professionals. Aust Health Rev. 2011;35(3):284–9.
2. Bettocchi C, et al. Emergencies in andrology. In: Mirone V, editor. Clinical uro-andrology. New York: Springer; 2015. p. 277–83.
3. Ferna A, et al. European urology male erectile dysfunction and health-related quality of life. Eur Urol. 2003;44:245–53.
4. Broderick GA, et al. Priapism: pathogenesis, epidemiology, and management. J Sex Med. 2010;7:476.
5. El-Bahnasawy MS, et al. Low-flow priapism: risk factors for erectile dysfunction. BJU Int. 2002;89:285.
6. Roghmann F, et al. Incidence of priapism in emergency departments in the United States. J Urol. 2013;190(4):1275–80.
7. Cherian J, et al. Medical and surgical management of priapism. Postgrad Med J. 2006;82(964):89–94.
8. Nelson JH, et al. Priapism: evolution of management in 48 patients in a 22-year series. J Urol. 1977;117:455.
9. Sood S, et al. Priapism associated with atypical antipsychotic medications: a review. Int Clin Psychopharmacol. 2008;23(1):9–17.
10. Porst H, et al. The rationale for prostaglandin E1 in erectile failure: a survey of worldwide experience. J Urol. 1996;155:802.
11. Rezaee ME, et al. Are we overstating the risk of priapism with oral phosphodiesterase type 5 inhibitors? J Sex Med. 2020;17:1579.

12. James Johnson M, et al. Which patients with ischaemic priapism require further investigation for malignancy? Int J Impot Res. 2020;32:195.
13. Ingram AR, et al. An update on non-ischemic priapism. Sex Med Rev. 2020;8(1):140–9.
14. Salonia A, et al. Guidelines on sexual and reproductive health. Arnhem: EAU Guidelines Office; 2021.
15. Vreugdenhil S, et al. Ischemic priapism as a model of exhausted metabolism. Physiol Rep. 2019;7:e13999.
16. Hakim LS, et al. Evolving concepts in the diagnosis and treatment of arterial high flow priapism. J Urol. 1996;155:541.
17. Zacharakis E, et al. Penile prosthesis insertion in patients with refractory ischaemic priapism: early vs delayed implantation. BJU Int. 2014;114:576.
18. Ateyah A, et al. Intracavernosal irrigation by cold saline as a simple method of treating iatrogenic prolonged erection. J Sex Med. 2005;2:248.
19. Wen C, et al. Management of ischemic priapism with high-dose intracavernosal phenylephrine: from bench to bedside. J Sex Med. 2006;3:918.
20. Burnett AL, et al. Standard operating procedures for priapism. J Sex Med. 2013;10:180.
21. Ramstein JJ, et al. Clinical outcomes of periprocedural antithrombotic therapy in ischemic priapism management. J Sex Med. 2020;17:2260.
22. Ralph DJ, et al. The immediate insertion of a penile prosthesis for acute ischaemic priapism. Eur Urol. 2009;56:1033.
23. Laroche JP, et al. Mondor's disease: what's new since 1939? Thromb Res. 2012;130:56–8.
24. Hashimoto T, et al. Atypical penile Mondor's disease occurring on the ventral aspect of the penis. J Dermatol. 2020;47(2):e58–60.
25. Öztürk H. Penile Mondor's disease. Basic Clin Androl. 2014;24:5.
26. Amano M, et al. Mondor's disease: a review of the literature. Intern Med. 2018;57:2607–12.
27. Wild J, et al. Penile Mondor's disease—an understated entity. Urol Case Rep. 2020;31:101176.
28. Choe JM. Paraphimosis: current treatment options. Am Fam Physician. 2000;62(12):2623–6, 2628
29. Herzog LW, Alvarez SR. The frequency of foreskin problems in uncircumcised children. Am J Dis Child. 1986;140(3):254–6.
30. Palmisano F, Gadda F, Spinelli MG, Montanari E. Glans penis necrosis following paraphimosis: a rare case with brief literature review. Urol Case Rep. 2018;16:57–8.
31. Pohlman GD, Phillips JM, Wilcox DT. Simple method of paraphimosis reduction revisited: point of technique and review of the literature. J Pediatr Urol. 2013;9(1):104–7.
32. Cahill D, Rane A. Reduction of paraphimosis with granulated sugar. BJU Int. 1999;83(3):362.
33. Anand A, Kapoor S. Mannitol for paraphimosis reduction. Urol Int. 2013;90(1):106–8.
34. Hayashi Y, Kojima Y, Mizuno K, Kohri K. Prepuce: phimosis, paraphimosis, and circumcision. ScientificWorldJournal. 2011;11:289–301.
35. Sato Y, Takagi S, Uchida K, Shima M, Tobe M, Haga K, Honama I, Hirobe M. Long-term follow-up of penile glans necrosis due to paraphimosis. IJU Case Rep. 2019;2(4):171–3.
36. Mydlo JH. Surgeon experience with penile fracture. J Urol. 2001;166(2):526–9.
37. Llarena R, Villafruela A, Azurmendi I, et al. Fractura de pene con rotura asociada de uretra. Arch Esp Urol. 2006;59(7):732–6.
38. Serrano A, Golbano JM, González-Peramato P, et al. Fractura de pene: evaluación diagnóstica y actitudes terapéuticas. Revisión de la literatura. Arch Esp Urol. 2001;54(8):803–10.
39. Morey AF, Rozanski TA, Wein AJ. Genital and lower urinary tract trauma. In: Wein AJ, Kavoussi LR, Novick AC, Partin AW, Peters CA, editors. Campbell-Walsh urology. 9th ed. Philadelphia: Saunders Elsevier; 2007. Chapter 88.
40. Gontero P, Muir GH, Frea B. Pathological findings of penile fractures their surgical management. Urol Int. 2003;71:77–82.
41. Bertolotto M, Calderan L, Cova MA. Imaging of penile traumas—therapeutic implications. Eur Radiol. 2005;15(12):2475–82.
42. Bertolotto M, Mucelli RP. Nonpenetrating penile traumas: sonographic and doppler features. AJR. 2004;183:1085–9.

43. Uder M, Gohl D, Takahashi M, et al. MRI of penile fracture: diagnosis therapeutic follow-up. Eur Radiol. 2002;12:113–20.
44. Martínez-Piñeiro L, Ríos E, de la Peña JJ. Traumatismos de uretra y genitales. In: Jiménez Cruz JF, Rioja Sanz LA, Rioja Sanz C, Allona Almagro A, editors. Tratado de Urología. 2nd ed. Barcelona: Prous Science; 2006. p. 1615–39.
45. Kamdar C, Mooppan UM, Kim H, et al. Penile fracture: preoperative evaluation and surgical technique for optimal patient outcome. BJU Int. 2008;102:1640–4.
46. Muntener M, Suter S, Hauri D, et al. Long-term experience with surgical and conservative treatment of penile fracture. J Urol. 2004;172(2):576–9.
47. Mazaris EM, Livadas K, Chalikopoulos D, et al. Penile fractures: surgical approach with a midline ventral incision. BJU Int. 2009;104:520–3.
48. Zargooshi J. Penile fracture in Kermanshah, Iran: the long-term results of surgical treatment. BJU Int. 2002;89:890–4.
49. Bhat AL, Kumar A, Mathur SC, et al. Penile strangulation. Br J Urol. 1991;68:618–21.
50. Silberstein J, Grabowski J, Lakin C, et al. Penile constriction devices: case report, review of the literature, and recommendations for extrication. J Sex Med. 2008;5:1747–57.
51. Ivanovski O, Stankov O, Kuzmanoski M, et al. Penile strangulation: two case reports and review of the literature. Sex Med. 2007;4:1775–80.
52. Vahasarja VJ, Hellstrom PA, Serlo W, et al. Treatment of penile incarceration by the string method: 2 case reports. J Urol. 1993;149:372–3.
53. Noh J, Kang TW, Heo T, et al. Penile strangulation treated with the modified string method. Urology. 2004;64:591.
54. Perabo FG, Steiner G, Albers P, et al. Treatment of penile strangulation by constricting devices. Urology. 2002;59:137.
55. Santucci RA, Deng D, Carney J. Removal of metal penile foreign body with a widely available emergency-medical-services-provided air-driven grinder. Urology. 2004;63:1183–4.
56. Burnett AL, Bivalacqua TJ. Priapism: current principles and practice. Urol Clin North Am. 2007;34:631–42.
57. Martín M, López J, Pérez M, et al. Lesión de los cuerpos cavernosos por arma de fuego. Presentación de un caso y revisión de la literatura. Actas Urol Esp. 2009;33(10):1138–40.
58. Husmann DA, Boone TB, Wilson WT. Management of low velocity gunshot wounds to the anterior urethra: the role of primary repair versus urinary diversion alone. J Urol. 1993;150:70–2.
59. Bandi G, Santucci RA. Controversies in the management of male external genitourinary trauma. J Trauma. 2004;56:1362–70.
60. Morey AF, Metro MJ, Carney KJ, et al. Consensus on genitourinary trauma: external genitalia. BJU Int. 2004;94:507–15.
61. Wessels HB. Genital skin loss: unified reconstructive approach to a heterogenous entity. World J Urol. 1999;17:107–14.
62. Wyatt JP, Scobie WG. The management of penile zip entrapment in Children. Injury. 1994;25:59.
63. Flowerdew R, Fishman IJ, Churchill BM. Management of penile zipper injury. J Urol. 1977;117:671.
64. Mydlo JH. Treatment of a delayed zipper injury. Urol Int. 2000;64:45–6.
65. Gomes CM, Ribeiro-Filho L, Giron AM, et al. Genital trauma due to animal bites. J Urol. 2000;165:80–3.
66. Goldstein EJC. Bites. In: Mandell GL, Bennet JE, Dolin R, editors. Principles and practice of infectious diseases. Philadelphia: Churchill Livingstone; 2000. p. 3202.
67. Van der Horst C, Martínez Portillo FJ, Seif C, et al. Male genital injury: diagnostics and treatment. BJU Int. 2004;93:927–30.
68. Font B, Segura F. Infecciones por bacilos gramnegativos causadas por mordeduras y arañazos de animales. In: Farreras P, Rozman C, editors. Medicina Interna. 15th ed. Madrid: Elsevier; 2005. p. 2293–6.

69. De Lagausie P, Jehanno P. Six years follow-up of a penis replantation in a child. J Pediatr Surg. 2008;43:E11–2.
70. Jezior JR, Brady JD, Schlossberg SM. Management of penile amputation injuries. World J Surg. 2001;25(12):1602–9.
71. Rashid M, Sarwar SU. Avulsion injuries of the male external genitalia: classification and reconstruction with the customised radial forearm free flap. Br J Plast Surg. 2005;58(5):585–92.
72. Burgher SW. Acute scrotal pain. Emerg Med Clin North Am. 1998;16:781–809, vi
73. Brandes SB, Chelsky MJ, Hanno PM. Adult acute idiopathic scrotal edema. Urology. 1994;44:602–5.
74. Jefferson RH, Perez LM, Joseph DB. Critical analysis of the clinical presentation of acute scrotum: a 9 year experience at a single institution. J Urol. 1997;158:1198–200.
75. McAndrew HF, Pemberton R, Kikiros CS, et al. The incidence and investigation of acute scrotal problems in children. Pediatr Surg Int. 2002;18:435–7.
76. Zhao LC, Lautz TB, Meeks JJ, Maizels M. Pediatric testicular torsion epidemiology using a national database: incidence, risk of orchiectomy and possible measures toward improving the quality of care. J Urol. 2011;186(5):2009–13.
77. Liang T, Metcalfe P, Sevcik W, Noga M. Retrospective review of diagnosis and treatment in children presenting to the pediatric department with acute scrotum. AJR Am J Rentgenol. 2013;200(5):W444–9.
78. Callewaert PR, Van Kerrebroeck P. New insights into perinatal testicular torsion. Eur J Pediatr. 2010;169(6):705–12.
79. Nguyen L, Lievano G, Ghosh L, Radhakrishnan J, Fornell L, John E. Effect of unilateral testicular torsion on blood flow and histology of contralateral testes. J Pediatr Surg. 1999;34(5):680–3.
80. Kapoor S. Testicular torsion: a race against time. Int J Clin Pract. 2008;62:821–7.
81. Benjamin K. Scrotal and inguinal masses in the newborn period. Adv Neonatal Care. 2002;2:140–8.
82. Eaton SH, Cendron MA, Estrada CR, et al. Intermittent testicular torsion: diagnostic features and management outcomes. J Urol. 2005;174:1532–5.
83. Nelson CP, Williams JF, Bloom DA. The cremasteric reflex: a useful but imperfect sign in testicular torsion. J Pediatr Surg. 2003;38:1248–9.
84. Baker LA, Sigman D, Mathews RI, Benson J, Docimo SG. An analysis of clinical outcomes using color doppler testicular ultrasound for testicular torsion. Pediatrics. 2000;105(3 pt 1):604–7.
85. Waldert M, Klatte T, Schmidbauer J, Remzi M, Lackner J, Marberger M. Color Doppler sonography reliably identifies testicular torsion in boys. Urology. 2010;75(5):1170–4.
86. Wu HC, Sun SS, Kao A, Chuang FJ, Lin CC, Lee CC. Comparison of radionuclide imaging and ultrasonography in the differentiation of acute testicular torsion and inflammatory testicular disease. Clin Nucl Med. 2002;27(7):490–3.
87. Mushtaq I, Fung M, Glasson MJ. Retrospective review of paediatric patients with acute scrotum. ANZ J Surg. 2003;73:55–8.
88. Whitaker RH. Diagnoses not to be missed. Torsion of the testis. Br J Hosp Med. 1982;27:66–9.
89. Sessions AE, Rabinowitz R, Hulbert WC, Goldstein MM, Mevorach RA. Testicular torsion: direction, degree, duration and disinformation. J Urol. 2003;169(2):663–5.
90. Favorito LA, Cavalcante AG, Costa WS. Anatomic aspects of epididymis and tunica vaginalis in patients with testicular torsion. Int Braz J Urol. 2004;30(5):420–4.
91. Haynes BE, Haynes VE. Manipulative detorsion: beware the twist that does not turn. J Urol. 1987;137(1):118–9.
92. Korkut M, Icoz G, Dayangac M, Akgun E, Yeniay L, Erdogan O, et al. Outcome analysis in patients with Fournier's gangrene. Report of 45 cases. Dis Colon Rectum. 2003;46:649–52.
93. Sorensen MD, Krieger JN, Rivara FP, Klien MB, Hunter W. Fournier's gangrene: population-based epidemiology and outcomes. J Urol. 2009;181:2120–6.
94. Ersay A, Yilmaz G, Akgun Y, Celik Y. Factors affecting mortality of Fournier's gangrene: review of 70 patients. ANZ J Surg. 2007;77:43–8.

95. Eke N. Fournier's gangrene: a review of 1726 cases. Br J Surg. 2000;87:718–28.
96. Koukouras D, Kallidonis P, Panagopoulos C, Al-Aown A, Athanosopoulos A, Rigopoulos C, et al. Fournier's gangrene, a urologic and surgical emergency: presentation of multi-institutional experience with 45 cases. Urol Int. 2011;186:167–72.
97. Morpurgo E, Galandiuk S. Fournier's gangrene. Surg Clin North Am. 2002;82:1213–24.
98. Barreda JT, Scheiding MM, Fernandez CS, Campana JMC, Aguilera JR, Miranda EF, et al. Fournier's gangrene. A retrospective study of 41 cases. Cir Esp. 2010;87:218–23.
99. Chennamsetty A, Khourdaji I, Burks F, Killinger KA. Contemporary diagnosis and management of Fournier's gangrene. Ther Adv Urol. 2015;7(4):203–15.
100. Benizri E, Fabiani P, Migliori G, Chevallier D, Peyrottes A, Raucoules M, Amiel J, Mouiel J, Toubol J. Gangrene of the perineum. Urology. 1996;47:93.
101. Morua AG, Lopez JAA, Garcia JDG, Montelongo RM, Geurra LSG. Fournier's gangrene: our experience in 5 years, bibliography review and assessment of the Fournier's gangrene severity index. Arch Esp Urol. 2009;67(7):532e40.
102. Saenz EV, Martınez P, Magro H, Ovalle MV, Vega JM, Tostado JFA. Experience in management of Fournier's gangrene. Tech Coloproctol. 2002;6(1):5e10.
103. Sherman J, Solliday M, Paraiso E, Becker J, Mydlo JH. Early CT findings of Fournier's gangrene in a healthy male. Clin Imaging. 1998;22(6):425e7.
104. Sharif HS, Clark DC, Aabed MY, Aideyan OA, Haddad MC, Mattson TA. MR imaging of thoracic and abdominal wall infection: comparison with other imaging procedures. Am J Roentgenol. 1990;154(5):989e95.
105. Wong CH, Khin LW, Heng KS, Tan KC, Low CO. The LRINEC (Laboratory Risk Indicator for Necrotizing Fasciitis) score: a tool for distinguishing necrotizing fasciitis from other soft tissue infections. Crit Care Med. 2004;32:1535e41.
106. Roghmann F, von Bodman C, Löppenberg B, Hinkel A, Palisaar J, Noldus J. Is there a need for the Fournier's gangrene severity index? Comparison of scoring systems for outcome prediction in patients with Fournier's gangrene. BJU Int. 2012;110(9):1359–65.
107. Rivers E, Nguyen B, Havstad S, Ressler J, Muzzin A, Knoblich B, et al. Early goal directed therapy in the treatment of severe sepsis and septic shock. N Engl J Med. 2001;345:1368e77.
108. EAU guidelines on urological infections. 2021. https://uroweb.org/guideline/urological-infections/
109. Quatan N, Kirby RS. Improving outcomes in Fournier's gangrene. BJU Int. 2004;93:691.
110. Chao WN, et al. Impact of timing of surgery on outcome of Vibrio vulnificus related necrotizing fasciitis. Am J Surg. 2013;206:32–9.
111. Creta M, Longo N, Arcaniolo D, Giannella R, Cai T, Cicalese A, De Nunzio C, Grimaldi G, Cicalese V, De Sio M, Autorino R, Lima E, Fedelini P, Marmo M, Capece M, La Rocca R, Tubaro A, Imbimbo C, Mirone V, Fusco F. Hyperbaric oxygen therapy reduces mortality in patients with Fournier's Gangrene. Results from a multiinstitutional observational study. Minerva Urol Nefrol. 2020;72(2):223–8.

Peyronie's Disease and Penile Curvature

6

Giorgio Ivan Russo, Christian Di Gaetano,
Alberto Costa Silva, and Afonso Morgado

Abstract

Peyronie's Disease is a common acquired connective tissue disorder of the tunica albuginea characterized by the presence of a localized fibrotic plaque that reduces the elasticity of tunica albuginea itself leading to penile curvature, shortening or narrowing, painful erection and sexual discomfort. Epidemiological data on Peyronie's disease are limited, it is not a rare disease; the prevalence in general population is between 0.3% to 13.1%, but can increase in some specific sub-populations. The etiology of Peyronie's disease is still unknown and unclear, but the most accredited theory is that it could be a wound-healing disorder caused by repetitive microvascular injury or trauma to the tunica albuginea. The diagnosis of Peyronie's disease should be based on a comprehensive medical and sexual history and a detailed physical examination. Assessment of penile deformity and curvature in the erect state should be performed whit ICI (intra cavernous injection) or vacuum devices. There is no a consensus about the optimal therapeutical approach to the disease, the specific pathophysiology of Peyronie's disease still remains unknown. In the early stage of Peyronie's disease medical treatment is often employed, when there are symptoms but should not be fibrotic or calcific plaque. Non-surgical treatments for Peyronie's disease aim to treat patients in the acute and chronic phases of disease. Surgery remains to this day the gold stan-

G. I. Russo (✉)
Urology Section, University of Catania, Catania, Italy

Policlinico Universitario Gaspare Rodolico, Urology Unit, University of Catania, Catania, Italy

C. Di Gaetano
Urology Section, University of Catania, Catania, Italy

A. C. Silva · A. Morgado
Serviço de Urologia, Centro Hospitalar Universitário São João, Porto, Portugal

© The Author(s), under exclusive license to Springer Nature
Switzerland AG 2022
S. Sarikaya et al. (eds.), *Andrology and Sexual Medicine*, Management of Urology,
https://doi.org/10.1007/978-3-031-12049-7_6

dard, and is the treatment option that can most rapidly and reliably correct a penile deformity. Although surgical treatment is reliable, it is not without potential complications that are not as infrequent as both surgeon and patient would desire Surgical treatment options for Peyronie's disease can be categorized into one of three types: tunical shortening procedures, tunical lengthening procedures and penile prosthesis implantation, with or without adjunct straightening techniques.

Introduction

Peyronie's Disease (PD) is a common acquired connective tissue disorder of the tunica albuginea (TA) characterized by the presence of a localized fibrotic plaque that reduces the elasticity of TA itself leading to penile curvature (PC), shortening or narrowing, painful erection and sexual discomfort [1]. Symptoms of PD are reported to create physically and psychologically devastating problems for the patient, the partner and the relationship alike; it could be considered not only a patient's disease but a couple disease. The etiology of PD is still unknown and unclear, but the most accredited theory is that it could be a wound-healing disorder caused by repetitive microvascular injury or trauma to the TA [2]. There are different therapeutic options for the treatment of PD, non-surgical (oral, topical, injectable, mechanical, or combined therapies) and surgical, the choice of which depends on the degree of curvature and the intensity of the symptoms [3].

Epidemiology

Epidemiological data on PD are limited and the results can range because inclusion of patients with different comorbidities within the study population. The onset age of PD is between 45 and 60 years [4]; *Mulhall et al.* reported, in a review of 1500 patients, that 53.5 years was the age of presentation of disease [5].

PD is not a rare disease, it is estimated that the prevalence in general population is between 0.3% to 13.1%, but can increase in some specific sub-populations [6]. The biggest study to analyze the prevalence of PD was performed by *Schwarzer et al.* [7], in which 8000 men in Germany were recruited through the administration of a questionnaire, and a total of 4432 (55.4%) responded; the results showed a prevalence of 3.2% of PD, much higher than other previous studies. Furthermore, the prevalence age-related was 1.5% in the group aged 30–39, 3% in those 40–49 and 50–59, 4% in those 60–69; the highest prevalence was 6.5% in men >70 years. In the United States the prevalence of PD is reported to be between 0.4% and 3.2% [8]. In an Italian multicenter population-based epidemiological survey was found a larger rate of prevalence of PD (7.1%) [9]. In a Japanese study the prevalence of PD was lower than the other studies (0.6%) in healthy Japanese men, which suggests a possible racial difference [10].

It is possible that these reported data of prevalence of PD are falsely low and the occurrence of PD could be higher due patients' disinclination to report an embarrassing condition to their physician. In addition, associations were pointed out between PD and aging, hypertension, diabetes and self-reported ED [11]. *El-Sakka et al.*, in a population study with 1440 male patient with erectile dysfunction (ED), assessed that prevalence of PD in ED patients were higher than general population (7.9%); moreover 11.8% had mild, 38.3% had moderate and 49.9% had severe ED [12]. The prevalence of PD in diabetic patients with ED was investigated by *Arafa et al.*; they evaluated 206 diabetic patients and 42 (20.3%) had PD [13]. The prevalence of PD was evaluated in 532 men presenting for prostate cancer screening: a palpable penile plaque was found in 48 men (8.9%): of these men 32 (6%) reported noticing PC [5]. An association between PD and Dupuytren's disease (DD) was recorded and reported for the first time in 1828; according to a single-center study in Dutch, PD patients showed coexisting DD in 20% of cases [14].

Penile Anatomy And Peyronie's Disease

The penile rigidity depends by the corpora cavernosa, that are surrounded by the TA. The latter is a multilayered structure composed of type-1 collagen oriented with an inner circular and outer longitudinal layer interlaced with elastin fibers separated by an incomplete septum; this is anchored into the inner circular layer and maintains the structural integrity of the tunica [15, 16]. Microvascular trauma to the anchor sites may be one of the triggers leading to PD [17].

Intracavernous pillars reinforce the structure which anchor the TA across the corpora cavernosa at the 2 to 6 o'clock and 10 to 6 o'clock positions, and with finer pillars at the 5 and 7 o'clock positions. The longitudinal layer of the TA is thinnest at the 3 and 9 o'clock positions and it is absent between the 5 and 7 o'clock positions of the corpora [18]. *Pryor and Ralph* evaluated that 60% to 70% of plaques are located on the dorsal aspect of the penis and they are usually associated with the septum [19].

Etiology

The etiology of PD is unknown and still debated, but it could involve abnormal wound healing and development of a fibrotic plaque, not too dissimilar to that of a keloid scar [20]. Penile trauma is considered the major risk factor of PD [2] and it could be caused by surgical treatments or accidents, or may be due to repetitive trauma during sexual intercourse. Collagen synthesis is increased in respect to its breakdown, but also the excessive deposition of type I and III collagen reduces the elasticity of the TA, limiting lengthening and causing PC [18].

The first study to suggest a genetic origin in PD was reported by *Willscher et al.* who noted a genetic transmission mode via HLA-B7 cross-reacting group [21]. Many others hypotheses about genetic etiology of PD have been proposed: elevated levels of transforming growth factor-β1 (TGF-β1), caused by a single nucleotide polymorphism, leading to activation of collagen I synthesis [22]; duplication of chromosome 7 and 8 and deletion of chromosome Y [23]; over expression of gene pleitrophin (PTN/OSF-1) that leads to fibroblast proliferation [24]; epigenetic regulation by histone deacetylases (HDAC), in particular epigenetics modification involves HDAC inhibition [25].

Other studies have suggested a possible role of hypogonadism in PD. *Moreno and Morgentaler* found that 74.4% of patients with PD presented low testosterone levels (<300 ng/dL); furthermore, low testosterone levels were related with PC as compared with eugonadal patients [26]. Instead, *Kirby et al.* found no correlation between low testosterone levels and higher rate of PC [27].

In literature many studies reported risk factors that included comorbidity conditions such as advancing age, obesity, dyslipidemia, diabetes, atherosclerosis and psychosomatic disorders [28, 29]. *Usta et al.* reported that 68% of patients with PD had at least one of the comorbidity and hypertension and smoking were the most frequently comorbidities associated [30]. *Kadioglu et al.* reported at least one risk factor for systemic vascular disease in 53.7% of patients with PS, with DM and hypercholesterolemia that were the most common [11]. *Pavone et al.* reported percentages statistically significant of smokers patients with PD (40%), otherwise the percentage between the not smokers is significantly lower (26%); in the same way they reported a significantly association between PD and blood hypertension [31]. In *Bjekic's et al.* case control study, diabetes and hypertension are significant related to PD [28].

Pathogenesis

Many theories for the pathogenesis of PD have been proposed.

The theory mainly accepted by the authors is trauma or microtrauma to the TA, especially during sexual intercourse in susceptible individuals. Microtrauma leads to inflammation, disruption of the elastic fibers, deposition of fibrin, a potent chemoattractant, with the attraction of inflammatory cells and mediators (macrophage, neutrophils, mast cells, cytokines, and fibroblast) [32].

Some authors reported a possible role of the immune system. Peyronie's patients showed increased levels of elastin antibodies (anti-tropoelastin and anti-α-elastin) [33].

An oxidative damaged-based genesis of PD is demonstrated considering an imbalance between nitric oxide (NO) and reactive oxygen species (ROS); an increase in the level of inducible nitric oxide synthase (iNOS) can be detected after injection of TGF-β1. NO causes the creation of peroxynitrite, associated with the release of ROS, that lead to the enhanced activity of fibroblast and fibrogenesis [34].

Cantini et al. evaluated overexpression of myostatin (member of TGF-β family) in PD plaques; it induced new plaque upon administration and condensed the already formed plaque of TGF-β1 [35].

Course of Disease

Generally, PD is characterized by two consecutives phases: an acute inflammatory phase followed by a chronic phase.

The acute phase is characterized by penile pain and a progressive increase in plaque size or PC. The duration of this phase is 12 months from the onset of the disease. If left untreated in this phase, PD deteriorates. *Mulhall et al.* demonstrated that PC worsened in almost half of the cohort (246), while 12% of patients improved in terms of degree of curvature, 40% remained stable and 48% worsened during the follow-up period (1 year without treatment) [36].

The chronic phase is a period of stability with the absence of penile pain in which PC and plaque size remain the same; it is generally accepted to be 12 months after the onset of the disease [37].

Clinical Aspects

The most frequent presenting symptoms of patients with PD include penile pain, erectile deformity and palpable plaque, as well as ED [19, 38]. Not all patients experience pain or are able to palpate a plaque. Pain, in the acute phase, can occur in the flaccid condition with plaque palpation, with erection, or during intercourse. Chronic phase is characterized by pain resolution, but in some patients pain may persist as a "torque" when a strong erection occurs [39]. Type of curvature influences sexual activity: patients with dorsal curvature, up to 60 degrees, could not have impairment in sexual activity but patients with ventral or lateral curvature may have more difficult with intromission because of discomfort.

Patient's estimates of curvature are unreliable. *Bacal et al.* reported that 50% of patients overestimated their degree of curvature by an average of 20 degrees [40].

Kelami, in 1983, introduced classification of curvature by degrees: mild <30°, moderate between 31° and 60° and severe >60° [41].

Penile deformity is usually defined by the orientation of the plaque. Patients with simple dorsal plaque usually tend to have dorsal curvature; transverse or spiraling scars, partial or circumferential, could lead to varying degrees of curvature including hourglass deformity [19].

Diagnosis

The diagnosis of PD should be based, as with all medical conditions, on a comprehensive medical and sexual history and a detailed physical examination [42].

In particular, the interview should focus on symptoms of the acute phase (pain, deformity and palpable plaque) and on erectile dysfunction. Penile pain is present in the early phase (6 months) and resolve spontaneously for the 90% of patients in the first year from the onset [19, 36].

The patient should be asked about personal or family history of other fibrotic disorders including Dupuytren's or Ledderhose disease.

Correlation between ED and PD has been demonstrated in 55% of the patients. Administration of International Index of Erectile Function (IIEF) questionnaires and use of duplex ultrasonography may be performed in case of ED suspicion. Ultrasonography is also a useful tool for the plaque size and placement measurements [42].

Penile deformity causes distress in patients documented by mental health questionnaires showing depression in 48% of patients [43]. PD questionnaire (PDQ) is a recent validated tool to evaluate not only structural changes of the penile conformity bat also how PD affects psychological condition of the patients. The questionnaire has 15 items divided in three domains: Peyronie's psychological and physical symptoms, penile pain and the effects of PD symptoms [44].

The value of a photograph of the erect penis is controversial but can be useful during the initial consultation; it should be taken by the patient from above and from the side in the erect state.

The penis should be examined on stretch to asses and identify the Peyronie's plaque. The location of the plaque is important, but measurement of the plaque is inaccurate; furthermore there is no evidence that a size reduction is associated with curvature reduction [45].

The stretched penile length (SPL) is also a parameter to measure. It should be measured from the pubis to the corona dorsally. The consistence of the plaque should be also recorded: "rock hard", a sign of calcification but it will need to be confirmed with ultrasonography (hyperdensity of the plaque with shadowing behind) [46]. It is demonstrated that the previous notion according which calcification is an indicator of chronic phase is untrue, because it can occur early after the onset of the scarring process [45]; it is most likely the result of genetic subtypes in which there is the activation of osteoblastic activity [47].

Levin et al. published a calcification grading system: no calcification, grade 1 (<0.3 cm), grade 2 (0.3–1.5 cm) and grade 3 (>1.5 cm or multiple plaques ≥1.0 cm) [43].

Assessment of penile deformity and curvature in the erect state should be performed whit ICI (intra cavernous injection) or vacuum devices. *Ohebshalom et al.* demonstrated that the use of vasoactive agents is the most accurated method to assess the PC, especially in patients with ED [48]. Furthermore several studies demonstrated that the preoperative erectile function (EF) correlates with post-operative results [43, 49].

Oral Treatment

The specific pathophysiology of PD still remains unknown. Despite the published recommendations, there is no a consensus about the optimal therapeutical approach to the disease. Medical treatment is often employed in the early stage of PD, when there are symptoms but should not be fibrotic or calcific plaque [50]. It is important to recognize that there are few randomized control trials (RCT) available about oral therapy in PD.

Potaba

Potassium aminobenzoate (Potaba) is a member of the vitamin B complex. *Zarafonetis and Horrax* demonstrated mechanism of action: in fibroblast cell cultures potassium aminobenzoate can reduce the formation of collagen. It is believed that this drug, increasing monoamine oxidase activity (MAO), decreases serotonin levels; results are an enhancement of the endogenous antifibrotic properties of tissues [51].

Mechanism of action involves three different patterns: increased oxygen uptake, increased activity of MAO and decreased fibrogenesis, and glycosaminoglycan secretion.

Weidner et al., in a randomized double-blind placebo-controlled trial of 103 patients with noncalcified plaque, reported positive outcomes on penile plaque size but no effect in penile deviation or penile pain [52].

The most suggested therapeutic approach is based on 4 g in three times daily.

Vitamin E

Vitamin E is one of the oldest described oral treatments for the treatment of PD and the most commonly oral treatment prescribed, due to its low cost and the lack of side effects.

It is a fat-soluble vitamin and a natural antioxidant and inhibits fibrosis by acting as a scavenger of ROS, known to be increased during the acute and proliferative phases of wound healing.

Several well-designed studies have demonstrated no significant improvement in pain, curvature, and plaque size when compared with placebo [42]. *Gelbard et al.* compared treatment with vitamin E with the natural history of PD with no differences between the two groups in terms of curvature, pain, or the ability to have intercourse [53]. In a randomized double-blind placebo-controlled study of a total of 236 men with PD vitamin E administration did not show benefit [54].

The most commonly suggested dose is based on 400 UI once or twice daily dosage. Possible adverse events include nausea, vomiting, diarrhea, headache and dizziness.

Colchicine

Colchicine is a drug commonly used for treatment of acute gout attacks; it seems to have three hypothetic mechanisms of action: anti-inflammatory effect due to inhibition cytokine release from leukocytes, inhibits collagen synthesis and subsequent fibrosis by inhibiting neutrophil microtubules [55]. Three prospective studies without control groups revealed an improvement in penile pain, plaque size and PC with oral colchicine. *Akkus et al.* reported that colchicine resolved penile pain in 78%, plaque size in 50% and PC in 38% of patients [56]. *Kadioglu et al.* showed that colchicine improved penile pain in 95% and penile deformity in 30% of cases [57]. The combination of colchicine and vitamin E also improved PC in 27% and 40% of patients at 3 and 6 months follow-up [58].

The most common drug-related adverse effects include gastrointestinal effects (nausea, vomiting, diarrhea).

Tamoxifen

Tamoxifen is a selective estrogen receptor modulator (SERM) with tissue-specific activities depending on tissue-specific estrogen receptor expression. Proposed mechanism of Tamoxifen in PD is the modulation of TGF-β secretion from fibroblast; higher concentrations of TGF-β in the cellular environment inhibit the inflammatory response, with macrophage deactivation and T-lymphocyte suppression.

Ralph et al. demonstrated that Tamoxifen was effective in improving penile pain, plaque size and PC [59]. This results were not confirmed in a subsequent randomized placebo-controlled trial [60].

Carnitine

L-carnitine is a trimethylamine molecule that naturally occurring as a metabolic intermediate; it facilitates entry of long-chain fatty acids into oxidative energy cycle, inhibiting acetyl coenzyme-A to help repair of damaged cells.

Biagiotti and Cavallini compared L-carnitine (1 g twice daily) with tamoxifen (20 mg twice daily) in a RCT involving 48 patients in the early stage of PD. They reported that L-carnitine was significantly more effective than tamoxifen in terms of PC and penile pain improvement [61].

The same group documented that the combination of L-carnitine with intralesional verapamil injections resulted in better outcomes compared with verapamil and tamoxifen association [62].

Pentoxifylline

Pentoxifylline is a non-specific phosphodiesterase (PDE) inhibitor that has been shown to block the TGF-β1-mediated pathway of inflammation and increase fibrinolytic activity.

In vitro studies reported that pentoxifylline increases cyclic adenosine monophosphate levels and reduces collagen I expression, compared to placebo [63].

Brant et al. reported positive results on use of pentoxifylline on PD patients [64]. The same group showed that pentoxifylline was able to stabilize or decrease calcium content in PD plaque [65].

The most common side effects include nausea, vomiting, dyspepsia, malaise, flushing, dizziness, headache and hypotension.

PDE-5 Inhibitors

PDE5 inhibitors increase the levels of cGMP, inhibit collagen synthesis and induce fibroblast and myofibroblast apoptosis.

Chung et al. reported data about patients with an isolated septal scar without signs of penile deformity treated with tadalafil 2.5 mg daily for 6 months; 69% of patients had resolution of the septal scar [38].

A more recent RCT by *Palmieri et al.* showed that combination of tadalafil with extracorporeal shockwave therapy (ESWT) improves IIEF and quality-of-life (QoL) scores, but did not alter PC and plaque size [66].

Intralesional Injection Therapies

Non-surgical treatments for PD aim to treat patients in the acute and chronic phases of disease. Surgery is still the gold treatment for patients with stable disease. The rationale of intralesional injection therapies is based on fibrotic and inflammatory etiopathology of the disease.

Verapamil

Verapamil is calcium channel-blocker that interferes with extracellular matrix production and decreases collagen and TGF-β production, and also increases collagenase activity.

Several comparative trials viewed at the clinical potential of verapamil in PD.

Rehman et al. compared, in a placebo controlled-study, verapamil 10 mg to saline injection; it demonstrated significant improvement in PC, EF and reduction of plaque size [67].

Shirazi et al., in a randomized placebo-controlled trial, using verapamil versus placebo in 80 patients, did not demonstrated significant verapamil effective in any of the endpoints measured (plaque size, PC, penile pain and EF) [68].

Additional three study investigated, in a randomized setting, verapamil + transdermal electromotive administration; unfortunately they were not able to show a significant reduction in PC [69–71].

Verapamil was compared with hyaluronic acid in a study by *Favilla et al.* [72]. They were able to demonstrate a significant improvement in PC in patients treated with hyaluronic acid.

Currently, the published data for verapamil injection or transdermal electromotive administration verapamil are limited with lack or control groups and statistical analysis. To date there is no recommendation to verapamil application outside clinical trial-setting, and so it is no recommended by the EAU guidelines.

Interferon α-2B

Interferon α-2B decreases fibroblast proliferation, extracellular matrix production and collagen production from fibroblasts improving the wound-healing process.

In a randomized placebo-controlled trial with 103 patients who underwent interferon, was reported a significant improvement in curvature and reduction in pain [73].

Kendirci et al. reported a statistically improvement in PC in patients treated with interferon α-2B compared to placebo, but not for plaque size [74].

A retrospective study detected no differences between interferon α-2B versus interferon α-2B + penile traction in terms of PC or penile length [75].

Overall, interferon α-2B seems to improve only limitedly PC, so it is not recommended by EAU guidelines for the treatment of PD.

Hyaluronic Acid

A comparative non-placebo controlled non-randomized retrospective study has been compared hyaluronic acid injection versus no treatment. They reported that hyaluronic acid could stabilize PC at 6-months follow-up and decrease PC at 12-months follow-up (9.1°); hyaluronic acid injections also reduced plaque size and improved EF, evaluated through IIEF score administration [76].

Two prospective single arm studies reported improvement of PC and EF, reduction of plaque size and penile pain but no formal statistical analysis was performed [77, 78].

The quality of available evidence is too low to recommend the usage of hyaluronic acid in clinical practice.

Clostridium Collagenase

Collagenase clostridium histolyticum (CCH) (Xiapex®) is the first approved non-surgical treatment for PD. It was licensed in December 2013 from Food and Drug Administration (FDA) and subsequently by European Medicines Agency (EMA). It is produced by the bacterium *C. histolyticum* and consists of a mixture of class I and III collagenase that selectively degrades collagen types I and III, which are elevated in PD.

The first analysis of this drug in vitro was performed by *Gelbard et al.*, who demonstrated that CCH reduced plaque size, sparing arteries, nerves and elastic tissues [79].

The phase I prospective, randomized, double-blind, placebo-controlled study was performed with 49 men with PD; the treatment group showed a significant improvement in plaque size and penile deformity [80].

In a phase IIb randomized, double-blind, placebo-controlled trial, 147 patients with PD were enrolled to evaluate the safety and the efficacy of CCH. Patients were randomized in four groups to receive CCH or placebo (3:1) and penile modelling (1:1). Patients receiving CCH and penile modelling had a significant improvement in PC and decrease in symptoms, compared with placebo [81].

Safety and efficacy of CCH was established by two large phase 3 trials named IMPRESS (Investigation for Maximal Peyronie Reduction Efficacy and Safety Studies) I and II [82, 83]. A total of 417 and 415 subjects with stable disease (>12 months) and PC between 30° and 90° degrees were enrolled. The treatment groups were given up to four cycles of treatment at six-weekly intervals; each cycle consisted of two injections of 0.58 mg CCH, two injections per cycle separated by 24–72 h with the second injection followed 24–72 h later by penile modeling. Data revealed that men treated with CCH showed an improvement in PC of 34% ($-7.0°$ ± 14.8°), compared with 18.2% (-9.3 ± 13.6) of the control-group ($p < 0.0001$). There was an additional improvement in PDQ and IIEF.

Levine et al. carried out a phase III clinical trial with 347 patients where they reported a significant improvement of PC of 34% (18.3 ± 14.02) and PDQ score; subgroup analysis reported an improvement of PC of 34% in patients with curvature between 30° and 60°, and a 37% improvement in 60°–90° group [84].

IMPRESS I and II reported adverse events in CCH injection in 84.2% of participants, compared with 36.3% in the control group. The most common complication were confined to penis or groin, and in 79% of case did not require any invasive intervention; they were penile bruising, including hematoma (80% vs. 26%), penile swelling (55% vs. 3.2%) and penile pain (45% vs. 9.3%). Three corporal ruptures were recorded.

In 2017 Ralph's team developed a new modified protocol for CCH injections in order to reduce number of injections, number of visits, cost and duration of treatment [85]. London protocol consisted of three 0.9 mg CCH injections at 4-weeks intervals. This allows a better distribution of the drug among the plaque; furthermore, in the trial protocol, inflammatory swelling after injection made second injection after 1–3 days less precise. In this protocol physician penile modelling is replaced by home penile stretching by the use of vacuum pump in order to reduce the number of patients hospital accesses. Overall, the London protocol consists of a total of three injections over four visits (including assessment) with a duration of treatment of 12 weeks, in comparison to IMPRESS protocol consisting of eight injections, 14 visits and a duration of treatment of 24 weeks. The results of this protocol are comparable to the IMPRESS trial in terms of PC improvement, IIEF domain score and PDQ bother, pain, psychological and physical symptoms domain scores.

There is no unanimous consent regarding the management of the acute phase of PD. *Cocci et al.* evaluated the advantages and the effects of using a single intralesional injection of CCH in patients with the active phase of PD. Overall, 84 patients aged older than 18 years with the acute phase of PD were enrolled. They demonstrated an improvement at the 3-month evaluation in terms of PC, Visual Analogue Scale (VAS) score at rest and during sexual intercourse, mean IIEF-5 score, PDQ-PS, PDQ-PP and PDQ-BD, with the benefit persisting also after 6 months. These preliminary results suggest the effectiveness of this therapeutic option [86].

A retrospective study evaluated the efficacy CCH PD patients with atypical deformities. In the study were enrolled 65 patients that underwent modified treatment protocol (London protocol); patients were instructed to follow a strict routine, with daily penile modeling and stretching at home. Results demonstrated that median changes of PC were −20.0° in ventral PC, −20.0° in hourglass and −15.0° in shortening PC; furthermore, treatment success was not influenced by characteristics of curvature. In conclusion, CCH could represent an effective therapeutic option for the conservative management of patients with atypical PC [87].

In 2019, a systematic review and a network meta-analysis was performed by *Russo et al.* in order to compare the efficacy of different classes of intralesional therapy (CCH, hyaluronic acid, verapamil, and interferon α-2β). Outcomes of the study are the mean change in PC and in EF. Considering PC improvement, CCH showed better outcomes compared with other drugs. When considering improvement in EF, hyaluronic acid, verapamil and interferon α-2β showed a slight increase when compared with CCH. Moreover, verapamil and interferon α-2β showed slightly worse mean change in comparison to hyaluronic acid, whereas interferon α-2β was worse than verapamil. It was not possible compare other specific outcomes (penile pain, plaque size, patient satisfaction), because of the lack of homogeneity across relevant studies. CCH and interferon α-2β showed the best outcome in terms of PC, whereas hyaluronic acid was most efficient in relation to EF [88].

During September and October 2019, there was a lack of Xiapex® in Europe; on November fourth 2019, the company gave notice that Xiapex® is being withdrawn from the European market and it will be exclusively available in the USA [89].

Other Treatments

Penile Traction and Vacuum Devices

Penile traction therapy is a new therapeutic option for PD. Traction, at a cellular level, alters gene expression and encourages cell proliferation; it can also trigger scar remodeling. This process is called *mechanotransduction*, in which mechanical stimuli are converted into chemical responses [90]. Histological staining following traction therapy demonstrated reorganization and remodeling of collagen fibers into uniform packed fibrils parallel to the axis of mechanical strain [88].

An in vitro experimental study performed in order to determine the cellular effects of penile traction using primary Peyronie's cell cultures, demonstrated significant alteration in ultrastructure of the collagen tissue: a significant decrease in ASMA, an increase in metalloproteinases involved in collagen degradation; receptor for AMS, heat shock protein 47 (HSP47) and TGF-β1 receptors were not upregulated [89].

The first study on penile traction therapy was performed by *Levine et al.* [91]. The authors use penile traction on 10 men in which prior medical therapy had failed. They reported a reduction of curvature in all men up to 45°; average reduction was 33%, but this outcome was not statistical significant due to the small sample size. Moreover, all men reported improvement in penile length (0.5–2.5 cm), with no adverse events documented. Results were maintained at 6 months after completion of therapy. The IIEF domain score increased from 18.3 to 23.6.

Gontero et al. performed a phase 2 prospective study on 15 PD patients with a minimum of 12 months history of PS and PC not exceeding 50°. Patients performed penile traction form a minimum of 5 h per day, up to a maximum of 9 h. PC decreased from 31° to 27° at 6 months, which was not statistically significant. However, there was a significant improvement in stretched and flaccid penile length (1.3 and 0.83 cm, respectively). Results were maintained at 12 months [92].

A prospective non-randomized study assessed efficacy of penile traction to PD patients in the acute phase [93]. In this trial, 55 patients, who underwent penile traction for 6–9 h a day for 6 months, were compared with 41 patients also in the acute phase who did not. Mean duration of use was 4.6 h per day. In the interventional group, the PC decreased from 33° at baseline to 15° at 6 months and 13° at 9 months, with a mean decrease of 20° ($p < 0.05$). Additionally, pain scores decreased with treatment while EF and erection hardness improved. Furthermore, the need for surgery was reduced in 40% of patients and simplified the complexity of the surgical procedure (from grafting to plication) in one of every three patients.

The role of penile traction in the management of patients with PD in the stable phase was assessed by *Moncada et al.* [94]. A total of 93 patients with stable PD and no erectile dysfunction were followed for a period of 12-weeks and half of them was treated with *PeniMaster-PRO* (a novel vacuum device that apply the force over the entire glans in order to decrease patient discomfort). Patients in the interventional group were instructed to use the device for 3–8 h daily for 12 consecutively weeks. Patients treated experienced an improvement of PC of 31.2° ($p < 0.001$) at 12 weeks, representing a 41.1% improvement from baseline, which significantly correlates with the number of hours use of the device. The treatment also improved EF and penile length and girth.

Penile vacuum pump therapy is a relatively novel option for patients with PD. The technique uses mechanical forced induced by vacuum for lengthening and widening of the tunica albuginea in order to reduce PC in erection. *Raheem et al.* performed a single-arm observational study to assess the efficacy of vacuum erection device to mechanically straighten the penis in 41 patients with PD. Subjects wore the vacuum device for 10 min twice daily, without the constriction ring, for 12 weeks. Of the 31 patients who completed the study, 21 demonstrated PC reduction by 5° to 25°, three had a worsening of the curvature and in seven the curvature remained the same from the baseline. At the end of the study 51% of patients were satisfied of the outcome and wanted no further treatments, 49% went on to surgical correction [95].

Shockwave Therapy

Shockwave therapy causes mechanical stress and microtrauma in the tissues: direct damage to the penile plaque and increases the vascularity of the targeted area, which leads to the induction of an inflammatory reaction, lysis of the plaque and removal by macrophages [96].

First randomized placebo-controlled trial was presented by *Palmieri et al.* In this study, 100 patients with acute stage of PD were recruited and randomized to receive shockwave therapy (n = 50) or placebo (n = 50). After 12 weeks of treatment were not significantly differences in PC and plaque size between the two groups. At 24 weeks follow-up were noted significant differences in mean plaque size and mean curvature degree, but not clinically meaningful [97].

A second study by *Chitale et al.* employed 36 patients with PD in a stable phase. Patients were randomized to receive shockwave therapy (n = 16) or sham therapy (n = 16). At 6-months follow-up no statistically differences were noted in term of plaque size, PC, IIEF-5 score and VAS [98].

Recently *Hatzichristodoulou et al.* performed a placebo-controlled, prospective randomized single-blind study. 102 PD patients were randomly assigned (n = 51) to shockwave or placebo therapy. After therapy, penile pain decreased in 85% of patients in the shockwave therapy group and in 48.0% of patients in the placebo group, which showed significant difference. No differences were noted in plaque size and deviation angle [99].

In the last RCT, 100 men with PD and ED were randomized to receive Shockwave therapy alone once a week (n = 50) or shockwave therapy + tadalafil 5 mg (n = 50). After 12 and 24 weeks, penile pain during erection was alleviated in both groups compared with baseline. Plaque size and PC were not significantly different in the two groups. In addition, EF was improved more in the combination group [66].

Laser, Radiation and Iontophoresis Therapy

Laser therapy in PD must be used in a nonsurgical modality, energy should be reduced in order to minimize heating effects. The precise biological mechanism of use of laser in PD is still unclear. Has been reported that it causes an increase of cellular effects (collagen and protein synthesis, cell granular decrease, cell proliferation, membrane potential, phagocytosis, ATP synthesis) [100]. Furthermore, local vasodilation cause increase in tissue oxygenation that can also relieve pain.

Studies about laser therapy on PD are small, with methodologically high risk of bias and, above all, relative contradictive. Although it seem to relieve pain in acute phase of disease, decrease of PC or reduction of plaque size seem to temporally. This treatment seems to be not useful in patients with hourglass deformity, complex or ventral deformity and in calcified plaques. Laser-therapy is not approved for treatment of PD, it remains only inside of clinical studies.

Radiation therapy is an empirical treatment for PD, based on studies about Dupuytren's contraction. Historically low-dose of radiations have been used to treat painful erections in patients in the early stages of disease.

Multiple studies have demonstrated varied success in terms of penile pain, PC, plaque size and EF; but the absence of validate means of measuring penile, the limited relevance of plaque size reduction and variable improvement in penile pain are a real problem [101–103]. Considering association with negative collateral effects, this treatment is not recommended in PD.

Iontophoresis of electromotive drug administration (EMDA) is an effective and painless method to deliver medication to a localized tissue area through the use of a constant current. Advantages of this technique include improved onset time and a rapid offset time. In PD patients this technique is used for the transdermal administration of drugs [104].

Many studies confirmed success of association of gel or topical drugs and iontophoresis and EMDA [69–71, 105]. It is a treatment that offers a new option for patients who are distressed by PD but do not want to undergo surgical correction and prefer to avoid intralesional injection therapy.

Combination Therapy

In PD patients single therapies provide limited efficacy. In this setting, combination of two or more conservative treatments may improve symptoms.

A systematic review and meta-analysis has been performed to explore the effects of available conservative combination therapies for active and stable PD. Overall, 13 studies on active PD and 10 on stable PD (1962 participants) were included. In patients with active or stable PD, the available evidence is inconclusive to support the use of any combination treatment modality. Comparing the effects of CCH plus adjunctive mechanical therapies (penile traction or vacuum pump) versus CCH monotherapy on penile curvature and length in patients with stable PD, CCH and adjunctive mechanical therapies resulted in an additional decrease of 0.3° in penile curvature and in an increase of 0.5 cm in penile length [106].

The available combination treatment modalities do not improve symptoms further compared with monotherapy and should not be implemented in patients with active or stable PD. Further high-quality randomized trials combining only recommended treatments are mandatory.

Surgical Treatment

After the resolution of the acute phase, Peyronie's disease (PD) often leaves the patient scarred with a penile deformity that may interfere with sexual intercourse and impact his/their satisfaction with sexual life. Spontaneous resolution of

Peyronie's penile deformity is known to be infrequent, and conservative treatment (when even possible) has some limitations that reduce its appeal or applicability. Thus, men who wish to resolve their penile deformity will more often than not seek surgical treatment. Surgery remains to this day the gold standard, and is the treatment option that can most rapidly and reliably correct a penile deformity.

Although surgical treatment is reliable, it is not without potential complications that are not as infrequent as both surgeon and patient would desire, which may impair the patient's and couple's satisfaction with treatment. Before considering surgical treatment, it is paramount to ensure that it is indicated and, if so, when it can be performed. Not every patient with a penile curvature or deformity will desire, or need, a surgical correction.

Surgical treatment is only indicated for patients who report clinically a significant penile deformity that precludes satisfactory sexual intercourse and/or causes pain for themselves or their partner. Some authors would also consider a curvature or deformity that causes distress (as a result of the appearance of the erect penis) as an indication for surgical treatment; however, the authors of this chapter are not in agreement with this latter indication.

It is fundamental to define what is meant by a "significant deformity". Historically it has been defined by expert opinion as a penile curvature of more than 30 degrees or of a "complex" curvature. By "complex", authors usually mean a hinge or hourglass deformity, which may not cause a significant curvature but can nonetheless impair axial stability during penetration. A simple penile curvature of less than 30 degrees should never be casually regarded as the obvious cause of sexual distress, and other causes (such as penile dysmorphic disorder) should be rigorously examined and excluded before considering the surgical correction of such curvature at the behest of a patient.

As mentioned before, spontaneous resolution in the natural progression of PD is infrequent; however, worsening of curvature after diagnosis can happen in up to 48% of patients [36]. Thus, failure to wait for curvature stabilization is a known cause for early recurrence after surgical correction. It is agreed by expert opinion that patients must have stable condition for at least 3, and as much as 9, months after the onset of PD before considering surgical treatment. In the past, these timeframes were longer (from at least 6 months to more than 12 months after the onset), but in the last decade a shorter compromise between the natural progression of PD and patient distress with waiting has been established.

How to Select the Right Surgical Procedure for the Individual Patient?

Rather than curvature correction *per se*, patient's and couple's satisfaction is the ultimate goal of the surgical correction of a penile deformity. To achieve this goal the correct selection of surgical techniques is paramount. Three important factors should be considered, in this order: erectile function, stretched or erect penile length, and the degree of penile curvature and/or type of penile deformity. No matter how straight a penis may look, a soft erection (or no erection at all) or a perceived short penis will often be a cause for patient's dissatisfaction after a "successful" intra-operative curvature correction.

Questionnaires (such as the International Index of Erectile Function) can be used to exclude concomitant erectile dysfunction (ED), and if there is any doubt regarding patient's erectile function a penile doppler ultrasound or an intracavernous injection test should be performed to exclude vasculogenic ED. Therefore, all candidates must have intact erectile function, or ED responsive to phosphodiesterase 5 inhibitors, so that postoperative ED will be less likely [107].

For PD surgical treatment, a definition for "short" penile length has been suggested by expert opinion as an erect penile length less than 8 cm. It is important to measure the penis reliably and consistently so measurements can be compared over time. Penile length should be recorded, but also how the measurement was performed (e.g., stretched/erect, symphysis pubis/base of penile shaft, dorsal/ventral). Stretched penile length is an excellent surrogate for erect penile length (and pharmacologically induced erect penile length and stretched penile length are both good predictors of post-inflatable prosthesis penile length). The authors suggest measuring the penis dorsally from the symphysis pubis to the tip of the glans, and to also note how many centimeters are buried beneath pubic adiposity. For practicality this is usually performed under stretch, but if a penile doppler ultrasound or intracavernous injection test is indicated, we also measure penile length after intracavernous injection of the vasoactive agent in the same manner.

If during patient assessment a "short" penile length is noted, a shortening tunical procedure will most likely even further decrease penile length, compromising sexual intercourse. Apart from a man's (and sometimes also their partner's) subjective complaints of a shortened penis, a "short" penile shaft can be easily displaced from the introitus under pelvic thrust.

Surgical Techniques

Surgical treatment options for PD can be categorized into one of three types: tunical shortening procedures, tunical lengthening procedures and penile prosthesis implantation (PPI), with or without adjunct straightening techniques (if residual curvature is noted) [108].

For practical purposes, the reader can consider that a penile curvature has two sides: the convex or longer side, usually not affected by the disease; and the concave or shorter side, which is impacted by Peyronie's plaque and fibrosis.

Tunical Shortening Procedures

Tunical shortening procedures are a group of surgical techniques that have in common the contraction of the corpora cavernosa at the convex side of the curvature, thus shortening the healthy side of the corpora to match the restriction in elasticity on the opposing side. The reduction in penile length thus caused is usually at least 1 mm per 10 degrees of desired curvature correction [109]. The downside of such techniques is that penile shortening will always result, and it may be symptomatic and cause dissatisfaction with treatment.

These procedures can be considered for men without complex deformity, non-severe curvature or ED, and an adequate penile length. Numerous different techniques have been described and can be classified as either excisional, incisional, or plication techniques [110–112].

Excisional techniques will incise and excise the tunica, usually in the form of an ellipse with two imaginary points as its co-vertexes, and then close the tunical defect transversally. The first of these techniques was described for the first time in 1965 by Dr. Reed Nesbit in congenital curvatures [113], while Pryor and Fitzpatrick first described the use of the procedure for PD [114]. This is known as the Nesbit technique, and has become a successful option for the treatment of both congenital and acquired penile curvatures, such as PD. The authors hazard to state that this is still the standard technique for tunical shortening. The drawback of this technique has been the concern for veno-occlusive dysfunction due to tunical incision. Some modifications of the original technique have been described, such as partial-thickness excision (not entering the corpus cavernosum) to avoid the latter concern of ED.

Incisional techniques will incise the line between the two imaginary points and then transversally close the defect, following the Heineke-Mikulicz principle. The more popular method has been the Yachia technique, on which the authors have been trained and still use to this date. It was initially described by Lemberger in 1984 [115], and later popularised by Yachia in 1990 when he reported a case-series of 10 patients [116].

Plication techniques will directly suture the two points without incising or excising the tunica albuginea, and thus may limit the potential damage to the veno-occlusive mechanism, preventing postoperative ED [117, 118]. The first described plication technique was the Essed-Schroeder in 1985, in which one or two parallel plications using figure-of-eight sutures to bury the knot were placed [119]. Currently, use of 16 or 24-dot techniques (made widespread by Gholami and Lue) are gaining popularity [120]. In these techniques, two pairs of Lembert-like sutures are placed along the entire penile shaft and are progressively tensioned under penile erection until complete curvature correction is achieved. It has the appealing advantage of allowing the correction of virtually any dorsal and/or lateral curvature with the same technique (only varying tensioning). One disadvantage of the plication technique is that it implies the use of non-absorbable sutures, and knot palpation is known to be a cause for patient dissatisfaction.

The Baskin-Duckett technique, originally described for ventral congenital curvatures [121], and the Levine modification [122] are types of tunica albuginea plications (TAP) in which the incisional principle is used in part, combined with plication. In these techniques, the tunica albuginea is only partially incised (incision shapes and locations may vary depending on the actual technique), not entering the corpus cavernosa, and then the two imaginary points are sutured together as in a regular plication technique.

There is no universally recommended or clearly superior tunical shortening technique. Most have been reported as retrospective case-series, without standardized reporting or comparison with other techniques. In general, tunical shortening techniques allow complete penile straightening in more than 85% of patients. Recurrence of the curvature is uncommon, and the use of non-absorbable sutures or longer-lasting absorbable sutures may reduce its risk. Penile hypoesthesia is uncommon and usually transitory, lasting between 3 and 6 months. The risk of postoperative ED is very low. As previously described, penile shortening will inevitably occur, and it's the most commonly patient-reported adverse outcome for these procedures [110].

Tunical Lengthening Procedures

Tunical lengthening procedures consist of plaque incision, with or without plaque excision, at the concave side of the curvature. It creates a tunica defect that will need to be covered with a graft. This technique thus achieves penile straightening by increasing the length of the "short" concave side.

Depending on the type and location of the curvature different incisional techniques can be applied. The more popular incisional techniques are the I, H and Y incisions. All of these incisions have in common a transverse incision along with the point of maximal curvature. This incision will usually involve half, or almost half, of the circumference of the tunica, with its lateral endings then differing between the incision types. The I incision is the base incision that leaves an ellipsoid defect, and it can be modified so that a perpendicular incision is added to each side, allowing the defect to gain a more quadrilateral shape (which will, in turn, ease the measurement of the defect and trimming of the graft material). The Y incision is also a valuable modification if an hourglass deformity is present. The base I incision will terminate in a Y in each side allowing for tunical enlargement and correction of both the deformity hourglass deformity and curvature. In cases of extreme or complex curvatures, more than one incision may be needed. The use of geometric principles introduced by Paulo Egydio may help to determine the minimal shape and size of the incision to achieve curvature correction [123].

Several grafts have been tried and tested, but the ideal one is yet to be found. The ideal graft should be readily available, cost-effective, easy to use, flexible, resistant to traction, not prone to infection, contraction or ED, cause minimal morbidity if the graft is harvested, and have good host tolerance if not autologous [110]. Grafts can be autologous (taken from the patient, such as the dermis, dorsal penile vein, fascia lata, tunica vaginalis, tunica albuginea or buccal mucosa), allogeneic (also of human origin but from a deceased donor, such as the pericardium, fascia lata or dura mater), xenogeneic (extracted from non-human animal species and tissues, such as bovine pericardium, porcine small intestinal submucosa, bovine and porcine dermis, or TachoSil®), and synthetic grafts (these include Dacron® and Gore-Tex® meshes) [124–126]. Lowsley and Boyce in 1950 experimented with an operation for the management of PD and were the first authors to perform plaque excision and grafting with fat for the treatment of PD, followed by Horton and Devine, in 1974, using a dermal skin graft. Since then, many grafts have been used and are currently in use. Dermal grafts have lost prominence in the last two decades due to their tendency to contract and cause late curvature recurrence. Vein grafts have the theoretical advantage of endothelial-to-endothelial contact when grafted to underlying cavernosal tissue. The saphenous vein has been the most used vein graft, as the superficial penile dorsal vein has a limited size that can be harvested. Moreover, vein grafts often require extensive and laborious graft preparation before suturing to the tunical defect can be performed. The tunica vaginalis has also been used in the past, due its low risk of contraction and its low metabolic requirements; however, it is quite thin and may be prone to aneurism. In recent years, the buccal mucosa (which has historically been one of the most if not the most used autologous graft in urethroplasty) has been applied to penile curvatures, so far with favourable short- and medium-term results.

The drawback of the use of autologous grafts is the added morbidity and surgery time from graft harvesting, so allografts have also been explored. Allografts offer the same biological stability and mechanical resistance as do autologous grafts, with the advantage of being ready-to-use and having no added morbidity. Cost-effectiveness may depend on local pricing. Cadaveric dura mater is no longer in use, but cadaveric fascia lata, temporalis fascia and pericardium (Tutoplast©) are currently in use, with the latter being the most used.

Xenografts have been trending in the last two decades and are by now the most favored option by genitourinary surgeons, as they are ready-to-use. Small intestinal submucosa (formerly Surgisis® and now Biodesign®), a type I collagen-based xenogenic graft derived from the submucosal layer of the porcine small intestine, has been shown to promote tissue-specific regeneration and angiogenesis, and supports host cell migration, differentiation and growth of endothelial cells, resulting in tissue structurally and functionally like the original. The four-layer version of Biodesign® has ideal mechanical resistance, but it is necessary to add an extra 20% in graft length and width to accommodate its tendency to undergo later contraction. The authors are well versed in this graft and has used it in the past [127].

Although first described in 2002 [128], only in the last decade with Hatzichristodoulou's publications has collagen fleece (TachoSil©) been gaining interest [129–131]. Its use in PD has two major advantages: decreased operating time, as no suturing is required after proper application, and it has an additional hemostatic effect. According to Hatzichristodoulou's popularized technique, the collagen fleece should be moistened in physiological saline before being molded to the tunical defect, and care should take to ensure that an overlapping margin of at least 5 mm is achieved in all borders, with no suture recommended. The authors currently uses this graft and prefer to first mold the graft to the tunical defect and only then moisten it with a sponge embedded in physiological saline (If previously moistened the graft can become too fragile and may easily rupture). Initially, it was widely thought that collagen fleece could not be used for ventral curvatures, but this has been refuted by Hatzichristodoulou [132], although in a limited sample. Other xenografts in current use are bovine pericardium.

Synthetic grafts should be avoided presently, as better options are now clearly available. Synthetic grafts have shown an increased risk of infection, secondary graft inflammation that can cause significant tissue fibrosis, significant graft contracture, and can even possibly cause allergic reactions. The authors are only familiar with its use for PPI for gender-affirming surgery and have no experience with its used for tunical lengthening corporoplasty.

As a whole, tunical lengthening procedures can be considered as an option for patients with significant penile shortening, severe curvature (>60°) and/or complex deformities such as hourglass or hinge effects without underlying ED. Barring synthetic grafts, graft selection should be based on availability and surgeon's experience, as there is a lack of randomized controlled trials comparing grafts. Although very heterogeneous populations and methods are used, results seem to be comparable between grafts. Complete penile straightening is achieved in more than 85% of patients, along with a 1–1.5 cm gain in penile length, but overall these techniques have shown a higher risk of ED than tunical shortening procedures due to veno-occlusive dysfunction, as well as higher rates of penile hypo-aesthesia.

In conclusion, autologous grafts present the disadvantage of added morbidity and increased operative time due to graft harvesting. Allografts and xenografts have been trending in the last two decades, although their added cost can be prohibitive in some countries. Almost all grafts still require graft suturing to the tunical defect and this surgical step (although straightforward) is usually time-consuming and in some cases, such as in the presence of an ossified plaque, can also be challenging. The sole exception are collagen fleeces, which do not require suturing and have shown a significant reduction in operative time when compared with other grafts [133]. This characteristic of collagen fleece is the driver of its uptrend.

Penile Prothesis Implant

For patients with PD and ED unresponsive to medical therapy, PPI is required, and if needed must be combined with tunical lengthening procedures.

Patients with ED and less than 30° of curvature or an hourglass deformity may be treated with prothesis implantation alone, not requiring any additional measures. Regular cycling of the penile prothesis will gradually straighten the penis and resolve its deformity. Intraoperatively, when the curvature exceeds 30° and is not ventral, manual modeling (the so-called "Wilson's maneuver", or forcefully bending the clamped inflated penile prothesis in the opposite direction of the curvature for at least 90 straight seconds two times) may result in sufficient straightening of the penis [134, 135]. This maneuver has a 3–5% risk of urethral perforation, most likely due to distal extrusion of cylinders at the fossa navicularis [39]. If after two attempts the curvature remains greater than 30°, additional maneuvers should be considered to optimize straightening. Further curvature correction can be achieved either by lengthening the shorter side of the shaft with relaxing tunical incisions or by shortening the longer side with plications; usually tunical lengthening is preferred is this case as ED is not a concern, and penile shortening is a common complain of patients with PD.

Tunical lengthening combined with PPI has similar principles to the aforementioned techniques, and those can also be applied in this setting allowing up to a 2 cm gain in penile length; yet as ED and veno-occlusive dysfunction are not an issue in this setting, more advanced incisional patterns can be applied to allow a farther gain in penile length (between 2 and 4 cm). The first of these techniques was the Sliding technique [136], which involved both dorsal neurovascular bundle and urethral dissection, tunical incision in a specific pattern and tunical "sliding" until maximal length of the neurovascular bundle and urethra were achieved, then use of a double ventral-dorsal porcine small intestinal submucosal graft. This technique was later modified by Paulo Egydio—the Modified Sliding Technique, also known as MoST [136]—to optimize surgical time and avoid graft placement: only the tunica was incised and the corpus cavernosa was only separated dorsally from the tunica, allowing the corpus to cover the ventral defect, while the dorsal defect was only covered with Buck's fascia. Later, the same author added a dorsal incision to split the dorsal gap into two smaller ones to avoid cylinder herniation—the technique known as Multiple-Slit Technique (MuST) [136]. These modifications allowed a significant shortening of operative time but, unfortunately, these techniques have an increased risk of glans necrosis, a very rare but devastating complication. It is believed that extensive combined dissection of the urethra and neurovascular bundle can be a risk factor for glans necrosis, and the latter author has adjusted his MuST technique to the Tunical Expansion Procedure (TEP). In this, no mobilization of the urethra is required and combined dorso-ventral tunical incisions are replaced by multiple 5–8 mm incisions along the tunical shaft to permit tunical lengthening [136, 137]. This technique also promises an average penile lengthening of 3.5 cm. Other modifications of these more popular techniques have also been described, but the authors believe that advanced tunical lengthening procedures should only be performed in a high-volume center as care to precise detail is critical to avoid complications and ensure patient satisfaction.

Adjuvant Procedures

Circumcision

Historically, circumcision has was recommended during curvature corrections, especially if phimosis was present. However, not every patient will have phimosis, and it is known that even a "minor" adjuvant procedure such as a circumcision can be a cause of patient dissatisfaction. A decade ago, Prof. David Ralph's group published a case series that showed that, in patients with normal foreskins, if no circumcision was performed during tunical procedures a secondary circumcision was only required in 0.8% of patients [136]. Our experience has shown us that circumcision can safely be avoided, but that transitory edema of the foreskin with difficult retraction may last between 3 to 6 months. The decision for secondary circumcision should be delayed until after this timeframe.

Other alternatives to avoid circumcision are alternative surgical incisions (to the standard subcoronal incision), like the median incision along the penile shaft or, for combined PPI, everting the penile shaft through the traditional penoscrotal incision.

The authors further recommend that if circumcision is routinely performed or is deemed necessary, it should be discussed beforehand with the patient.

Penile Cosmetic Surgeries

Although not well documented in published literature, penile cosmetic surgeries such as suspensory ligament resection, with or without V-Y plasty, or ventral phalloplasty/scrotoplasty, are sometimes combined with tunical procedures to enhance the flaccid penile length in response to patient's complaining of penile shortening. It is important to note that these techniques do not increase penile length when erect, and in the absence of symptomatic dorsal suprapubic web or ventral scrotal web they should not be performed. These techniques are out of the scope of this chapter and will not be further discussed.

Surgical Technique

The authors will describe their standard approach for a dorsal or dorso-lateral penile curvature in a patient without clinically significant ED and in whom the placement of a penile prothesis is not intended. Trichotomy is performed at the table and the skin is prepared with an iodopovidone solution. Antibiotic prophylaxis is usually limited to a single-dose first-generation cephalosporin given just before surgical incision. The authors recognize that possibly no antibiotic prophylaxis is warranted as this is a clean procedure. Thromboprophylaxis is performed according to individual patients' thrombotic risk.

For a standard tunical procedure, a subcoronal incision 1 cm below the coronal sulcus is performed. At this point, if circumcision is to be routinely performed or if significant phimosis is identified, excessive foreskin is resected. Dartos' fascia is incised circumferentially until Buck's fascia is identified, and complete degloving of the entire penile shaft is performed along this fascia. Buck's fascia is incised bilaterally by two longitudinal para-urethral incisions. It is important to note that distally the neurovascular bundle fans out, and care should be taken to not incise Buck's fascia at this point. *Tips and tricks*: If a collagen fleece graft is planned, care should be taken to leave at least a 1-cm margin from the urethra edge, as this will ease graft placement and Buck's fascia closure. If a pure lateral curvature is present and a tunical shortening procedure is planned, Buck's fascia can be open just unilaterally opposite to the curvature.

At this point, an artificial saline erection is induced, and penile curvature axis is noted. If a plication tunical procedure is planned, an artificial erection can be induced before incision is performed with an intracavernous vasoactive agent such as alprostadil (this will ease the correct tensioning of plication suture and avoid the need for artificial saline). If a tunical shortening procedure is planned, then at this point tunical plication, incision or excision is performed. *Tips and tricks*: In case tunical excision or incision was chosen, Allis clamps can be used to simulate tunical shortening and curvature correction. The Allis jaws will leave the tunica albuginea marked and these marks can be used as a reference for incision or excision. The use of non-absorbable sutures or longer-lasting absorbable sutures may reduce recurrence of the curvature and should be preferred.

On the other hand, if a tunical lengthening procedure is planned, the dorsal neurovascular bundle is mobilized, taking care not to use traction as it can cause postoperative penile hypoesthesia. Bipolar cautery should be preferred during this step. Once again, it should be noted that the neurovascular bundle fans out distally and should only be detached from the tunica and not cut at this time-point. The penile shaft is clamped using a rubber band or bladder catheter, and an artificial erection is performed, noting the pole of the penile curvature. A perpendicular line to the penile shaft is marked at the pole of the curvature using a pen. A semi-circumferential I, H or Y incision is performed along this line using the pole of the curvature as its midpoint. An H incision is the most versatile incision as its edges can be prolonged to allow further tunical lengthening. A formula proposed by Egydio can be used to calculate the minimum dimensions required for complete curvature correction [136]. As an alternative, the surgeon can extend the H edges proximally and distally until the penile shaft matches the neurovascular bundle length. Usually, an Y incision is reserved for an hourglass deformity and will also ease girth restoration. The incision edges can then be trimmed so a quadrilateral shape is formed, and the tunical defect width and length are measured. The graft is cut to size, and if the chosen graft is known to be at risk of postoperative contraction, an extra 20% should be added to noted measurements. The graft is used to cover the tunical defect and is sutured. *Tips and tricks:* Suture can be performed in quadrants, and if two surgeons are present two simultaneous sutures can be performed on opposite sides. This can significantly reduce penile clamp time. If a collagen fleece is used, no suture is required and a simple I incision is usually sufficient.

After the graft is sutured, an artificial erection is repeated, and residual curvature is assessed. If a residual curvature is present, it is usually mild and can be corrected with an additional tunical shortening procedure. The penile clamp is removed, and Buck's fascia is closed bilaterally. The Dartos is approximated at the original sub-coronal incision, and the foreskin is closed using either separate or continuous fast-reabsorbing sutures.

A compressive dressing is applied to the penile shaft, its distal edges fixed to the coronal sulcus using spare sutures, leaving the urethral meatus clear of the dressing. The dressing is left in place between 2 to 7 days to prevent significant penile hematoma and edema. If only a tunical shortening procedure was performed a compressive bandage can de left in place for just a day and there is no need for suture.

Postoperative Cares

Postoperative care is especially important for tunical lengthening procedures, as penile rehabilitation is paramount for success. Patients can be safely discharged on the same or the next day with the dressing in place. An appointment is scheduled the week after for dressing removal and wound care. If no significant complications are noted, the patient is started on daily tadalafil 5 mg and is instructed on how to perform penile massage (gentle penile stretching and contralateral bending for 30 min a day. After 4 weeks the patient is reassessed, and if no complication is noted sexual intercourse may be resumed. At this point the patient is questioned regarding spontaneous erection rigidity and residual penile curvature, and counseled regarding penile hypoesthesia if present. At 3 months of follow-up patient is assessed regarding their ability to successfully resume sexual function, and if not then reasons for lack of success are explored. If the patient was able to satisfactorily resume sexual intercourse tadalafil is stopped at this time point.

Complications

Although generally safe, surgical correction of PD can have some complications. However, the authors will not describe complications of PPI here because it exceeds the objective of this chapter.

Persistence and Recurrence of Curvature

The failure to fully correct curvature is one of the most common complications, and is probably due to surgical failure. Recurrence likely results from failure to wait until the disease has stabilized, reactivation of previously stable disease, or the use of early absorbable sutures. There are no studies proving the superiority of any one technique with regards to preventing curvature recurrence. Residual curvature may be acceptable if of minimal magnitude. If excessive, however, it may be considered poor surgical technique and can result in patient dissatisfaction [109, 136]. Up to 22% of recurrent curvatures are severe and surgery may again be necessary [111]. Rehabilitation programs based on penile traction, penile massage and phosphodiesterase 5 inhibitors may reduce the risk of penile curvature recurrence and shortening [138]. If necessary, revision surgery should be carried out after complete healing, stabilization of the curvature and assessment of erectile function. By consensus, it should occur at least 6 months after the initial procedure.

Erectile Dysfunction

De novo ED is the Achilles heel of PD surgery, having a higher incidence (around 20–36%) in grafting procedures [139–141]. It's multifactorial, with the main contributors involving disruption of the veno-occlusive mechanism in the case of graft procedures. Also, neurovascular bundle damage during its mobilization, psychogenic etiology, and even circumcision are risk factors [111, 142]. For those who do not already have it, PPI can be a solution in patients who have developed de novo refractory ED, being executed in a delayed fashion.

Glans Necrosis

Glans necrosis has never been reported after tunical shortening procedures. Although rare it can occur in up to 2.4% of patients submitted to concomitant tunical lengthening and PPI, and it is a feared complication [143]. It is usually associated with advanced tunical lengthening (such as "sliding" techniques) or coincident distal urethral injury repair, and both have been identified as intra-operative risk factors. The presence of preoperative comorbidities such as atherosclerotic cardiovascular disease, diabetes mellitus, smoking, previous prosthesis explanation, and previous radiation therapy are other postulated risk factors [144, 145]. Immediate prosthesis removal is recommended in the presence of risk factors as expectant management often leads to significant glans loss.

Other Complications

Grafting procedures can also result in bulging/ballooning, promoting a new penile deformity in 12.5% of patients, being severe in only 3% [111]. Although uncommon, this may also arise following plication procedures. Correction is made by excision of the dilated tunical segment and subsequent graft insertion.

Almost three-quarters of patients also report the feeling of palpation of surgical knots, but pain is only present in 4–6% [111, 146, 147]. This occurs typically when non-absorbable sutures are used. It can be diminished with the use of long-lasting absorbable sutures, that provide suture tension for a long enough time to be effective while being eventually absorbed in weeks to months.

Glans hyposthesia results from neuropraxia, but infiltration of Peyronie's plaque into the neurovascular bundle structures has also been proposed as a possible cause [118]. It is usually transient, with resolution within 12 months from surgery.

Conclusion

Surgical treatment of PD has high rates of success but it is not devoid of complications. It is paramount to first ensure that the patient really needs surgical treatment, and if so then erectile function, penile length and the severity of the curvature should be taken into account to select the surgical technique. Some techniques, such as advanced tunical lengthening procedures, are more complex and can have devastating complications, and thus we counsel that these should be performed only by experienced genito-urinary reconstructive surgeons in high-volume centers. Being a theme of the intimacy of the man and the couple, it is imperative to carefully explain the procedure to the patient to avoid false expectations, dissatisfaction with outcomes, and possible medico-legal issues to the surgeon.

References

1. Taylor FL, Levine LA. Peyronie's disease. Urol Clin N Am. 2007;34(4):517–34.
2. de Rose AF, Mantica G, Bocca B, Szpytko A, van der Merwe A, Terrone C. Supporting the role of penile trauma and micro-trauma in the etiology of Peyronie's disease. Prospective observational study using the electronic microscope to examine two types of plaques. Aging Male. 2020;23(5):740–5.
3. Capoccia E, Levine LA. Contemporary review of Peyronie's disease treatment. Curr Urol Rep. 2018;19(7):51.
4. Tal R, Hall MS, Alex B, Choi J, Mulhall JP. Peyronie's disease in teenagers. J Sex Med. 2012;9(1):302–8.
5. Mulhall JP, Creech SD, Boorjian SA, Ghaly S, Kim ED, Moty A, et al. Subjective and objective analysis of the prevalence of Peyronie's disease in a population of men presenting for prostate cancer screening. J Urol. 2004;171(6 Part 1):2350–3.
6. DiBenedetti DB, Nguyen D, Zografos L, Ziemiecki R, Zhou X. A population-based study of Peyronie's disease: prevalence and treatment patterns in the United States. Adv Urol. 2011;2011:1–9.
7. Schwarzer U, Sommer F, Klotz T, Braun M, Reifenrath B, Engelmann U. The prevalence of Peyronie's disease: results of a large survey. BJU Int. 2001;88(7):727–30.
8. Lindsay MB, Schain DM, Grambsch P, Benson RC, Beard CM, Kurland LT. The incidence of Peyronie's disease in Rochester, Minnesota, 1950 through 1984. J Urol. 1991;146(4):1007–9.
9. la Pera G, Pescatori ES, Calabrese M, Boffini A, Colombo F, Andriani E, et al. Peyronie's disease: prevalence and association with cigarette smoking. Eur Urol. 2001;40(5):525–30.
10. Shiraishi K, Shimabukuro T, Matsuyama H. The prevalence of Peyronie's disease in Japan: a study in men undergoing maintenance hemodialysis and routine health checks. J Sex Med. 2012;9(10):2716–23.
11. Kadioglu A, Sanli O, Akman T, Canguven O, Aydin M, Akbulut F, et al. Factors affecting the degree of penile deformity in Peyronie disease: an analysis of 1001 patients. J Androl. 2011;32(5):502–8.
12. El-Sakka AI. Prevalence of Peyronie's disease among patients with erectile dysfunction. Eur Urol. 2006;49(3):564–9.
13. Arafa M, Eid H, El-Badry A, Ezz-Eldine K, Shamloul R. The prevalence of Peyronie's disease in diabetic patients with erectile dysfunction. Int J Impot Res. 2007;19(2):213–7.
14. Nugteren HM, Nijman JM, de Jong IJ, van Driel MF. The association between Peyronie's and Dupuytren's disease. Int J Impot Res. 2011;23(4):142–5.
15. Gentile V, Modesti A, la Pera G, Vasaturo F, Modica A, Prigiotti G, et al. Ultrastructural and immunohistochemical characterization of the tunica albuginea in Peyronie's disease and veno-occlusive dysfunction. J Androl. 1996;17(2):96–103.
16. Kelly DA. Penises as variable-volume hydrostatic skeletons. Ann N Y Acad Sci. 2007;1101(1):453–63.
17. Devine CJ Jr, Somers KD, Jordan GH, Schlossberg SM. Proposal: trauma as the cause of the Peyronie's lesion. J Urol. 1997;157(1):285–90.
18. Brock G, Hsu GL, Nunes L, von Heyden B, Lue TF. The anatomy of the tunica albuginea in the normal penis and Peyronie's disease. J Urol. 1997;157(1):276–81.
19. Pryor JP, Ralph DJ. Clinical presentations of Peyronie's disease. Int J Impot Res. 2002;14(5):414–7.

20. Somers KD, Dawson DM. Fibrin deposition in Peyronie's disease plaque. J Urol. 1997;157(1):311–5.
21. Willscher MK, Cwazka WF, Novicki DE. The association of histocompatibility antigens of the B7 cross-reacting group with Peyronie's disease. J Urol. 1979;122(1):34–5.
22. Awad MR, El-Gamel A, Hasleton P, Turner DM, Sinnott PJ, Hutchinson IV. Genotypic variation in the transforming growth factor-beta1 gene: association with transforming growth factor-beta1 production, fibrotic lung disease, and graft fibrosis after lung transplantation. Transplantation. 1998;66(8):1014–20.
23. Somers KD, Winters BA, Dawson DM, Leffell MS, Wright GL, Devine CJ, et al. Chromosome abnormalities in Peyronie's disease. J Urol. 1987;137(4):672–5.
24. Imai S, Kaksonen M, Raulo E, Kinnunen T, Fages C, Meng X, et al. Osteoblast recruitment and bone formation enhanced by cell matrix–associated heparin-binding growth-associated molecule (HB-GAM). J Cell Biol. 1998;143(4):1113–28.
25. Thiagalingam S, Cheng KH, Lee HJ, Mineva N, Thiagalingam A, Ponte JF. Histone deacetylases: unique players in shaping the epigenetic histone code. Ann N Y Acad Sci. 2003;983(1):84–100.
26. Moreno SA, Morgentaler A. Original research—Peyronie's disease: testosterone deficiency and Peyronie's disease: pilot data suggesting a significant relationship. J Sex Med. 2009;6(6):1729–35.
27. Kirby EW, Verges D, Matthews J, Carson CC, Coward RM. Low testosterone has a similar prevalence among men with sexual dysfunction due to either Peyronie's disease or erectile dysfunction and does not correlate with Peyronie's disease severity. J Sex Med. 2015;12(3):690–6.
28. Bjekic MD, Vlajinac HD, Sipetic SB, Marinkovic JM. Risk factors for Peyronie's disease: a case-control study. BJU Int. 2006;97(3):570–4.
29. Casabé A, Bechara A, Cheliz G, de Bonis W, Rey H. Risk factors of Peyronie's disease. What does our clinical experience show? J Sex Med. 2011;8(2):518–23.
30. Usta MF, Bivalacqua TJ, Jabren GW, Myers L, Sanabria J, Sikka SC, et al. Relationship between the severity of penile curvature and the presence of comorbidities in men with Peyronie's disease. J Urol. 2004;171(2):775–9.
31. Pavone C, D'Amato F, Dispensa N, Torretta F, Magno C. Smoking, diabetes, blood hypertension: possible etiologic role for Peyronie's disease? Analysis in 279 patients with a control group in Sicily. Arch Ital Urol Androl. 2015;87(1):20.
32. Al-Thakafi S, Al-Hathal N. Peyronie's disease: a literature review on epidemiology, genetics, pathophysiology, diagnosis and work-up. Transl Androl Urol. 2016;5(3):280–9.
33. Stewart S, Malto M, Sandberg L, Colburn KK. Increased serum levels of anti-elastin antibodies in patients with Peyronie's disease. J Urol. 1994;152(1):105–6.
34. Bivalacqua TJ, Champion HC, Leungwattanakij S, Yang DY, Hyun JS, Abdel-Mageed AB, et al. Evaluation of nitric oxide synthase and arginase in the induction of a Peyronie's-like condition in the rat. J Androl. 2001;22(3):497–506.
35. Cantini LP, Ferrini MG, Vernet D, Magee TR, Qian A, Gelfand RA, et al. Profibrotic role of myostatin in Peyronie's disease. J Sex Med. 2008;5(7):1607–22.
36. Mulhall JP, Schiff J, Guhring P. An analysis of the natural history of Peyronie's disease. J Urol. 2006;175(6):2115–8.
37. Hellstrom WJ, Bivalacqua TJ. Peyronie's disease: etiology, medical, and surgical therapy. J Androl. 2000;21(3):347–54.
38. Chung E, DeYoung L, Brock GB. The role of PDE5 inhibitors in penile septal scar remodeling: assessment of clinical and radiological outcomes. J Sex Med. 2011;8(5):1472–7.
39. Levine LA, Larsen SM. Surgery for Peyronie's disease. Asian J Androl. 2013;15(1):27–34.
40. Bacal V, Rumohr J, Sturm R, Lipshultz LI, Schumacher M, Grober ED. Correlation of degree of penile curvature between patient estimates and objective measures among men with Peyronie's disease. J Sex Med. 2009;6(3):862–5.
41. Kelâmi A. Classification of congenital and acquired penile deviation. Urol Int. 1983;38(4):229–33.

42. Ralph D, Gonzalez-Cadavid N, Mirone V, Perovic S, Sohn M, Usta M, et al. The management of Peyronie's disease: evidence-based 2010 guidelines. J Sex Med. 2010;7(7):2359–74.
43. Levine LA, Greenfield JM. Establishing a standardized evaluation of the man with Peyronie's disease. Int J Impot Res. 2003;15(S5):S103–12.
44. Hellstrom WJG, Feldman R, Rosen RC, Smith T, Kaufman G, Tursi J. Bother and distress associated with Peyronie's disease: validation of the Peyronie's disease questionnaire. J Urol. 2013;190(2):627–34.
45. Levine LA, Burnett AL. Standard operating procedures for Peyronie's disease. J Sex Med. 2013;10(1):230–44.
46. Hauck E. Diagnostic value of magnetic resonance imaging in Peyronie's disease—a comparison both with palpation and ultrasound in the evaluation of plaque formation. Eur Urol. 2003;43(3):293–300.
47. Vernet D, Nolazco G, Cantini L, Magee TR, Qian A, Rajfer J, et al. Evidence that osteogenic progenitor cells in the human tunica albuginea may originate from stem cells: implications for Peyronie disease1. Biol Reprod. 2005;73(6):1199–210.
48. Ohebshalom M, Mulhall J, Guhring P, Parker M. Measurement of penile curvature in Peyronie's disease patients: comparison of three methods. J Sex Med. 2007;4(1):199–203.
49. Taylor FL, Abern MR, Levine LA. Predicting erectile dysfunction following surgical correction of Peyronie's disease without inflatable penile prosthesis placement: vascular assessment and preoperative risk factors. J Sex Med. 2012;9(1):296–301.
50. Chung E, Ralph D, Kagioglu A, Garaffa G, Shamsodini A, Bivalacqua T, et al. Evidence-based management guidelines on Peyronie's disease. J Sex Med. 2016;13(6):905–23.
51. Zarafonetis CJD, Horrax TM. Treatment of Peyronie's disease with potassium para-aminobenzoate (potaba). J Urol. 1959;81(6):770–2.
52. Weidner W, Hauck EW, Schnitker J. Potassium paraaminobenzoate (POTABA™) in the treatment of Peyronie's disease: a prospective, placebo-controlled, randomized study. Eur Urol. 2005;47(4):530–6.
53. Gelbard MK, Dorey F, James K. The natural history of Peyronie's disease. J Urol. 1990;144(6):1376–9.
54. Safarinejad MR, Hosseini SY, Kolahi AA. Comparison of vitamin E and propionyl-L-carnitine, separately or in combination, in patients with early chronic Peyronie's disease: a double-blind, placebo controlled, randomized study. J Urol. 2007;178(4):1398–403.
55. Yafi FA, Pinsky MR, Sangkum P, Hellstrom WJG. Therapeutic advances in the treatment of Peyronie's disease. Andrology. 2015;3(4):650–60.
56. Akkus E, Breza J, Carrier S, Kadioglu A, Rehman J, Lue TE. Is colchicine effective in Peyronie's disease? A pilot study. Urology. 1994;44(2):291–5.
57. Kadioğlu A, Tefekli A, Köksal T, Usta M, Erol H. Treatment of Peyronie's disease with oral colchicine: long-term results and predictive parameters of successful outcome. Int J Impot Res. 2000;12(3):169–75.
58. Akman T, Sanli O, Uluocak N, Akbulut F, Nane I, Demir S, et al. The most commonly altered type of Peyronie's disease deformity under oral colchicine treatment is lateral curvature that mostly shifts to the dorsal side. Andrologia. 2011;43(1):28–33.
59. Ralph DJ, Brooks MD, Bottazzo GF, Pryor JP. The treatment of Peyronie's disease with tamoxifen. Br J Urol. 1992;70(6):648–51.
60. Teloken C, Rhoden EL, Grazziotin TM, da Ros CT, Sogari PR, Souto CAV. Tamoxifen versus placebo in the treatment of Peyronie's disease. J Urol. 1999;162(6):2003–5.
61. Biagiotti G, Cavallini G. Acetyl-L-carnitine vs tamoxifen in the oral therapy of Peyronie's disease: a preliminary report. BJU Int. 2001;88(1):63–7.
62. Cavallini G, Biagiotti G, Koverech A, Vitali G. Oral propionyl-l-carnitine and intra-plaque verapamil in the therapy of advanced and resistant Peyronie's disease. BJU Int. 2002;89(9):895–900.
63. Shindel AW, Lin G, Ning H, Banie L, Huang YC, Liu G, et al. Pentoxifylline attenuates transforming growth factor-β1-stimulated collagen deposition and elastogenesis in human

tunica albuginea-derived fibroblasts part 1: impact on extracellular matrix. J Sex Med. 2010;7(6):2077–85.

64. Brant WO, Dean RC, Lue TF. Treatment of Peyronie's disease with oral pentoxifylline. Nat Clin Pract Urol. 2006;3(2):111–5.

65. Smith JF, Shindel AW, Huang YC, Clavijo RI, Flechner L, Breyer BN, et al. Pentoxifylline treatment and penile calcifications in men with Peyronie's disease. Asian J Androl. 2011;13(2):322–5.

66. Palmieri A, Imbimbo C, Creta M, Verze P, Fusco F, Mirone V. Tadalafil once daily and extra-corporeal shock wave therapy in the management of patients with Peyronie's disease and erectile dysfunction: results from a prospective randomized trial. Int J Androl. 2012;35(2):190–5.

67. Rehman J, Benet A, Melman A. Use of intralesional verapamil to dissolve Peyronie's disease plaque: a long-term single-blind study. Urology. 1998;51(4):620–6.

68. Shirazi M, Haghpanah AR, Badiee M, Afrasiabi MA, Haghpanah S. Effect of intralesional verapamil for treatment of Peyronie's disease: a randomized single-blind, placebo-controlled study. Int Urol Nephrol. 2009;41(3):467–71.

69. Greenfield JM, Shah SJ, Levine LA. Verapamil versus saline in electromotive drug administration for Peyronie's disease: a double-blind, placebo controlled trial. J Urol. 2007;177(3):972–5.

70. Mehrsai AR, Namdari F, Salavati A, Dehghani S, Allameh F, Pourmand G. Comparison of transdermal electromotive administration of verapamil and dexamethasone versus intra-lesional injection for Peyronie's disease. Andrology. 2013;1(1):129–32.

71. Montorsi F, Salonia A, Guazzoni G, Barbieri L, Colombo R, Brausi M, et al. Transdermal electromotive multi-drug administration for Peyronie's disease: preliminary results. J Androl. 2000;21(1):85–90.

72. Favilla V, Russo GI, Zucchi A, Siracusa G, Privitera S, Cimino S, et al. Evaluation of intralesional injection of hyaluronic acid compared with verapamil in Peyronie's disease: preliminary results from a prospective, double-blinded, randomized study. Andrology. 2017;5(4):771–5.

73. Hellstrom WJG, Kendirci M, Matern R, Cockerham Y, Myers L, Sikka SC, et al. Single-blind, multicenter, placebo controlled, parallel study to assess the safety and efficacy of intralesional interferon α-2b for minimally invasive treatment for Peyronie's disease. J Urol. 2006;176(1):394–8.

74. Kendirci M, Usta MF, Matern RV, Nowfar S, Sikka SC, Hellstrom WJG. The impact of intra-lesional interferon α-2b injection therapy on penile hemodynamics in men with Peyronie's disease. J Sex Med. 2005;2(5):709–15.

75. Yafi FA, Pinsky MR, Stewart C, Sangkum P, Ates E, Trost LW, et al. The effect of duration of penile traction therapy in patients undergoing intralesional injection therapy for Peyronie's disease. J Urol. 2015;194(3):754–8.

76. Gennaro R, Barletta D, Paulis G. Intralesional hyaluronic acid: an innovative treatment for Peyronie's disease. Int Urol Nephrol. 2015;47(10):1595–602.

77. Lamprakopoulos A, Zorzos I, Lykourinas M. The use of betamethasone and hyaluronidase injections in the treatment of Peyronie's disease. Scand J Urol Nephrol. 2000;34(6):355–60.

78. Zucchi A, Costantini E, Cai T, Cavallini G, Liguori G, Favilla V, et al. Intralesional injection of hyaluronic acid in patients affected with Peyronie's disease: preliminary results from a prospective, multicenter, pilot study. Sex Med. 2016;4(2):e85–90.

79. Gelbard MK, Walsh R, Kaufman JJ. Collagenase for Peyronie's disease experimental studies. Urol Res. 1982;10(3):135–40.

80. Gelbard MK, James K, Riach P, Dorey F. Collagenase versus placebo in the treatment of Peyronie's disease: a double-blind study. J Urol. 1993;149(1):56–8.

81. Gelbard M, Lipshultz LI, Tursi J, Smith T, Kaufman G, Levine LA. Phase 2b study of the clinical efficacy and safety of collagenase clostridium histolyticum in patients with Peyronie disease. J Urol. 2012;187(6):2268–74.

82. Gelbard M, Goldstein I, Hellstrom WJG, McMahon CG, Smith T, Tursi J, et al. Clinical efficacy, safety and tolerability of collagenase clostridium histolyticum for the treatment of

Peyronie disease in 2 large double-blind, randomized, placebo controlled phase 3 studies. J Urol. 2013;190(1):199–207.

83. Gelbard M, Hellstrom WJG, McMahon CG, Levine LA, Smith T, Tursi J, et al. Baseline characteristics from an ongoing phase 3 study of collagenase clostridium histolyticum in patients with Peyronie's disease. J Sex Med. 2013;10(11):2822–31.

84. Levine LA, Cuzin B, Mark S, Gelbard MK, Jones NA, Liu G, et al. Clinical safety and effectiveness of collagenase clostridium histolyticum injection in patients with Peyronie's disease: a phase 3 open-label study. J Sex Med. 2015;12(1):248–58.

85. Abdel Raheem A, Capece M, Kalejaiye O, Abdel-Raheem T, Falcone M, Johnson M, et al. Safety and effectiveness of collagenase clostridium histolyticum in the treatment of Peyronie's disease using a new modified shortened protocol. BJU Int. 2017;120(5):717–23.

86. Cocci A, di Maida F, Russo GI, Capogrosso P, Francesco L, Rizzo M, et al. Efficacy of collagenase clostridium histolyticum (Xiapex®) in patients with the acute phase of Peyronie's disease. Clin Drug Investig. 2020;40(6):583–8.

87. Cocci A, di Maida F, Russo GI, di Mauro M, Cito G, Falcone M, et al. How atypical penile curvature influence clinical outcomes in patients with Peyronie's disease receiving collagenase *Clostridium Histolyticum* therapy? World J Mens Health. 2020;38(1):78.

88. Russo GI, Cacciamani G, Cocci A, Kessler TM, Morgia G, Serefoglu EC, et al. Comparative effectiveness of intralesional therapy for Peyronie's disease in controlled clinical studies: a systematic review and network meta-analysis. J Sex Med. 2019;16(2):289–99.

89. Cocci A, Russo GI, Salamanca JIM, Ralph D, Palmieri A, Mondaini N. The end of an era: withdrawal of Xiapex (clostridium histolyticum collagenase) from the European market. Eur Urol. 2020;77(5):660–1.

90. Alenghat FJ, Ingber DE. Mechanotransduction: all signals point to cytoskeleton, matrix, and integrins. Sci STKE. 2002;2002(119):pe6.

91. Levine LA, Newell M, Taylor FL. Penile traction therapy for treatment of Peyronie's disease: a single-center pilot study. J Sex Med. 2008;5(6):1468–73.

92. Gontero P, di Marco M, Giubilei G, Bartoletti R, Pappagallo G, Tizzani A, et al. Original research—Peyronie's disease: use of penile extender device in the treatment of penile curvature as a result of Peyronie's disease. Results of a phase II prospective study. J Sex Med. 2009;6(2):558–66.

93. Martínez-Salamanca JI, Egui A, Moncada I, Minaya J, Ballesteros CM, del Portillo L, et al. Acute phase Peyronie's disease management with traction device: a nonrandomized prospective controlled trial with ultrasound correlation. J Sex Med. 2014;11(2):506–15.

94. Moncada I, Krishnappa P, Romero J, Torremade J, Fraile A, Martinez-Salamanca JI, et al. Penile traction therapy with the new device 'Penimaster PRO' is effective and safe in the stable phase of Peyronie's disease: a controlled multicentre study. BJU Int. 2019;123(4):694–702.

95. Raheem AA, Garaffa G, Raheem TA, Dixon M, Kayes A, Christopher N, et al. The role of vacuum pump therapy to mechanically straighten the penis in Peyronie's disease. BJU Int. 2010;106(8):1178–80.

96. Gholami SS, Gonzalez-Cadavid NF, Lin CS, Rajfer J, Lue TF. Peyronie's disease: a review. J Urol. 2003;169(4):1234–41.

97. Palmieri A, Imbimbo C, Longo N, Fusco F, Verze P, Mangiapia F, et al. A first prospective, randomized, double-blind, placebo-controlled clinical trial evaluating extracorporeal shock wave therapy for the treatment of Peyronie's disease. Eur Urol. 2009;56(2):363–70.

98. Chitale S, Morsey M, Swift L, Sethia K. Limited shock wave therapy vs sham treatment in men with Peyronie's disease: results of a prospective randomized controlled double-blind trial. BJU Int. 2010;106(9):1352–6.

99. Hatzichristodoulou G, Meisner C, Gschwend JE, Stenzl A, Lahme S. Extracorporeal shock wave therapy in Peyronie's disease: results of a placebo-controlled, prospective, randomized, single-blind study. J Sex Med. 2013;10(11):2815–21.

100. Basford JR. Low-energy laser therapy: controversies and new research findings. Lasers Surg Med. 1989;9(1):1–5.

101. Incrocci L, Wijnmaalen A, Slob AK, Hop WCJ, Levendag PC. Low-dose radiotherapy in 179 patients with Peyronie's disease: treatment outcome and current sexual functioning. Int J Radiat Oncol Biol Phys. 2000;47(5):1353–6.

102. Incrocci L, Hop WCJ, Slob AK. Current sexual functioning in 106 patients with Peyronie's disease treated with radiotherapy 9 years earlier. Urology. 2000;56(6):1030–3.

103. Viljoen IM, Goedhals L, Doman MJ. Peyronie's disease—a perspective on the disease and the long-term results of radiotherapy. S Afr Med J. 1993;83(1):19–20.

104. Hatzichristodoulou G. Konservative Therapie der Induratio penis plastica—update 2015. Urologe. 2015;54(5):641–7.

105. di Stasi SM, Giannantoni A, Stephen RL, Capelli G, Giurioli A, Jannini EA, et al. A prospective, randomized study using transdermal electromotive administration of verapamil and dexamethasone for Peyronie's disease. J Urol. 2004;171(4):1605–8.

106. Pyrgidis N, Yafi FA, Sokolakis I, Dimitriadis F, Mykoniatis I, Russo GI, et al. Assessment of conservative combination therapies for active and stable Peyronie's disease: a systematic review and meta-analysis. Eur Urol Focus. 2021; https://doi.org/10.1016/j.euf.2021.12.003.

107. Chung E, Clendinning E, Lessard L, Brock G. Five-year follow-up of Peyronie's graft surgery: outcomes and patient satisfaction. J Sex Med. 2011;8(2):594–600.

108. Hatzimouratidis K, Eardley I, Giuliano F, Hatzichristou D, Moncada I, Salonia A, et al. EAU guidelines on penile curvature. Eur Urol. 2012;62(3):543–52.

109. Langston JP, Carson CC. Peyronie disease: plication or grafting. Urol Clin N Am. 2011;38(2):207–16.

110. Salonia A. Sexual and reproductive health EAU guidelines. 2022. https://uroweb.org/guideline/sexual-and-reproductive-health/#10.

111. Osmonov D, Ragheb A, Ward S, Blecher G, Falcone M, Soave A, et al. ESSM position statement on surgical treatment of Peyronie's disease. Sex Med. 2022;10(1):100459.

112. Nehra A, et al. Peyronie's disease: AUA guideline. J Urol. 2015;194(3):745–53.

113. Nesbit RM. Congenital curvature of the phallus: report of three cases with description of corrective operation. J Urol. 1965;93(2):230–2.

114. Pryor JP, Fitzpatrick JM. A new approach to the correction of the penile deformity in Peyronie's disease. J Urol. 1979;122(5):622–3.

115. Lemberger RJ, Bishop MC, Bates CP. Nesbit's operation for Peyronie's disease. Br J Urol. 1984;56(6):721–3.

116. Yachia D. Modified corporoplasty for the treatment of penile curvature. J Urol. 1990;143(1):80–2.

117. Seveso M, Melegari S, de Francesco O, Macchi A, Romero Otero J, Taverna G, et al. Surgical correction of Peyronie's disease via tunica albuginea plication: long-term follow-up. Andrology. 2018;6(1):47–52.

118. Nooter RI, Bosch JLHR, Schroder FH. Peyronie's disease and congenital penile curvature: long-term results of operative treatment with the plication procedure. Br J Urol. 1994;74(4):497–500.

119. Essed E, Schroeder FH. New surgical treatment for peyronie disease. Urology. 1985;25(6):582–7.

120. Gholami SS, Lue TF. Correction of penile curvature using the 16-DOT plication technique: a review of 132 patients. J Urol. 2002;167(5):2066–9.

121. Baskin LS, Duckett JW. Dorsal tunica albuginea plication for hypospadias curvature. J Urol. 1994;151(6):1668–71.

122. Levine LA. Penile straightening with tunica albuginea plication procedure. In: Peyronie's disease. Totowa, NJ: Humana Press; 2007. p. 151–9.

123. Egydio PH, Lucon AM, Arap S. A single relaxing incision to correct different types of penile curvature: surgical technique based on geometrical principles. BJU Int. 2004;94(7):1147–57.

124. Valente P, Gomes C, Tomada N. Small intestinal submucosa grafting for Peyronie disease: outcomes and patient satisfaction. Urology. 2017;100:117–24.

125. Kovac JR, Brock GB. Surgical outcomes and patient satisfaction after dermal, pericardial, and small intestinal submucosal grafting for Peyronie's disease. J Sex Med. 2007;4(5):1500–8.

126. Fernández-Pascual E, Manfredi C, Torremadé J, Ibarra FP, Geli JS, Romero-Otero J, et al. Multicenter prospective study of grafting with collagen fleece TachoSil in patients with Peyronie's disease. J Sex Med. 2020;17(11):2279–86.

127. Morgado A, Morgado MR, Tomada N. Penile lengthening with porcine small intestinal submucosa grafting in Peyronie's disease treatment: long-term surgical outcomes, patients' satisfaction and dissatisfaction predictors. Andrology. 2018;6(6):909–15.

128. Lahme S. Collagen fleece for defect coverage following plaque excision in patients with Peyronie's disease. Eur Urol. 2002;41(4):401–5.

129. Sokolakis I, Pyrgidis N, Hatzichristodoulou G. The use of collagen fleece (TachoSil) as grafting material in the surgical treatment of Peyronie's disease. A comprehensive narrative review. Int J Impot Res. 2022;34:260–8.

130. Hatzichristodoulou G. Evolution of the surgical sealing patch TachoSil® in Peyronie's disease reconstructive surgery: technique and contemporary literature review. World J Urol. 2020;38(2):315–21.

131. Hatzichristodoulou G, Osmonov D, Kübler H, Hellstrom WJG, Yafi FA. Contemporary review of grafting techniques for the surgical treatment of Peyronie's disease. Sex Med Rev. 2017;5(4):544–52.

132. Hatzichristodoulou G. Introducing the ventral sealing technique using collagen fleece for surgical therapy of patients with ventral Peyronie's curvature: initial experience. Int J Impot Res. 2018;30(6):306–11.

133. Farrell MR, Abdelsayed GA, Ziegelmann MJ, Levine LA. A comparison of hemostatic patches versus pericardium allograft for the treatment of complex Peyronie's disease with penile prosthesis and plaque incision. Urology. 2019;129:113–8.

134. Wilson SK, Delk JR. A new treatment for Peyronie's disease: modeling the penis over an inflatable penile prosthesis. J Urol. 1994;152(4):1121–3.

135. Wilson SK. Surgical techniques: modeling technique for penile curvature. J Sex Med. 2007;4(1):231–4.

136. Rolle L, Ceruti C, Timpano M, Sedigh O, Destefanis P, Galletto E, et al. A new, innovative, lengthening surgical procedure for Peyronie's disease by penile prosthesis implantation with double dorsal-ventral patch graft: the "sliding technique". J Sex Med. 2012;9(9):2389–95.

137. Egydio P. MP39–04 an innovative strategy for non-grafting penile enlargement: the Egydio paradigm for tunica expansion procedures (TEP). J Urol. 2020;203(Suppl. 4):e578.

138. Rybak J, Papagiannopoulos D, Levine L. A retrospective comparative study of traction therapy vs. no traction following tunica Albuginea plication or partial excision and grafting for Peyronie's disease: measured lengths and patient perceptions. J Sex Med. 2012;9(9):2396–403.

139. Hatzichristodoulou G. Grafting techniques for Peyronie's disease. Transl Androl Urol. 2016;5(3):334–41.

140. Wimpissinger F, Parnham A, Gutjahr G, Maksys S, Baierlein M, Stackl W. 10 years' plaque incision and vein grafting for Peyronie's disease: does time matter? J Sex Med. 2016;13(1):120–8.

141. Kalsi J, Minhas S, Christopher N, Ralph D. The results of plaque incision and venous grafting (Lue procedure) to correct the penile deformity of Peyronie's disease. BJU Int. 2005;95(7):1029–33.

142. Kim D, Pang MG. The effect of male circumcision on sexuality. BJU Int. 2007;99(3):619–22.

143. Wilson SK, Mora-Estaves C, Egydio P, Ralph D, Habous M, Love C, et al. Glans necrosis following penile prosthesis implantation: prevention and treatment suggestions. Urology. 2017;107:144–8.

144. Yildirim A, Basok EK, Basaran A, Tokuc R. Gangrene of the distal penis after implantation of malleable penile prosthesis in a diabetic patient. Adv Ther. 2008;25(2):143–7.

145. Weiner DM, Lowe FC. Surgical management of ischemic penile gangrene in diabetics with end stage atherosclerosis. J Urol. 1996;155(3):926–9.

146. van der Horst C, Martínez Portillo FJ, Melchior D, Bross S, Alken P, Juenemann KP. Polytetrafluoroethylene versus polypropylene sutures for Essed-Schroeder tunical plication. J Urol. 2003;170(2):472–5.
147. Mobley EM, Fuchs ME, Myers JB, Brant WO. Update on plication procedures for Peyronie's disease and other penile deformities. Ther Adv Urol. 2012;4(6):335–46.

Reconstructive Andrologic Surgery

7

Patrick Gordon, Wai Gin Lee, and David Ralph

Abstract

Reconstructive andrology is a branch of surgery dedicated to the return of normal form and function of the external male genitalia that is aesthetically pleasing to the patient. In sexually active patients this is particularly challenging to ensure good aesthetics, preserve erogenous sensation while maintaining erectile tissue adequate for penetrative intercourse. This can be due to congenital or acquired conditions. By far the most common procedure (indeed in all surgery) is circumcision. In this chapter, we will not deal with this, but how to manage some common complications related to this and other more common reconstructive procedures. Gender affirmation surgery will be covered in another chapter.

Principles of Reconstructive Surgery

One of the main principles of reconstruction is to provide skin coverage of the organs without compromising their function and form. Often a wide range of options exist, with the simplest if possible being chosen. Wherever possible skin should be closed primarily, if tissue doesn't allow this then first choice should be a local flap from surrounding tissue. If local tissue can't be used then for larger tissue defects free grafts requiring microvascular anastomosis may be required.

P. Gordon · W. G. Lee · D. Ralph (✉)
University College London Hospitals, London, UK
e-mail: patrick.gordon3@nhs.net; waigin.lee@nhs.net; david@andrology.co.uk

© The Author(s), under exclusive license to Springer Nature
Switzerland AG 2022
S. Sarikaya et al. (eds.), *Andrology and Sexual Medicine*, Management of Urology,
https://doi.org/10.1007/978-3-031-12049-7_7

151

For skin-only coverage autologous skin grafts can be used. The vast majority being split thickness skin grafts (STSG) containing epidermis and part of the dermis only, so have limited nutrient requirement to survive period of plasmatic imbibition before blood vessels develop (capillary inosculation) within 36-h. Here an air dermatome is used to harvest skin from a donor site of varying thickness (0.16 of an inch most commonly used). For larger areas once harvested the STSG can be passed through a mesher. This makes multiple rows of small cuts to expand the surface area for varying ratios (1:1.5, 1:3). Meshed grafts tend to contract more but provide excellent cosmesis on the scrotum. They are then sutured in place (including central quilting sutures to allow haematoma to be evacuated through the needle puncture as well as further securing the graft), with compressive dressings for a period of time (7–10 days) to allow optimum take of the graft. Donor sites can usually be dressed simply and will re-epithelialise. STSG advantages are ease of access, simple dressings to donor site, high percentage of graft take, large areas can be covered (especially with use of a mesher) and good cosmesis (especially for penile or scrotal skin with no subdermal fat). The disadvantages are they can contract significantly.

Full thickness skin grafts (FTSG) contain the epidermis and entire dermis (including hair follicles so take from non-hair baring areas) which provides more mechanical strength (resistant shear force, less shrinkage/contracture), generally better function and cosmesis. Area to be excised is measured and marked then excised using a scalpel. Fat is then stripped and the graft is then sutured in place with compression dressings the same as a STSG. Disadvantages are that deeper donor site that will require closure, and greater neovascularisation requirements.

Ultimately patients and procedures being undertaken in reconstructive andrology are becoming more challenging and complex. As such patients should be managed in high volume centres with experienced clinicians working in a multidisciplinary team. By discussing complex cases in this manner amongst experienced nursing, urologists, plastics, vascular, radiology, dermatology, microbiology, psychiatry, pain management, patients can benefit from improved outcomes.

Hidradenitis Suppurativa

Hidradenitis Suppurativa (HS) is an autoimmune chronic inflammatory skin condition that affects apocrine gland-bearing skin in the axillae, groin and lower back. It causes chronic abscesses that constantly exude purulent discharge leading to sinuses, fistulae and scarring [1].

HS often presents at puberty and leads to significant psychological distress. Associations and risk factors include family history, smoking, diabetes/metabolic syndrome and other common skin disorders (acne, psoriasis). It has a strong association with inflammatory bowel disease and patients should be evaluated by a gastroenterologist to rule out perineal Crohn's disease.

HS is characterised clinically by:

- Typical distribution (groin/perineum, axilla, mammary folds, lower back)
- Painful firm papules, abscesses and nodules
- Draining sinuses/fistulae linking inflammatory lesions
- Hypertrophic and atrophic scars
- Swabs for bacteriology are typically negative

Complications of HS can include:

- Secondary infection
- Psychological effects and negative impact on quality-of-life
- Squamous cell carcinoma
- Anaemia of chronic disease

Treatment starts with weight loss if overweight and antibiotics (if secondary infection). Immunosuppression becomes the mainstay of treatment, including newer agents like monoclonal antibodies [2]. Surgery is reserved to remove heavily inflamed and diseased areas that can potentially lead to secondary malignancies. Wounds can be left to heal by secondary intention, but larger areas will require skin grafting (surgical techniques discussed later in chapter) or flaps. Graft site should be clear of disease and infection prior to successful grafting, which may require several trips to the operating theatre. Patients should be managed carefully as a team (Dermatologists, surgeons, Microbiologists) to optimise medical therapy before and after grafting. With this, good results can be achieved as illustrated below (Fig. 7.1).

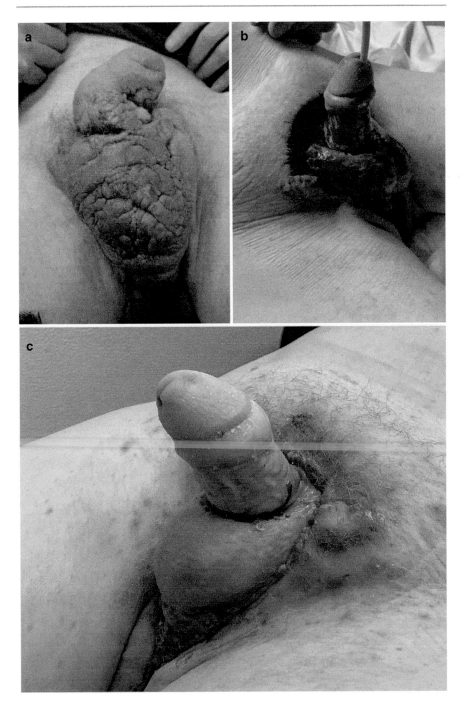

Fig. 7.1 Photos show the same patient with HS. (**a**) Pre-surgery. (**b**) After debridement. (**c**) 1-month post-surgery (STSG penile shaft, 1:3 meshed SSTG scrotum) with acceptable results

Fournier's Gangrene

Fournier's gangrene (FG) is a rare form of necrotising fasciitis affecting the perineal, genital, and perianal regions. It is a life-threatening condition carrying a mortality of 20–40% [3]. It is rare and primarily affects men, but can be seen in women (ratio 10:1) [4]. Patients are often immunosuppressed or diabetic and tend to have multiple co-morbidities leading to impaired blood supply to the genitals. Pathogens tend to be a polymicrobial flora, with the synergistic effect of anaerobes and aerobes leading to the rapid spread of infection along the fascial planes.

Diagnosis is clinical and is based on the typical rapidly progressing skin changes (erythema rapidly turning into crepitus/gas and necrosis) seen in a systemically unwell patient. Treatment is urgent radical debridement of all dead tissue up to a bleeding margin in conjunction with patient resuscitation and broad-spectrum antibiotics. Further relook in theatre 24–48 h often required to sure all dead/infected tissue removed. Any patient deterioration requires prompt wound review.

Multiple debridement's (on average 3) lead to large skin defects that require reconstruction in certain patients [5]. Closure of these skin defects may be by secondary intention or may require the use of STSG or tissue flaps once the wound is healthy and free of infection.

Genital Lymphoedema

This is a rare condition that can be extremely debilitating to patients and difficult to manage. Lymphoedema is the abnormal collection of lymphatic fluid due to lymphatic obstruction. It can occur across the body, and in the genitals, it can be isolated to the penis or scrotum or both. It is classed as primary (or idiopathic) due to abnormal lymphatic development or more commonly it is secondary to other causes such as iatrogenic (surgery or radiotherapy), malignancy, and infection (parasitic or venereal). The disease process needs to involve both inguinal lymphatic chains, due to the bilateral lymph drainage of the genitals. Rare inflammatory disorders such as vasculitis, sarcoidosis and Crohn's disease can also be a cause so careful attention should be paid to the medical history [6].

Patients can suffer regular superimposed infections in the form of cellulitis which result in further inflammation and subsequent formation of collagen deposition. This further impairs existing lymphatic drainage leading to progressive swelling and fibrosis of the overlying skin, worsening the patient's symptoms and morbidity.

Proposed management should first identify and treat the underlying pathology, if possible. Treatment aims to restore sexual and voiding function with the best possible cosmetic results. If identified early, conservative measures can have good results. When conservative measures such as compression garments, elevation and massage fail to reduce swelling and infection, surgery to excise the diseased skin and subcutaneous tissue is required. Surgery to restore lymphatic drainage has poor results [7].

Excision of skin and subcutaneous tissue is the primary goal, Buck's fascia is never involved. Surgical procedures may include circumcision to improve voiding (note the inner prepuce rarely involved due to separate drainage via dorsal neurovascular bundle into pudendal system), partial or total scrotectomy with or without skin grafting (FTSG or STSG). FTSG have the advantage of reduced contracture and improved elasticity, but with the disadvantages of needing a larger donor site and increased risk of loss. STSG are easier to harvest and manage, but can contract significantly. Hence, STSG should be used with caution on the penile shaft. Scrotal reconstruction can often be achieved by primary closure due to the unaffected lateral scrotal tissue (tend to have separate lymphatic drainage). Penile wound defects can be covered using STSG quilted in place with a compression bandage for 7-days. In combined penoscrotal oedema, the scrotum should be managed first as it can lead to spontaneous resolution of the penile lymphoedema.

Preputioplasty

Phimosis is a condition where the foreskin (or prepuce) of the penis cannot be retracted and the inner prepuce may be fused to the glans. In adults, this tends to be due to lichen sclerosus (LS) unlike in the paediatric population. LS is an inflammatory scarring dermatosis affecting genital skin in both sexes [7] This progressive slow-growing disease leads to contraction and adhesions of the mucosa causing painful narrowing of the prepuce and can spread proximally through the urethral meatus causing urethral strictures. As well as causing difficulty in voiding and pain during erections the chronic inflammation increases the risk of developing malignancy [8]. As such, circumcision is recommended as steroid creams may have little benefit in the adult population.

Preputioplasty is an alternative to circumcision for men with phimosis who wish to preserve their foreskin. The aim is to release the constricting band in the foreskin. It's rarely used in adult's due to the primary driver for disease progression being active LS which tends to require a full circumcision (to excise all abnormal skin). Several techniques are used, being variations on gaining length but cutting vertically and closing longitudinally (Fig. 7.2). This can leave the distal edges of the foreskin uneven (so called 'Fish mouth' appearance), patients should be counselled for this as a cosmetic outcome.

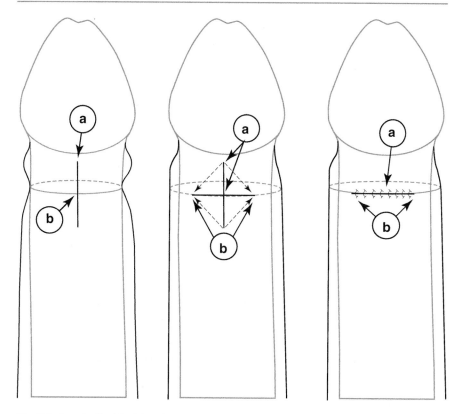

Fig. 7.2 Longitudinal incision through skin to Buck's fascia, which is then closed transversely. Can be single or multiple. Post-operatively, patients should be encouraged to mobilise the skin as comfort allows

Foreskin Restoration (Reversal of Circumcision)

There is a growing group of men who suffer body image issues following their circumcision performed in childhood and they may seek restorative procedures. Patients may complain of loss of glans sensation, reduced sexual arousal and increased glans sensitivity during exercise [9] Using scrotal skin as a staged, transferred flap can achieve good cosmetic results (Fig. 7.3) but patients should be warned it will take several operations over 1–2 years to achieve.

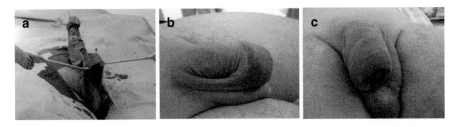

Fig. 7.3 These images show the steps for foreskin restoration. (**a**) Graft site prepared and the penile shaft is buried in anterior scrotum. (**b, c**) Over several stages the scrotal skin is slowly divided in stages to allow new blood supply to develop on the penile shaft with good cosmetic end result

Aesthetic Revision Surgery of the Male Genitalia

Appearance of the male genitalia is strongly linked with self-esteem and sexual identity. Increasing exposure to pornographic material can lead some men to develop thoughts of inadequacy with their own genitalia (even when it is acceptable to their partner). Aesthetic surgery of the male genitalia serves to restore or correct these perceived deficiencies. It is important prior to any procedure that the patient's expectations and goals are discussed and documented in detail to avoid unrealistic expectations and exclude underlying psychiatric issues. If necessary, these patients should be assessed by a mental health professional. A thorough history of erectile, orgasmic and urinary function should be documented. Below we briefly summarise some of the procedures that can be offered.

Penile Lengthening

Division of the suspensory ligament may improve penile length in the flaccid state. This can be achieved through a small incision above the penopubic junction in the midline. Some surgeons after dividing the ligament place a spacer in the form of a testicular prosthesis to stop the ligament re-attaching (which can further shorten the penis) [10]. The length gained afterwards is variable, and if too much of the ligament is divided the penis can become unstable in the erect state.

Penile Girth Enhancement

Procedures offering increased penile girth are increasingly common. The most common being autologous fat injection above Buck's fascia. Results vary depending on practitioner experience, and the number of tunneling sites required. Complications include infections, asymmetric fat distribution, nodule formation and erectile dysfunction due to corporal fibrosis. When removing asymmetric fat or nodules, care should be taken not to remove too much fat as this can result in lymphedema. Dermal fillers like hyaluronic acid can be used as an alternative.

Dermal grafts are sheets that can be circumferentially wrapped around Bucks fascia to increase girth with a smooth texture. Various incisions can be used with grafts being secured proximally and distally. Complications include unsightly scar sites, infection, skin loss and scar contracture resulting in penile shortening. The graft may also migrate. Allografts can also be used with a similar risk of complications. Removing these grafts can damage the neurovascular bundle and lead to severe penile shortening.

Penoscrotal Transposition

Penoscrotal transposition is a rare external genitalia anomaly resulting in a partial or complete positional exchange between the penis and the scrotum. In rare and extreme cases, the shaft comes out in the perineum (raises the question of penile agenesis or ambiguous genitalia), but more commonly, in incomplete cases the shaft emerges from the scrotum. It has a strong association with chordee, hypospadias and potentially life-threatening congenital abnormalities, so at diagnosis there should be a high index of suspicion for other abnormalities [10]. The embryological sequence responsible for this malformation remains unclear; however, it has been suggested that an abnormal positioning of the genital tubercle in relation to the scrotal swellings during the critical fourth to fifth week of gestation could affect the migration of the scrotal swellings [11].

Basic principles of surgical repair are to move the scrotal skin posterior, and penis anterior. This relies on the creation of rotational flaps to mobilise the scrotum downwards (Glenn & Anderson) or transpose the penis to an opening created in the skin through tunneling (McIlvoy & Harris). This may be in a single, or more commonly, staged procedure. Urethral reconstruction may also be required with associated hypospadias. Complications may include fistulae, dehiscence, flap necrosis, lymphoedema and testicular injury but good cosmesis is possible (Fig. 7.4).

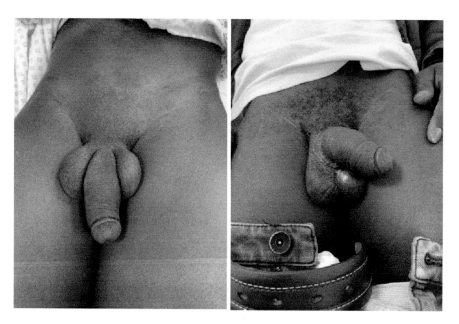

Fig. 7.4 Images show a mild form of penoscrotal transposition that was corrected in a single stage procedure

Genital Foreign Body

Self-mutilation of the genitals is rare with an unknown incidence. Reasons may relate to body dysmorphia, psychiatric/personality/gender identity disorders or substance misuse. Insults can vary from cutting, to full amputation or strangulation with various objects. Immediate management may require control of bleeding in the case of amputation and patient resuscitation. Management depends on the timing of injury, severity of injury and mental state of the patient. Reconstruction should aim to restore voiding and sexual function by replicating as close to normal anatomy as possible. Total penile amputation can be re-planted with the appropriate microsurgical expertise and timely presentation/intervention (within 13 h). Division of suspensory ligament may also avoid the need for perineal urethrostomy by increasing functional penile length.

Management of these patients should be multidisciplinary involving a psychiatrist and support workers. Patients with ongoing ideations of self-harm will require psychiatric treatment to prevent further self-harm to any subsequent surgical reconstruction.

Injection of silicone (other substances such as paraffin or vaseline have been described) into the penile shaft fat for augmentation (either by the patient himself or an often unregulated practitioner) has been reported for over 50 years. Silicone can exist in liquid and solid forms and has used for several cosmetic treatments. Several complications have been reported:

- Pain
- Migration
- Tissue induration
- Erythema

More severe granulomatous reactions (so called siliconoma) may present as recurrent infections/cellulitis, ulceration, nodules and regional lymph node enlargement (Fig. 7.5a). Damage to vasculature can result in tissue necrosis. Histologically, the granulomatous response is characterised by the presence of large numbers of histiocytes and giant Langerhans' cells [12]. Once injected, the only treatment is excision of the affected tissues with the overlying skin because the skin is usually adherent to the dense inflammatory granulomatous tissue (Fig. 7.5b). Skin grafting is usually required for wound closure (Fig. 7.5c).

Buried Penis

Buried penis in an increasingly common problem due to increasing rates of obesity although it can also be caused by severe LS, radical circumcision and lymphoedema. The penis is a normal size, but the shaft is trapped below the pubic skin (Fig. 7.6a). Burying of the penile shaft leads to difficulty in voiding leading to skin breakdown and difficulties in sexual function. Undiagnosed urethral strictures should also be considered in these patients who have voiding difficulty. Patients should be encouraged to

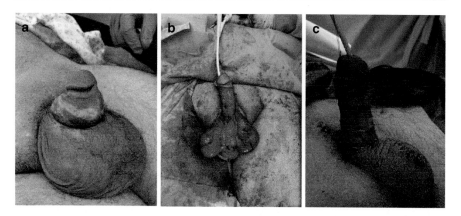

Fig. 7.5 (**a**) Serial Images above from same patient presenting with a siliconoma. (**b**) Affected tissue was excised while protecting the testes and penile shaft. (**c**) STSG applied to the penile shaft with primary closure of the scrotum

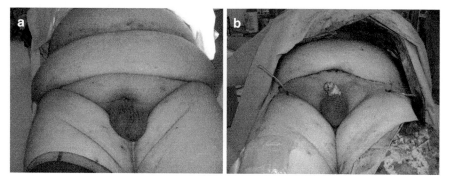

Fig. 7.6 (**a**) Patient with severe buried penis due to suprapubic fat pad. (**b**) FTSG was used to resurface the penile shaft after unburying

lose weight (with a target weight agreed). They will require the support of their family doctor, dietician and, in some cases, bariatric surgeon. Patients often have significant comorbidities and so require careful pre-operative evaluation. In motivated patients who have met their target weight, surgery can then be offered with significant improvements in quality of life achieved.

There are several surgical techniques and options vary depending on the quantity and quality of penile, pubic and scrotal skin. The primary step is to mobilise and release the penis from underlying scar tissue. The suprapubic fat pannus is then excised (panniculectomy) to further increase exposure. During dissection care should be taken to identify and protect the spermatic cord bilaterally, with dissection down to the level of the rectus fascia. The patient should be marked pre-operatively while both lying and standing so the patient knows how much tissue is being removed and to prevent 'dog ears' following closure.

The suprapubic skin is anchored to the rectus fascia along with the base of penis to reform the penopubic angle (Fig. 7.6b). The final stage once penis correctly secured and overhanging fat pannus removed is to cover any skin defects. Local flaps (scrotal flaps) can be used. Alternatively, STSG or FTSG can be used because they are easily harvested, and will match penile shaft skin with little subcutaneous fat. STSG also lack hair follicles and have better take. Drain should be left on either side to prevent seroma formation.

A select group will benefit from a malleable penile prosthesis. This is indicated in men with co-existing erectile dysfunction. If required this can be exchanged for an inflatable implant at a later date, but an inflatable device should be avoided at the time of unburying surgery due to the risk of wound breakdown and infection.

Peri-operative risks increase with rising body mass index and poor diabetic control [13]. They include increasing length of hospital stay, delayed healing, wound breakdown/infection, seroma formation and graft loss.

References

1. Zouboulis CC, Del Marmol V, Mrowietz U, Prens EP, Tzellos T, Jemec GBE. Hidradenitis suppurativa/acne inversa: criteria for diagnosis, severity assessment, classification and disease evaluation. Dermatology. 2015;231(2):184–90.
2. Saunte DM, Jemec GB. Hidradenitis suppurativa: advances in diagnosis and treatment. JAMA. 2017;318(20):2019–32.
3. García Marín A, Turégano Fuentes F, Cuadrado Ayuso M, et al. Predictive factors for mortality in Fournier's gangrene: a series of 59 cases. Cir Esp. 2015;93(1):12–7.
4. Eke N. Fournier's gangrene: a review of 1726 cases. Br J Surg. 2000;87(6):718–28.
5. Koukouras D, Kallidonis P, Panagopoulos C, et al. Fournier's gangrene, a urologic and surgical emergency: presentation of a multi-institutional experience with 45 cases. Urol Int. 2011;86:167–72.
6. Garaffa G, Christopher N, Ralph DJ. The management of genital lymphoedema. BJU Int. 2008;102(4):480–4.
7. Osmonov D, Hamann C, Eraky A, Kalz A, Melchior D, Bergholz R, Romero-Otero J. Preputioplasty as a surgical alternative in treatment of phimosis. Int J Impot Res. 2021;1:1–6.
8. Mohd Mustapa MF, Exton LS, Bell HK, et al. Updated guidance for writing a British Association of Dermatologists clinical guideline: the adoption of the GRADE methodology 2016. Br J Dermatol. 2017;176:44–51.
9. Alter GJ. Penile enlargement surgery. Tech Urol. 1998;4(2):70–6.
10. Pinke LA, Rathbun SR, Husmann DA, Kramer SA. Penoscrotal transposition: review of 53 patients. J Urol. 2001;166(5):1865–8.
11. Bloom DA, Wan J, Key D. Disorders of the male external genitalia and inguinal canal. In: Kelalis PP, King LR, Belman AB, editors. Clinical pediatric urology, vol. 2. 3rd ed. Philadelphia: Saunders; 1992. p. 1015–49.
12. Pasternack FR, Fox LP, Engler DE. Silicone granuloma treated with etanercept. Arch Dermatol. 2005;14:13–5.
13. Cooper JM, Paige KT, Beshilan JM, Downey DL, Thirlby RC. Abdominal panniculectomies: high patient satisfaction despite significant complication rates. Ann Plast Surg. 2008;61:188–96.

Transmasculine Gender Affirmation Surgery

8

Wai Gin Lee, David Ralph, and Nim Christopher

Abstract

Transmasculine gender affirmation surgery (GAS) is evolving rapidly due to surgical and socioeconomic advances over recent decades. Important innovations include the use of free or pedicled sensate tissue flaps with integrated urethra coupled with an improved understanding of how best to offer inclusive care. Shared decision making with an individualised approach for care; coupled with novel customised urological prosthetics are encouraging developments and will likely lead to improved outcomes and satisfaction. The prospect of further innovation in techniques for penile allotransplantation and tissue bio-engineering are tantalising goals for the future.

Introduction

Gender affirmation surgery (GAS) is a modular series of procedures that aligns a person's physical appearance more closely with their experienced gender identity. The procedures are "modular" because not all individuals will want, require, or qualify for every intervention.

Transmasculine genital gender affirmation surgery (GAS) is evolving rapidly due to surgical and socioeconomic advances over recent decades. There has been a 20-fold increase in the number of individuals referred for assessment at the gender identity clinic in Amsterdam between 1980 and 2015 [1]. Genital GAS has doubled from an average of 11 procedures a year prior to 2011 to an average of 22

W. G. Lee (✉) · D. Ralph · N. Christopher
University College London Hospitals NHS Foundation Trust, London, UK

St Peter's Andrology Centre, London, UK
e-mail: waigin.lee@nhs.net

Table 8.1 Summary of procedures constituting gender affirmation surgery

GAS		Options
Genital (bottom surgery)	Penile reconstruction	Phalloplasty
		Metoidioplasty (meta)[a]
	Adjunctive procedures	Urethral lengthening (join-up)
		Scrotoplasty
		Glansplasty (glans sculpting)
		Clitoral transposition (burying of clitoris)
	Removal of "female" organs	Hysterectomy
		Salpingo-oophorectomy
		Vaginectomy (colpectomy)
Non-genital	Chest reconstruction (top surgery)	Long scar (double incision)
		Short scar
	Facial masculinisation	
	Vocal cord surgery	Rarely required

[a]Colloquial or alternative terms in parentheses

procedures a year since 2015 [2]. GAS is also requested at an increasingly younger age [3] possibly because information on transgender identities has become much more accessible via the internet and social acceptance has improved.

Broadly speaking, GAS can be classified as genital or non-genital procedures. In transmasculine persons (see definitions below), genital GAS encompasses penile reconstruction with or without adjunctive procedures and removal of the "female" organs (Table 8.1). Non-genital GAS usually refers to chest reconstruction (masculinisation) but can include other procedures (Table 8.1).

Urologists traditionally played an important role in genital GAS given the anatomical region and the need for reconstruction of the urinary tract and for insertion of urological prosthetics. However, a specialist andrologist with an understanding of reconstructive surgical principles and microsurgery may be best placed to comprehensively address the surgical needs of transmasculine individuals.

The advanced and diverse techniques required for transmasculine GAS cannot be adequately discussed within a chapter. The following chapter will introduce important concepts of transmasculine GAS to whet the appetite of the reader. The reader may then choose to pursue more in-depth reading and training at an appropriate centre, if desired.

Definitions and Terminology

Clinicians who intend to work within the field of GAS must have some understanding of the terminology that underpins inclusive care [4]. *Sex assigned at birth* (e.g., assigned male at birth, AMAB; assigned female at birth, AFAB) refers to the sex assigned to a newborn by a clinician. *Gender identity* is one's psychological sense of one's gender (a spectrum between female, male and "other"). "Other" includes *non-binary* persons who may identify with both genders, a gender different to male or female, outside the gender binary or as not having a gender altogether [5].

Transgender is an umbrella term for individuals whose sex assigned at birth do not match their gender identity. This mismatch is termed *gender incongruence*, which may lead to psychological distress or *gender dysphoria*. *Sexual orientation* is a separate concept that refers to the type of person one is sexually and/or emotionally attracted to. *Transmasculine* is defined as those who identify as being part of the male or masculine half of the spectrum and may therefore seek some form of masculinising GAS.

Genital Gender Affirmation Surgery

Genital GAS (in the properly selected patient) ameliorates gender dysphoria [6] and improves the psychological functioning of transmasculine persons [7]. The role of the clinician is to empower shared decision making given the multitude of options available to the individual. The options need to be balanced against the potential for morbidity (especially if a donor site is required) and unsatisfactory results [8].

Genital GAS should be offered in accordance with the World Professional Association for Transgender Health Standards of Care. The seventh version was published in 2011 [9] and the eighth version completed public review in early 2022 and will likely be published in the spring of 2022. Currently, one would need to have persistent and well-documented gender dysphoria with the capacity for informed consent and be of the age of majority in one's country to qualify. Additionally, physical and mental health should be stable, and the individual should have lived for more than a year in a congruent gender role while on testosterone therapy.

Penile Reconstruction

The options for penile reconstruction are phalloplasty or metoidioplasty [10]. Phalloplasty offers the most complete genital transformation with a full size neophallus and the ability to engage in penetrative intercourse. Metoidioplasty reconstructs a small penis without the need of a donor site. The small penis retains full tactile and erogenous sensation with the ability for natural erections.

Phalloplasty: A Historical Overview

The term phalloplasty originates from the Greek words phallos (penis-like) and plastos (to mould/sculpt). The first phalloplasty was performed by Nikolaj Bogoraz on a 23-year-old man AMAB following traumatic partial penile amputation (for infidelity) in 1936 [11]. The neophallus was reconstructed in stages using a tubed pedicled graft from the abdomen with rib cartilage as a phallic stiffener. Urethroplasty was achieved using a tubed scrotal flap.

Fig. 8.1 Tube-within-a-tube urethra with urethral stent

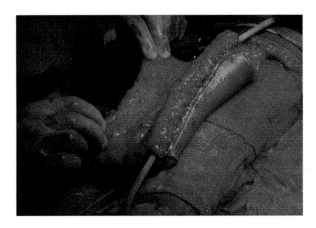

Over 10 years later, Laurence Michael Dillon (born Laura Maude Dillon) was the first transman to undergo phalloplasty requiring 13 operations over 4 years (1946–9). The technique pioneered by his New Zealand-born surgeon in London, Sir Harold Gillies, was to combine two tubed abdominal flaps. The first flap was tubularised forming the neo-urethra and a second flap then enclosed the first as a composite neo-phallus [12]. The Gillies phalloplasty remained the preferred technique for several decades despite subsequent advances including the first pedicled flap (1972) and the first free flap (1982) phalloplasty [13].

The sensate radial forearm free (RFF) flap with integrated (tube-within-a-tube) urethra developed by Chang and Hwang in 1984 further revolutionised phalloplasty [14]. Urethral reconstruction within the neo-phallus was historically achieved by prelaminated urethra (grafted tissue tubed over a catheter and buried in an epifascial tunnel) or by skin tube urethra where both long edges are incised, undermined and tubularised [15]. These were usually performed over two or more stages. The novel "tube-within-a-tube" design offered a better vascularised skin tube urethra reconstructed in a single stage (Fig. 8.1). This technique reduced the rate of urethral complications from 75% to 43% [16].

Contemporary Phalloplasty Techniques

Modern phalloplasty techniques utilise local or distant tissue flaps to reconstruct a neo-phallus. Distant flaps are raised as free flaps (requires microsurgery) or pedicled flaps (retains the native blood supply). The choice of flap is decided by multiple factors including patient donor site preference, preferred aesthetic and functional outcome, patient factors (degree of hirsutism and previous surgery or self-harm) and surgical expertise. The RFF flap remains the most common flap for phalloplasty although the anterolateral thigh (ALT) (pedicled or free) flap, musculocutaneous latissimus dorsi (free) flap and abdominal (pedicled) flap are common alternatives (Table 8.2).

Characteristics of the common flaps are summarised in Table 8.3. RFF flap is popular because of the constant vascular anatomy with a long pedicle facilitating

Table 8.2 Contemporary options for flap design based on donor site

Donor site	Flap design		
	Tube-in-tube	Phallus only	Urethra only
Radial forearm [14]	√	√	√
Anterolateral thigh [17]	√	√	
Abdomen [16]		√	
MLD [18]		√	√
Ulnar forearm [19]			√

MLD, musculocutaneous latissimus dorsi

Table 8.3 Comparison of flap characteristics and outcomes following phalloplasty

Flap	Sensation	Visible donor site scar	Genital skin color match	Urethral segment hair removal	Bulky
RFF	Best	Yes	No	No	No
ALT	Yes	No	Yes	Yes	Yes
MLD	Poor	No	No	NA	Yes
AF	Variable	No	Yes	NA	Yes

RFF, radial forearm free; ALT, anterolateral thigh; MLD, musculocutaneous latissimus dorsi; NA, not applicable; AF, abdominal

Fig. 8.2 Radial forearm free flap phalloplasty with associated donor site

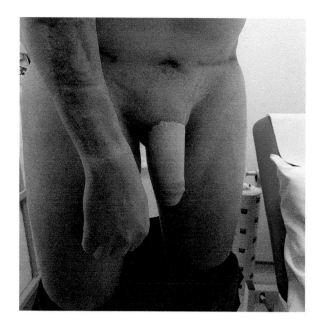

microvascular anastomosis and a hairless urethral segment. The resultant neophallus looks good and offers excellent sensation in 90% of patients [20]. A visible and large donor site is the primary disadvantage and can be viewed as stigmatising by some transmasculine individuals (Fig. 8.2).

The abdominal (pedicled) flap is ideal for those who prefer a phallus-only procedure with a shorter operative and recovery time. It should be considered in individuals with multiple co-morbidities that may complicate free flap phalloplasty. However, a composite RFF flap urethroplasty is required if standing micturition is desired [21].

Metoidioplasty

Metoidioplasty is performed by lengthening the hypertrophied clitoris following testosterone stimulation to form a small penis (Fig. 8.3). The surgical principles to reconstruct a small penis was first described in 1973 by Durfee and Rowland [22]. The term "metoidioplasty" was coined several years later in 1989 by Laub and Lebovic from the Greek words "meta" (change), "aidion" (male genitalia), and "plasty" (formation). The term "micropenis" has negative connotations and should be avoided.

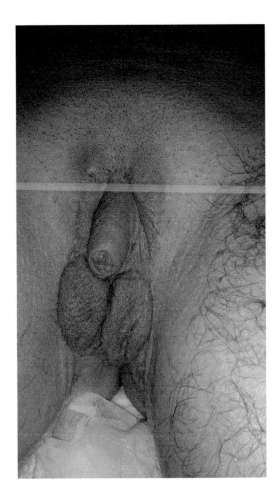

Fig. 8.3 Metoidioplasty with urethral lengthening, vaginectomy and scrotoplasty

A metoidioplasty normally measures between 4.8–10.2 cm (mean 5.6 cm) making it best suited for those of smaller build (body mass index $\leq$25 kg/m^2) but some techniques may achieve 6–12 cm (mean 8.7 cm) [23]. Most will be able to void while standing (87–100%) but many will continue to void in a cubicle (rather than at a urinal) [24]. Penetrative intercourse may rarely be possible. In a series of 813 cases, urethral fistulae and strictures occurred in 8.85% and 1.70% respectively while 99% of 655 individuals were satisfied with the cosmesis [25].

Penile Allotransplantation

Penile vascularised composite allotransplantation (VCA) may eventually offer the ideal approach for penile reconstruction. The ability to reconstruct "like-with-like" may allow natural erections and improve penile sensation (erogenous and tactile) and cosmesis. Techniques remain in their infancy even though the first penile VCA was performed 16 years ago in 2006 [26].

To date, only five cases have been reported in men AMAB but the most recent case (South Africa, 2017) has not been published in a peer-reviewed journal. The first case from 2006 required elective explant on day 14 primarily for psychosocial reasons [26]. Full urinary and sexual function was restored in the other three reported cases [27–29].

Penile VCA for genital GAS may also be technically feasible [30] but there are many anatomical, philosophical, and ethical concerns to be addressed before this may be considered. The lack of an established recipient bed in the female pelvis (tunica albuginea, corpora cavernosa and corpora spongiosum) will add further complexity to the technique. All patients to date have suffered iatrogenic or traumatic loss of their penis. Organ donors may be less accepting of GAS. The risks and costs of lifetime immunosuppression and monitoring also needs to be balanced against the more readily available option of phalloplasty. Eventually, tissue bioengineering may address some of these concerns once the many challenges to develop and apply 3D bioprinting in clinical practice have been surmounted.

Adjunctive Procedures

Staging of Surgery

The optimal timing and sequence of adjunctive procedures have not been clarified. Some centres combine phalloplasty with urethral lengthening (joining the phallus urethra to native urethra), glansplasty (fashioning a glans for the neophallus), clitoral transposition (repositioning or burying the clitoris), scrotoplasty (reconstruction of a neoscrotum) and removal of some/all of the "female" reproductive organs (hysterectomy, salpingo-oophorectomy and vaginectomy) in one stage. Other centres perform phalloplasty and the other procedures in two stages.

Combining all the above procedures reduces the number (and cost) of admissions but at the expense of longer operating times and the potential for escalating complications leading to major loss of the reconstruction [31]. Furthermore, urethral complications are common and will be symptomatic while awaiting repair. If urethral lengthening is staged, the fistula or stricture will remain asymptomatic (not leak) and can be repaired routinely at the time of the planned "second" stage with the use of adjacent tissue that may have been sacrificed if reconstruction was completed in one stage.

Penile and Testicular Prosthesis Insertion

The insertion of an erectile device with testicular prosthesis is always performed as a separate stage to the initial reconstruction. An interval of at least 6 months is recommended to allow the neophallus to heal and mature. A para-scrotal or infrapubic approach can be used and commercially available inflatable penile prostheses (IPP) are currently adapted for use in this cohort [32]. Satisfaction with the erectile devices is good and most can engage in penetrative intercourse (>80%) [33].

The pump of the device acts as a testis in one hemiscrotum and a testicular prosthesis is inserted on the contralateral side (Fig. 8.4). Malleable penile prostheses are not recommended due to the high risk of erosion. Polyethylene terephthalate

Fig. 8.4 Fully inflated erectile device with contralateral testicular prosthesis in situ

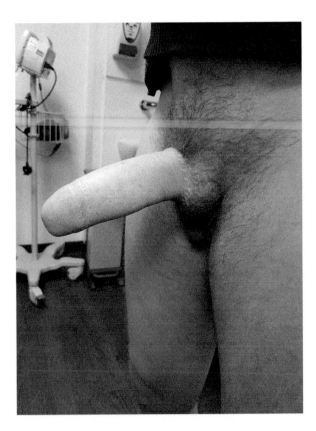

(Dacron) graft or hernia mesh is used to anchor the penile prosthesis cylinders to the pubis and tip of the neophallus due to the lack of corpora cavernosa.

The first erectile devices tailored for transmasculine persons (ZSI-475 FTM and ZSI-100 FTM, Zephyr Surgical Implants, Switzerland) are promising because they preclude the need for a cap and sock fashioned using either mesh, polyethylene, or polytetrafluoroethylene [34, 35]. However, numbers implanted, and reported outcomes (with short follow-up) are still limited, necessitating further studies. The devices are also not FDA-approved in the United States.

Non-genital Gender Affirmation Surgery

Chest Reconstruction

Chest masculinisation or "top surgery" is the most common surgical procedure for transmasculine persons. The 2015 U.S. Transgender Survey reported that most transmen (97%) and non-binary individuals AFAB (73%) had either had top surgery or desired it in the future [36]. They bind and conceal their breasts daily with tight wraps and restrictive garments while awaiting surgery.

The WPATH SOC do not stipulate that adults commence testosterone therapy prior to chest reconstruction (in contrast to genital GAS) [9]. The SOC advises adolescents who request top surgery to have lived an "ample" time as male with testosterone therapy for at least one year although this is also not a pre-requisite.

Briefly, the goal of mastectomy is to provide a smooth masculine chest contour while minimising and hiding scars along anatomic lines [37]. Techniques to achieve this can be divided into long scar ("double incision") techniques (more commonly performed) or short scar techniques including peri-areolar, circum-areolar or other skin resection patterns around the areola [38]. Adjunctive techniques like liposuction may also be combined with excision of the gland. An aesthetic male nipple areolar complex is also reconstructed. The nipples may be transferred as free grafts or on a pedicle.

Chest reconstruction have high satisfaction rates (up to 88%) and nipple sensitivity was rated as "good" or "very good" in 80% of breasts [38]. Individuals reported better body satisfaction, self-esteem and body image-related quality of life with reduced situational body dysphoria (e.g., while changing or showering) [39]. Interestingly, physicians rated the appearance after surgery more poorly than the patients themselves [40].

Other Non-genital Procedures

Vocal Cord Surgery

Voice is one of the most obvious dimorphic traits in humans. A low pitch voice plays a central role in masculine gender presentation. Individuals are least satisfied with their voice (compared to other traits) prior to transitioning but are most

Table 8.4 Options for facial masculinisation surgery in transmasculine persons

Facial unit	Facial aesthetic subunit	Surgical options
Upper face	Forehead	Forehead lengthening or augmentation
	Brow	Supra-orbital ridge augmentation
Mid face	Maxilla	Maxillary augmentation
	Nose	Rhinoplasty preader grafts
Lower face	Chin	Genioplasty
	Thyroid cartilage	Augmentation with bone graft

satisfied of the perceived change with testosterone therapy [41]. These changes coupled with vocal therapy are usually adequate and vocal cord surgery is rarely indicated [42] unlike for transfeminine persons.

Facial Masculinisation Surgery

Aesthetic procedures to further masculinise the face are not usually required (as opposed to the transfeminine population). The AMAB facial skeleton is larger, squarer and more angulated with sharp lines and a stronger jaw when compared to those AFAB [43]. The supraorbital ridge is more prominent and projects anterior to the eyes.

If desired, surgical options are available as summarised in Table 8.4 [44].

Summary

Transmasculine GAS is a complex field, and clinical practice continues to evolve rapidly. Key milestones include the advent of free and pedicled sensate flaps with integrated urethra and the development of a customised erectile device for the neophallus. The understanding of why, when, and how genital GAS is offered continues to improve. Functional and esthetic outcomes are acceptable but there is significant opportunity for improving techniques and outcomes in all aspects of GAS.

References

1. Wiepjes CM, Nota NM, de Blok CJM, Klaver M, de Vries ALC, Wensing-Kruger SA, et al. The Amsterdam Cohort of Gender Dysphoria Study (1972–2015): trends in prevalence, treatment, and regrets. J Sex Med. 2018;15(4):582–90.
2. Al-Tamimi M, Pigot GL, Elfering L, Ozer M, de Haseth K, van de Grift TC, et al. Genital gender-affirming surgery in transgender men in the Netherlands from 1989 to 2018: the evolution of surgical care. Plast Reconstr Surg. 2020;145(1):153e–61e.
3. Aydin D, Buk LJ, Partoft S, Bonde C, Thomsen MV, Tos T. Transgender surgery in Denmark From 1994 to 2015: 20-year follow-up study. J Sex Med. 2016;13(4):720–5.
4. Turban JL, Ehrensaft D. Research review: gender identity in youth: treatment paradigms and controversies. J Child Psychol Psychiatry. 2018;59(12):1228–43.
5. Galupo MP, Pulice-Farrow L, Pehl E. "There is nothing to do about it": nonbinary individuals' experience of gender dysphoria. Transgend Health. 2021;6(2):101–10.

6. Van De Grift TC, Elaut E, Cerwenka SC, Cohen-Kettenis PT, De Cuypere G, Richter-Appelt H, et al. Effects of medical interventions on gender dysphoria and body image: a follow-up study. Psychosom Med. 2017;79(7):815–23.
7. Wernick JA, Busa S, Matouk K, Nicholson J, Janssen A. A systematic review of the psychological benefits of gender-affirming surgery. Urol Clin North Am. 2019;46(4):475–86.
8. Rachlin K. Factors which influence individual's decisions when considering female-to-male genital reconstructive surgery. Int J Transgenderism. 1999;3(3):97.
9. Coleman E, Bockting W, Botzer M, Cohen-Kettenis P, DeCuypere G, Feldman J, et al. Standards of care for the health of transsexual, transgender, and gender-nonconforming people, version 7. Int J Transgend. 2012;13(4):165–232.
10. Lee WG, Christopher N, Ralph DJ. Penile reconstruction and the role of surgery in gender dysphoria. Eur Urol Focus. 2019;5(3):337–9.
11. Bogoraz N. Über die volle plastische Wiederherstellung eines zum Koitus fähigen Penis (Peniplastica totalis). Zentralbl Chir. 1936;22:1271–6.
12. Nair R, Sriprasad S. Sir Harold Gillies: pioneer of phalloplasty and the birth of uroplastic surgery. J Urol. 2010;183(4S):e437.
13. Zurada A, Salandy S, Roberts W, Gielecki J, Schober J, Loukas M. The evolution of transgender surgery. Clin Anat. 2018;31(6):878–86.
14. Chang TS, Hwang WY. Forearm flap in one-stage reconstruction of the penis. Plast Reconstr Surg. 1984;74(2):251–8.
15. Hage JJ, Bouman FG, Bloem JJ. Preconstruction of the pars pendulans urethrae for phalloplasty in female-to-male transsexuals. Plast Reconstr Surg. 1993;91(7):1303–7.
16. Bettocchi C, Ralph DJ, Pryor JP. Pedicled pubic phalloplasty in females with gender dysphoria. BJU Int. 2005;95(1):120–4.
17. Felici N, Felici A. A new phalloplasty technique: the free anterolateral thigh flap phalloplasty. J Plast Reconstr Aesthet Surg. 2006;59(2):153–7.
18. Djordjevic ML, Bumbasirevic MZ, Vukovic PM, Sansalone S, Perovic SV. Musculocutaneous latissimus dorsi free transfer flap for total phalloplasty in children. J Pediatr Urol. 2006;2(4):333–9.
19. Lee HB, Hur JY, Song JM, Tark KC. Long anterior urethral reconstruction using a sensate ulnar forearm free flap. Plast Reconstr Surg. 2001;108(7):2053–6.
20. Garaffa G, Christopher NA, Ralph DJ. Total phallic reconstruction in female-to-male transsexuals. Eur Urol. 2010;57(4):715–22.
21. Garaffa G, Ralph DJ, Christopher N. Total urethral construction with the radial artery-based forearm free flap in the transsexual. BJU Int. 2010;106(8):1206–10.
22. Durfee R, Rowland W. Penile substitution with clitoral enlargement and urethral transfer. In: Laub DR, Gandy P, editors. Proceedings of the second interdisciplanary symposium on gender dysphoria syndrome. Palo Alto: Stanford University Press; 1973. p. 181–3.
23. Cohanzad S. Extensive metoidioplasty as a technique capable of creating a compatible analogue to a natural penis in female transsexuals. Aesthet Plast Surg. 2016;40(1):130–8.
24. Bizic MR, Stojanovic B, Joksic I, Djordjevic ML. Metoidioplasty. Urol Clin North Am. 2019;46(4):555–66.
25. Bordas N, Stojanovic B, Bizic M, Szanto A, Djordjevic ML. Metoidioplasty: surgical options and outcomes in 813 cases. Front Endocrinol (Lausanne). 2021;12:760284.
26. Hu W, Lu J, Zhang L, Wu W, Nie H, Zhu Y, et al. A preliminary report of penile transplantation. Eur Urol. 2006;50(4):851–3.
27. Cetrulo CL Jr, Li K, Salinas HM, Treiser MD, Schol I, Barrisford GW, et al. Penis transplantation: first US experience. 2018;1(5):983–8.
28. van der Merwe A, Graewe F, Zuhlke A, Barsdorf NW, Zarrabi AD, Viljoen JT, et al. Penile allotransplantation for penis amputation following ritual circumcision: a case report with 24 months of follow-up. Lancet. 2017;390(10099):1038–47.
29. Szafran AA, Redett R, Burnett AL. Penile transplantation: the US experience and institutional program set-up. Transl. 2018;7(4):639–45.

30. Selvaggi G, Wesslen E, Elander A, Wroblewski P, Thorarinsson A, Olausson M. En bloc surgical dissection for penile transplantation for trans-men: a cadaveric study. Biomed Res Int. 2018;2018:6754030.
31. Monstrey S, Hoebeke P, Selvaggi G, Ceulemans P, Van Landuyt K, Blondeel P, et al. Penile reconstruction: is the radial forearm flap really the standard technique? Plast Reconstr Surg. 2009;124(2):510–8.
32. Lee WG, Christopher N, Ralph D. IPP in neophallus. In: Moncada-Iribarren I, Martinez-Salamanca JI, Lledo-Garcia E, Mulcahy JJ, editors. Textbook of urogenital prosthetic surgery. Madrid, Spain: Editorial Médica Panamericana S.A.; 2020. p. 213–31.
33. Falcone M, Garaffa G, Gillo A, Dente D, Christopher AN, Ralph DJ. Outcomes of inflatable penile prosthesis insertion in 247 patients completing female to male gender reassignment surgery. BJU Int. 2018;121(1):139–44.
34. Verla W, Goedertier W, Lumen N, Spinoit AF, Waterloos M, Waterschoot M, et al. Implantation of the ZSI 475 FTM erectile device after phalloplasty: a prospective analysis of surgical outcomes. J Sex Med. 2021;18(3):615–22.
35. Neuville P, Morel-Journel N, Cabelguenne D, Ruffion A, Paparel P, Terrier J-E. First outcomes of the ZSI 475 FtM, a specific prosthesis designed for phalloplasty. J Sex Med. 2019;16(2):316–22.
36. The Report of The U.S. Transgender Surgery 2015. National Center for Transgender Equality. https://www.ustranssurvey.org/reports2015. Accessed February 2022.
37. Donato DP, Walzer NK, Rivera A, Wright L, Agarwal CA. Female-to-male chest reconstruction: a review of technique and outcomes. Ann Plast Surg. 2017;79(3):259–63.
38. Wolter A, Diedrichson J, Scholz T, Arens-Landwehr A, Liebau J. Sexual reassignment surgery in female-to-male transsexuals: an algorithm for subcutaneous mastectomy. J Plast Reconstr Aesthet Surg. 2015;68(2):184–91.
39. van de Grift TC, Kreukels BP, Elfering L, Ozer M, Bouman MB, Buncamper ME, et al. Body image in transmen: multidimensional measurement and the effects of mastectomy. J Sex Med. 2016;13(11):1778–86.
40. Oles N, Darrach H, Landford W, Garza M, Twose C, Park CS, et al. Gender affirming surgery: a comprehensive, systematic review of all peer-reviewed literature and methods of assessing patient-centered outcomes (part 1: breast/chest, face, and voice). Ann Surg. 2022;275(1):e52–66.
41. Hodges-Simeon CR, Grail GPO, Albert G, Groll MD, Stepp CE, Carre JM, et al. Testosterone therapy masculinizes speech and gender presentation in transgender men. Sci. 2021;11(1):3494.
42. McNeill EJ. Management of the transgender voice. J Laryngol Otol. 2006;120(7):521–3.
43. Colebunders B, Brondeel S, D'Arpa S, Hoebeke P, Monstrey S. An update on the surgical treatment for transgender patients. Sex Med Rev. 2017;5(1):103–9.
44. Sayegh F, Ludwig DC, Ascha M, Vyas K, Shakir A, Kwong JW, et al. Facial masculinization surgery and its role in the treatment of gender dysphoria. J Craniofac Surg. 2019;30(5):1339–46.

Transfeminine Gender Affirmation Surgery

9

S. C. Morgenstern and M. Sohn

Abstract

Transpersons, who experience a discrepancy between the gender assigned at birth and the perception of gender identity seem a common phenomenon throughout the ages and in all cultures and centuries and should not be seen as pathological. The dramatic rise in prevalence over the last decades, however, has led to a marked increase in the demand for surgical reassignment and consequently the need for multidisciplinary, highly specialised centres and professionals.

While for some transgender persons, hormonal and surgical body modifications are not needed to achieve comfort with their identity, for many others surgical gender reassignment is essential and medically necessary.

The goals of male-to-female genital reassignment surgery for transwomen include orchiectomy, the creation of a sensitive neoclitoris with the ability to provide sexual sensation, a neovulva and a neovagina which should allow penetration.

For genital reassignment surgery the pedicled penile skin inversion is the most commonly used technique. In the absence of sufficient penile shaft skin length an augmentation with full thickness skin flaps or vaginoplasty using bowel segments (e.g., sigmavagina) have been established as techniques of choice (Sohn and Morgenstern, German National Guidelines for Transgender Care, 2023, in press).

The commonest complications include a diverted urinary stream, stenosis of the introitus and the neovagina, and lifelong neovaginal self-dilatation is often indicated.

S. C. Morgenstern (✉) · M. Sohn
Unit for Reconstructive Urology and Gender Reassignment Surgery, Clinic for Urology,
Agaplesion Markus Krankenhaus, Frankfurt, Germany
e-mail: saskia.morgenstern@agaplesion.de

The capability of achieving orgasm, functional and aesthetical satisfaction, as well as overall satisfaction with a drastic improvement of well-being, has been proven by many studies and the regret rate is lower than 1% (Wiepjes et al., J Sex Med 15(4):582–90, 2018).

Introduction

This chapter provides an up-to-date overview of male-to-female-transgender genital affirmation surgery based on a systematic literature review with a focus on perioperative treatment strategies and surgical techniques for this challenging, but for the people affected truly life changing, treatment.

In andrology and sexual medicine many practitioners are increasingly confronted with gender nonconformity. This may be the result of the drastic rise of prevalence over the last decades, an increased presence in media, or a growing number of specialised centres with a consequently higher need for training opportunities [1]. An over 40 years cohort study from one of Europe's largest transgender centres shows a 20-fold increase of people appling for transgender healthcare with an estimated prevalence of transwomen (male-to female transgender) of 1:3800 and 1:5200 for transmen (female-to-male-transgender). Even though the total number is continuously rising, the percentage of individuals deciding for surgery after starting hormone therapy has stayed stable at 74.7% of the transwomen, and 83.8% of the transmen. The same applies to the regret rate after gender reassignment surgery which was found to be equally low (0.6% for transwomen, 0.3% for transman) [2].

Despite being a relatively small percentage of our patients, the adequate care for this subgroup is especially challenging. Not only are they usually affected by a long ordeal, often facing multiple emotional and social stigmatisms and obstructions until they receive adequate treatment, but the treatment itself can include various, highly complex surgeries and requires a very strict, lifelong self-management by the patient. Involved practitioners can only follow so-called standards of care, as no evidence based surgical treatment algorithms exist due to insufficient available data. Despite this the overall satisfaction rate after male-to-female genital reassignment surgery is reported as high as up to 92% [3, 4] and regrets are reported as under 1% [2].

In 2010 the World Professional Association for Transgender Health (WPATH) stated that "the expression of gender characteristics, including identities, that are not stereotypically associated with one's assigned sex at birth is a common and culturally diverse human phenomenon [that] should not be judged as inherently pathological or negative." [5]. Despite gender nonconformity including a broad spectrum of partly overlapping variants with changing nomenclatures, the following article is using the term male-to-female transgender or transwoman for a person who experience themselves as female despite a male karyotype. Even if there are no valid epidemiological data, the global prevalence of male-to-female transgender was previously estimated by the WPATH in 2012 as 1:11,900 to 1:45,000 and for female-to-male transgender 1:30,000 to 1:200,000 [5]. Whereas the already mentioned large, longitudinal study from the Amsterdam group estimated a 20-fold increase in the prevalence over the last 40 years, a shift towards adolescent transperson and estimate a prevalence of transwomen (male-to female transgender) 1:3800 and 1:5200 for transmen (female-to-male transgender) [2]. It remains unclear to which extent these numbers from the Netherlands can be applied to other countries [1, 6–9].

It is worth emphasising, that only some gender-nonconforming persons undergo all stages of surgical gender-reassignment as described in the following chapter. The individual perception of the discrepancy of the gender assigned by birth/genetics and the inner gender identity of a person may lead to a very wide range of individualized processes. Body modifications such as hormonal and or surgical treatment are not needed for some persons to achieve comfort with their identity [5]. In the Amsterdam study in 2010 only 65% of all persons who applied for transgender health care underwent hormonal therapy, and 74.7% of the transwomen, and 83.8% of the transmen who started hormonal therapy proceeded to surgery [2].

Various options for male-to-female gender reassignment surgery exists, and there is a broad individual span of which body-transforming options are medically indicated for the individual person [5]. This ranges from the so called "top-surgery", e.g., augmentation of the breast, facial feminization procedures like modifications of the forehead, cheeks, nose, chin, the angle of the mandible and the upper lip and voice surgery by chondrolaryngoplasty procedures [10]. Nevertheless, this chapter focuses on genital reassignment. Figure 9.1 provides intraoperative before and after pictures of one of the most commonly used techniques of male-to-female gender reassignment while Fig. 9.2 shows the 6-month postoperative result.

The authors also emphasize that transgender surgery puts the performing surgeon in the unique position, where highly elective, often irreversible procedures with a high likelihood of risk and long-term complications are carried out on a

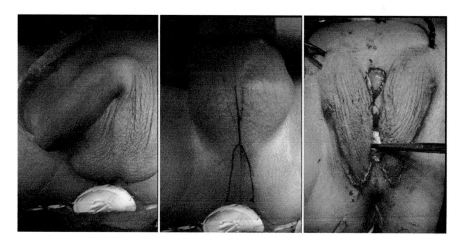

Fig. 9.1 Male-to- female genital reassignment surgery (penoscrotal inversion vaginoplasty technique), pre- and postoperative findings

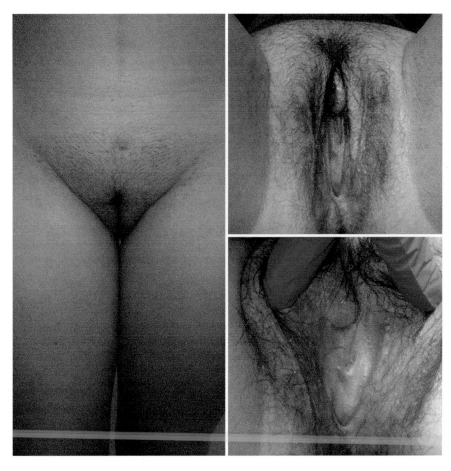

Fig. 9.2 6-month postoperative result of male-to- female genital reassignment surgery (single stage penoscrotal inversion vaginoplasty technique)

physically healthy body. Therefore, an extensive, multidisciplinary preoperative counselling and preparation, a very careful patient selection and best possible treatment standards are crucial [5, 8, 10].

Perioperative Management

Preoperative Requirements and Criteria

Being a highly elective surgery with an irreversible physical, psychological and social impact on the person's life, the preoperative selection and preparation is highly complex. The process of being cleared for surgical body modifications usually takes many months or years.

Multidisciplinary Team

The mandatory multidisciplinary approach to transgender care comprises psychological and mental therapy by mental health professionals trained in this field, hormonal therapy by endocrinologists or other specially trained medical professionals, and surgical therapy by surgical professionals with an expertise in this area. Additional voice and communication therapy, e.g., by speech therapists may also be beneficial [5].

Having previously mentioned that surgical options are not required for some transgender persons, it should be stated, that for many others surgical gender reassignment is essential and medically necessary to achieve comfort with their gender identity [5]. For genital reassignment surgery the responsible surgeon may be a urologist, a plastic surgeon or a general surgeon, or even other surgical specialties when adequate training, expertise and experience in the field of genitourethral surgery has been acquired [11–14].

Criteria for Genital Reassignment Surgery

Even noting the lack of evidence based surgical guidelines, the World Professional Association for Transgender Health provides clinical guidance and effective pathways in their "Standards of Care (SOC) for the Health of Transsexual, Transgender, and Gender Nonconforming People", which is seen as a broadly and globally followed standard in transgender care. For each group of body-assigning surgery different criteria are applied and country-specific modifications on these criteria exist. The criteria defined by the WPATH for genital reassignment surgery for male-to-female transgender persons are as follows:

1. Persistent, well-documented gender dysphoria (two referral letters from qualified mental health professionals who have independently assessed the person)
2. Capacity to make a fully informed decision and to consent for treatment
3. Age of majority in the given country
4. If significant medical or mental health concerns are present, they must be well controlled
5. 12 continuous months of hormone therapy as appropriate to the patient's gender goals (unless hormones are not clinically indicated for the individual) [5]

If above mentioned criteria are met, the generally substantial cost for the surgical procedures are often covered by the governmental/national health insurance in many countries. A letter of approval for cost coverage by the persons' health insurance provider is mandatory in many transgender centres prior to surgery.

A controlled HIV or Hepatitis infection is not a contraindication for genital reassignment surgery, and there is no upper age limit [15]. Nevertheless, higher age, obesity, and cardiovascular comorbidities all increase the risk of pre- and postoperative complications. Therefore, careful preoperative counselling and the best possible reduction of risk factors prior to surgery are crucial. Furthermore, it maybe rational not to proceed through all potential genital reassignment surgical steps in individual cases. There is an ongoing controversy in regards to the minimum age required for genital reassignment surgery. A current study, carried out amongst

WPATH-associated US-American surgeons showed that 11 out of 20 surgeons are performing genital reassignment surgery on under 18 years old trans persons [16]. Nevertheless, the authors recommend, in line with the WPATH recommendation, not to operate on underage persons.

Fertility

Prior to the surgery the potential wish for fertility preserving measures must be discussed with the person [5, 17], especially given the global trend of continually younger trans persons seeking surgical gender affirmation [2]. It may be necessary, for example, to temporally put on-hold hormonal therapy to increase spermatogenesis/sperm quality for potential future in vitro fertilisation measurements [17]. Nevertheless, the trans person should be aware, that long-term hormonal therapy can lead to a severe decrease of fertility. A histology study shows a complete spermatogenesis in only in 24.07% of transwomen [18]. Until now more than 40 transplantations of the uterus (with a subsequent number of 12 vital birth) has been performed globally, and even though this has not been put into practise yet, uterus transplantation may also become a future option for transwomen [19].

Pre- and Postoperative Course

Counseling and Compliance Strategies

The performing surgeon is not only responsible to assure whether the above-mentioned criteria are fulfilled, they must undertake extensive discussions of the procedure and postoperative course. This must take place at a minimum of 24 h prior to surgery and should be carefully documented. It should include the different surgical techniques with their advantages and disadvantages, limitations, risks and possible complications, including the surgeons own complication rates and his/her own before-and-after photographs. Ideally the person should receive written information material prior to the consultation and should be given sufficient time for individual questions in order to achieve well-informed, shared decision-making, ensuring that the person is in a position to give informed consent [5].

The authors emphasize that it is beneficial, for further patient compliance and general satisfaction, to focus in this context on the following additional aspects: the expected period of immobilisation and pain, pain relieving strategies, gaining realistic expectation of outcomes, the need for patients postoperative self-management of the wounds, the need for disciplined neovaginal care/self-dilatations with its impact on social/work life, and individual strategies to "get-used-to" the new genital in a functional and sexual way. If possible/wanted the discussions should include the person's partner(s).

Perioperative Patient Management

The positioning in the operating room is dependent on the surgical technique but usually the person is placed in a lithotomy position. The authors prefer to place the person's legs in slings, as they have been formerly used extensively for the perineal

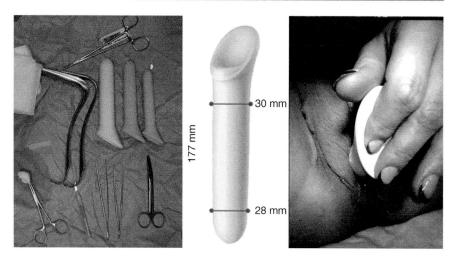

Fig. 9.3 Equipment for postoperative care in week 1 and patients' self- management by frequent self- dilatation of the neovagina using a medical silicon dilatator

prostatectomy. This allows temporary extension to an extreme lithotomy position, providing excellent access for surgical steps such as the dissection of the neovaginal cavity. Shaving, draping, antiseptic skin preparation and antibiotic prophylaxis usually follows the local hygienic protocols, and there is some controversy about the need for preoperative bowl preparation. The procedure is usually carried out under general anaesthesia with the need for relaxation, and usually the patient is able to be transferred back to the ward after the surgery without the need for intermediate or intensive care observation. Systemic and physical prophylaxis of deep venous thrombosis is recommended.

Depending on the surgeon's technique and experience, usually a bedrest of 5–7 days is required to allow the neovaginal-space holder and the compression dressings to stay in place. Urinary diversion is usually performed via a suprapubic catheter and left in place for the first days.

In our department, the surgeon removes the dressings and the space holder on postoperative day 5 to inspect the progress of wound healing on the vulva as well as the neovaginal cavity using gynaecological specula. At this stage the transwoman is extensively counselled in self-care (see below) and starts daily self-dilation of the neovagina using silicon based medical dilators. This is performed four times a day for 30 min (see Fig. 9.3), followed by vaginal showering and wound disinfection.

Patient Self-Management, Follow Up and Cancer Screening

Patient Self-Management

During the inpatient stay in the authors department, the transwomen are trained in frequent genital hygiene and regular vaginal dilations. The latter must be carried out by the patient in order to maintain vaginal depth and width on a lifelong basis and might be reduced if regular penetrative sexual intercourse is performed. They also receive consultation about the axis and the dimensions of the neovagina which, due to the male pelvis, differs from a biological vagina. This is important for the patient and their partner(s) as this might affect sexual intercourse [5].

Follow Up

In 2009, Monstrey et al. showed that long-term postoperative care and follow-up after surgical treatment for gender persons are associated with good surgical and psychosocial outcomes [5]. It seems beneficial to use standardised questionnaires during the routine follow up appointments by the surgeons whenever possible. Published in 2020, "The Operated Male-to-Female Sexual Function Index" (oMt-FSFI) is the first validated questionnaire for assessment of key sexual function after male-to-female gender affirming surgery [20].

Routine Check-Ups and Cancer Screening

Routine check-ups, including endocrinology monitoring and cancer screening, are usually performed outside the authors department by specialised office physicians.

Screening for prostate cancer, the only remaining male-specific organ in a transwoman with full genital reassignment surgery, remains particular challenging as diagnostics are limited and healthcare providers are often not specifically trained. In 2021 the British Journal of Urology International published recommendations based on a review of all (yet not extensive) data until January 2021. This identified 10 cases of prostate cancer in transgender women worldwide. For transwomen who underwent hormonal therapy and genital reassignment surgery, it is recommended to perform a multiparametric MRI if PSA is over 1 ng/mL and a biopsy if it shows a PIRADS >3 [21].

Surgical Techniques for Male-to-Female Genital Reassignment

Even though various options for male-to-female gender reassignment surgery may be indicated for transwoman to achieve comfort with her gender/identity (e.g., augmentation of the breast, facial feminization, voice surgery, etc.), we focus in the following on the surgical options for genital reassignment:

Basic Principles of Male-to-Female Genital Reassignment

Genital reassignment surgery for transwomen can be carried out in a single stage or a staged manner. Dependent to the persons needs and anatomical features, the surgical steps should include orchiectomy, the creation of a sensitive neoclitoris with the ability to provide sexual sensation, a neovulva and a neovagina which should allow penetration. In up to 84% of primary attempted single staged approaches there is a need for secondary corrective procedures [4, 22–24].

Abraham [25] was the first to describe an intentional gender affirmation surgery for a transperson and in 1956 Burou, a French gynaecologist, invented and applied the first vaginoplasty technique using an inverted pedicle penile skin flap [10]. Karim et al. [26] defined the goals of male-to-female genital reassignment surgery for transwomen, which are still in use today: The creation of a feminine perineo-genital complex, which satisfies the functional and aesthetical needs of the person while leading to a minimum of operative scarring. The neomeatus should allow a seated micturition with a caudal facing, unobstructed urinary stream and be free of stenosis or fistulae. The neovagina should ideally be coated by hair free, elastic and moist epithelium with a depth of a minimum of 10 cm and a width of at least 3 cm. Neovulva and neovagina should allow satisfying sexual stimulation during sexual activity [17].

Bilateral inguinal orchiectomy, a central part of male to female gender reassignment surgery, is commonly performed during the main genital reassignment surgery. For individual reasons transwomen may wish to undergo only the orchiectomy without proceeding to a genital reassignment [27]. In these cases, an orchiectomy, either with two separate inguinal incisions or via a single, longitudinal scrotal incision, can be performed in a separate procedure prior the vaginoplasty [17]. This generally does not affect the outcome of potential future vagino- and vulvoplasty procedures, if requested on a later stage [23]. Preservation of the testes is not recommended, as it leads to the need of continuation of androgen suppressive hormonal therapy [17].

Orchiectomy, Vagino-, Clitorido-, Labio- and Vulvoplasty- Techniques

Due to the lack of evidence based, randomized, controlled studies and very inhomogeneous data, no evidence based standards on surgical transgender care currently exist. A review of current published data, including the authors experience in up to 30 years in genital reassignment for transwomen illustrated with own operating pictures, provides the following overview of outcomes, complications and available techniques, while focus on the most commonly used techniques in our centre:

Incision According to the Preferred Vaginoplasty Technique

The incision is based on the preferred surgical technique for neovaginal lining. The most commonly used technique for vaginal lining worldwide involves the use of inverted penile skin with or without extension through pedicled or free scrotal skin. When a pedicled scrotal flap is used, it can also be correctly referred to as the peno-scrotal inversion technique [17]. The individual patient's hair status and the extent of pedicled scrotal flap will determine the possible need for preoperative epilation treatment [28].

If a free scrotal skin graft is used, it can be thinned and defatted by hand, taking the hair follicles with it. Thus, in the majority of cases, an inverted y-shaped perineoscrotal incision will be made, with extension into the ventral penile shaft if necessary.

Orchiectomy

After dissection of the testicles and spermatic cords and tracing them to the inguinal canal, bilateral orchiectomy is usually carried out by identifying the testicular cord at the level of the external inguinal ring. Separate ligations of the deferens duct and the testicular vessels are performed and the proximal stumps are placed into the inguinal canal [23].

Perineal Dissection and Urethral Preparation

For further dissection, it is recommended to use a self-holding hook system (e.g., Scott retractor). Exposure of the centrum tendineum is recommended as a starting point for subsequent dissection and preparation of the neovaginal cavity. The bulbo-spongiosus and ischiocavernosi muscles can then be dissected and resected. The next step is mobilization of the urethra and the surrounding corpus spongiosum from the corpora cavernosa and dissection in the distal region. If the penile inversion technique is used, further dissection is then performed between Colle's and Buck's fascia distally to the glans.

Creation of the Neoglans and Dissection of the Neurovascular Bundle

Since the beginning of the 1990s [29], the formation of a neoclitoris from the dorsal vascular nerve bundle and part of the glans has been one of the standard techniques for primary genital approximation in a male-to-female transperson. For this purpose, the entire glans or parts of the glans together with the dorsal vascular nerve bundle are dissected from the corpora cavernosa to the pelvic floor. Whether the dorsal vascular nerve bundle is dissected directly over the corpora or with the inclusion of a dorsal strip of the tunica is optional [30], as is how much distal prepuce remains on the glans (see clitoroplasty). The corpora cavernosa can then be dissected and resected directly over the pubic bones as close as possible. It is recommended to resect the corpora cavernosa as completely as possible to avoid later potential constriction of the introitus during sexual arousal by still present proximal corpora remnants [17, 31]. The same applies for the bulb of the corpus spongiosus, for which partial resection is therefore recommended.

Creation of the Neovaginal Cavity

For the creation of the neovaginal cavity, the pelvic floor is sharply opened in the area of the centrum tendineum and a layer in the retroprostatic prerectal space is sought and dilated, ideally following the sheets of Denonvillier's fascia. The dissection can be performed under digital rectal control if a rectal shield was sutured in at the beginning of the operation. Whether a partial incision of the levator fibres is required on both sides may depend on the individual anatomical conditions of the pelvic inlet [31, 32]. Usually a vaginal depth of 14–15 cm and a width of 4 cm can be created by his manner (see Fig. 9.4).

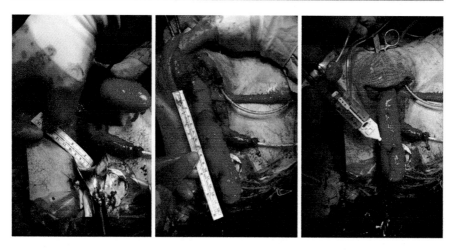

Fig. 9.4 Neovaginal cavity measurement and neovaginal sleeve, fibrinogenic glue is used prior to the invagination

Vaginoplasty

Despite the penoscrotal inversion technique for lining the neovaginal cavity being the most commonly used technique in male-to-female transgender persons, there are several other vaginoplasty techniques available. These range from lengthening of the penile skin lining with pedicled peritoneal lobes, laparoscopically harvested vascular pedicled intestinal parts (ileum, sigmoid) and experimental free grafts (e.g., amnion [14], oral mucosa [33, 34], dermal allograft [35, 36]). The following focuses on the two most used and reported techniques, the penoscrotal inversion-plasty (PI) and the vascularised bowel-segment vaginoplasty, where ileum or sigma parts are used to create the neovagina.

Penoscrotal Inversionplasty (PI)

The penile or penoscrotal inversionplasty continues to be, worldwide, the most frequently performed surgical technique for the creation of a neovaginal lining in male-to-female transgender as part of primary surgery. It is also the most widely published technique, including long-term postoperative outcomes [4, 17, 24, 28, 32, 37–44]. Depending on the individual hair type and extent of scrotal inversion, preoperative epilation treatment might be sensible and necessary [28, 32].

A systematic literature review from 2015 evaluated 216 publications on vaginoplasty, of which 13 studies allowed for outcome analysis. The cited studies show a vaginal depth between 10–13.5 cm with a width between 3 and 4 cm. The cited studies also include techniques using portions of the urethra or free scrotal additional skin grafts (see below).

A "true" penoscrotal inversionplasty, creating the entire neovagina from that skin alone, can only be performed if sufficient penile length is available. A lack of penile shaft skin can be the result of previous circumcision, a hypoplastic penis due to previous hormonal puberty blockers or if parts of the penile shaft skin are used for the formation of the small labia and the foreskin of the neoclitoris. To extend the inverted penile skin tube, augmentation with free scrotal skin grafts (with or without pedicled urethral strip—so-called "combined method"—[41, 45]), or single stage or staged extensions using bowel segments have been published [46, 47]. The preferred surgical technique differs considerably between the groups of authors.

The augmentation with free full-thickness skin grafts, predominantly obtained from excess scrotal skin, is one of the most commonly used and followed up technique to extend insufficient penile inversion vaginoplasty (see below). Figure 9.5 shows the neovaginal augmentation with a carefully defatted free full-thickness skin graft, where special care must also be taken to remove potential hair follicles.

Currently, several centres favour the inclusion of a urethral strip in the vaginal lining also from the point of view of allowing potential moistening of the neovagina [45, 48–50]. The potential benefit of the additional use of urethral strips has not yet

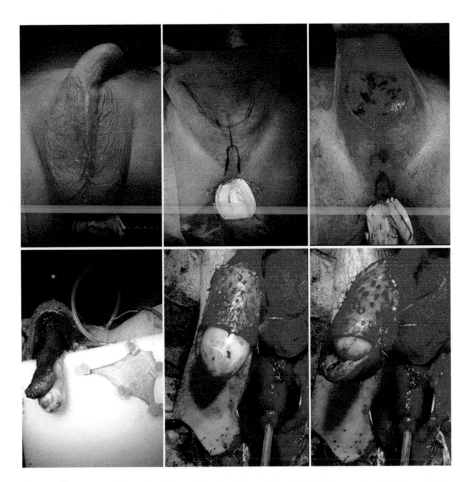

Fig. 9.5 Penoscrotal inversionplasty - skin incision and free full- thickness scrotal skin graft for neovaginal augmentation

been demonstrated by prospective studies compared with penoscrotal inversion alone. The concept itself also seems debatable, as the urethelium does not contain mucous producing cells.

A study from Amsterdam prospectively compared the results of lengthening penile inversionplasty using free scrotal skin grafts with the isolated penile inversion technique. With penile length measured intraoperatively 11 cm and below, a free scrotal skin graft was used as an extension of the neovaginal lining, if above 11 cm an isolated penile inversionplasty was performed. In both groups there was an equal slight shrinkage of the neovagina within the first postoperative weeks, but the measured vaginal length stayed equal with or without scrotal skin graft extension on postoperative week 3 and year one. This shows that the additional use of free full-thickness skin grafts did not significantly affect the shrinkage of neovaginal length. Also sensitivity and subjective satisfaction rates did not differ significantly between the treatment methods, so lengthening of the vaginal lining with free scrotal skin grafts can be recommended for short penile length [51]. Recently, a study of 41 patients also highlighted the potential of lengthening the penile skin tube with robotically harvested pedicled peritoneal flaps [52]. In a retrospective study of 475 patients, a high success rate for sufficient vaginal lining and vaginal volume was found with a median follow-up of 7.8 years, and free scrotal extension of the penile skin tube was always performed in relatively short penises. Only 2.9% of patients required performance of a repeat vaginoplasty for atresia or shrinkage of the primary neovagina [53]. These results were confirmed by a study of 240 patients from Philadelphia published in 2019. Here, extension of the penile cutaneous tube by free scrotal grafts and inclusion of a urethral strip in the penile skin graft were also performed. With a rather short follow-up of 3 months, the stenosis rate of the neovaginal cavity was 2.1% [54]. The methodology of combined techniques for vaginal lining has been more standardized in Thailand, and has now been published in over 3000 patients, with systematic follow-up studies available in nearly 400 patients [55].

Vascularised Bowel: Segment Vaginoplasty (Ileum/Sigma)

The laparoscopic harvest of vascularized sigmoid or ileum segments for neovaginal linings is about to established as a valuable option to counter the increase of hypoplastic genitalia after puberty-blocking hormonal therapy in young transwoman as well a salvage vaginoplasty technique. After failed primary neovaginal creation from penile or penoscrotal skin graft, laparoscopically assisted sigmoid neovaginal creation is now the method of choice, which usually requires general surgeons to be added to the interdisciplinary team. Advantages of vaginoplasty techniques using intestinal parts are the lack of need for bougienage, as well as the intestinal secretions moistening-effect on the neovaginal cavity as well as the possibility to achieve sufficient depth and adequate width of the vaginal cavity when sigmoid parts are used. To avoid stenosis of the introitus, special care is required while creating the anastomosis of the sigmoid wall with the external skin, and a life-long self-dilatation of the introitus is needed in many cases.

First experiences with pedicled intestinal parts for reconstruction of the vagina were already made between 1892 and 1904 in patients with vaginal atresia. The first mention of neovaginal creation from intestinal parts in male-to-female transgender dates back to 1974 [49]. A large case series of 86 patients was published in 2011, but only 27 patients with male-to-female transgender identity were included [56]. In all cases, a rectosigmoid segment of 8–11 cm in length was used. All 27 patients had previously received a neovaginal device with inverted penile skin, but this had resulted in vaginal stenosis. A follow-up of 47 months showed a satisfactory result in 80%. The procedure was performed via a combined transabdominal and perineal approach. In 2016, another study involving secondary vaginoplasties after failed primary creation was published by the Amsterdam team on 24 patients. This was a long-term follow-up study with a mean follow-up of almost 30 years, as all patients were operated on between 1970 and 2000. The long-term follow-up showed that 79% had to undergo at least one further follow-up operation, mostly due to the development of introitus stenosis and a high functional and aesthetic satisfaction rate was shown [57]. In the same year, the same group published their first results after primary creation of a sigmoid neovagina in 31 young patients with an average age of 19 years at the time of surgery. The reason for choosing the surgical procedure in all cases was a pronounced penoscrotal hypoplasia with an average penile skin length of 7 cm. In 84% of the patients, puberty-blocking medication and opposite-sex hormone administration had been performed previously. In 30 of 31 cases, creation of a sigmoid neovagina was performed, and in one case, removal of a terminal ileal segment was performed due to insufficient mobilization of the sigmoid segment [58]. In all cases, the operation was performed in combination of a perineal approach and a laparoscopic transabdominal approach in cooperation with an appropriately laparoscopically trained general surgeon. Again, the postoperative results after one-year follow-up were very satisfactory, so that total laparoscopic vaginoplasty with pedicled bowel was recommended as a satisfactory alternative for patients with hypoplastic penoscrotal genitals. In the same year, there was another publication of now 63 laparoscopic sigmoid vaginoplasties by the same team [59].

A multicentre study on the use of ileum as a vaginal liner was published in 2018 with the aim of identifying whether the ileum or sigmoid are suitable for creation of a neovagina in primary or secondary surgery. In five patients, remodelling of the removed ileum segment into a U-pouch was performed, and in the remaining 27 patients, a simple ileum segment was used as a vaginal liner. In all cases, isolation and dissection of the ileum segment was again performed laparoscopically [60]. At a median follow-up of 35 months, subsequent introitus stenosis was found in 12.5% of patients. The rates of other complications were similar to those of sigmoid neovaginal insertion, with 29 of 32 patients having a history of failed neovaginal insertion. A systematic review from Gothenburg showed a high success rate of vaginoplasty from pedicled intestinal grafts using laparoscopic techniques, in 34 selected studies [61]. Another systematic review comparing the complications and outcome of vaginoplasty after penile or penoscrotal inversion or sigmoid neovagina in male-to-female transperson was published from the Mayo Clinic in Rochester. The results of 3716 patients from the 46 studies reviewed show that both techniques have specific advantages and disadvantages, but are able to reproduce reliable results with high subjective satisfaction in those undergoing the procedure [40].

It should be noted that the most extensive experience with this surgical technique has not been in male-to-female transperson, but in patients with vaginal agenesis [62]. There are numerous studies for bowel segment vaginoplasty in vaginal agenesia, some with a very high number of cases, on the successful performance of laparoscopically assisted creation of sigmaneovaginas [63–66].

Clitoridoplasty, Labioplasty and Vulvoplasty

From an aesthetic point of view, there is no consensus on the ideal appearance of a female vulva [67]. Accordingly, there are a variety of surgical techniques for aesthetic procedures in gynaecology patients. In male-to-female transgender, an aesthetically pleasing and functionally-sensory satisfactory vulva should be achieved as part of primary genital reassignment [68]. This can be achieved in single-stage or multi-staged procedures, but a key point of vulvaplasty is the creation of a sensitive, orgasm-capable clitoris. This has become an established part of primary genital approximation since the early 1990s [29, 69].

For the dissection and visualization of a neoclitoris, it is necessary to use a portion of the glans while preserving the dorsal vascular nerve bundle as completely as possible (see Fig. 9.6). This can be dissected under magnifying glass magnification between the tunica albuginea of the corpora cavernosa and Buck's fascia from the corpora cavernosa to the base of the penis, after previously dissecting the penile skin between Colle's fascia and Buck's fascia as a pedunculated flap of skin for lining the neovaginal cavity and/or shaping the external genitalia.

Alternatively, as preferred by some authors, a strip of tunica albuginea can be left on the vascular nerve bundle, which significantly reduces the duration of surgery [30]. This facilitates preservation of the nervous and vascular structures of the dorsal vascular nerve bundle but results in some volume increase, which may complicate subsequent placement of the vascular nerve bundle. In several studies, regardless of the technique used to prepare the dorsal vascular/nerve bundle, the neoclitoris and vulva showed good pressure and vibratory sensitivity, as well as orgasmic capacity between 80% and 90% [30, 70, 71]. In all the techniques described, urethra and corpus spongiosum are dissected from the corpora cavernosa down to the pelvic floor [4, 28, 31, 72, 73].

If the procedure is intended to be performed in a single-staged fashion as part of the primary genital surgery, the clitoro-labial complex should then be shaped simultaneously. Various techniques currently exist for this purpose but have yet to be compared in comparative studies [28, 45, 47, 48, 50, 54, 55, 73–77]. Some groups use pedicled flaps of scrotal skin to create the vulvar as shown in Fig. 9.7.

Also (in non-circumcised patients) parts of the inner foreskin can be left on the vascular nerve bundle as pedicled flaps, and these foreskin flaps are sutured bilaterally around the reduced glans as small labia. From caudally, a strip of the shortened dorsal urethral wall can be sutured to the underside of the clitoris in a pedicled fashion as a vestibule substitute to achieve a moistening effect (which is pathophysiological debatable as urothelium does not produce moisture itself) and a natural aspect of the neovestibule [17, 45, 50, 55, 75]. Even if such reconstruction of the clitoro-labial complex is intended to be performed single-staged as part of primary

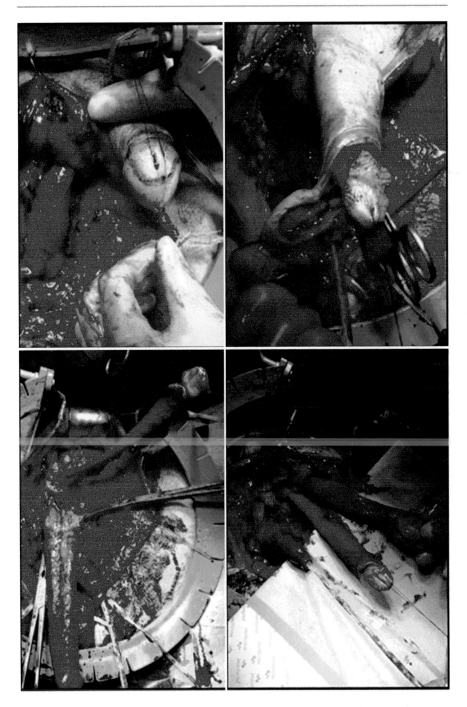

Fig. 9.6 Creation of the neoclitoris by using a part of the glans and preserving the entire neuro-vascular bundle

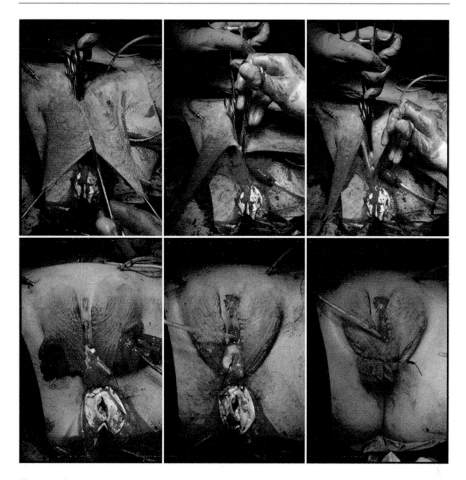

Fig. 9.7 Creation of the neovulva by using scrotal skin flaps

genital reassignment, secondary revision surgery to correct the clitoro-labial complex can often be expected [22, 31, 45].

Alternatively, a staged creation of the outer genitalia may be performed, in which case the clitoro-labial complex may be reconstructed including a female mons pubis [22, 31, 78–80]. An anterior commissure of the labia majora can, therefore, be achieved with the subsequent excision of an onion-shaped infrapubic skin area, with formation of a clitoridal prepuce, while also resulting in shaping of the labia minora, the so called mons-pubis-plasty [4, 37, 44] (see Fig. 9.8).

Complications and Outcomes

Despite the detailed numbers for specific complications and outcomes subsequent to the various surgical techniques provided in section "Orchiectomy, Vagino-,

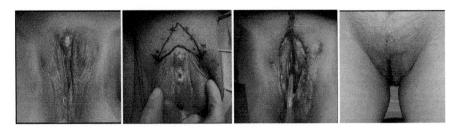

Fig. 9.8 Mons-pubis-plasty

Clitorido-, Labio- and Vulvoplasty- Techniques", the following section summarizes the most frequent complications and provides an overview about general outcomes.

Complications

Given that male-to-female genital reassignment surgery requires separation and reassembling of the entire urogenital complex, the spectrum of subsequent complications is broad, yet not life threatening, with as yet no reported mortal invents during that procedure [81].

Reported complications range from complete or partial necrosis of the neovulva, neovagina, vesico- or recto- neovaginal fistulae, neomeatal stenosis, and neovaginal shrinkage. Despite surgical techniques for creating a neovagina are functionally and aesthetically excellent, there are cases of anorgasmia reported, and a second stage labiaplasty may be needed for cosmesis [5].

Rectal Complications

Injuries of the rectum, which can be caused while dissecting the neovaginal cavity, are reported with a rate of up to 4.5% [41]. Closed commonly in a two-layer fashion, this doesn't usually lead to the need for bowel diversion or to significant long-term complications, even though the risk of developing recto-neovaginal fistulae is increased [82]. In the event of recto-vaginal fistula as a long-term complication, however, a staged repair with a temporary bowel diversion may be necessary.

Urethral Complications

While intraoperative urethral complications can occur in up to 4%, they usually can be repaired instantly and only leads to a prolonged catheterization [53, 79].

Postoperative urinary retention is usually caused by temporally swelling and doesn't require active treatment, and urinary incontinence is a very rare phenomenon and mostly self-limiting.

A diverted urinary stream appears to be the most common complication with a range of 5.6–33%. If caused by a neomeatal stenosis this can be repaired with a simple meatotomy/meatoplasty [81], if more complex techniques like a Y-V Plasty are recommended [83].

Neovulvar Complications

Scar tissue formation can lead to a stenotic introitus in up to 12% of cases [81], and can usually be released by procedures such as modifications of a V-Y-plasty. Swelling of potentially remaining parts of the spongiosus body during sexual arousal can lead to obstruction of the introitus of the neovagina. If present, in the authors' experience, a paraneomeatal T shape incision allows access to identify, mobilize and resect the hypertrophic part of the spongiosus remnants.

Neovaginal Complications

Most commonly because of inadequate dilations, neovaginal stenosis can occur in about 7% [81]. In penoscrotal inversionplasties augmented with full thickness scrotal skin grafts, a repeat vaginoplasty for atresia or shrinkage of the primary neovagina can be needed in 2.9% [53].

If intestine is used for the creation of the neovagina (sigmavagina), the additional morbidity of bowel surgery (such as anastomotic leakage) needs to be taken in consideration. In addition, the patient needs to be aware of the mucous—and smell production of the used segment. This can be discomforting, and in severe cases the retention of mucous can lead to chronic infection up to diversion colitis (which requires topic treatment or even surgical resection [84]. In order to prevent this, as well as to prevent sigmocutaneous stenosis, the patient needs to dilate and shower the sigmoidal neovagina on a regular basis. Also regular neovaginoscopies as cancer prevention is needed, as the malignancy rate is reported as 3% [85].

Outcomes

Various groups with high numbers of patients have shown a strongly positive effect of the genital reassignment surgery on subjective wellbeing and sexual function [42, 86–88]. The overall subjective satisfaction rate after male-to-female genital reassignment surgery ranged from 80% [42] to as high as 92% [3]. A retrospective study also reported 72% of transwomen to be very satisfied with the cosmetic respective functional outcome of the surgery [89] and the patients reported less stigmatism in public [5]. In several studies, regardless of the surgical technique used, the neoclitoris and vulva showed good pressure and vibratory sensitivity, as well as orgasmic capacity between 80% and 90% [30, 70, 71]. In regards to vaginal depth, a study from Amsterdam showed equivalent results if free scrotal skin grafts are used to augment the neovagina for short penile length [51]. A systematic review comparing the complications and outcome of vaginoplasty with penile/penoscrotal inversion or sigmoid neovagina in male-to-female from the Mayo Clinic in Rochester on 3716 patients from 46 studies, showed that both techniques had specific advantages and disadvantages, but that they delivered reliable results with high subjective satisfaction in those undergoing the procedures [40].

Regrets are reported as extremely rare and range from 1–1.5% of transwomen in older studies [5] to only 0.6% in the before mentioned more recent over 40 years' cohort study from one of Europe's largest transgender centre [2].

Conclusion

The discrepancy between the gender assigned at birth and the perception of gender identity seams a common phenomenon over all cultures, centuries and ages and should not be seen as pathological. There is a drastic rise in prevalence over the last decades, with a consequent increase in the number of persons seeking surgical reassignment, while regret rates stay stable [2]. For persons who seek surgical body modifications (which is only a subgroup of transgender persons) there are strict protocols to be followed prior to the complex, and often staged surgeries [5].

For genital reassignment surgery, the pedicled penile skin inversion technique is the most commonly used technique globally [90]. This technique, however, is limited to cases with adequate penile shaft skin. This has become to be a more frequent challenge for transgender surgeons, especially since there is a trend towards transwomen presenting with hypoplastic genitalia after puberty-blocking hormonal therapy, and also the increased importance of the clitoro-labial complex in recent years, where often parts of the penile skin are used for the formation of the small labia and the foreskin of the neoclitoris. Accordingly, vaginoplasty techniques using bowel segments like the sigmavagina are growing in relevance, especially when there is also not enough excess scrotal skin to enlarge the depth of a invaginated penile skin neovagina with a scrotal full thickness skin graft.

The most common complications include a diverted urinary stream and stenosis of the introitus and the neovagina, which is often a result of inadequate self-dilatation.

The capability of achieving orgasm, functional and aesthetical satisfaction as well as overall satisfaction with a drastic improvement of well-being and a decrease of stigmatism is proven by many studies, and the regret rate is lower than 1% [2].

The increased need for transgender health care, as well as the mandatory overlapping work of medical, psychological, social and therapeutic professions, and the complexity of the perioperative requirements and the surgical procedures, raises the need for multidisciplinary, highly specialised centres and professionals.

References

1. Morgenstern SC, Sohn M. Prothetik nach Genitalaufbau bei Transmännern. Urologe. 2021;60:722–31.
2. Wiepjes CM, et al. The Amsterdam Cohort of Gender Dysphoria Study (1972–2015): trends in prevalence, treatment, and regrets. J Sex Med. 2018;15(4):582–90.
3. Löwenberg H, et al. Komplikationen, subjektive Zufriedenheit und sexuelles Erleben nach geschlechtsangleichender Operation bei Mann-zu-Frau-Transsexualität. Z Sex Forsch. 2010;23(4):328–47. https://doi.org/10.1055/s-0030-1262718.
4. Heß J, et al. Geschlechtsangleichung von Mann zu Frau. Urologe. 2020;59:1348–55.
5. Coleman E, Bockting W, Botzer M, Cohen-Kettenis P, DeCuypere G, Feldman J, et al. Standards of care for the health of transsexual, transgender, and gender-nonconforming people, version 7. Int J Transgend. 2012;13(4):165–232. https://doi.org/10.1080/15532739.2011.700873.
6. De Graaf NM, Carmichael P, Steensma D, et al. Evidence for a change in the sex ratio of children referred for gender dysphoria: data from the gender identity development service in London (2000–2017). J Sex Med. 2018;15:1381–3.

7. Jacobsson J, Andreasson M, Kölby L, et al. Patients priorities regarding female-to-male gender affirmation surgery of the genitalia: a pilot study of 47 patients in Sweden. J Sex Med. 2017;14:857–64.

8. Sohn M, Rieger U, Morgenstern SC. "Operative Verfahren der Angleichung von Frau zu Mann" in: Michel MS, Thüroff JW, Janetschek G, Wirth M (Hrsg.) "Die Urologie", 2nd edition, Springer Verlag GmbH Berlin Heidelberg. 2023, in press. Series ISSN 2625-3461. Series E-ISSN 2625-350X.

9. Meyer G, Mayer M, Mondorf A, Herrmann E, Bojunga J. Increasing normality-persisting barriers: current socio-demographic characteristics of 350 individuals diagnosed with gender dysphoria. Clin Endocrinol. 2020;92(3):241–6.

10. Ettner R, Monstrey S, Coleman E, editors. Principles of transgender medicine and surgery. 2nd ed. New York: Routledge; 2016.

11. Smith JR, et al. Are surgical residents prepared for fellowship training in gender confirming surgery? J Sex Med. 2017;14:1066–7.

12. Falcone M, et al. A single center analysis on the learning curve of male-to-female penoscrotal vaginoplasty by multiple surgical measures. Urology. 2017;99:234–9.

13. Schechter LS, et al. Gender confirmation surgery: guiding principles. J Sex Med. 2017;14:852–6.

14. Seyed-Forootan K, et al. Autologous fibroblast seeded amnion for reconstruction of neovagina in male-to-female reassignment surgery. Aesthet Plast Surg. 2018;42:491–7.

15. Rossi NR, et al. Operative Geschlechtsangleichung im Alter. Urologe. 2012;51:1414–8.

16. Milrod C, et al. Age is just a number: WPATH-affiliated surgeons experiences and attitudes, toward vaginoplasty in transgender females under 18 years of age in the United States. J Sex Med. 2017;14:624–34.

17. Colebunders B, et al. Male to female gender reassigment surgery. In: Ettner R, et al., editors. Transgender medicine and surgery. 2nd ed. New York: Routledge; 2016. p. 250–78.

18. Schneider F, et al. Testicular functions and clinical characterization of patients with GD undergoing, sex reassignment surgery. J Sex Med. 2015;12:2190–200.

19. Jones BP, et al. Uterine transplantation in transgender women. BJOG. 2018;126:152–6. https://doi.org/10.1111/1471-0528.15438.

20. Vedovo F, et al. Operated male-to-female sexual function index: validity of the first questionnaire developed to assess sexual function after male-to-female gender affirming surgery. J Urol. 2020;204(1):115–20. https://doi.org/10.1097/JU.0000000000000791.

21. Bertoncelli Tanaka M, et al. Prostate cancer in transgender women: what does a urologist need to know? BJU Int. 2022;129(1):113–22. https://doi.org/10.1111/bju.15521.

22. Imbimbo C, et al. A report from a single institutes 14-year experience in treatment of male-to-female transsexuals. J Sex Med. 2009;6:2736–45.

23. Sohn MH, et al. Operative Genitalangleichung bei Mann-zu-Frau Transsexualität: Gibt es Leitlinien oder Standards? Handchir Mikrochir Plast Chir. 2013;45:207–10.

24. Lawrence A. Patient reported complications and functional outcomes of male-to-female sex reassignment surgery. Arch Sex Behav. 2006;35:717–27.

25. Abraham F, et al. Genitalumwandlungen an zwei männlichen Transvestiten. Z Sexualwiss Sexualpolit. 1931;18:223–6.

26. Karim RB, Hage JJ, Mulder JW. Neovaginoplasty in male transsexuals: review of surgical techniques and recommendations regarding eligibility. Ann Plast Surg. 1996;37(6):669–75. PMID: 8988784.

27. Jiany D, et al. Does depth matter? Factors affecting choice of vulvoplasty over vaginoplasty as gender-affirming, genital surgery for transgender women. J Sex Med. 2018;15:902–6.

28. Chen ML, et al. Overview of surgical techniques in gender-affirming genital surgery. Transl Androl Urol. 2019;8:191–208.

29. Eldh J, et al. Construction of an neovagina with preservation of the glans penis as a clitoris in male transsexuals. Plast Reconstr Surg. 1993;91:895–900.

30. Hess J, et al. Modified preparation of the neurovascular bundle in male-to-female transgender patients. Urol Int. 2016;96:354–9.

31. Sohn HM, et al. Genitalangleichende operation. Urologe. 2017;56:1246–55.
32. Reed HM, et al. Aesthetic and functional male-to-female genital and perineal surgery: feminizing vaginoplasty. Semin Plast Surg. 2011;25:163–74.
33. Dessy LA, et al. The use of cultured autologous oral epithelial cells for vaginoplasty in male-to-female transsexuals: a feasibility, safety and advantageousness clinical pilot study. Plast Reconstr Surg. 2014;133:158–61.
34. Grimsby G, et al. The use of autologous buccal mucosa crafts in vaginal reconstruction. Curr Urol Rep. 2014;15:428–33.
35. Stany MP, et al. The use of acellular dermal allograft for vulvovaginal reconstruction. Int J Gynecol Cancer. 2010;20:1079–81.
36. Miyahara Y, et al. Less invasive new vaginoplasty using laparoscopy, atelocollagen sponge, and hand-made mould. Kobe J Med Sci. 2013;58:138–44.
37. Sohn M, et al. Operative Angleichung des Geschlechts. In: Beier KM, Bosinski HAG, editors. Sexualmedizin. München: Elsevier; 2021. p. 419–28.
38. Frey JD, et al. A historical review of gender-affirming medicine: focus on genital reconstruction surgery. J Sex Med. 2017;14:991–1002.
39. Colebunders B, et al. An update on the surgical treatment for transgender patients. Sex Med Rev. 2017;5(1):103–9. https://doi.org/10.1016/j.sxmr.2016.08.001.
40. Manrique OJ, et al. Complications and patient-reported outcomes in male-of-female vaginoplasty–where are we today: a systematic review and meta-analysis. Ann Plast Surg. 2018;80:684–90.
41. Horbach SER, et al. Outcome of vaginoplasty in male-to-female transgenders: a systematic review of surgical techniques. J Sex Med. 2015;12:1499–512.
42. Sohn M, et al. Gender identity disorders: diagnostic and surgical aspects. J Sex Med. 2007;4:1193–208.
43. Heß J, et al. Zufriedenheit mit der Mann-zur Frau geschlechtsangleichenden operation. Dtsch Ärztebl. 2014;111:795–801.
44. Selvaggi G, et al. Gender reassignment surgery: an overview. Nat Rev Urol. 2011;8:274–81.
45. Zavlin D, et al. Male-to-female sex reassignment surgery using the combined vaginoplasty technique: satisfaction of transgender patients with aesthetic, functional, and sexual outcomes. Aesthet Plast Surg. 2018;42(1):178–87. https://doi.org/10.1007/s00266-017-1003-z.
46. Chokrungvaronont P, et al. Sex reassignment surgery in Thailand. J Med Assoc Thail. 2004;87:1402–8.
47. Kaushik N, et al. Sigma-lead male-to-female gender affirmation surgery: blending cosmesis with functionality. Plast Reconstr Surg Glob Open. 2019;7(4):e2169. https://doi.org/10.1097/GOX.0000000000002169.
48. Perovic SV, et al. Vaginoplasty in male-to-female transsexuals using penile skin and urethral flap. Int J Transgend. 2005;8:43–64.
49. Bizic M, et al. An overview of neovaginal reconstruction options in male-of-female transsexuals. ScientificWorldJournal. 2014;2014:638919. https://doi.org/10.1155/2014/638919.
50. Trombetta C, et al. La neouretroclitoridoplastica secondo to petrovic. Urologia. 2011;78:267–73.
51. Buncamper ME, et al. Penile inversion vaginoplasty with or without additional full-thickness skin graft: to graft or not to graft? Plast Reconstr Surg. 2017;139(3):649e–56e. https://doi.org/10.1097/PRS/0000000000003108.
52. Jacoby A, et al. Robotic davydov peritoneal flap vaginoplasty for augmentation of vaginal depth in feminizing vaginoplasty. J Urol. 2019;201(6):1171–6. https://doi.org/10.1097/JU.0000000000000107.
53. Buncamper ME, et al. Surgical outcome after penile inversion vaginoplasty: a retrospective study of 475 transgender women. Plast Reconstr Surg. 2016;138(5):999–1007. https://doi.org/10.1097/PRS.0000000000002684.
54. Levy JA, et al. Male-to-female gender reassignment surgery: an institutional analysis of outcomes short-term complications and risk factors for 240 patients undergoing penile inversion vaginoplasty. Urology. 2019;131:228–33.

55. Wangjiraniran B, et al. Male-to-female vaginoplasty: preecha's surgical technique. J Plast Surg Hand Surg. 2015;49(3):153–9. https://doi.org/10.3109/2000656X.2014.967253.
56. Djordjevic ML, et al. Rectosigmoid vaginoplasty: clinical experience and outcomes in 86 cases. J Sex Med. 2011;8:3487–94.
57. Van der Sluis WB, et al. Long-term follow-up of transgender women after secondary intestinal vaginoplasty. J Sex Med. 2016;13:702–10.
58. Bouman MB, et al. Patient-reported esthetic and functional outcomes of primary total laparoscopic intestinal vaginoplasty in transgender women with penoscrotal hypoplasia. J Sex Med. 2016;13:1438–44.
59. Bouman MB, et al. Total laparoscopic sigmoid vaginoplasty. Fertil Steril. 2016;106:e22–3.
60. Van der Sluis WB, et al. Ileal vaginoplasty as vaginal reconstruction in transgender women and patients with disorders of sex development: an international, multicentre, retrospective study on surgical characteristics and outcomes. BJU Int. 2018;121(6):952–8.
61. Georgus K, et al. Bowel vaginoplasty: a systematic review. J Plast Surg Hand Surg. 2018;52(5):265–73.
62. Kim SK, et al. Is rectosigmoid vaginoplasty still useful? Arch Plast Surg. 2017;44:48–52.
63. Nowier A, et al. Surgical and functional outcomes of sigmoid vaginoplasty among patients with variants of disorders of sex development. Int Braz J Urol. 2012;38:380–8.
64. Yang B, et al. Vaginal reconstruction with sigmoid colon in patients with congenital absence of vagina and menses retention: a report of treatment experience in 22 young women. Int Urogynecol J. 2013;24:155–60.
65. Chen-Xi Z, et al. Laparoscopic and gasless laparoscopic sigmoid colon vaginoplasty in women with vaginal agenesis. Chin Med J. 2012;125:203–8.
66. Kisku S, et al. Bowel vaginoplasty in children and young women: an institutional experience with 55 patients. Int Urogynecol J. 2015;26:1441–8.
67. Clerico C, et al. Anatomy and aesthetics of the labia minora: the ideal vulva? Aesthet Plast Surg. 2017;41:714–9.
68. Ralph D, et al. Trauma, gender reassignment and penile augmentation. J Sex Med. 2010;7:1657–67.
69. Hage JJ, et al. Sculpturing the neoclitoris in vaginoplasty for male-to-female transsexuals. Plast Reconstr Surg. 1994;93:358–64.
70. Le Breton M, et al. Genital sensory detection thresholds and patient satisfaction with vaginoplasty in male-to-female transgender women. J Sex Med. 2017;14:274–81.
71. Selvaggi G, et al. Genital sensitivity after sex reassignment surgery in transsexual patients. Ann Plast Surg. 2007;58:427–33.
72. Selvaggi G, et al. Gender identity disorder: general overview and surgical treatment for vaginoplasty in male-to-female transsexuals. Plast Reconstr Surg. 2005;116:135–45.
73. Perovic S, et al. Genitoplasty in male-to-female transsexuals. Curr Opin Urol. 2009;19:571–6.
74. Cocci A, et al. Male-to-female gender affirming surgery: modified surgical approach for the glans reconfiguration in the neoclitoris (M-shape neoclitorolabioplasty). Arch Ital Urol Androl. 2019;91:119–24.
75. Opsomer D, et al. Creation of clitoral hood and labia minora in penile inversion vaginoplasty in circumcised and uncircumcised transwomen. Plast Reconstr Surg. 2018;142:729–33.
76. Giraldo F, et al. Corona glans clitoroplasty and urethropreputial vestibuloplasty in male-to-female transsexuals: the vulval aesthetic refinement by the Andalusia Gender Team. Plast Reconstr Surg. 2004;114(6):1543–50.
77. Soli M, et al. Male-to-female gender reassignment: modified surgical technique for creating the neoclitoris and mons veneris. J Sex Med. 2008;5:210–6.
78. Krege S, et al. Male-to-female transsexualism: a technique results and long-term follow up in 66 patients. BJU Int. 2001;88:396–402.
79. Rossi NR, et al. Gender reassignment surgery—a 13 year review of surgical outcomes. Int Braz J Urol. 2012;38:97–107.

80. Hage JJ, et al. Secondary corrections of the vulva in male-to-female transsexuals. Plast Reconstr Surg. 2000;106:350–9.
81. Hadj-Moussa M, et al. Feminizing genital gender-confirmation surgery. Sex Med Rev. 2018;6(3):457–468.e2. https://doi.org/10.1016/j.sxmr.2017.11.005.
82. van der Sluis WB, et al. Clinical characteristics and management of neovaginal fistulas after vaginoplasty in transgender women. Obstet Gynecol. 2016;127(6):1118–26. https://doi.org/10.1097/AOG.0000000000001421.
83. Riechardt S, et al. European Association of urology guidelines on urethral stricture disease part 3: management of strictures in females and transgender patients. Eur Urol Focus. 2021; https://doi.org/10.1016/j.euf.2021.07.013.
84. van der Sluis WB, et al. Diversion neovaginitis after sigmoid vaginoplasty: endoscopic and clinical characteristics. Fertil Steril. 2016;105(3):834–839.e1. https://doi.org/10.1016/j.fertnstert.2015.11.013.
85. Bouman M-B, et al. Intestinal vaginoplasty revisited: a review of surgical techniques, complications, and sexual function. J Sex Med. 2014;11(7):1835–47. https://doi.org/10.1111/jsm.12538.
86. De Cuypere G, et al. Sexual and physical health after sex reassignment surgery. Arch Sex Behav. 2005;34(6):679–90. https://doi.org/10.1007/s10508-005-7926-5.
87. Gijs L, et al. Surgical treatment of gender dysphoria in adults and adolescents: Recent developments, effectiveness, and challenges. Annu Rev Sex Res. 2007;18:178–84. https://doi.org/10.1080/10532528.2007.10559851.
88. Klein C, Gorzalka BB. Sexual functioning in transsexuals following hormone therapy and genital surgery: a review. J Sex Med. 2009;6(11):2922–39.; quiz 2940-1. https://doi.org/10.1111/j.1743-6109.2009.01370.x.
89. Hess J, et al. Satisfaction with male-to-female gender reassignment surgery. Dtsch Arztebl Int. 2014;111(47):795–801. https://doi.org/10.3238/arztebl.2014.0795.
90. Sohn M, Morgenstern SC. S2K-Leitlinie Geschlechtsangleichende chirurgische Maßnahmen bei Geschlechtsinkongruenz und Geschlechtsdysphorie, Kapitel Feminisierende Maßnahmen. German National Guidelines for Transgender Care. 2023, in press.

Penile Rehabilitation: Current Challenges and Future Perspectives

10

Nicolò Schifano, Paolo Capogrosso,
and Francesco Montorsi

Abstract

Radical prostatectomy (RP) represents the treatment of choice to manage clinically-localized prostate cancer (PCa). However, the risk of postoperative functional side effects including urinary incontinence (UI) and erectile dysfunction (ED) remains non-negligible. The pathophysiology of post-RP ED primarily involves three factors which almost inevitably occur after RP: neural damage, vascular damage, and damage to the penile smooth muscle. Due to post-RP neuroapraxia, the penis remains in a condition of unantagonized flaccidity, with the metabolic balance being shifted in favour of collagenisation which eventually exerts a permanent detrimental effect on erectile function (EF). Preoperative EF-levels, the patients' fitness and surgical-technique associated factors represent the main predictors to estimate the likelihood to recover after RP. Penile rehabilitation aims to prevent corporal smooth muscle alterations through the means of obtaining reasonably frequent erections in order to enable the patient to re-engage in sexual activity but also to re-establish his preoperative sexual function. The rehabilitation-protocol should be tailored according to the individuals' features and their estimated likelihood to recover. PDE5Is exert a favourable effect on both the EF-levels during the treatment and on the structure of the corpora cavernosa, even though they have failed to show an improvement of spontaneous EF-recovery vs. placebo. The concomitant use of vacuum erection devices (VEDs) may offer some advantages in terms of patients' satisfaction and compli-

N. Schifano · F. Montorsi (✉)
Università Vita-Salute San Raffaele, Milan, Italy

Unit of Urology; URI; IRCCS Ospedale San Raffaele, Milan, Italy
e-mail: montorsi.francesco@hsr.it

P. Capogrosso
ASST Sette Laghi—Circolo e Fondazione Macchi Hospital, Varese, Italy

S. Sarikaya et al. (eds.), *Andrology and Sexual Medicine*, Management of Urology,
https://doi.org/10.1007/978-3-031-12049-7_10

ance with the rehabilitation vs. PDE5I-monotherapy. Intracavernous Injections (ICIs) present with high and immediate levels of effectiveness, but should be reserved to PDE5I-refractory cases due to their inconvenient modality of administration. A number of novel rehabilitation options, including the use of Low Intensity Extracoroporeal Shock Wave Therapy (LI-SWT) and the use of stem cells, are currently under investigation in both the preclinical and clinical settings. Penile rehabilitation protocols should be initiated as early as feasible after RP. Patients should routinely associate drugs with sexual stimulation, with or without the involvement of the partner. Moreover, the comprehensive sexual well-being of the couple should be considered with a specific attention toward the occurrence of sexual dysfunctions other than ED, thus including low sexual desire and orgasmic dysfunction.

Introduction

Prostate cancer (PCa) represents one of the most frequent diagnosed malignancies in Europe and in the United States [1]. Radical prostatectomy (RP) is the treatment of choice to manage clinically localized PCa, providing indeed excellent oncologic outcomes in the long-term [2].

However, the risk of significant post-surgical side effects has to be taken into account. Even though significant progresses have been made aiming to ensure a minimally-invasive surgical approach, the risk of postoperative urinary incontinence [3] (UI) and erectile dysfunction (ED) remains non-negligible, with a detrimental impact on the patient's well-being [2, 4]. Over the last decades, PCa has been more and more often diagnosed at younger ages, hence the increased importance of focusing on post-operative sexual function.

It is difficult to provide an accurate estimate of the real prevalence of ED after RP based on the existing literature, due to the remarkable heterogeneity of the populations in study, the different modalities of data collection and reporting, and the discrepancies in definitions of a normal erectile function (EF) after RP [5]. Postoperative ED is however a relatively common sequela after RP, with rates ranging between 19% and 78% [6].

In this context, penile rehabilitation has been proposed as a strategy to enhance the recovery of EF after surgery for PCa and reducing the risk of permanent ED.

Pathophysiology

The pathophysiology of post-RP ED pathophysiology primarily involves three different factors: neural damage, vascular damage, and damage to the smooth muscle of the penis [7].

The erection of the penis can be considered a neurovascular event, and this indeed requires the integrity of both the neural and the vascular mechanisms. In the flaccid state the smooth muscles of the corporal sinusoids of the penis are tonically contracted, allowing only a small amount of arterial flow. The penis receives its innervation from the cavernous nerves which originate from the pelvic plexus. Sexual stimulation triggers the release of neurotransmitters from the cavernous nerve terminals, which initiate the erectile cascade. The endothelial cells in the sinusoidal veins of the corpora cavernosa of the penis produce nitric oxide, which elicits an intracellular pathway resulting in decreased intracellular calcium levels and subsequent corporal smooth muscle relaxation [8]. The relaxation of the smooth muscle of the corpus cavernosum in turn triggers the veno-occlusive mechanisms which maintain the erection [9].

The neurovascular bundle, which contains the cavernous nerves, runs along the anterolateral aspect of the prostate [10]. Due to the anatomical proximity of the neurovascular bundles and prostate, levels of injury to erectile nerves during the RP are unfortunately unavoidable, even when the neurovascular bundle is meticulously dissected during surgery [7]. Cavernous nerves are damaged due to a range of different mechanisms, including: the stretching of the cavernous nerves during prostate mobilisation, the possible thermal injury from electrocautery, the inflammation which inevitably occurs after surgical manipulation, and/or neural ischemia secondary to the damage of the vascular supply to erectile nerves. Erectile dysfunction becomes clinically evident immediately after RP, due to a phenomenon of temporary loss of function of the cavernous nerves owing to blockage of nerve conduction called neuropraxia [11]. The full recovery from neuropraxia may take up to 3 years after the insult [12–14].

It has been widely documented that significant functional and structural/anatomical changes arise from neuropraxia, with the corporal smooth muscle and the endothelium being exposed to the detrimental effect of tissue hypoxia [15]. Penile corporal oxygenation is maintained at adequate and physiologic levels whilst the penis undergoes through the erectile cycle on a regular basis [7]. In the flaccid state, the corporal $pO2$ is 35–40 mmHg [16], with this resulting in the upregulation of some fibrogenic cytokines such as TGF-b [7]. Increased levels of TGF-b lead to augmented collagenic deposition and alterations in smooth muscle-to-collagen ratios, which is capable of eventually causing penile fibrosis which in turn induces venous leak [7]. Iacono et al. [17] have shown that as early as 2 months after RP there is significant increase of the collagenic deposition in the erectile tissues. Erect penis is oxygenated with a $pO2$ which is instead typically increased to the 75–100 mmHg range [16]. In-vitro studies have shown that higher oxygenation levels upregulate the production of endogenous prostaglandins as well as cyclic AMP exerting a favourable pro-erectile effect [18].

Due to postoperative neuroapraxia, the penis remains in a state of unantagonized flaccidity, with the metabolic balance being shifted in favour of collagenisation thus causing the impairment of the elasticity of the corpora cavernosa. These inelastic corporal sinusoids fail to exert their compressive action on the subtunical venules, eventually leading to the venous leak (e.g., corpora-veno-occlusive dysfunction, or venogenic erectile dysfunction) development [7].

Mulhall and Graydon [19] have shown that more than half of the men had venous leak after RP. In a similar study, the incidence of early venous leak (e.g., less than

4 months after RP) was about 10% and increased to approximately 35% between 8 and 12 months after RP and thereafter to 50% 12 months after surgery [13].

Vascular injury is another factor that contributes to the occurrence of post-RP ED. Levels of possible damage to the accessory pudendal arteries (APAs) may occur during RP [20]. Although the incidence of these arteries is variable based on literature [20–25], they typically lie above the levator ani where they are prone to surgical damage; their origin may be variable as they may arise from the femoral, obturator, vesical, or iliac artery. Breza et al. [20] described in details the arterial anatomy of 10 cadavers, with the APAs being observed in seven of them where they provided the major source of arterial inflow into the penis.

Factors Influencing the Likelihood to Recover Erectile Function

Briganti et al. described three categories of risk to estimate the likelihood of post-RP ED based on the patient-associated preoperative features [26]. First, those men who present with a good preoperative EF have an high expectancy of preserving it after surgery. Preoperative EF represents in fact the main predictor of ED-risk after RP [26–29]. Second, the younger and healthier individuals show higher recovery rates as compared to their older and sicker counterparts [26–28, 30–33]. The likelihood to achieve satisfactory EF after RP is very low among those patients having a pre-existent severe ED [26–29, 34]. Finally, the modality/extension of the nerve-sparing approach, the surgical technique (open, laparoscopic, robotic-assisted), and the surgical experience of the operator may also have a substantial impact on the likelihood to recover after RP [35, 36]. According to a recent meta-analysis, the preservation of the neuro-vascular bundle is not significantly associated with worse oncological outcomes, whilst it leads to better EF- and urinary continence- (UC) recovery [37]. Another recent meta-analysis [38] has identified that robot-assisted RP (RARP) results in better functional outcomes, thus including EF-recovery, when compared to laparoscopic and open techniques.

Rationale of Penile Rehabilitation

The concept of penile rehabilitation, first suggested by Montorsi et al. [39] in the late 1990s, involves the use of any medication or device after RP to maximize EF recovery. Its main purpose is to prevent corporal smooth muscle alterations through the means of obtaining reasonably frequent erections in order to enable the patient to re-engage in sexual activity but also to re-establish his preoperative EF levels [7]. More recently a more comprehensive definition of this concept has been suggested, describing penile rehabilitation as the use of any drug, intervention, procedure or device to promote male sexual function after any type of insult to the function of the penis [40] (e.g., including also modifications in girth, length, and curvature of the penile shaft). While this most typically happens with RP, any possible insult to the normal physiology of EF, as those associated with Peyronie's disease, penile fracture, priapism, radical pelvic surgery or trauma, may benefit from an attempt of penile rehabilitation [40].

Penile Rehabilitation Protocols and Their Tailoring to the Patient

Salonia et al. [6] distinguished five main categories of penile rehabilitation treatment: phosphodiesterase type 5 inhibitors (PDE5Is), intracavernosal injections (ICIs), intraurethral and topical alprostadil, vacuum erectile device (VED) therapy, and testosterone therapy. The penile rehabilitation practice patterns among the American Urological Association (AUA) members were analyzed by Tal et al. [41]. They found that penile rehabilitation was adopted in the majority of cases (e.g., 89%) after RP, with PDE5Is being indeed the overall preferred option.

For those younger and fitter patients having a normal preoperative EF, physicians should prefer in the first instance the less invasive penile rehabilitation protocols, such as oral treatment with PDE5Is [42]. Those relatively more invasive protocols such as the use of intracavernosal injections (ICIs) and their combination with VED should be offered as second-line options [43] and reserved to patients with preoperative ED who would benefit from a more aggressive management. For those cases where any available penile rehabilitation strategy has failed or when severe preoperative ED was documented, a penile implant surgery should be offered given their favourable success profile [44]. Novel therapies such as low-intensity shock wave therapy (LISWT) and stem cells' treatments should be offered as experimental modalities [45].

The most commonly used penile rehabilitation protocols are summarized in Table 10.1.

Table 10.1 Penile rehabilitation protocols commonly used in clinical practice

Treatment	Suggested protocol
Sildenafil 50–100 mg	On demand (at least 3 times per week)
Vardenafil 10–20 mg	On demand (at least 3 times per week)
Tadalafil 5–20 mg	Daily (5 mg) On demand (at least 3 times per week—10 to 20 mg)
Intracavernous injection of Alprostadil 5–20 µg	On demand (at least 3 times per week)
Vacuum erection device	On demand (at least 3 sessions per week)
Combination treatments	PDE5is 3 times per week + on demand Alprostadil Alprostadil 3 times per week + on demand/daily PDE5i Daily Tadalafil + on demand higher dosage PDE5i Vacuum erection device + PDE5i/Alprostadil

PDE5is, phosphodiesterase type 5 inhibitors

The Importance of Preoperative Counseling

In the preoperative setting, patients are typically too optimistic regarding their expectation of getting back to their preoperative EF [46]. The occurrence of post-RP ED should be discussed with every RP-candidate, given that levels of temporary EF-loss occur most invariably, and permanent ED may also happen in some. Counseling the patient with regards to the expected timing of EF recovery and to the uncertainty of the extent of recovery is of crucial importance. Patients should also be informed regarding the predictors of EF-recovery and should be aware of all the available penile rehabilitation strategies along with their possible limitations. In order to build realistic expectations, patients should be aware that currently there is no conclusive evidence that penile rehabilitation can facilitate the recovery of unassisted erections after surgery. Finally, the possible occurrence of additional sexual side-effects should be discussed by the physician, thus including anejaculation, reduced libido, orgasmic dysfunction, climacturia, and penile morphometric alterations [47].

Timing to Start Penile Rehabilitation

Penile rehabilitation should be started as early as possible during the postoperative course [36, 48], with some studies supporting to commence the patient on PDE5Is when the catheter is removed [43]. Mulhall et al. [49] showed a significantly more consistent improvement in the International Index of Erectile Function (IIEF)-EF domain score for the early penile rehabilitation group (e.g., rehabilitation started <6 months after surgery) when compared to the delayed group (e.g., rehabilitation started >6 months after surgery). They documented also that more patients in the early group achieved satisfactory unassisted erections and PDE5I-assisted erections vs. the delayed group at 2 years after RP (e.g., 58% vs. 30%). Since PDE5Is are the least invasive option, they can be prescribed early after surgery [42, 43]. VED and ICIs may instead be considered not earlier than one month after RP [39, 50, 51].

Phosphodiesterase Type 5 Inhibitors

In a survey [52] over 95% of the International Society for Sexual Medicine (ISSM) members routinely prescribed PDE5Is to their RP patients. Although the available clinical studies [53–63] reported conflicting results regarding the actual efficacy of rehabilitation protocols based on PDE5Is (Table 10.2), preclinical data [64–75] strongly support the beneficial effects of this strategy.

Indeed, the vast majority of clinical studies presented with significant methodological limitations thus including the lack of randomization, a suboptimal duration of the rehabilitation protocol and significant dropout rates [76]. Among

Table 10.2 Summary of the randomized clinical trials of PDE5Is-based penile rehabilitation protocols

Study	Cases (n)	Study design	Patients' features	Rehabilitation protocol and timing of outcome assessment	Main findings
Padma-Nathan et al. [57]	Sil 50 mg OaD (23), Sil 100 mg OaD (28), placebo (25)	Double-blinded RCT	Age 18–70 y, preoperatively potent, BNS	Started 4 wk after RP, EDT at 36 wk, 8 wk DFW	EF recovery[a] ($P = 0.02$), 27% Sil, 4% placebo
Montorsi et al. [56]	Vard OaD (137), Vard PRN (141), placebo (145)	Double-blinded double-dummy RCT	Age 18–64 y, preoperatively potent, BNS	Started 14 d after RP, EDT at 9 mo, 2 mo DFW, 2-mo Vard OaD OL	IIEF-EF score > 22 at EDT, 48.2% Vard PRN ($P < 0.0001$ vs. placebo), 32% Vard OaD, 24.8% placebo; IIEF-EF score > 22 at DFW ($P > 0.05$ all comparisons), 29.1% Vard PRN, 24.1% Vard OaD, 29.1% placebo
Mulhall et al. [58]	Ava 200 mg (94), Ava 100 mg (90), placebo (87)	Double-blinded RCT	Age 18–70 y, history of ED after BNS	Started _6 mo after RP, EDT at 12 wk	IIEF-EF score change at EDT ($P < 0.01$ all comparisons), 5.2 Ava 200 mg, 3.6 Ava 100 mg, 0.1 placebo
Pavlovich et al. [59]	Sil OaD placebo PRN (50), Sil PRN placebo OaD (50)	Double-blinded RCT	Age < 65 y, preoperatively potent, UNS or BNS	Started 1 d after RP, EDT at 12 mo, 1 mo DFW	Recovery of baseline IIEF-EF score at EDT ($P = 0.4$), 63% Sil PRN, 57% Sil OaD; recovery of baseline IIEF-EF score at DFW ($P = 0.01$), 65% Sil PRN, 47% Sil OaD
Montorsi et al. [55]	Tad OaD (139), Tad PRN (143), placebo (141)	Double-blinded double-dummy RCT	Age < 68 y, baseline IIEF-EF score >22, BNS	Started within 6 wk after RP, EDT at 9 mo, 6-wk DFW, 3-mo OL	IIEF-EF score _ 22 at DFW, 20.9% Tad OaD ($P = 0.6$ vs. placebo), 16.9% Tad PRN ($P = 0.7$ vs. placebo), 19.1% placebo

(continued)

Table 10.2 (continued)

Study	Cases (n)	Study design	Patients' features	Rehabilitation protocol and timing of outcome assessment	Main findings
Mulhall et al. [60]	Tad OaD (139), Tad PRN (143), placebo (141)	Double-blinded double-dummy RCT	Age < 68 y, baseline IIEF-EF score >22, BNS	Started within 6 wk after RP, EDT at 9 mo, 6-wk DFW, 3-mo OL	Patients' return to baseline IIEF-EF score at EDT (*P* value not provided), 22.3% Tad OaD, 11.3% Tad PRN, 7.8% placebo; patients' return to baseline IIEF-EF score at DFW (*P* value not provided), 12.2% Tad OaD, 9.2% Tad PRN, 11.4% placebo
Moncada et al. [61]	Tad OaD (139), Tad PRN (143), placebo (141)	Double-blinded double-dummy RCT	Age < 68 y, baseline IIEF-EF score >22, BNS	Started within 6 wk after RP, EDT at 9 mo, 6-wk DFW, 3-mo OL	Time to EF recovery during DBT (for 25% of patients), Tad OaD 5.8 mo (*P* = 0.03 vs. placebo), Tad PRN 9 mo (*P* = 0.01 vs. placebo), placebo 9.3 mo
Brock et al. [62]	Tad OaD (139), Tad PRN (143), placebo (141)	Double-blinded double-dummy RCT	Age < 68 y, baseline IIEF-EF score >22, BNS	Started within 6 wk after RP, EDT at 9 mo, 6-wk DFW, 3-mo OL	Stretched penile length at EDT, Tad OaD -2.2 mm (*P* = 0.03 vs. placebo), Tad PRN -7.9 mm (*P* = 0.3 vs. placebo), placebo −6.3 mm
Montorsi et al. [63]	Tad OaD (139), Tad PRN (143), placebo (141)	Double-blinded double-dummy RCT	Age < 68 y, baseline IIEF-EF score >22, BNS	Started within 6 wk after RP, EDT at 9 mo, 6-wk DFW, 3-mo OL	Predictors for recovery of EF: high preoperative IIEF-SD score, high preoperative IIEF score on item 15, robotic surgery, NS score, Tad OaD

AVA, avanafil; BNS, bilateral nerve-sparing procedure; DBT, double-blinded treatment; DFW, drug-free washout period; ED, erectile dysfunction; EDT, end of study treatment; EF, erectile function; IIEF, International Index of Erectile Function; IIEF-EF, International Index of Erectile Function erectile function domain; IIEF-SD, International Index of Erectile Function sexual desire domain; NS, nerve-sparing; OaD, once daily; OL, open-label treatment; PDE5Is, phosphodiesterase type 5 inhibitors; PRN, on demand; RCT, randomized clinical trial; RP, radical prostatectomy; Sil, sildenafil; Tad, tadalafil; UNS, unilateral nerve sparing procedure; Vard, vardenafil

[a]Defined as a score higher than 8 on questions 3 and 4 of the IIEF and a "yes" response to the question, "Over the past 4 weeks, have your erections been good enough for satisfactory sexual activity?"

these studies, those trials with a more robust statistical validity have failed to demonstrate any meaningful advantage of penile rehabilitation with PDE5is in terms of achieving a recovery of unassisted erections as compared to placebo [76]. A recent meta-analysis [77] found that PDE5I-administration is indeed capable of increasing EF-levels during the treatment, even though the analysis of the available evidence did not support the improved recovery of spontaneous EF.

Although PDE5I-rehabilitation protocols were not proven to be effective in facilitating the spontaneous return to the preoperative EF, these medications have been proven significantly effective in preserving both the structure of the corpora cavernosa and the penile length after RP [55]. For these reasons, clinical guidelines still suggest the use of PDE5is in the early post-operative phase since this strategy is in any case considered better than leaving the cavernous tissues untreated after surgery [36, 49, 78]. Nowadays, none of the available randomized controlled trials (RCTs) definitively demonstrated a superiority of the once daily administration of PDE5-Is compared to the on-demand (at least three times per week) administration protocols (Table 10.1) [79]. Tadalafil might have the best profile for its use in the penile rehabilitation setting due to his long half-life [80–82]. Of note, overall discontinuation rates of PDE5Is after RP are as high as 72.6% at 18 months follow-up [83], due to a range of reasons including treatment effect below expectations, loss of interest in sex, psychological factors, EF recovery and concerns about their cardiovascular safety.

Intracavernosal Injections

The use of ICIs with alprostadil was the first proposed protocol to enhance EF recovery after RP. This treatment has been associated with high and immediate levels of effectiveness, especially in terms of penile hardness. Montorsi et al. [39] reported data of 27 post-RP patients who were submitted ICIs of prostaglandin-E1, 2–3 times per week. At 6-month follow up, 67% of treated men showed levels of recovered EF, compared to only 20% in the control group. Similarly, Mulhall et al. [84] showed that performing ICIs 3 times per week after RP could lead to a 52% return of functional erection at 18 months follow-up as compared to only 19% in the control group. However, ICIs have been historically associated with low patients compliance due to their inconvenient modality of administration: in their series Polito et al. [85] observed that out of 430 patients who were offered a protocol of postoperative ICIs for sexual rehabilitation, 157 (36.5%) refused to enter the protocol, and 18.6% dropped out of treatment over the first 6 months.

Two alternative molecules typically used for ICI therapy are papaverine (e.g., non-selective phosphodiesterase enzyme type 5 inhibitor) and phentolamine (e.g., a nonselective alpha-adrenergic antagonist) [86]. Bimix combines papaverine and phentolamine, whereas Trimix consists of Bimix components and alprostadil combined [86].

Intraurethral Alprostadil

Alprostadil can be administered in the form of an intraurethral suppository or in the form of a topical cream [87]. The main limitation with the use of this topical treatment after RP, particularly in the first postoperative year, is the frequent occurrence of penile pain. Raina et al. [88] described their experience with 54 patients using intraurethral alprostadil after RP. Although the treatment showed levels of beneficial effect on their assisted EF, the compliance with the treatment was only 63% after a mean follow-up period of about 2 years. All of the patients reported penile pain being associated with the use of the medication.

Vacuum Erection Device

VED therapy is based on the use of a mechanical device that utilizes a negative pressure of approximately 150–200 mmHg to increase the penile blood inflow in order to obtain on-demand erections [89]. Its use in the penile rehabilitation is however controversial [90], although the European Association of Urology (EAU) guidelines suggest VED as an option to be considered when standard oral PDE5I-treatment fails [91].

Indeed, oral PDE5Is alone are not always effective in the post-RP setting and may be associated with adverse effects and significant dropout rates. The concomitant use of a VED may increase the patient's compliance with the treatment and satisfaction and may offer advantages to monotherapy when dealing with penile shortening after RP [92, 93].

There are several possible drawbacks associated with the VED use, including instability at the base of the penis, a cyanotic appearance and a cooler erection [94]. Vacuum therapy is not suitable for penile rehabilitation purpose before the urethral catheter removal [94].

Novel Penile Rehabilitation Options

Currently, a number of innovative treatments aimed to improve EF recovery after RP are under investigation in both the preclinical and clinical setting.

Low Intensity Extracorporeal Shock Wave Therapy

Pre-clinical studies suggest that LI-SWT may induce cellular microtrauma at the level of the cavernous bodies, which in turn stimulates the release of several cytokines and angiogenic factors including the vascular endothelial growth factor (VEGF) and the endothelial nitric oxide synthase (eNOS), thus promoting tissue-neovascularization [95]. To date, few clinical studies have investigated the effect of LI-SWT in the post-operative setting. Zewin et al. reported data of 128 post nerve-sparing radical cystoprostatectomy subjects [96]. All patients were allocated to one of three groups: LI-SWT; PDE5i; and control. During the follow-up, 16% more patients in the LI-SWT group showed satisfactory EF recovery levels as compared to the control group. Although the difference was not statistically significant ($P = 0.14$), the results were still considered of clinical relevance. In a second study, Frey et al. [97] reported data of 16 patients with mild to severe ED after 12 months since RP. All patients were treated with a 6-week course of LI-SWT and then re-assessed at 1- and 12-month after treatment with no other erectogenic aids allowed during the study period. Results showed a significant improvement in terms of EF recovery, as assessed with the IIEF-EF. As the authors correctly pointed out, it is possible that even better results could be achieved if the treatment is given at an earlier stage after surgery, thus preventing penile fibrosis.

Baccaglini et al. [98] conducted the first RCT aimed at describing the efficacy and safety related with early PDE5Is-introduction with or without LI-SWT on EF-recovery after RP. The treatment protocol was started 6 weeks after RP for a period of 8 weeks. The median IIEF-5 scores at 4 months after surgery in the intervention group (e.g., PDE5is + LI-SWT) were significantly higher than those in the control group (12.0 vs. 10.0, $P = 0.006$). However, the study failed to reach the primary clinical endpoint considering a 4-point difference between the two treatment arms.

The current guidelines are still cautious regarding the adoption of LI-SWT after RP. Further studies are needed to better identify the efficacy of this approach in this setting, including the definition of the optimal shock wave energy delivery strategies.

Stem Cells

In their landmark study, Bochinski et al. [99] showed that stem cells were able to preserve EF in a rat model of neurogenic impotence when injected into the corpora cavernosa. Kendirci et al. [100] and Albersen et al. [101] subsequently published two milestone studies that validated further these results.

Stem cells are classified according to their differentiation potential in totipotent, pluripotent, multipotent, progenitor or precursor cells [44]. The most convenient method of stem-cell administration for ED-treatment is represented by intracavernosal injection [102].

Adult mesenchymal stem cells (MSCs) are multipotent stem cells which are able to differentiate into specific subtypes of mesenchymal cells. They can release in a paracrine-fashion a wide spectrum of trophic factors and cytokines. They can exert an in-vivo beneficial influence when injected in the corpora cavernosa even if they do not engraft in the target tissue and/or they do not differentiate locally [103, 104]. This conclusion was based on the observations that a partial recovery of EF was observed after injection of cell lysate from adipose-tissue-derived stem cells (ADSC) and the limited presence of stem cells engrafted in the corpus cavernosum [101].

One of the most promising strategies in post-RP penile rehabilitation setting is represented by the intracavernous injection of bone marrow-mononuclear cells

(BM-MNCs). Following a range of preclinical encouraging results, a few phase 1 and 2 clinical trials are currently ongoing [105]. The BM-MNCs are an heterogeneous population of cells, which include mesenchymal stem cells, endothelial progenitor cells, and haematopoietic stem cells. These progenitor cells may exert anti-apoptotic, neurotrophic, and angiogenic effects. Yiou et al. [106] selected 12 post-RP patients with localized PCa and whose ED had proved to be unresponsive to medical treatments. Patients were divided into four groups and were treated with escalating BM-MNC dosages. Compared to baseline levels, a significant improvement in terms of intercourse satisfaction and EF were observed at the 6-month follow up. Interestingly, clinical benefits were also associated with improvement of peak systolic velocity at the level of the cavernous arteries and with increased penile nitric oxide release.

Further, larger randomized studies are needed to better define the real efficacy of the stem cell-based approaches for addressing ED after RP.

Sexual Rehabilitation Beside Penile Rehabilitation

Rehabilitation of post-RP sexual function has primarily been focused on facilitating the recovery of the EF. However, other sexual function domains contribute to a successful sexual recovery.

Non-penetrative Intercourse

In those cases when penetrative sex is not possible due to the erections being not firm enough, the patient and the couple should be invited to engage at least in non-penetrative intercourse through the means of oral sex and mutual masturbation. Couples who identify alternative ways of being sexual in the presence of ED report lower sexual distress and higher compliance with rehabilitation protocols [107].

Ejaculatory Complaints

Besides the recovery of EF, the preservation of a normal orgasmic function (OF) is crucial [108].

Urinary incontinence (UI) during sex (e.g., climacturia), dysorgasmia (e.g., painful orgasm) and anorgasmia can also severely impair orgasmic function following RP [109]. Dysorgasmia has a prevalence ranging from 3% to 18% after RP [110] while climacturia could affect up to 30% of patients after surgery [111]. Treatment options for painful orgasm could include the use of tamsulosin to reduce the contraction of the bladder neck responsible for the painful sensation [110]. Likewise, for climacturia patients may be invited to void before sexual intercourse or to apply penile tension loop during sexual activity; moreover, the optimization of UC with pelvic floor muscle training could reduce the risk of urine leakage [110].

Penile Morphometric Changes

Radical prostatectomy could result in penile shrinkage as documented in both open and robotic series [112–114], with penile length losses of up to 2 cm at 12 months in open RP [112, 113]. Those studies investigating this issue in the RARP setting documented a return to baseline penile length at 1 year after surgery [115, 116].

A treatment/preventative measure option to be considered is the adoption of a PDE5Is-based rehabilitation protocol, especially with the use of tadalafil, which has been proven beneficial in reducing significantly the length and girth-loss in both the flaccid and erect state at 3 and 6 months postoperatively after nerve-sparing RP [55, 62].

Moreover, the post RP patient is exposed to an increased risk of developing penile curvature and morphometric alterations due to Peyronie's disease (PD) [117], which has shown a prevalence of 15.9% after surgery [118].

Psychological Factors

Post-RP ED may typically cause a diminished feeling of masculinity. Moreover, the psychological impact of receiving a PCa diagnosis may also affect a patient's mental state. These factors could significantly affect the couple's sexual functioning after surgery. In this context, a psychological support exerts a favorable effect on patients' adherence to penile rehabilitation protocols. A RCT involving 189 couples showed that, after RP, patients in the peer support groups had higher sexual functioning levels when compared to men attending the usual care groups [119].

Canada et al. reported that sexual counseling intervention at 3-month reduced patients' distress and increased both partners' perceived levels of sexual functioning, with an increase of penile rehabilitation protocol adherence from 31% at baseline to 49% at the 6-month follow-up [120].

Penile Rehabilitation After Surgery Other Than Radical Prostatectomy

Radical Cystoprostatectomy

EF recovery after RC ranged between 14% and 80% [121]. Nerve sparing RC approaches might improve functional outcomes according to literature, although rehabilitation programs remain necessary to optimize recovery [122]. Continent patients receiving orthotopic neobladder reconstructions showed better EF-outcomes when compared to incontinent patients and to those undergoing other forms of urinary diversion [123], even though these findings may be due to the orthotopic diversion being typically offered to generally healthier and younger patients, who have a higher likelihood to recover their pre-existent EF. The concept of sexuality preserving cystectomy was introduced by Horenblas et al. [124], with a surgical approach characterized by the preservation of the vas, the prostate, and the seminal vesicles. The majority of men undergoing this modified-approach experienced a prompt return of a normal EF after surgery. However, this technique presents with significant oncological concerns in leaving the prostatic urethra in place.

Rectal Surgery

Erecetile dysfunction is also prevalent among patients undergoing rectal cancer surgery, ranging between 10% to 60% [125]. Abdomino-perineal resection (APR) presents with a higher risk of postoperative ED than low anterior resection procedure [126]. The colostomy made after APR may also alter the patients' self-perceived body image and may increase the rate of postoperative sexual dysfunctions [127]. Surgical experience may also influence ED rates with series from high-volume cancer centers reporting lower rates of ED [128]. Rehabilitation protocols often require a multidisciplinary approach for these patients which should comprise psychological support for both the patient and the partner along with the use of pharmacological agents [129]. Among the available medications, the efficacy of sildenafil was demonstrated in a study where 32 patients treated with rectal resection were randomized to medical treatment or placebo [130]. Erectile function improved in 80% of patients receiving sildenafil compared to 17% of patients treated with placebo [130].

Conclusions

Despite the improvements of surgical techniques and of penile rehabilitation protocols, ED remains still a common finding after RP. To date, there is no standardized rehabilitation protocol after RP owing to the controversial evidence regarding the efficacy of any treatment for restoring a baseline spontaneous EF after surgery.

However, the adherence to these rehabilitation treatments has to be encouraged, as they have been proven beneficial in maintaining the penile structure intact. Penile rehabilitation protocols should be initiated as early as feasible after surgery and RP-candidates should receive appropriate preoperative counseling regarding the available penile rehabilitation regimens. The rehabilitation-strategy of choice should be tailored on the patient's specific individual features and likelihood to recover.

Moreover, patients should be carefully counselled regarding the importance to associate drug treatment with sexual stimulation, which should be performed routinely with or without the involvement of the partner. Last, the comprehensive sexual well-being of the couple should be considered with a specific attention toward the occurrence of sexual dysfunctions other than ED and including impaired sexual desire and orgasmic dysfunction.

References

1. Siegel R, Ma J, Zou Z, Jemal A. Cancer statistics, 2014. CA Cancer J Clin. 2014;64:9–29.
2. Schiavina R, et al. Survival, Continence and Potency (SCP) recovery after radical retropubic prostatectomy: a long-term combined evaluation of surgical outcomes. Eur J Surg Oncol. 2014;40:1716–23.
3. Schifano N, Capogrosso P, Tutolo M, Dehò F, Montorsi F, Salonia A. How to prevent and manage post-prostatectomy incontinence: a review. World J Mens Health. 2021;39(4):581–97.
4. Mullins JK, et al. The impact of anatomical radical retropubic prostatectomy on cancer control: the 30-year anniversary. J Urol. 2012;188:2219–24.
5. Salonia A, et al. Prevention and management of post prostatectomy erectile dysfunction. Transl Androl Urol. 2015;4:421–37.
6. Salonia A, et al. Sexual rehabilitation after treatment for prostate cancer—part 2: recommendations from the Fourth International Consultation for Sexual Medicine (ICSM 2015). J Sex Med. 2017;14:297–315.
7. Mulhall JP. Penile rehabilitation following radical prostatectomy. Curr Opin Urol. 2008;18:613–20.
8. Kim N, et al. Oxygen tension regulates the nitric oxide pathway. Physiological role in penile erection. J Clin Invest. 1993;91:437–42.
9. Minhas S, Blecher G, Almekaty K, Kalejaiye O. Does penile rehabilitation have a role in the treatment of erectile dysfunction following radical prostatectomy? F1000Research. 2017;6:1–12.
10. Walz J, Graefen M, Huland H. Surgical anatomy of the prostate in the era of radical robotic prostatectomy. Curr Opin Urol. 2011;21:173–8.
11. Clavell-Hernández J, Wang R. The controversy surrounding penile rehabilitation after radical prostatectomy. Transl Androl Urol. 2017;6:2–11.
12. Wang R. Penile rehabilitation after radical prostatectomy: where do we stand and where are we going? J Sex Med. 2007;4(4 Pt 2):1085–97. https://doi.org/10.1111/j.1743-6109.2007.00482.x.
13. Mulhall JP, et al. Erectile dysfunction after radical prostatectomy: hemodynamic profiles and their correlation with the recovery of erectile function. J Urol. 2002;167:1371–5.
14. Walsh PC. Patient-reported urinary continence and sexual function after anatomic radical prostatectomy. J Urol. 2000;164:242.
15. User HM, Hairston JH, Zelner DJ, McKenna KE, McVary KT. Penile weight and cell subtype specific changes in a postradical prostatectomy model of erectile dysfunction. J Urol. 2003;169:1175–9.
16. Dean RC, Lue TF. Physiology of penile erection and pathophysiology of erectile dysfunction. Urol Clin North Am. 2005;32:379–95.
17. Iacono F, et al. Histological alterations in cavernous tissue after radical prostatectomy. J Urol. 2005;173:1673–6.
18. Moreland RB, et al. O2-dependent prostanoid synthesis activates functional PGE receptors on corpus cavernosum smooth muscle. Am J Physiol Heart Circ Physiol. 2001;281:552–8.
19. Mulhall JP, Graydon RJ. The hemodynamics of erectile dysfunction following nerve-sparing radical retropubic prostatectomy. Int J Impot Res. 1996;8:91–4.
20. Breza J, Aboseif SR, Orvis BR, Lue TF, Tanagho EA. Detailed anatomy of penile neurovascular structures: surgical significance. J Urol. 1989;141:437–43.
21. Benoit G, Droupy S, Quillard J, Paradis V, Giuliano F. Supra and infralevator neurovascular pathways to the penile corpora cavernosa. J Anat. 1999;195(Pt 4):605–15.
22. Droupy S, et al. Assessment of the functional role of accessory pudendal arteries in erection by transrectal color doppler ultrasound. J Urol. 1999;162:1987–91.
23. Polascik TJ, Walsh PC. Radical retropubic prostatectomy: the influence of accessory pudendal arteries on the recovery of sexual function. J Urol. 1995;154:150–2.

24. Rogers CG, Trock BP, Walsh PC. Preservation of accessory pudendal arteries during radical retropubic prostatectomy: surgical technique and results. Urology. 2004;64:148–51.

25. Secin FP, et al. Anatomy of accessory pudendal arteries in laparoscopic radical prostatectomy. J Urol. 2005;174:523–6; discussion 526.

26. Briganti A, et al. Choosing the best candidates for penile rehabilitation after bilateral nerve-sparing radical prostatectomy. J Sex Med. 2012;9:608–17.

27. Briganti A, et al. Predicting erectile function recovery after bilateral nerve sparing radical prostatectomy: a proposal of a novel preoperative risk stratification. J Sex Med. 2010;7:2521–31.

28. Briganti A, et al. Prediction of sexual function after radical prostatectomy. Cancer. 2009;115:3150–9.

29. Gacci M, et al. Original article: clinical investigation factors predicting continence recovery 1 month after radical prostatectomy: results of a multicenter survey. Int J Urol. 2011;18:700–8.

30. Gandaglia G, et al. How to optimize patient selection for robot-assisted radical prostatectomy: functional outcome analyses from a tertiary referral center. J Endourol. 2014;28:792–800.

31. Abdollah F, et al. Prediction of functional outcomes after nerve-sparing radical prostatectomy: results of conditional survival analyses. Eur Urol. 2012;62:42–52.

32. Gallina A, et al. Erectile function outcome after bilateral nerve sparing radical prostatectomy: which patients may be left untreated? J Sex Med. 2012;9:903–8.

33. Teloken PE, et al. Defining the impact of vascular risk factors on erectile function recovery after radical prostatectomy. BJU Int. 2013;111:653–7.

34. Harris CR, Punnen S, Carroll PR. Men with low preoperative sexual function may benefit from nerve sparing radical prostatectomy. J Urol. 2013;190:981–6.

35. Ficarra V, et al. Systematic review and meta-analysis of studies reporting potency rates after robot-assisted radical prostatectomy. Eur Urol. 2012;62(3):418–30. https://doi.org/10.1016/j.eururo.2012.05.046.

36. Salonia A, et al. Prevention and management of postprostatectomy sexual dysfunctions. Part 1: choosing the right patient at the right time for the right surgery. Eur Urol. 2012;62:261–72.

37. Nguyen LN, et al. The risks and benefits of cavernous neurovascular bundle sparing during radical prostatectomy: a systematic review and meta-analysis. J Urol. 2017;198:760–9.

38. Du Y, et al. Robot-assisted radical prostatectomy is more beneficial for prostate cancer patients: a system review and meta-analysis. Med Sci Monit. 2018;24:272–87.

39. Montorsi F, et al. Recovery of spontaneous erectile function after nervesparing radical retropubic prostatectomy with and without early intracavernous injections of alprostadil: results of a prospective, randomized trial. J Urol. 1997;158(4):1408–10. https://doi.org/10.1016/S0022-5347(01)64227-7.

40. Hakky TS, et al. Penile rehabilitation: the evolutionary concept in the management of erectile dysfunction. Curr Urol Rep. 2014;15:393.

41. Tal R, Teloken P, Mulhall JP. Erectile function rehabilitation after radical prostatectomy: practice patterns among AUA members. J Sex Med. 2011;8(8):2370–6. https://doi.org/10.1111/j.1743-6109.2011.02355.x.

42. Segal RL, Bivalacqua TJ, Burnett AL. Current penile-rehabilitation strategies: clinical evidence. Arab J Urol. 2013;11:230–6.

43. Jo JK, et al. Effect of starting penile rehabilitation with sildenafil immediately after robot-assisted laparoscopic radical prostatectomy on erectile function recovery: a prospective randomized trial. J Urol. 2018;199:1600–6.

44. Castiglione F, Ralph DJ, Muneer A. Surgical techniques for managing post-prostatectomy erectile dysfunction. Curr Urol Rep. 2017;18:90.

45. Lima TFN, Bitran J, Frech FS, Ramasamy R. Prevalence of post-prostatectomy erectile dysfunction and a review of the recommended therapeutic modalities. Int J Impot Res. 2021;33:401–9.

46. Symon Z, et al. Measuring patients' expectations regarding health-related quality-of-life outcomes associated with prostate cancer surgery or radiotherapy. Urology. 2006;68:1224–9.

47. Schifano N, Cakir OO, Castiglione F, Montorsi F, Garaffa G. Multidisciplinary approach and management of patients who seek medical advice for penile size concerns: a narrative review. Int J Impot Res. 2021;34(5):434–51. https://doi.org/10.1038/s41443-021-00444-5.

48. Mulhall JP, Bella AJ, Briganti A, McCullough A, Brock G. Erectile function rehabilitation in the radical prostatectomy patient. J Sex Med. 2010;7:1687–98.

49. Mulhall JP, Parker M, Waters BW, Flanigan R. The timing of penile rehabilitation after bilateral nerve-sparing radical prostatectomy affects the recovery of erectile function. BJU Int. 2010;105:37–41.

50. Nandipati K, Raina R, Agarwal A, Zippe CD. Early combination therapy: intracavernosal injections and sildenafil following radical prostatectomy increases sexual activity and the return of natural erections. Int J Impot Res. 2006;18:446–51.

51. Köhler TS, et al. A pilot study on the early use of the vacuum erection device after radical retropubic prostatectomy. BJU Int. 2007;100:858–62.

52. Teloken P, Mesquita G, Montorsi F, Mulhall J. Post-radical prostatectomy pharmacological penile rehabilitation: practice patterns among the international society for sexual medicine practitioners. J Sex Med. 2009;6:2032–8.

53. McCullough AR, et al. Recovery of erectile function after nerve sparing radical prostatectomy and penile rehabilitation with nightly intraurethral alprostadil versus sildenafil citrate. J Urol. 2010;183:2451–6.

54. Bannowsky A, Schulze H, van der Horst C, Hautmann S, Jünemann K-P. Recovery of erectile function after nerve-sparing radical prostatectomy: improvement with nightly low-dose sildenafil. BJU Int. 2008;101:1279–83.

55. Montorsi F, et al. Effects of tadalafil treatment on erectile function recovery following bilateral nerve-sparing radical prostatectomy: a randomised placebo-controlled study (REACTT). Eur Urol. 2014;65(3):587–96. https://doi.org/10.1016/j.eururo.2013.09.051.

56. Montorsi F, et al. Effect of nightly versus on-demand vardenafil on recovery of erectile function in men following bilateral nerve-sparing radical prostatectomy. Eur Urol. 2008;54(4):924–31. https://doi.org/10.1016/j.eururo.2008.06.083.

57. Padma-Nathan H, et al. Randomized, double-blind, placebo-controlled study of postoperative nightly sildenafil citrate for the prevention of erectile dysfunction after bilateral nerve-sparing radical prostatectomy. Int J Impot Res. 2008;20(5):479–86. https://doi.org/10.1038/ijir.2008.33.

58. Mulhall JP, et al. A phase 3, placebo controlled study of the safety and efficacy of avanafil for the treatment of erectile dysfunction after nerve sparing radical prostatectomy. J Urol. 2013;189:2229–36.

59. Pavlovich CP, et al. Nightly vs on-demand sildenafil for penile rehabilitation after minimally invasive nerve-sparing radical prostatectomy: results of a randomized double-blind trial with placebo. BJU Int. 2013;112(6):844–51. https://doi.org/10.1111/bju.12253.

60. Mulhall JP, et al. Effects of tadalafil once-daily or on-demand vs placebo on return to baseline erectile function after bilateral nerve-sparing radical prostatectomy—results from a randomized controlled trial (REACTT). J Sex Med. 2016;13(4):679–83. https://doi.org/10.1016/j.jsxm.2016.01.022.

61. Moncada I, et al. Effects of tadalafil once daily or on demand versus placebo on time to recovery of erectile function in patients after bilateral nerve-sparing radical prostatectomy. World J Urol. 2015;33(7):1031–8. https://doi.org/10.1007/s00345-014-1377-3.

62. Brock G, et al. Effect of tadalafil once daily on penile length loss and morning erections in patients after bilateral nerve-sparing radical prostatectomy: results from a randomized controlled trial. Urology. 2015;85:1090–6.

63. Montorsi F, et al. Exploratory decision-tree modeling of data from the randomized REACTT trial of tadalafil versus placebo to predict recovery of erectile function after bilateral nerve-sparing radical prostatectomy. Eur Urol. 2016;70:529–37.

64. Ferrini MG, et al. Vardenafil prevents fibrosis and loss of corporal smooth muscle that occurs after bilateral cavernosal nerve resection in the rat. Urology. 2006;68:429–35.

65. Vignozzi L, et al. Effect of chronic tadalafil administration on penile hypoxia induced by cavernous neurotomy in the rat. J Sex Med. 2006;3:419–31.
66. Ferrini MG, et al. Fibrosis and loss of smooth muscle in the corpora cavernosa precede corporal veno-occlusive dysfunction (CVOD) induced by experimental cavernosal nerve damage in the rat. J Sex Med. 2009;6:415–28.
67. Özden E, et al. Effect of sildenafil citrate on penile weight and physiology of cavernous smooth muscle in a post-radical prostatectomy model of erectile dysfunction in rats. Urology. 2011;77:761.e1–7.
68. Hatzimouratidis K, et al. Phosphodiesterase type 5 inhibitors in postprostatectomy erectile dysfunction: a critical analysis of the basic science rationale and clinical application. Eur Urol. 2009;55:334–47.
69. Kovanecz I, et al. Long-term continuous sildenafil treatment ameliorates corporal veno-occlusive dysfunction (CVOD) induced by cavernosal nerve resection in rats. Int J Impot Res. 2008;20:202–12.
70. Lagoda G, Jin L, Lehrfeld TJ, Liu T, Burnett AL. FK506 and sildenafil promote erectile function recovery after cavernous nerve injury through antioxidative mechanisms. J Sex Med. 2007;4:908–16.
71. Hlaing SM, et al. Sildenafil promotes neuroprotection of the pelvic ganglia neurones after bilateral cavernosal nerve resection in the rat. BJU Int. 2013;111:159–70.
72. Sirad F, et al. Sildenafil promotes smooth muscle preservation and ameliorates fibrosis through modulation of extracellular matrix and tissue growth factor gene expression after bilateral cavernosal nerve resection in the rat. J Sex Med. 2011;8:1048–60.
73. Kovanecz I, et al. Chronic daily tadalafil prevents the corporal fibrosis and veno-occlusive dysfunction that occurs after cavernosal nerve resection. BJU Int. 2008;101:203–10.
74. Mulhall JP, et al. The functional and structural consequences of cavernous nerve injury are ameliorated by sildenafil citrate. J Sex Med. 2008;5:1126–36.
75. Lysiak JJ, et al. Tadalafil increases Akt and extracellular signal-regulated kinase 1/2 activation, and prevents apoptotic cell death in the penis following denervation. J Urol. 2008;179:779–85.
76. Clavell-Hernandez J, Ermec B, Kadioglu A, Wang R. Perplexity of penile rehabilitation following radical prostatectomy. Turk J Urol. 2019;45:77–82.
77. Liu C, Lopez DS, Chen M, Wang R. Penile rehabilitation therapy following radical prostatectomy: a meta-analysis. J Sex Med. 2017;14:1496–503.
78. Kaiho Y, Yamashita S, Arai Y. Optimization of sexual function outcome after radical prostatectomy using phosphodiesterase type 5 inhibitors. Int J Urol. 2013;20:285–9.
79. Gandaglia G, et al. Penile rehabilitation after radical prostatectomy: does it work? Transl Androl Urol. 2015;4:110–23.
80. Smith WB 2nd, et al. PDE5 inhibitors: considerations for preference and long-term adherence. Int J Clin Pract. 2013;67:768–80.
81. Montorsi F, et al. Earliest time to onset of action leading to successful intercourse with vardenafil determined in an at-home setting: a randomized, double-blind, placebo-controlled trial. J Sex Med. 2004;1:168–78.
82. Castiglione F, Nini A, Briganti A. Penile rehabilitation with phosphodiesterase type 5 inhibitors after nerve-sparing radical prostatectomy: are we targeting the right patients? Eur Urol. 2014;65:673–4.
83. Salonia A, et al. Acceptance of and discontinuation rate from erectile dysfunction oral treatment in patients following bilateral nerve-sparing radical prostatectomy. Eur Urol. 2008;53:564–70.
84. Mulhall JP, et al. The use of an erectogenic pharmacotheraphy regimen following radical prostatectomy improves recovery of spontaneous erectile function. J Sex Med. 2005;2(4):532–40; discussion 540–2. https://doi.org/10.1111/j.1743-6109.2005.00081_1.x.
85. Polito M, D'anzeo G, Conti A, Muzzonigro G. Erectile rehabilitation with intracavernous alprostadil after radical prostatectomy: refusal and dropout rates. BJU Int. 2012;110: 1–4.

86. Kim P, Clavijo RI. Management of male sexual dysfunction after cancer treatment. Urol Oncol. 2020; https://doi.org/10.1016/j.urolonc.2020.08.006.

87. Hatzimouratidis K, et al. Pharmacotherapy for erectile dysfunction: recommendations from the Fourth International Consultation for Sexual Medicine (ICSM 2015). J Sex Med. 2016;13:465–88.

88. Raina R, et al. Long-term efficacy and compliance of MUSE for erectile dysfunction following radical prostatectomy: SHIM (IIEF-5) analysis. Int J Impot Res. 2005;17:86–90.

89. Yuan J, et al. Vacuum therapy in erectile dysfunction—science and clinical evidence. Int J Impot Res. 2010;22:211–9.

90. Basal S, Wambi C, Acikel C, Gupta M, Badani K. Optimal strategy for penile rehabilitation after robot-assisted radical prostatectomy based on preoperative erectile function. BJU Int. 2013;111:658–65.

91. Hatzimouratidis K, et al. Guidelines on male sexual dysfunction: erectile dysfunction and premature ejaculation. Eur Urol. 2010;57:804–14.

92. Sun L, Peng F-L, Yu Z-L, Liu C-L, Chen J. Combined sildenafil with vacuum erection device therapy in the management of diabetic men with erectile dysfunction after failure of first-line sildenafil monotherapy. Int J Urol. 2014;21:1263–7.

93. Zippe CD, Pahlajani G. Vacuum erection devices to treat erectile dysfunction and early penile rehabilitation following radical prostatectomy. Curr Urol Rep. 2008;9:506–13.

94. Qin F, Wang S, Li J, Wu C, Yuan J. The early use of vacuum therapy for penile rehabilitation after radical prostatectomy: systematic review and meta-analysis. Am J Mens Health. 2018;12:2136–43.

95. Capogrosso P, et al. Low-intensity shock wave therapy in sexual medicine-clinical recommendations from the European Society of Sexual Medicine (ESSM). J Sex Med. 2019;16:1490–505.

96. Zewin TS, et al. Efficacy and safety of low-intensity shock wave therapy in penile rehabilitation post nerve-sparing radical cystoprostatectomy: a randomized controlled trial. Int Urol Nephrol. 2018;50:2007–14.

97. Frey A, Sønksen J, Fode M. Low-intensity extracorporeal shockwave therapy in the treatment of postprostatectomy erectile dysfunction: a pilot study. Scand J Urol. 2016;50(2):123–7. https://doi.org/10.3109/21681805.2015.1100675.

98. Baccaglini W, et al. The role of the low-intensity extracorporeal shockwave therapy on penile rehabilitation after radical prostatectomy: a randomized clinical trial. J Sex Med. 2020;17:688–94.

99. Bochinski D, et al. The effect of neural embryonic stem cell therapy in a rat model of cavernosal nerve injury. BJU Int. 2004;94:904–9.

100. Kendirci M, et al. Transplantation of nonhematopoietic adult bone marrow stem/progenitor cells isolated by p75 nerve growth factor receptor into the penis rescues erectile function in a rat model of cavernous nerve injury. J Urol. 2010;184:1560–6.

101. Albersen M, et al. Injections of adipose tissue-derived stem cells and stem cell lysate improve recovery of erectile function in a rat model of cavernous nerve injury. J Sex Med. 2010;7:3331–40.

102. Lin C-S, et al. Stem cell therapy for erectile dysfunction: a critical review. Stem Cells Dev. 2012;21:343–51.

103. Castiglione F, et al. Intratunical injection of human adipose tissue-derived stem cells prevents fibrosis and is associated with improved erectile function in a rat model of Peyronie's disease. Eur Urol. 2013;63:551–60.

104. Castiglione F, et al. Adipose-derived stem cells counteract urethral stricture formation in rats. Eur Urol. 2016;70:1032–41.

105. Capogrosso P, Montorsi F, Salonia A. Phase I and phase II clinical trials for the treatment of male sexual dysfunction—a systematic review of the literature. Expert Opin Investig Drugs. 2018;27(7):583–93.

106. Yiou R, et al. Safety of intracavernous bone marrow-mononuclear cells for postradical prostatectomy erectile dysfunction: an open dose-escalation pilot study. Eur Urol. 2016;69:988–91.

107. Beck AM, Robinson JW, Carlson LE. Sexual values as the key to maintaining satisfying sex after prostate cancer treatment: the physical pleasure-relational intimacy model of sexual motivation. Arch Sex Behav. 2013;42:1637–47.
108. Du K, et al. Orgasmic function after radical prostatectomy. J Urol. 2017;198:407–13.
109. Barnas JL, et al. The prevalence and nature of orgasmic dysfunction after radical prostatectomy. BJU Int. 2004;94:603–5.
110. Capogrosso P, Ventimiglia E, Cazzaniga W, Montorsi F, Salonia A. Orgasmic dysfunction after radical prostatectomy. World J Mens Health. 2017;35:1–13.
111. Capogrosso P, et al. Orgasmic dysfunction after robot-assisted versus open radical prostatectomy. Eur Urol. 2016;70:223–6.
112. Gontero P, et al. New insights into the pathogenesis of penile shortening after radical prostatectomy and the role of postoperative sexual function. J Urol. 2007;178:602–7.
113. Savoie M, Kim SS, Soloway MS. A prospective study measuring penile length in men treated with radical prostatectomy for prostate cancer. J Urol. 2003;169:1462–4.
114. Carlsson S, et al. Self-perceived penile shortening after radical prostatectomy. Int J Impot Res. 2012;24:179–84.
115. Engel JD, Sutherland DE, Williams SB, Wagner KR. Changes in penile length after robot-assisted laparoscopic radical prostatectomy. J Endourol. 2011;25:65–9.
116. Kadono Y, et al. Changes in penile length after radical prostatectomy: investigation of the underlying anatomical mechanism. BJU Int. 2017;120(2):293–9. https://doi.org/10.1111/bju.13777.
117. Segal R, Burnett AL. Erectile preservation following radical prostatectomy. Ther Adv Urol. 2011;3:35–46.
118. Tal R, et al. Peyronie's disease following radical prostatectomy: incidence and predictors. J Sex Med. 2010;7:1254–61.
119. Chambers SK, et al. A randomised controlled trial of a couples-based sexuality intervention for men with localised prostate cancer and their female partners. Psychooncology. 2015;24:748–56.
120. Canada AL, Neese LE, Sui D, Schover LR. Pilot intervention to enhance sexual rehabilitation for couples after treatment for localized prostate carcinoma. Cancer. 2005;104:2689–700.
121. Schlegel PN, Walsh PC. Neuroanatomical approach to radical cystoprostatectomy with preservation of sexual function. J Urol. 1987;138:1402–6.
122. Miyao N, et al. Recovery of sexual function after nerve-sparing radical prostatectomy or cystectomy. Int J Urol. 2001;8:158–64.
123. El-Bahnasawy MS, Ismail T, Elsobky E, Alzalouey EI, Bazeed MA. Prognostic factors predicting successful response to sildenafil after radical cystoprostatectomy. Scand J Urol Nephrol. 2008;42:110–5.
124. Horenblas S, Meinhardt W, Ijzerman W, Moonen LF. Sexuality preserving cystectomy and neobladder: initial results. J Urol. 2001;166:837–40.
125. Banerjee AK. Sexual dysfunction after surgery for rectal cancer. Lancet. 1999;353:1900–2.
126. Keating JP. Sexual function after rectal excision. ANZ J Surg. 2004;74:248–59.
127. Nishizawa Y, et al. Male sexual dysfunction after rectal cancer surgery. Int J Color Dis. 2011;26:1541–8.
128. Havenga K, et al. Male and female sexual and urinary function after total mesorectal excision with autonomic nerve preservation for carcinoma of the rectum. J Am Coll Surg. 1996;182:495–502.
129. Eveno C, Lamblin A, Mariette C, Pocard M. Sexual and urinary dysfunction after proctectomy for rectal cancer. J Visc Surg. 2010;147:e21–30.
130. Lindsey I, George B, Kettlewell M, Mortensen N. Randomized, double-blind, placebo-controlled trial of sildenafil (viagra) for erectile dysfunction after rectal excision for cancer and inflammatory bowel disease. Dis Colon Rectum. 2002;45:727–32.

Pathophysiology and Clinical Aspects of Sexual Dysfunction in Women

11

Ozhan Ozdemir and Gulsum Gulcan Kocamis

Abstract

Female sexual dysfunction is a prevalent problem in the general community; however, it has not been studied as extensively as male sexual dysfunction. In this article we summarize the pathophysiology, classification and treatment of female sexual dysfunction.

Pathophysiology and Clinical Aspects of Sexual Dysfunction in Women

Female sexual dysfunction (FSD) is a common condition and often taken for granted in the general population. FSD is characterized as a disease that causes full-size non-public distress due to sexual desire, orgasm, arousal, and sexual ache [1]. According to Basson et al. "It is a multifactorial, age-related, progressive problem" [2]. From 35% up to 45% of ladies realize that they have got a problem of low sexual desire. The diagnosis of the disease, clinical and surgical treatment, lack of expertise to control this life experience, and physical and mental distress increases the incidence and severity of sexual problems. Thus, physicians are required to be capable of discovering such sexual problems and recognizing whether or not to provide a remedy to patients.

The determinant factors of sexual health are complicated and multifactorial. The feeling of oneself as a sexual being, one's normal fitness state, a sense of well-being, and one's prior sexual experiences are all regarded as intrapersonal factors. For

O. Ozdemir (✉) · G. G. Kocamis
Department of Obstetrics and Gynecology, Gulhane School of Medicine, University of Health Sciences, Ankara, Turkey
e-mail: ozhan.ozdemir@sbu.edu.tr

© The Author(s), under exclusive license to Springer Nature Switzerland AG 2022
S. Sarikaya et al. (eds.), *Andrology and Sexual Medicine*, Management of Urology, https://doi.org/10.1007/978-3-031-12049-7_11

219

partnered individuals, these features also apply to the partners. Interpersonal factors, on the other hand, include the period and nature of the relationship, conversation patterns, and the diversity and type of ongoing lifestyles, occasions and stressors [3].

The birth of a child and retirement are two examples of somehow positive life events that might contribute to sexual dysfunction. Sexuality includes a wide variety of expressions of intimacy and is essential to self-identification with strong cultural, biological, and psychological components. The reason is that lots of women see their sexuality as a key quality of life problem, the obstetrician-gynecologist plays a critical role in examining sexual function. Furthermore, gynecologic disorder procedures and therapeutic interventions can affect sexual response. The clinician has to make no longer presumptions or judgments about the woman's conduct, and when counseling patients have to hold on thoughts the possibility of cultural and private variation in sexual practices.

Female Pelvic Anatomy

The female sexual anatomy is consisted of the mons pubis, the vulva which contains the labia majora, labia minora, interlabial area, and clitoris. The inner genitalia include the vestibule, periurethral glans, and vagina, as well as the uterus, fallopian tubes, and ovaries. The arousal is triggered by genital vasocongestion, which is driven by increased sympathetic nervous system activity. The introitus is exposed when the vulva swells; the vagina lengthens and dilates; the outer part of the vagina tightens; the clitoris lengthens and dilates; and the uterus rises above the levator plate.

The stimulation of the pelvic nerves relaxes smooth muscles and decreases the resistance inside the arteries, resulting in improved blood flow to the clitoris. This blood flowing is caused by an active neurogenic dilation of the sinusoidal blood spaces, which leads to the corpora cavernosa of the clitoris to emerge as engorged, and the clitoris will have regularly greater prominence. It has been indicated that the vulvar systems emerge as engorged; however, they are not erected due to the fact that the thinner tunica in women does not entice venous blood, and it consequently pools with chronic influx and outflow. Furthermore, increased strain within the capillaries of the genital vasculature and fluid transudation via the sub-epithelium of the vaginal walls cause vaginal lubrication. Secretions are a combination of androgen-structured vulvar glands that release mucin and aquaporin channels inside the vaginal mucosa, resulting in a blood serum transudate. Nipple erection, skin flushing, and elevations in heart rate, blood pressure, and breathing rate are all extragenital changes associated with arousal [4].

Physiology of Female Sexual Response

A woman's sexual response is determined in part by neurobiological factors. The factors including hormones and neurochemicals influence the brain and signal transmission between the central nervous system and the erogenous zone to arouse sexual desire. Sexual responses are believed to be influenced by excitatory and inhibitory pathways in the brain, including the hypothalamus and limbic system affecting both excitatory and inhibitory mechanisms, and the cortex and midbrain affecting inhibitory mechanisms [5]. Studies based primarily on animal models have shown that the balance or sum of inhibitory and excitatory signals determines an individual's sexual response that is called as "sexual tipping point" [6, 7].

It is believed that hypoactive sexual desire disorder may be caused by a hypoactive excitatory factor, a hyperactive inhibitory factor, or both of them. Imaging studies indicated that women having hypoactive sexual desire disorder had high level of activation in the medial frontal gyrus and right inferior gyrus when compared to women without sexual dysfunction, confirming hyperfunction inhibition in women experiencing hypoactive sexual desire disorder [8].

Increased autonomic nervous system activity as well as tachycardia, skin flushing, and vaginal lubrication, are all physiological components of a woman's sexual reaction. Moreover, the sexual response cycle also involves a number of neurotransmitters. Norepinephrine, dopamine, oxytocin, and serotonin via 5-hydroxytryptamine (5HT) 1A and 2C are considered to have positive sexual influences. Serotonin, prolactin, and γ-aminobutyric acid (GABA) via most other receptors are thought to negatively affect the cycle negatively [9].

Traditional Model: Masters, Johnson and Kaplan found that a normal woman's sexual response cycle is consisted of four stages: arousal, stabilization, orgasm, and resolution [10].

- Desire: The sexual desire of women and men is known as libido. A balance between dopamine stimulation and serotonin inhibition maintains this desire. The threshold of reaction is decided with the aid of using androgens, in particular, testosterone. This is valid for both women and men.
- Arousal: This stage is mediated by parasympathetic connections with the pelvic organs resulted in vascular engorgement. Women's arousal tends to be slower and more receptive to touch and mental stimuli, and it is demonstrated by vaginal lubrication. Men's arousal is usually faster and more responsive to visual stimuli and is manifested by penis erection.
- Plateau: This step involves progression and intensification of the excitement phase. The length of this phase can be changeable. The neural pathway and physiologic mechanism are the same as excitement.
- Orgasm: This step is mediated by sympathetic connections, resulting in reflex tonic-clonic pelvic floor muscle contractions followed by uterine contractions. Women have greater individual differences in orgasm than men. A unique feature of women is their ability to have multiple orgasms in a row.
- Resolution: This step is manifested by a go back to the basal physiologic state with reversal of vasocongestion and muscle tension. Resolution can be quicker for men and slower for women.

Intimacy-Based Model: An alternative sexual response model illustrates an intimacy-based motivation, integral sexual stimuli, and the psychological and biological components governing the processing of those stimuli [10].

Sexual Dysfunction and Hormonal Influences

There are many factors to consider when identifying the source of sexual dysfunction. Medical and surgical conditions that can cause sexual dysfunction varies from anatomical processes to lower urinary tract problems such as endocrine disorders, malignant neoplasms including breast and ovarian cancer, inflammatory diseases such as fibromyalgia and rheumatoid arthritis, and neurological conditions. In addition, numerous acquired issues such as delivery, hormonal changes, menopause, trauma, breastfeeding, and so on can result in sexual dysfunction. Depression and anxiety are among psychological factors which can be counted as possible causes of sexual dysfunction.

Factors affecting individuals' lifestyle, such as eating junk food and being overweight, loss of exercise, smoking, alcohol, and drug abuse, can similarly contribute to psychosocial elements of age, education, income, and ethnicity. Other miscellaneous elements consist of preceding records of sexual abuse, sexual orientation, kind of sexual practices, terrible attitudes closer to sex, and negative body image [11].

Another cause of sexual dysfunction is an estrogen deficiency. Estradiol is the main female sex hormone in women, which allows maintaining the integrity of the vaginal mucosal epithelium and promotes lubrication. Estrogen has a crucial role in regulating sexual function and the production of nitric oxide in the vagina and clitoris. It also has a vasoprotective and vasodilating effect on the vagina. A sharp decrease in estrogen levels, vaginal lubrication, and decreased libido and frequency during menopause can lead to vaginitis. For safety reasons, postmenopausal estrogen therapy is not given at ovulatory levels, so co-administration of testosterone may benefit primarily through aromatization conversion to estrogen. A meta-analysis of sex hormone supplementation for the treatment of postmenopausal sexual dysfunction before a more recent transdermal testosterone study concluded that androgen therapy is only effective when administered in combination with estrogen, although some estrogen therapy has been associated with improved female sexual function [12].

A meta-analysis found that four out of five older estrogen-only studies that achieved similar estradiol levels at ovulation increased libido in postmenopausal women. Some approved studies combining postmenopausal estrogen therapy with testosterone therapy have associated a slight increase in libido [13].

Diagnosis

With the exception of substance/medication-induced sexual dysfunction, new categories (Diagnostic and Statistical Manual of Mental Disorders: DSM-5) contain duration and severity requirements. The subcategories of lifelong versus acquired, generic versus situational, and psychological versus mixed components have also been altered. Sexual dysfunction caused by a general medical problem and the subtype caused by psychological versus combined factors were all excluded.

The DSM-5 standards for sexual disorder require a minimal period of 6 months of signs and symptoms. These signs and symptoms need to be present from 75% up to 100% of the time for all diagnoses, except medication and substance-induced sexual disorder. This criterion removes the inclusion of people with moderate to slight signs and symptoms and renders the severity rating specifier pointless. In addition, the symptoms may create severe distress [14].

Treatment

There are many medications available to treat FSD which include hormones and different kinds of drugs. Nonetheless, not a single treatment has been accepted as the golden standard so far. Prior to the treatment, patients are required to be thoroughly evaluated for their medical condition and medication history causing sexual dysfunction. Estrogens, androgens, dopaminergic agonists, nitric oxide donors, prostaglandins, and a-melanocyte-stimulating hormones are widely used for the treatment of FSD. Females with reduced sexual desire are possibly respond well to androgens, estrogens, and dopamine receptor antagonists, while those with sexual arousal disorder may be more responsive to phosphodiesterase inhibitors and prostaglandins [1].

Transdermal Testosterone Therapy: Results show satisfactory sexual activity and an increase in libido. The risks (hirsutism, acne, virilization, and cardiovascular complications) must be weighed against the benefits of its use. It is recommended to monitor testosterone levels to avoid physiological treatment [15].

Sildenafil: Phosphodiesterase inhibitors can increase blood flow to the genitals but are generally not effective for treating arousal disorders. Sildenafil helps patients with sexual dysfunction due to SSRIs [15].

Bupropion: 300–400 mg of bupropion per day has been shown to increase sexual arousal and orgasm completion. Additionally, bupropion supplementation significantly improved critical factors of sexual function in women with SSRI-induced sexual dysfunction [15].

Flibanserin: Non-hormonal treatment for hypoactive sexual desire disorder (HSDD) in women. It is a serotonin 5HT receptor agonist and a 5HT receptor antagonist. The mechanism action for the treatment of HSDD is unknown. The recommended dose is 100 mg once daily at bedtime. Side effects include hypotension, syncope, and central nervous system depression. Drinking alcohol increases the risk of side effects and is contraindicated. This is mostly effective, and about 10% of women reported a "significant" or "very significant" improvement in their HSDD symptoms [15].

Ospermifene: Clinical trials have shown significant reductions in sexual pain, arousal, and desire [16].

Botulinum neurotoxin: Numerous studies have shown efficacy in reducing symptoms in a variety of conditions, including dyspareunia, vestibular pain, decreased arousal in persistent genital arousal, and the ability to withstand vaginal penetration [15].

Medical Device: The Eros Clitoral Therapy Device is a portable, FDA-approved medical device for the treatment of sexual arousal and orgasmic disorders in women. This appears to be useful for women with sexual arousal disorder. InterStim Therapy, which includes mild sacral nerve stimulation, was originally developed for the treatment of urinary incontinence and is currently being studied in sexual arousal disorders [17].

Patient Education: Information about vulvovaginitis and the anatomy of the pelvic floor can allow women to gain better understanding of the mechanisms and etiology of genital-pelvic pain and symptoms of penetration disorders. Self-care advice should suggest avoiding common vulvar contact irritants, including soaps, showers, tissues, scented products, and panty liners. Pointing out patients for inflammatory changes in the skin around the vulva and around the anus can help motivate them to refuse wipes or other irritants [18].

Dilation: Several prescription and over-the-counter medications are available that can self-dilate after radiation therapy or other trauma to relieve the vagina, release pelvic floor muscle trigger points, or correct vaginal stenosis. There is little literature on optimal strategies for the use of dilators.

Vaginal Fractional carbon dioxide (CO_2) Laser Treatment: The safety, efficacy, and value for money of vaginal fractionated carbon dioxide lasers for the treatment of vulvovaginal atrophy have not been adequately studied and have not been approved by the FDA. Even though previous studies demonstrate that there are some potential benefits in vulvovaginal atrophy, these studies were not placebo-controlled, and long-term results were not explained. Also, the cost of treatment is high compared to other options. In further studies, more data should analyze the effects and safety of this procedure, especially in the long-term treatment of vulvovaginal atrophy.Conflicts of InterestThe authors do not have a conflict of interest.

References

1. Raina R, Pahlajani G, Khan S, Gupta S, Agarwal A, Zippe CD. Female sexual dysfunction: classification, pathophysiology, and management. Fertil Steril. 2007;88(5):1273–84.
2. Basson R, Berman J, Burnett A, Derogatis L, Ferguson D, et al. Report of the international consensus development conference on female sexual dysfunction: definitions and classifications. J Urol. 2000;163(3):888–93.
3. Gershenson DM, Lentz GM, Valea FA, Lobo RA. Comprehensive gynecology. 8th ed. Philadelphia: Elsevier; 2022.
4. Quaghebeur J, Petros P, Wyndaele JJ, De Wachter S. Pelvic-floor function, dysfunction, and treatment. Eur J Obstet Gynecol Reprod Biol. 2021;265:143–9.
5. Simon JA, Kingsberg SA, Portman D, Williams LA, Krop J, Jordan R, et al. Long-term safety and efficacy of bremelanotide for hypoactive sexual desire disorder. Obstet Gynecol. 2019;134(5):909–17.

6. Perelman MA. The sexual tipping point: a mind/body model for sexual medicine. J Sex Med. 2009;6(3):629–32.

7. Kingsberg SA, Clayton AH, Pfaus JG. The female sexual response: current models, neurobiological underpinnings and agents currently approved or under investigation for the treatment of hypoactive sexual desire disorder. CNS Drugs. 2015;29(11):915–33.

8. Arnow BA, Millheiser L, Garrett A, Polan ML, Glover GH, Hill KR, et al. Women with hypoactive sexual desire disorder compared to normal females: a functional magnetic resonance imaging study. Neuroscience. 2009;158(2):484–502.

9. Casanova R, Chuang A, Goepfert AR, et al. Beckmann and Ling's obstetrics and gynecology. 8th ed. Chennai: Wolters Kluver; 2019.

10. Basson R. Female sexual response: the role of drugs in the management of sexual dysfunction. Obstet Gynecol. 2001;98(2):350–3.

11. Clayton AH, Margarita E, Juarez V. Female sexual dysfunction. Med Clin North Am. 2019;103(4):681–98.

12. Segraves RT, Clayton A, Croft H, Wolf A, Warnock J. Bupropion sustained release for the treatment of hypoactive sexual desire disorder in premenopausal women. J Clin Psychopharmacol. 2004;24(3):339–42.

13. Shifren JL, Davis SR, Moreau M, Waldbaum A, Bouchard C, DeRogatis L, et al. Testosterone patch for the treatment of hypoactive sexual desire disorder in naturally menopausal women: results from the INTIMATE NM1 Study. Menopause. 2006;13(5):770–9.

14. American Psychiatric Association. Diagnostic and statistical manual of mental disorders: DSM-5. Washington, DC: APA; 2013.

15. Simon JA, Clayton AH, Kim NN, Patel S. Clinically meaningful benefit in women with hypoactive sexual desire disorder treated with flibanserin. Sex Med. 2022;10(1):100476.

16. Pup LD, Sánchez-Borrego R. Ospemifene efficacy and safety data in women with vulvovaginal atrophy. Gynecol Endocrinol. 2020;36(7):569–77.

17. Wilson SK, Delk JR, Billups KL. Treating symptoms of female sexual arousal disorder with the Eros-Clitoral Therapy Device. J Gend Specif Med. 2001;4(2):54–8.

18. Melnik T, Hawton K, McGuire H. Interventions for vaginismus. Cochrane Database Syst Rev. 2012;12(12):CD001760.

Sexual Arousal and Sexual Pain Disorders in Women

12

Charmaine Borg, Lara Lakhsassi, and Peter J. de Jong

Abstract

Low or disrupted sexual arousal is discussed as a transdiagnostic-underlying denominator for women's sexual dysfunctions. The role of sexual arousal in attenuating the inhibitory aspects of sexual stimuli, as well as factors that weaken sexual arousal are described and clinical implications critically discussed. We put specific emphasis on the bidirectional relationship of sexual arousal and disgust/pain along with the role of disgust and pain expectancies in sexual dysfunctions. Thereby, we aimed to provide a critical evaluation of the treatment options for inhibited sexual arousal with focus on generic and specific interventions targeting disgust: a critical feature that thus far received only scant attention in the available literature.

Sexual Arousal

When an individual is—or, anticipates being—exposed to sexual stimuli of interest, be it imaginary or real, this will generally elicit sexual arousal, or sexual excitement. Sexual arousal or excitement is the physiological and/or psychological appetitive response that prepares one for a sexual encounter, typically referred to as feeling "turned on". Sexual motivation is accompanied by functionally related changes in cognitive, physiological, and behavioural response systems [1, 2]. As such, when a sex stimulus is considered appealing, or rewarding, and sexual arousal is elicited,

C. Borg (✉) · L. Lakhsassi · P. J. de Jong
Department of Clinical Psychology and Experimental Psychopathology, University of Groningen, Groningen, The Netherlands
e-mail: c.borg@rug.nl; l.lakhsassi@rug.nl; p.j.de.jong@rug.nl

© The Author(s), under exclusive license to Springer Nature Switzerland AG 2022
S. Sarikaya et al. (eds.), *Andrology and Sexual Medicine*, Management of Urology, https://doi.org/10.1007/978-3-031-12049-7_12

227

this will give rise to: (i) (cognitive) processing priority of such stimuli, thereby reducing access to attentional resources of potential distractors, (ii) selective activation of positive memory representations, (iii) pleasurable bodily sensations and/or feelings of sexual arousal, and (iv) increased motivation to pursue a sexual interaction or engage in sexual activity [3].

In the event where one subsequently engages in sexual activity, a positive feedback occurs where sexual arousal, pleasure, and motivation are continuously enhanced until the individual is sated, or, when orgasm is achieved. In turn, this feeling of satiety reciprocally incentivizes future sexual arousal and motivation to seek sexual contact [3].

In some cases, however, one may be exposed to sexual stimuli of interest and yet experience little to no sexual arousal—sometimes, even whilst wanting to be able to desire sex. For instance, if a sex stimulus is associated with negative memories of an earlier negative event, sexual arousal and motivation can be inhibited rather than facilitated [4, 5].

Consequently, the physiological and behavioural responses provide a different type of motivational feedback where future sexual arousal and motivation may not be incentivized [3].Weak sexual arousal, often 'inhibited' or disrupted sexual arousal is a common culprit in sexual dysfunctions, and, left untreated, may cause great personal and relationship distress. One may hypothesize that the overlap between various dysfunctions in women can be partially explained by an insufficient level of sexual excitement. In line with this thinking, it has been argued that inhibited sexual arousal can be seen as a major transdiagnostic factor in sexual dysfunctions in women, as defined in the Diagnostic and Statistical Manual, Version 5 (DSM 5; these are Sexual Interest and Arousal Disorder, Female Orgasmic disorder, and Genito-Pelvic Pain Penetration Disorder) [6, 7].This chapter, therefore, focuses on identifying the processes underlying (dys)functional sexual arousal as a potential transdiagnostic feature in various sexual problems and dysfunctions in order to delineate interventions aimed at promoting sexual health and emotional well-being. In this chapter we shall discuss the antecedent factors that hamper the full development of sexual arousal, as well as the consequences of having sex in the absence of sufficiently high sexual arousal—in women particularly. Genito-Pelvic Pain Penetration Disorder (GPPPD) will be used as a model to discuss the impact of inhibited sexual arousal and to outline treatment interventions that can be applied in sexual problems, with particular focus on interventions aimed at insufficient or inhibited sexual arousal.

Sexual Arousal as an Emotion

Sexual excitement or sexual arousal can be conceived as an emotion. To solidify this claim, let us consider fear, an intensely studied emotion; when a spider phobic individual is confronted with a spider, they experience automatic physiological fear responses, subjective feelings of fear and disgust, that support the concurrently elicited motivation to avoid and escape the stimulus in a way to create distance from the perceived threat. In this analogy, sexual excitement can be conceptualized as an emotion as well, not as part of the aversive motivational system that serves to avoid harmful outcomes ("punishment"), but rather as part of the appetitive motivational system that serves approach behaviour targeted to promote the experience of reward. Accordingly, in this chapter, sexual responses and behaviours have been conceptualised within the context of an incentive motivational model, which has long been applied to sexual motivation and behaviour [3, 8]. The starting point of this approach is: (i) the presence of a system that is sensitive to sexual stimuli, moderated by hormonal influences, neurotransmitters, and previous sexual experiences, (ii) that can be activated by the appraisal of sexual stimuli (iii) which will then result in an appetitive motivational state reflected in sexual arousal and an action tendency aimed at the acquisition of sexual gratification.

According to the incentive motivational model and other dominant models targeted at giving a backbone and an explanation to sexual behaviour and motivation—whether sexual arousal is facilitated or inhibited depends on a multitude of factors. That is, whether one is "turned on" or "turned off" depends on the sum total of all competing factors, each of which is based on one's past history/upbringing, sexual experiences, and natural individual proclivity toward inhibition or excitation and biological factors. Consequently, the opposing excitatory and inhibitory factors compete, the sum total of which ultimately tilt the scales toward the appetitive/approach or inhibition in a given sexual situation. In turn, this determines whether one will engage in sexual activity or—to a certain extent—inhibit themselves from it. Accordingly, sexual responses may be compromised when sexual inhibition outweighs sexual excitation; the two opposing processes generally inhibit one another [4], unless one remains in a state of ambivalence [3]. Thus, when one process is reduced, the other can be heightened. Likewise, when one is sexually aroused, excitatory stimuli typically become more salient while inhibitory stimuli are more attenuated [9, 10].

There are various factors that may inhibit the generation of sexual arousal and/or that can weaken its intensity. Among various factors inhibiting sexual arousal, such as organic factors and metabolic disorders, weak sexual arousal is frequently associated with negative thoughts and attitudes about sex (e.g., sex is sinful) and sexual stimuli (e.g., the ejaculate is sticky and disgusting) and an adverse emotional response, such as disgust, when confronted with such sexual cues. These may arise from a plethora of experiences, often including: having a conservative/religious upbringing where one holds the belief that any form of sex is unacceptable or sinful [11, 12], thereby creating a state of cognitive dissonance in moments where one unwillingly feels aroused or engages in sexual activity, or having a history of negative sexual experiences inclusive of feeling disrespected, not cared about, or abused. In consequence, confrontation with these cues or stimuli may trigger negative affective states, such as shame, guilt, anger, embarrassment, disgust, anxiety, or depression [7, 13].

Other common precursors may involve chronically high stress levels [14], performance anxiety [15] and as a consequence, distracted attention away from the sexual stimulus [14, 16]. In other words, rather than being associated with sexual gratification, sex stimuli may become associated with anxiety/stress, disgust and even aversion, among other negative emotions—all of which can interfere with subjective and genital sexual arousal [4, 17, 18].

Furthermore, it is important to consider relational dynamics in understanding how sexual arousal is influenced. For instance, an individual who is anxiously attached in their relationship may associate sex with maintaining the relationship, rather than with sexual pleasure. In such cases, their insecurity may be reflected in their sexual behaviour, causing their partner to down-regulate their sexual arousal in response, in turn enhancing the initial's partner's insecurity as they might misinterpret this response as a lack of interest [19]. In other cases, feeling criticized rather than accepted, or feeling that your sexual advances are rejected, could all weaken the generation of sexual arousal [20]. Indeed, there is increasing evidence suggesting that rejection or the feeling of not being an 'appropriate' or valued sexual partner can lead to self-rejection and self-disgust [21, 22]. In turn, this feeling of self-disgust may weaken the generation of sexual arousal resulting in a downward spiral that may give rise to persistent sexual problems.

Further, the quality of sex and its arousing features may be altered or weakened as a function of the duration of the relationship, when sex with the same partner becomes less novel and results in habituation. This area of research has been almost neglected in empirical investigations. However, there is some evidence suggesting that in the course of long-term relationships, heterosexual women tend to desire sexual activity less than men [23], which may not so much be indicative of a sex difference in capacity for sexual pleasure and sexual arousal, but rather may be due to mainstream sexual activities not being optimally tailored for women's sexual pleasure.

Besides, within the realms of relational dynamics, there are other perhaps more global factors that may have adverse effects on sexual arousal. For example, the level of knowledge on how to become aroused, insufficient experience and/or knowledge about one's own body or that of their partner, as well as poor communication skills. Although knowledge and communication about one's sexual wishes have been stressed as important qualities in sexual health, these are nonetheless usually not part of educational programs and books on sexual health [24]. Perhaps not unrelated, individuals may lack the motivation to become sexually aroused, which may be due to the various reasons previously mentioned (i.e., habituation in long-term relationships, or not allowing or recognizing oneself as a sexual being).

However, underlying the weak motivation to become sexually aroused, a prominent reason for the unwillingness or disinterest may be the lack of reinforcing sexual experiences [25]. For heterosexual women in particular, sexual activity, in most cultures, is less pleasurable than it is for men, and yet men and women do not differ in their capacity for sexual pleasure [26]. Hanging myths, such as that penile-vaginal intercourse is the ultimate goal for sexual pleasure surely do not help; without additional stimulation of the glans clitoris only about 25% to 30% of heterosexual women experience orgasm during intercourse [27], whereas over 90% of heterosexual men always orgasm during penile-vaginal intercourse. Clearly, then, sexual intercourse generally results in less gratifying experiences for women than for men.

This orgasm gap related to penile-vaginal intercourse is therefore highly relevant when discussing sexual arousal and sexual pleasure in women. Finally, weak sexual arousal may be strongly associated with other disorders and/or the treatment associated with it. For instance, it may be a by-product of a mental disorder (e.g., weaker sensitivity to potentially rewarding experiences or excessive worrying or rumination commonly reported in depressive disorders) or other medical/physical conditions (e.g., malignancies and metabolic disorders such as diabetes which due to neuropathy reduces the sensitivity of the perceptual system) that hinder sexual functioning, and/or pre-existing lack of sexual desire. Likewise, sexual arousal can be hindered by the medications used for treatment of these disorders, as is often the case with the treatment for major depression with selective serotonin reuptake inhibitors (SSRI's) [28, 29] or with antipsychotic medication, which may lower the sensitivity of the motivational system, potentially resulting in the absence of drive towards reward. Similar effects can be found with recreational drug use.

Disgust, and Its Relevance to Sex and Sexual Problems

Most of the factors considered so far in this chapter as prospectively interfering with sexual arousal are quite intuitive, and therefore prominent in the literature and used as key leads for improving treatment of sexual dysfunction. Thus, we would like to focus specifically on a factor that is less often recognized in sexual problems despite being inherent to sex: the feeling of disgust. In fact, disgust has been largely overlooked as a potential symptom in sexual problems and only in the last decade has it started gaining some attention in relation to sexual dysfunctions [18, 25, 30]. In the earlier sections we have already included a few examples of how disgust can appear in sexual problems; in the following sections, however, we would like to build a case on why and how disgust may be a critical element when considering sexual arousal-related dysfunctions and their treatment.

Disgust has been defined as a feeling of repulsion ensuing actual or vividly-imagined contact with a certain stimulus through taste, smell, touch or sight. This feeling consequently elicits inhibitory avoidance tendencies and defensive reflexes in order to protect us from the potential contaminant that this stimulus may contain [31, 32]. Indeed, in support of the view that disgust might serve to protect against contamination, it has been found that disgust responsivity is heightened in people with low immune status [33]. Accordingly, given that sexual stimuli and behaviors allow for ample pathogen exposure [34], it follows that sexual stimuli (e.g., vaginal fluid, saliva, the ejaculate) and behaviors also elicit disgust [35]. Evidently, disgust-induced avoidance may help prevent exposure to an infectious disease. However, such avoidance also interferes with the competing goals of sexual pleasure, reward, and procreation. In turn, other sex stimuli in mature individuals embody reproductive fitness (e.g., breasts and full lips in women, or broad shoulders and height in men), thereby counteracting sexual avoidance and instead eliciting sexual excitation and approach tendencies. So, while it seems that some sexual stimuli likely facilitate disgust and inhibition, other sexual stimuli likely facilitate sexual excitement [17].

Interestingly, sexual stimuli and behaviours seem to be prominently disgusting during the pre-pubertal stage of development, which explains why prepubertal children often feel disgusted when witnessing for example adults French-kissing and exchanging saliva, a potential contaminant [36, 37]. Once puberty has started, however, the hormonal changes trigger a natural inclination toward sexual excitation. Thus, as sexual stimuli begin to evoke sexual excitation and pleasure, a dual interaction between sexual arousal (i.e., excitatory) and disgust (i.e., inhibitory) manifests. Normally, sexual excitatory processes successfully outweigh the inhibitory ones, causing sex-relevant disgust to decrease, while sex-irrelevant disgust is stabilized or increased; accordingly, French-kissing becomes more appealing and rewarding [36]. In the event where disgust is not successfully moderated by sexual excitation, or its attenuation is delayed, however, sexual dysfunction may emerge. Here, individuals experience automatic feelings of repulsion by some sexual stimuli, or simply a dislike, sometimes accompanied by avoidance [32]. It is noteworthy that disgust and excitement-eliciting stimuli can be concurrently present and ambiguous [38]; the question of which process will prevail depends on the relative strength of the respective disgust and arousal associations. As alluded to earlier in this chapter, most factors involved in excitatory and inhibitory processes continuously vary and hold the potential for change in valence [39]. For example, a previously arousing stimulus might become aversive after an experience with sexual abuse or assault. On the flip side, a previously neutral stimulus could become erotic or even fetishized after a rewarding sexual experience. Thus, it is important to keep in mind that one is not "stuck" with these tendencies, and can work toward changing them if they wish to [5].

The Reciprocal Dynamics Between Sexual Arousal and Disgust

Evidently, feelings of disgust and sexual arousal in the sexual context may represent opposing needs; the need to avoid contamination and disease versus the need for pleasure and/or procreation. Once the latter need becomes more salient in the adolescent developmental stage, engagement in sexual activity is critical for a successful transition from sex-related disgust to sexual appetite, thereby kick-starting the sexual appetitive motivation system.

Similarly, there is a growing body of evidence indicating that sexual arousal may temporarily reduce the experience of sex-related disgust in both men [35, 40] and women [9]. Furthermore, sexual arousal has additionally been found to promote approach behavior toward initially disgusting stimuli [9]. This capacity for sexual arousal to inhibit disgust can help explain how individuals make initial contact and engage in (previously avoided) sexual behavior. Over time, repeated sexual behavior might very well result in weakening the disgust response toward sex-relevant stimuli and behaviours through habituation, thereby allowing more space for sexual arousal. Indeed, prolonged contact with initially disgusting stimuli has been shown to be an efficient strategy to reduce disgust [41].

That said, the motivation for initial sexual contact is largely motivated by the interaction between hormones and experience—with sexual reward as key factors involved in sexual motivation. In other words, sex hormones support the initial approach and, in turn, the subsequent reward may further contribute to the more approach behaviors. Over time, repeated exposure and prolonged contact (to sex-relevant disgust stimuli as well as sexual reward) allows for habituation of sex-relevant disgust responses, lowering the threshold for sexual approach behaviors, and strengthening excitatory processes especially when orgasm is reached.

Consequences of Having Sex in the Absence or Sufficiently High Sexual Arousal: Pain

When, for various reasons, sexual arousal is not sufficiently high, potential distractors and inhibitory factors associated with sex can remain at the forefront of one's attention during a sexual situation. Aside from feelings of disgust potentially arising in such a situation, one might also increasingly attend to other inhibitory factors, for instance, the painful friction associated with penile-vaginal penetration with little to no lubrication—as might occur in the event where the glans clitoris is not sufficiently stimulated prior to penetration (see Fig. 12.1, relationship '2'). The latter especially sheds light on the fact that sexual intercourse is not only sub-optimally tailored to reach sexual gratification in women, it may also be a source of pain [26] in the event where the woman is not sexually aroused enough to experience pleasure or orgasm prior to getting involved in penile-vaginal penetration [26]. Accordingly, studies have shown that women with GPPPD—largely defined by pain during

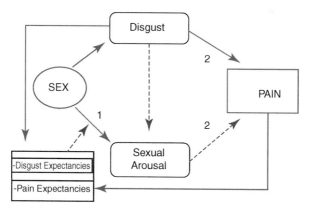

Fig. 12.1 Proposed relationships between sex, sexual arousal, disgust, pain, and pain/disgust expectancies that may help explain the development of sexual pain. (**1**) When one regularly experiences painful sex, pain and/or disgust expectancies may arise, which have inhibitory effects on sexual arousal. (**2**) Sex can elicit both sexual arousal and disgust; the former inhibits pain (see red arrow) while the latter facilitates it (see blue arrow). When sexual arousal is weakened by pain and/or disgust expectancies, there is more room for inhibitory factors (e.g., disgust) to become more salient

intercourse—often respond to erotic stimulation with disgust rather than sexual arousal [26, 42]. Moreover, they show a high prevalence of feeling disengaged and not experiencing erotic thoughts during sexual activity [11]. It thus plausibly follows that weak sexual arousal may be at the root of this (and other related) disorder(s) [25]. In regularly experiencing painful sex, pain expectancies and pain catastrophization may be elicited at the anticipation of future sexual encounters [43]. In turn, this expectancy may facilitate attention toward other inhibitory processes, thereby also undermining the development of sexual arousal (see Fig. 12.1, relationship '1'). This mechanism potentially changes sex stimuli from cues that activate the appetitive motivational system to cues that activate the aversive motivational system instead, thereby compromising the development of sexual arousal and reaching sexual gratification.

On top of this, weak sexual arousal can limit a woman's natural lubrication, altogether heightening the friction during penetration. Evidently, this process worsens pain expectancy, making it more likely that she will inadvertently tighten her pelvic floor muscles as a defense mechanism to penetration, thereby exacerbating the pain and allowing the vicious cycle to repeat itself [2, 7, 44, 45]. This process interferes with sexual activity becoming incentivized, resulting in a possible plummeting in sexual desire and detrimentally influencing the individual and their partner's sexual health and general well-being.

Keeping in mind the key role of sexual arousal in functional and pleasurable sex, a series of studies have investigated the influence of pain and disgust expectancies on sexual arousal. As expected, findings from classical conditioning studies involving acquired pain expectancy with certain sexual stimuli (CS+) and not with other sexual stimuli (CS−) revealed weaker subjective sexual arousal in response to the initially sexually arousing stimuli in both men and women following the acquisition of CS+ elicited pain expectancies. Correspondingly, it was further found that genital blood flow in women, as measured by a vaginal pulse amplitude (VPA) was also attenuated; although the same genital response was not found in men [46]. Interestingly, the findings also showed that pain expectancy can be quite tenacious in women with GPPPD, contrary to sexually asymptomatic women. Indeed, although subjective sexual arousal in women with GPPPD was reduced in response to the CS+, their genital response was differentially attenuated when faced with the safe CS− than with the threatening CS+. In fact, women with dyspareunia even showed strong pain expectancies toward the safe CS−, which had never before been paired with pain [47]. Similar studies have shown robust impacts of acquired disgust expectancies on sexual arousal measured on a VPA [5].

It is important to consider that all factors that undermine the development of high sexual arousal may lower the threshold for experiencing sexual pain, potentially leading to some sex stimuli eventually changing their motivational valence from appetitive and gratifying to aversive and threatening. Keeping in mind the current model of sexual pain and its persistence, we have designed a series of experiments to test the proposed relationships between pain, pain/disgust expectancies, and sexual arousal. We plan to build on the aforementioned model by dedicating our future set of studies to examining whether heightening sexual arousal might reduce (sexual) pain, and whether heightening disgust might increase pain sensitivity. To date, it has been established that sexual activity and orgasm in particular can reduce pain in women [48–50]. What has not yet been found, however, is whether sexual arousal—independent of stimulation or orgasm—can have a similar effect. In the context of sexual pain, it may be more crucial to first identify the potential influence of pre-coital sexual arousal on pain given its capacity to reduce inhibitory factors that contribute to pain during sex. This being said, previous studies aiming to answer this question have not (yet) found any pain modulating effect in women. It is noteworthy, however, that both studies propose that this may have been due to feelings of disgust having been inadvertently induced by the erotic stimuli among female participants [51, 52]. Accordingly, we have designed a replication study assessing the influence of sexual arousal and disgust on pain. This time we will additionally analyze if indeed the failure to find an analgesic effect in the erotic (sexual arousal eliciting) condition can be explained by the concurrent activation of disgust in women by the erotic materials (AsPredicted #87260, [53]). If the results would indeed demonstrate evidence of pain reduction (or pain facilitation in the context of disgust), these could potentially make critical targets for the treatment of GPPPD and related disorders.

Psychological Treatment for Inhibited Sexual Arousal

Naturally, a comprehensive assessment is always advised as a first step to diagnosing sexual problems, perhaps especially so for inhibited sexual arousal given its complexity. Treatment for inhibited or weakened sexual arousal focuses on the individual (and the response to sexual stimuli) as well as the relationship. In this chapter, the treatment section is split into two sections: (i) identifying and managing the inhibitory factors that occur in sex, and (ii) focusing on the lesser explored disgust-based interventions designed to allowing for the enhanced generation of sexual excitement.

Psychosexual-Education Targeting Factors Identified as Contenders to Sexual Arousal with Focus on the Relationship

Based on the two factors outlined above, treatment for inhibited sexual arousal requires a focus on the individual as well as the relationship in which the sexual problems have emerged. At the relationship level, it is important for the individual and their partner to express what they find pleasurable, to show flexibility in accepting and creating new experiences, and to show willingness in changing their 'old' sexual script. Not all individuals may feel able to do this right away, however; thus, it is essential to first foster a safe enough environment for this type of dialogue to take place by normalizing 'sex talk', and, if necessary, by re-framing any negative associations related to such conversation. This can be accomplished by educating the individuals on the empowering effect that such dialogue can have for the relationship. For instance, when a partner shares a potential sexual dislike, rather than responding with self-criticism, it can be quite empowering—even erotic—to respond with curiosity in order to better understand how to turn the partner 'on'. In turn, such an environment can gradually reduce potential fears relevant to disrupting the relationship cohesion by discussing sexual dissatisfaction or identifying a problem. Instead, it could encourage regular dialogue where wishes, fantasies, preferences, likes, and dislikes can be openly and erotically discussed, listened to, and understood [54].

In the event where the problem is a shortcoming in sexual technique in either partner, it could be recommended (in addition to openly communicating) to make use of erotic materials or readings [55], and to explore outside of one's comfort zone in order to allow for the creation of novel experiences. Similarly, in cases where one is not entirely sure of what they might or might not like, open communication and exploratory sensual touching exercises could be beneficial when combined and utilized for the purpose of discovery. Practicing open communication can further be encouraged beyond the sexual context given that interpersonal dynamics outside the bedroom may often have an indirect (negative) influence on intimacy in the bedroom.

Additionally, given that women with sexual problems hold stronger negative beliefs and negative self-schemas about themselves as sexual beings than women who are asymptomatic, CBT aimed at re-directing attention allocation toward the sexual stimuli—is an additional helpful treatment tool. In particular, CBT approaches (e.g., learning about pelvic floor awareness, general body awareness exercises, or guided masturbation) involving both partners appear to be most effective in enhancing knowledge of one's own body and bodily signals linked to sexual arousal, as well as that of their partner—fostering sexual pleasure and arousal.

At the individual level, it is crucial to assess personal thoughts and beliefs about sex. For instance, if the assessment shows that the patient holds certain sex-negative beliefs or myths, psychosexual education, a frequently used tool for such cases, may be necessary. Commonly held sexual myths include the following: (i) sex needs to be spontaneous for it to be pleasurable, (ii) men should always initiate sex and be ready for it, (iii) penile-vaginal intercourse is the ultimate 'goal' for sexual pleasure for both partners, (iv) only penile-vaginal sex is "real sex", and all women should be able to orgasm solely via penile-vaginal intercourse. Psychosexual education aims to restructure such beliefs and other similar unrealistic standards that might be interfering with the experience of sexual pleasure and excitement. In other words, it aims to debunk the myths, deflate their influence, and enhance sexual knowledge.

For instance, contesting the myth that sex ought to happen spontaneously in order to feel exciting, it might actually be helpful (and exciting) for some couples to schedule sex and incorporate it into their 'routine'; this is especially the case for couples who feel that they cannot find the time or energy for sex. Scheduled sex, when prioritized and kept to, can not only strengthen the couple's bond, but also be something exciting to look forward to. Accordingly, we are currently testing the impact of creative scheduled sex in long term couples in an online longitudinal study utilizing sex diaries in order to understand whether sexual creativity increases sexual arousal in couples that have been together long-term, and for which, perhaps the meaning of sex had become more negative (AsPredicted #88433), [56].

Regarding painful sex arising from weak sexual arousal, and perhaps related to the myths described above (myth #iii & #iv), it is often the case that women with GPPPD symptoms continue having sexual intercourse despite the pain it elicits [26, 44]. Whatever their rationalization for this may be (e.g., that their feelings of love and closeness outweigh those of pain; wanting to be 'normal'; simultaneously feeling arousal and pain; wanting to satisfy their partner) [26, 44], it may be wiser to temporarily stop and communicate about what might be more pleasurable before picking up with intercourse again, such that a sex-pain association can be intercepted and replaced with a sex-pleasure association, in turn reducing pain expectancy (and increasing arousal) in anticipation of sex. Indeed, continuing intercourse whilst ignoring pain may gradually hinder arousal and vaginal lubrication [44], as expected when the dual processes compete. In turn, this may cause the woman to feel tense, in turn exacerbating the pain. Again, it would be crucial here to communicate about pain and adaptive coping strategies. In fact, male partners who encourage coping strategies as well as sexual activity are associated with reduced pain and increased partner satisfaction. Conversely, men who get upset when painful sex occurs with their partner, or, on the flip side, men who are prone to avoiding sex due to being overly concerned with their partner, are both associated with increased pain [57, 58].

Disgust-Based Interventions for Enhancing Sexual Arousal

In cases where the inhibited sexual problems are related to feelings of disgust, 'traditional' sex therapy that does not address disgust might not be effective [25]. The acquired disgust expectancies when anticipating sex will understandably motivate sexual avoidance and withdrawal (i.e., safety behaviour), which may in turn be further emphasized by negative thoughts and beliefs about sex. Such situations often either result in complete avoidance of sex stimuli, or withdrawing some attention from sex stimuli such that one is only partially present, or 'in the moment', during sex. Although these safety behaviours might momentarily decrease levels of disgust, they also preclude exposure to prolonged physical contact, a necessary and effective requirement in countering disgust [17, 18].

Consistently, it is found that disgust is a perseverant emotion, one difficult to unlearn [41]—thereby earning itself the description of being a 'sticky emotion'. Attesting to this, in fact, is our recent study in which erotic stimuli were first paired with disgust stimuli, and later either paired with a positive stimulus instead (i.e., counter-conditioning) or shown without the disgust stimulus (i.e., extinction). The results have clearly shown that following the extinction and counterconditioning procedures, although sexual arousal was successfully restored, feelings of disgust and behavioural avoidance remained [5]. Similarly, emotion regulation strategies, designed to boost sexual arousal and reduce disgust are also not very helpful in the latter case; while sexual arousal can successfully be up-regulated, disgust is persistent [59]. The findings provide further evidence of disgust being a very resistant emotion. They further indicate that when the issue is disgust-related, targeting the enhancement of sexual arousal is not enough to reduce disgust [60].

This being said, disgust can be gradually reduced via repeated exposure involving direct and prolonged physical contact with the disgust stimulus, allowing for habituation and the eventual "unlearning" of disgust [41, 60, 61]. Habituation is key in establishing a lasting reduction in the disgust response. It is thus highly recommended to encourage the patient to routinely come into direct contact with her/his aversive and avoided stimuli (e.g., the ejaculate or vaginal fluid) until the automatic disgust response and urge to avoid—is significantly reduced [17]. Alongside habituation, it may also be helpful to include conceptual reorientation strategies [62]. This refers to a cognitive reframing technique in which the conceptualization and understanding of a (disgust) stimulus can eventually elicit a different response. When the core conceptualization of a disgust stimulus is, for instance, reoriented into perceiving it as something pleasurable, healthy, and functional (for more detailed examples, see [45], this can greatly influence one's response to it. For instance, rather than conceptualizing genital fluids as 'slimy', cognitive associations can be reoriented toward perceiving them helpful in reducing friction during intercourse, and in enhancing pleasure for both partners. In this sense, reframing techniques, inherent to CBT, are helpful not only in reducing avoidance and aversive responses; they may also promote pleasurable/rewarding or functional interpretations of these stimuli.

Conclusion

In this chapter we discussed sexual arousal in women, its role in attenuating the inhibitory aspects of some sexual stimuli, as well as factors that weaken sexual arousal. The bidirectional relationship of sexual arousal and disgust/pain was discussed, along with the role of disgust and pain expectancies in fuelling a cycle of sexual dysfunction. The chapter further aims at outlining the non-pharmacological treatment interventions for inhibited sexual arousal, with a special focus on reducing disgust responses to sex stimuli—an aspect of research that had gained only little attention in the last years.

It must be noted that while, in the last years, literature in this field of research has been increasing, at present, there is no single evidence-based intervention for dealing with accentuating sexual arousal. Rather we have various promising interventions that require additional research to solidify their efficacy. Finally, although there are increasingly recognized biomedically-oriented approaches targeting weakened sexual arousal, we would like to emphasize the importance of behavioural and psychological interventions in order to not only target symptoms, but also target the root of the symptoms and the factors that maintain them, thereby preventing the metaphorical root from growing again, and ultimately ensuring a longer-lasting result.

References

1. Everaerd W, Laan E, Both S. Sexual appetite, desire and motivation: energetics of the sexual system. Amsterdam: Royal Netherlands Academy of Arts and Sciences; 2001.

2. Borg C, de Jong PJ. Psychological approaches for low sexual arousal. In: McKay D, Abramowitz JS, Storch EA, editors. Treatments for psychological problems and syndromes. Hoboken, NJ: Wiley; 2017. p. 263–80.
3. Toates F. An integrative theoretical framework for understanding sexual motivation, arousal, and behavior. J Sex Res. 2009;46:168–93.
4. Borg C, Oosterwijk TA, Lisy D, Boesveldt S, de Jong PJ. The influence of olfactory disgust on (Genital) sexual arousal in men. PLoS One. 2019;14:e0213059.
5. Pawłowska A, Borg C, de Jong PJ, Both S. The effect of differential disgust conditioning and subsequent extinction versus counterconditioning procedures on women's sexual responses to erotic stimuli. Behav Res Ther. 2020;134:103714.
6. Williams JBW, First M. Diagnostic and statistical manual of mental disorders. Encyclopedia of social work. 2013. https://doi.org/10.1093/acrefore/9780199975839.013.104.
7. de Jong PJ, van Lankveld J, Elgersma HJ. Sexual problems. In: McKay D, Abramowitz JS, Taylor S, editors. Cognitive-behavioral therapy for refractory cases: turning failure into success. Washington, DC: American Psychological Association; 2010. p. 255–75.
8. Singer B, Toates FM. Sexual motivation. J Sex Res. 1987;23:481–501.
9. Borg C, de Jong PJ. Feelings of disgust and disgust-induced avoidance weaken following induced sexual arousal in women. PLoS One. 2012;7:e44111.
10. Borg C. Sex, disgust, and penetration disorders. Doctorate dissertation, Uitgeverij BOXpress, 's-Hertogenboscg. 2013.
11. Nobre PJ, Pinto-Gouveia J. Cognitive and emotional predictors of female sexual dysfunctions: preliminary findings. J Sex Marital Ther. 2008;34:325–42.
12. Borg C, de Jong PJ, Weijmar Schultz W. Vaginismus and dyspareunia: relationship with general and sex related moral standards. J Sex Med. 2011;8:223–31.
13. Carvalho J, Veríssimo A, Nobre PJ. Cognitive and emotional determinants characterizing women with persistent genital arousal disorder. J Sex Med. 2013;10:1549–58.
14. Hamilton LD, Meston CM. Chronic stress and sexual function in women. J Sex Med. 2013;10:2443–54.
15. Janssen E, Everaerd W, Spiering M, Janssen J. Automatic processes and the appraisal of sexual stimuli: toward an information processing model of sexual arousal. J Sex Res. 2000;37:8–23.
16. Barlow DH. Causes of sexual dysfunction: the role of anxiety and cognitive interference. J Consult Clin Psychol. 1986;54:140–8.
17. Borg C, Both S, ter Kuile MM, de Jong PJ. Sexual aversion. In: Hall KSK, Binik YM, editors. Principles and practice of sex therapy. New York: Guilford; 2020. p. 224–38.
18. Borg C, de Jong PJ. The realm of disgust in sexual behaviour. In: Powell PA, Consedine NS, editors. The handbook of disgust research. Cham: Springer; 2021. p. 159–72.
19. Dewitte M. On the interpersonal dynamics of sexuality. J Sex Marital Ther. 2014;40:209–32.
20. Graham CA, Sanders SA, Milhausen RR, McBride KR. Turning on and turning off: a focus group study of the factors that affect women's sexual arousal. Arch Sex Behav. 2004;33:527–38.
21. de Jong PJ, Borg C. Self-directed disgust: reciprocal relationships with sex and sexual dysfunction. In: Powell PA, Overton PG, Simpson J, editors. The revolting self: perspectives on the psychological and clinical implications of self-directed disgust. London: Karnac; 2018. p. 89–112.
22. Brouwer B, Borg C, de Jong PJ. Self-directed pathogen, sexual, and moral disgust in response to sex-related scenarios. 2022. (In preparation).
23. Klusmann D. Sexual motivation and the duration of partnership. Arch Sex Behav. 2002;31:275–87.
24. Kantor LM, Lindberg L. Pleasure and sex education: The need for broadening both content and measurement. Am J Public Health. 2020;110:145–8.
25. de Jong PJ, Peters ML. Sex and the sexual dysfunctions: the role of disgust and contamination sensitivity. In: Olatunji BO, McKay D, editors. Disgust and its disorders: theory, assessment, and treatment implications. Washington, DC: American Psychological Association; 2009. p. 253–70.

26. Laan ETM, Klein V, Werner MA, van Lunsen RHW, Janssen E. In pursuit of pleasure: a bio-psychosocial perspective on sexual pleasure and gender. Int J Sex Health. 2021;33:516–36.
27. Lloyd EA. The case of the female orgasm: bias in the science of evolution. Cambridge, MA: Harvard University Press; 2005.
28. Kalmbach DA, Kingsberg SA, Ciesla JA. How changes in depression and anxiety symptoms correspond to variations in female sexual response in a nonclinical sample of young women: a daily diary study. J Sex Med. 2014;11:2915–27.
29. Bartlik B, Kaplan P, Kaminetsky J, Roentsch G, Goldberg J. Medications with the potential to enhance sexual responsivity in women. Psychiatr Ann. 1999;29:46–52.
30. Borg C, Georgiadis JR, Renken RJ, Spoelstra SK, Weijmar Schultz W, de Jong PJ. Brain processing of visual stimuli representing sexual penetration versus core and animal-reminder disgust in women with lifelong vaginismus. PLoS One. 2014;9:e84882.
31. Curtis V, de Barra M, Aunger R. Disgust as an adaptive system for disease avoidance behaviour. Philos Trans R Soc Lond Ser B Biol Sci. 2011;366:389–401.
32. Oaten M, Stevenson RJ, Case TI. Disgust as a disease-avoidance mechanism. Psychol Bull. 2009;135:303–21.
33. Fessler DMT, Eng SJ, David Navarrete C. Elevated disgust sensitivity in the first trimester of pregnancy. Evol Hum Behav. 2005;26:344–51.
34. Kort R, Caspers M, van de Graaf A, van Egmond W, Keijser B, Roeselers G. Shaping the oral microbiota through intimate kissing. Microbiome. 2014;2:41.
35. Stevenson RJ, Case TI, Oaten MJ. Proactive strategies to avoid infectious disease. Philos Trans R Soc Lond Ser B Biol Sci. 2011;366:3361–3.
36. Borg C, Hinzmann J, Heitmann J, de Jong PJ. Disgust toward sex-relevant and sex-irrelevant stimuli in pre-, early, and middle adolescence. J Sex Res. 2019;56:102–13.
37. Oosterwijk TA, Borg C, van Dijk MWG. Age-related differences in self-reported disgust toward core disgust, sex-related, and food stimuli. J Adolesc. 2022;94(3):293–304.
38. Borg C, Pawłowska A, van Stokkum R, Georgiadis JR, de Jong PJ. The influence of sexual arousal on self-reported sexual willingness and automatic approach to models of low, medium, and high prior attractiveness. J Sex Res. 2020;57:872–84.
39. Perelman MA. Why the sexual tipping point is a "variable switch model". Curr Sex Health Rep. 2018;10:38–43. https://doi.org/10.1007/s11930-018-0148-3.
40. Ariely D, Loewenstein G. The heat of the moment: the effect of sexual arousal on sexual decision making. J Behav Decis Mak. 2006;19:87–98.
41. Bosman RC, Borg C, de Jong PJ. Optimising extinction of conditioned disgust. PLoS One. 2016;11:e0148626.
42. Borg C, de Jong PJ, Weijmar Schultz W. Vaginismus and dyspareunia: automatic vs. deliberate disgust responsivity. J Sex Med. 2010;7:2149–57.
43. Borg C, Peters ML, Weijmar Schultz W, de Jong PJ. Vaginismus: heightened harm avoidance and pain catastrophizing cognitions. J Sex Med. 2012;9:558–67.
44. Brauer M, Lakeman M, van Lunsen R, Laan E. Predictors of task-persistent and fear-avoiding behaviors in women with sexual pain disorders. J Sex Med. 2014;11:3051–63.
45. de Jong PJ, van Lankveld J, Elgersma HJ, Borg C. Disgust and sexual problems–theoretical conceptualization and case illustrations. Int J Cogn Ther. 2010;3:23–39.
46. Brom M, Laan E, Everaerd W, Spinhoven P, Both S. Extinction of aversive classically conditioned human sexual response. J Sex Med. 2015;12:916–35.
47. Both S, Brauer M, Weijenborg P, Laan E. Effects of aversive classical conditioning on sexual response in women with dyspareunia and sexually functional controls. J Sex Med. 2017;14:687–701.
48. Whipple B, Komisaruk BR. Elevation of pain threshold by vaginal stimulation in women. Pain. 1985;21:357–67.
49. Whipple B, Ogden G, Komisaruk BR. Physiological correlates of imagery-induced orgasm in women. Arch Sex Behav. 1992;21:121–33.
50. Komisaruk BR, Whipple B. Vaginal stimulation-produced analgesia in rats and women. Ann N Y Acad Sci. 1986;467:30–9.

51. Meagher MW, Arnau RC, Rhudy JL. Pain and emotion: effects of affective picture modulation. Psychosom Med. 2001;63:79–90.
52. Lakhsassi L, Borg C, Martusewicz S, Ploeg K, de Jong PJ. The influence of sexual arousal on subjective pain intensity during a cold pressor test in women. 2022. (In preparation) AsPredicted #36655.
53. Lakhsassi L, Borg C, de Jong PJ. The influence of sexual arousal and disgust on pain tolerance and subjective pain. 2022. (In preparation) AsPredicted #87260.
54. Brandenburg U, Bitzer J. The challenge of talking about sex: the importance of patient-physician interaction. Maturitas. 2009;63:124–7.
55. Leiblum S, Döring N. Internet sexuality: known risks and fresh chances for women. In: Cooper A, editor. Sex and the Internet: a guide for clinicians. New York: Routledge; 2002. p. 19–45.
56. Zorn T, Feilhauer L, Juhola E, Cox R, de Jong PJ, Borg C. Does sexual creativity enhance sexual and relationship satisfaction? Examining the effect of weekly creative sexual tasks in monogamous long-term couples. 2022. (In preparation) AsPredicted #88433.
57. Pukall CF, Goldstein AT, Bergeron S, Foster D, Stein A, Kellogg-Spadt S, Bachmann G. Vulvodynia: definition, prevalence, impact, and pathophysiological factors. J Sex Med. 2016;13:291–304.
58. Rosen NO, Bergeron S, Sadikaj G, Glowacka M, Delisle I, Baxter M-L. Impact of male partner responses on sexual function in women with vulvodynia and their partners: a dyadic daily experience study. Health Psychol. 2014;33:823–31.
59. van Overveld M, Borg C. Brief emotion regulation training facilitates arousal control during sexual stimuli. J Sex Res. 2015;52:996–1005.
60. Pawłowska A, Borg C, de Jong PJ. Up-regulating sexual arousal and down-regulating disgust while watching pornography: Effects on sexual arousal and disgust. J Sex Res. 2021;58:353–63.
61. Borg C, Bosman RC, Engelhard I, Olatunji BO, de Jong PJ. Is disgust sensitive to classical conditioning as indexed by facial electromyography and behavioural responses? Cogn Emot. 2016;30:669–86.
62. Rozin P, Fallon AE. A perspective on disgust. Psychol Rev. 1987;94:23–41.

Female Genito-Pelvic Pain and Penetration Disorders

Süleyman Eserdağ

Abstract

Vaginismus and dyspareunia were classified in DSM-V as female sexual dysfunctions in "Genito-Pelvic Pain and Penetration Disorders (GPPPD)," which describes persistent or recurrent difficulty/pain on sexual intercourse or penetration attempts. It is not easy to differentiate vaginismus, dyspareunia, and provoked vestibulodynia (PVD) because of their overlapping symptoms.

Gynecological examination and detailed anamnesis are important in diagnosing, grading, and designing treatment modalities. GPPPD treatments need a multidisciplinary team's multimodal approach, including gynecologist, psychiatrist, urologist, family consultant, sex therapist, psychologist, and physiotherapist.

This chapter shares my 20 years of knowledge and experience on vaginismus and dyspareunia treatments in light of literature.

It has not been easy for clinicians to clearly distinguish between vaginismus and dyspareunia problems, overlapping in terms of symptoms for years. Both genito-pelvic pain and penetration disorder (GPPPD) conditions contain many organic, psychological, cultural, and interpersonal interactions. Therefore, a holistic approach following the bio-psycho-social model is important in treatments.

GPPPD is a sexual problem that needs to be treated early. Otherwise, pain and anticipation of pain reflexively inhibit sexual arousal, thus decreasing vaginal lubrication, vulvar congestion, pelvic muscle relaxation, sexual pleasure, and satisfaction.

S. Eserdağ (✉)
Hera Clinic, Istanbul, Turkey

Obstetrics and Gynecology Department, Altınbaş University, Istanbul, Turkey
e-mail: suleyman@eserdag.com

© The Author(s), under exclusive license to Springer Nature
Switzerland AG 2022
S. Sarikaya et al. (eds.), *Andrology and Sexual Medicine*, Management of Urology,
https://doi.org/10.1007/978-3-031-12049-7_13

These circumstances make vestibular and vaginal mucosa more susceptible to micro-abrasions, resulting in additional genital pain and inflammation upon penetration attempts. Additionally, the emergence of low self-efficacy, avoidance, anxiety, and depression may intensify the experience of pain and perpetuate sexual dysfunction.

Vaginismus

Vaginismus is a common sexual dysfunction that strongly impairs the ability to experience sexual intercourse, detrimental to sexual and general health [1]. It negatively affects the quality of intimate relationships and reproductive capacity, leading to the nonconsummation of marriage. Furthermore, in cross-sectional research, vaginismus women have been reported to exhibit a high prevalence of psychopathological correlates, including depression, anxiety, low self-esteem [2], insecure attachment styles [3], histrionic/hysterical traits [4], and alexithymia [5].

Definitions

According to the Diagnostic and Statistical Manual of Mental Disorders, the fourth edition of the American Psychiatric Association text revision (DSM-IV-TR), vaginismus is separately included in the female sexual dysfunction category [6]. However, in the DSM-V classification in 2013, vaginismus and dyspareunia were classified as female sexual dysfunctions and included in the category of "Genito-Pelvic Pain and Penetration Disorders" (GPPPD), which describes persistent or recurrent difficulty/pain on sexual intercourse or penetration attempts [7].

According to the DSM-V, it has been described in the following criteria as [7]:

- Vaginal penetration during intercourse
- Marked vulvovaginal or pelvic pain during vaginal intercourse or penetration attempts
- Marked fear or anxiety about vulvovaginal or pelvic pain in anticipation of, during, or as a result of vaginal penetration
- Marked tensing or tightening of the pelvic floor muscles during attempted vaginal penetration

Vaginismus is defined as the inability to achieve vaginal penetration or experiencing extreme pain in the course of penetration due to the continuous spasmodic contraction of pelvic muscles in the outer 1/3 of the vagina during sexual intercourse [6]. It is one of the more common female psychosexual problems.

In vaginismus patients, the pelvic muscles, which normally operate entirely under the woman's control, strongly and involuntary contract during sexual intercourse just before the penile penetration, so causes the coitus to be impossible or painful [6, 8]. It can cause distress, relationship problems, fertility problems, and secondary sexual dysfunctions in partners.

According to Helen Singer Kaplan, vaginismus is an anxiety disorder; therefore, it is also referred to as "sexual phobia" or "fear of sexual intercourse" [9].

The International Classification of Diseases (ICD)-11 categorizes vaginismus either as a "sexual pain-penetration disorder" as HA20.

According to the ICD-11 sexual pain-penetration disorder is characterized by at least one of the following:

1. marked and persistent or recurrent difficulties with penetration, including due to involuntary tightening or tautness of the pelvic floor muscles during attempted penetration;
2. marked and persistent or recurrent vulvovaginal or pelvic pain during penetration;
3. marked and persistent or recurrent fear or anxiety about vulvovaginal or pelvic pain in anticipation of, during, or due to penetration.

The symptoms are recurrent during sexual interactions involving or potentially involving penetration, despite adequate sexual desire and stimulation, are not entirely attributable to a medical condition that adversely affects the pelvic area and results in genital and/or penetrative pain or to a mental disorder, are not entirely attributable to insufficient vaginal lubrication or post-menopausal/age-related changes, and are associated with clinically significant distress.

A recent consensus definition reflects these conclusions and defines vaginismus as: "Persistent or recurrent difficulties of the woman to allow vaginal entry of a penis, finger and/or any object, despite her expressed wish to do so". There is variable (phobic) avoidance, involuntary pelvic muscle contraction, and anticipation/fear/experience of pain. Structural or other physical abnormalities must be ruled out or addressed [8].

Historical Background

In 1547, Trotula of Salerno was thought to have provided the earliest description about vaginismus in her treatise on "*The Diseases of Women*", and described this phenomenon as "a tightening of the vulva so that even a woman who has been seduced may appear a virgin" [10].

In 1834, Huguier first described the syndrome. In 1859, Gynecologist Sims wrote: "*from personal experience, I can confidently assert that I know of no disease capable of producing so much unhappiness to both parties of the marriage contract, and I am happy to state that I know of no serious trouble that can be cured so easily, so safely and so certainly*" [11]. The use of graduated dilators, first described by Sims, in his 1861 publication, is likely the most commonly used treatment plan. Then the term was first coined in 1862 by him as well, and vaginismus has been conceptualized as a relatively infrequent but well understood and easily treatable female sexual dysfunction. While addressing the Obstetrical Society of London, Sims described vaginismus as "an involuntary spasmodic closure of the mouth of the vagina, attended with such excessive supersensitiveness as to form a complete barrier to coition" [12]. In 1970, Masters and Johnson provided a vivid clinical description of a typical vaginismic woman's behavior during a pelvic examination. Lamont, in 1978 classified vaginismus according to the patient's history and behavior during a gynecologic examination. To date, the involuntary muscle spasm remains the core element of the definition of vaginismus.

Prevalence

Although epidemiological data on vaginismus and dyspareunia patients are insufficient, clinical prevalence rates are between 5% and 17% [13]. Community estimates range from 0.5–1% [14]. Prevalence rates of 30% have been reported in primary care settings, increasing up to 42% in specialized clinics for female sexual disorders [15, 16]. While Master and Johnson stated that this problem is quite rare [17], some researchers underlined that it is a widespread sexual health problem [18].

Etiology

Etiological factors are primarily psychogenic. Negative sexual attitudes, lack of sexual education, psychological and/or physical traumas, and relationship difficulties have been reported in the literature [19, 20].

Tugrul and Kabakçi's reported that 85% of vaginismic women who applied for the treatment of vaginismus and 90% of their husbands evaluated their marriages as satisfactory [21]. Hawton and Catalan (n = 30) found that couples suffering from vaginismus have a significantly better relationship and communication when compared to other types of female sexual dysfunctions [22]. However, it remains unclear whether these are causes or consequences of vaginismus. It has frequently been reported to result from a bad couple relationship [23, 24].

In a recent study, the vaginismus patients described their spouses as extremely understanding-patient (74.7%), nervous-angry (10.6%), oppressive-conservative (2.5%), and prone to violence (1.9%) [25].

In clinical reports, partners of women with vaginismus have suffered from sexual dysfunction and had passive and unassertive personalities [26].

Vaginismus is also an anxiety disorder. Male partners feel like *"hitting a wall"* during the attempted intercourses, which is suggestive of spasm at the level of the introitus. At the same time, vaginismic women face a sort of "panic attack" reaction (crying, shaking, trembling, sweating, hyperventilating, having palpitations, nausea, vomiting, being faint) because of the sympathetic overactivity. Therefore, it is also called sexual phobia by some sexologists [9]. Most sexual phobias have been formed during childhood and puberty by environmental factors. The most frequent fears and "sexual myths" are related to the thoughts and misbeliefs that the woman will have too much pain during sexual intercourse, the vagina is narrow, there is a wall inside the vagina, the vagina is closed, the first night will be so difficult, painful, and bloody, the penis will penetrate the wrong place such as the bladder and anus, or the penis may be trapped inside the vagina. Some patients have such high anxiety that they fear dying during sexual intercourse. There is no initial problem of sexual reluctance in vaginismus, although this may develop over time, primarily due to the fear of pain and soreness. The sexual desire usually improves spontaneously when vaginismus is treated [27].

Finally, it should always be kept in mind that the spouses of vaginismic women can have primary or secondary sexual dysfunctions like premature ejaculation, erectile dysfunction, lack of sexual desire, etc., and should be evaluated during the vaginismus treatments [25].

Although the experience of sexual and/or physical abuse is generally considered a critical etiological factor in vaginismus, the empirical evidence is less conclusive. More extensive studies with matched control groups and well-validated definitions of abuse are required to resolve this issue [8].

The etiology of GPPPD has a multifactorial and complex interaction involving biological, psychological, and relational factors. What may initially be an adaptive nociceptive response resulting from peripheral tissue damage may gradually shift to neuropathic and/or inflammatory pain in the absence of acute injury. This maladaptive pain is harmful to sexual functioning, especially with increasing central nervous system involvement in pain sensitization. Thus, GPPPD should be evaluated from a biopsychosocial perspective and should never be viewed as a purely psychogenic problem.

Dyspareunia

Dyspareunia is defined as recurrent genital pain associated with sexual intercourse/penetration. Since we do not know precisely whether penetration pain is a cause or a result during sexual intercourse, it is often either considered together with vaginismus or cannot be differentiated. For this reason, many researchers felt diagnostic accuracy would be improved by combining both disorders into one unified category.

Dyspareunia is separately defined as a symptom of the genital system affecting females, caused by physical determinants in ICD-11 in the category as GA22 in "Noninflammatory disorders of female genital tract" parent. This symptom is characterized by recurrent genital pain or discomfort before, during, or after sexual intercourse or superficial or deep vaginal penetration related to an identifiable physical cause, not including lack of lubrication. Confirmation is by medical assessment of physical causes.

Etiology

Dyspareunia can be located in superficial (=introital, at the vaginal entrance), deep (in the pelvis), or sometimes both. Different conditions associated with/causative of superficial and deep dyspareunia are summarized in Table 13.1.

Table 13.1 Etiology of superficial and deep dyspareunia

Superficial pain
Inflammatory/dermatologic
• PVD (Provoked Vestibulodynia)
• Lichen sclerosus and lichen planus
• Hypertrophic vulvar dystrophies
• Granuloma fissuratum
• Chemical irritants (soaps, douches, etc.) and vulvar dermatitis
• Skin allergies (condom, semen, pads)
Superficial infectious
• Recurrent vulvovaginal candidiasis
• Sexually transmitted infections (herpes, trichomoniasis)
Neoplastic
• Paget disease
• Vulvar and vaginal intraepithelial neoplasms and premalignant lesions
• Pelvic neoplasms (cervical, uterine, ovarian, colon)
Neurologic
• Postherpetic neuralgia
• Nerve compression or injury (Pudendal nerve or genitofemoral nerve entrapment)
• Neuroma
Traumatic
• Female genital mutilation
• Obstetric lacerations and episiotomy scars
Structural
• Congenital abnormalities of the hymen (imperforate hymen, septate hymen)
• Müllerian agenesis
Iatrogenic
• Genital operations (Bartholin cyst excision, vaginoplasty, labiaplasty, vaginal hysterectomy)
• Cancer treatments: Chemotherapy and radiation
Hormonal
• Genitourinary syndrome (GUS) of Menopause
• Lactational amenorrhea
• Anorexia nervosa
• Hyperprolactinemia
• Oophorectomy
Psychogenic
• Vaginismus
• Female Sexual Interest/Arousal Disorder (FSIAD)
• Other psychopathologies (Somatization, depression, OCB)
Deep pain
• Endometriosis
• Leiomyoma
• Ovarian mass
• Pelvic adhesions

Table 13.1 (continued)

• Pelvic congestion syndrome
• Pelvic malignancies
• Chronic pelvic pain
• Skeletal and muscular diseases
• Gastrointestinal diseases (IBS, Inflammatory bowel diseases)
• POP (Pelvic organ prolapses)
• Uterine retroversion
Deep infectious
• PID (Pelvic inflammatory disease)
• UTI

PVD (Provoked Vestibulodynia) is the most frequent causative of dyspareunia in reproductive age, with a prevalence of 7% in the general population [28]. Friedrich firstly defined this condition in 1987, and these patients typically experience a very severe, sharp, burning pain upon vestibular touch or attempted vaginal entry [29]. However, underdiagnosed or ignored in most cases, it is diagnosed through the cotton-swab test, which consists of applying a cotton swab to various areas of the vulvar vestibule.

On the other hand, "vulvodynia" describes idiopathic chronic genital pain localized to the pudendal area with or without sexual contact. It cannot be classified as a female sexual dysfunction but can cause or contribute to female sexual dysfunction.

Pain Mechanism

Prolonged tissue damage triggered by a trauma, infection, or a chronicle irritant can lead to mast cell hyperactivation, resulting in over-production of inflammatory molecules and "neurotrophins". These neurotrophins can induce inflammation as well as the proliferation of peripheral nociceptors. With the involvement of nerve endings, sensitivity increases over time, and "hypersensitivity" develops. On the other hand, pain sensitivity after each stimulus also increases the person's expectation of psychogenic pain, called "allodynia". Thus, although hypersensitivity is prominent in patients with dyspareunia, allodynia is also added to the symptoms. The pelvic floor muscle tone also increases over time, and the situation enters a vicious circle [30]. With the "muscle memory" that occurs after each coit attempt, pain triggers contraction, and contraction triggers pain. Tissue biopsies from the posterior vestibulum have shown the presence of more free nerve endings in patients with vestibulodynia than in healthy individuals [31].

In a recent study, it has been concluded that the women with vaginismus had a lower threshold of pain, and the pain threshold decreased in higher grades of vaginismus [32].

Genetic predisposition also plays a vital role in exacerbating the autoimmune response and the formation of inflammation. For example, chronic diseases such as fibromyalgia, interstitial cystitis, and irritable bowel syndrome are more common in women with vulvodynia [33].

Long-term use of birth control pills may increase the risk of provoked vestibulodynia by lowering circulating estrogen and testosterone levels, making structural changes in the vulva, increasing chronic inflammation, or impairing vestibular mucosa histology [33]. In one study, these patients were shown to have a more sensitive mucosa to candida fungus [34].

In some vaginismic patients, the severe pain experienced after the sudden contraction caused by the lack of adequate wetting during the first intercourse, the general anxiety of the woman, ignorance, and the inexperience of the spouse, settles in the subconscious, and this fear proliferates over time and can turn into complete anxiety. In this condition known as "negative conditioning", many patients are so afraid that they have never had intercourse with their partners or do not dare to experience intercourse again once they had.

Management

A detailed anamnesis and gynecological examination play an important role in diagnosing GPPPD and determining the appropriate treatment method. *"One size does not fit all",* and treatments should be individualized according to the cause of vaginismus or dyspareunia, the grade of the problem, and the underlying psychological and/or organic factors. The aims of sexual treatments are pain relief, relaxation, and restoring sexual function with satisfaction.

The detailed anamnesis involves specific questions to clarify the patient's demographic, medical, psychological, and sexual background. Cultural context, past relationships, sexual education, and personal anatomy and physiology knowledge should be questioned. After this detailed anamnesis, the management continues with the gynecologic assessment in the dorsal lithotomy position. Prior to the gynecological evaluation, the patients should be informed of what would be done during the examination and be assured that they would not feel pain. It is important to give them time to prepare themselves psychologically and let them relax with the breathing exercises.

Eserdağ et al. first emphasized the importance of gynecological assessment for managing vaginismus patients and detailed its steps [35]. The gynecological examination starts with inspecting vulvar pathologies followed by the vulvar vestibule, hymen (septate hymen, cribriform hymen, etc.), the vaginal canal (septums), and contractions in introitus if possible, by gentle traction of labia majora. In addition, Bartholin cysts and abscesses, condylomas, herpes simplex lesions, vulvovaginitis, and pathologies such as lichen sclerosis may be diagnosed with the assessment. Different vulvar pathologies that cause GPPPD have been demonstrated in the Fig. 13.1a, b.

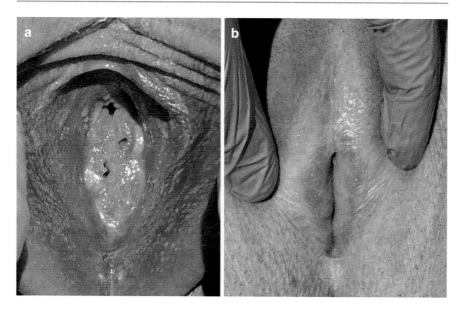

Fig. 13.1 Vulvar Pathologies. (**a**) Cribriform hymen (Left), (**b**) Lichen sclerosus (Right)

Grading

The degree of vaginismus is also important for management. Frequently, vaginismus patients are classified into the four degrees of severity as firstly defined by Lamont in 1978. According to the Lamont classification, the first-degree is perineal, and levator spasm relieved with reassurance, second-degree is perineal spasm maintained throughout the pelvic examination, third-degree is levator spasm, and elevation of buttocks, and fourth-degree is levator and perineal spasm, buttocks elevation, adduction, and retreat [36]. In 2011, Pacik redefined severe grade 5 vaginismus, including visceral response reaction to routine gynecologic examinations and spasm of the bulbocavernosus. These visceral responses manifest as crying, shaking, trembling, sweating, hyperventilating, experiencing palpitations or nausea, vomiting, going unconscious, wanting to jump off the table, or wanting to attack the doctor [37].

Our classification, the "Eserdag classification" system that we have been applying for more than 20 years is based on a gentle digital gynecologic evaluation after the genital inspection (Table 13.2). It is quite easy and objective to differentiate the four classes, which will guide the therapy.

Cognitive and Behavioral Therapies (CBT)

Vaginismus has been traditionally conceptualized as an easily treatable condition, mainly based on expert opinion. Cognitive and Behavioral Therapies (CBT) are the gold standard of the treatments. Cognitive therapies included giving information about genital anatomy, physiology, sexuality, first sexual experience and replacing

Table 13.2 The classification system of vaginismus based on a gynecological examination "Eserdag Classification" [38]

First-degree	Patient tolerates the examiner's index finger insertion into the vaginal canal, and involuntary vaginospasm is felt by the examiner
Second-degree	Patient tolerates insertion of the examiner's little finger to vaginal entry with difficulty and some anxiety
Third-degree	Patient demonstrates fear, cannot tolerate the examiner's finger in her vagina, and only allows the examiner to touch her vestibulum and vulva
Fourth-degree	Patient demonstrates tremendous fear, anxiety, and embarrassment, sometimes cries and elevates her buttocks, constricts her thighs, withdraws herself, contracts all her muscles (sometimes even her chin and toes), and does not allow the examiner even to touch her vulva or allows it with difficulty

unrealistic sexual myths in mind with factual knowledge. Behavioral therapies consist of pelvic exercises such as Kegel exercises, genital mirror exercises, breathing exercises, progressive relaxation, sensate focus exercises, and finally dilator and finger exercises.

Sensate focus is a series of structured touching activities to overcome anxiety and increase comfort with physical intimacy between the couples. They focus on touching rather than exerting performance. Intercourse is initially banned, and couples gradually use homework exercises to move through stages of intimacy to penetration.

Progressive relaxation consists of alternately tensing and relaxing groups of muscles in a prescribed sequence in the body. This is taught to women before self-fingering or insertion of vaginal trainers. Then, gradually increasing size, vaginal trainers (dilators) are inserted into the vagina for systematic desensitization. General management methods of the GPPPD have been summarized in the Table 13.3.

Pelvic Floor Physiotherapy

The aim of pelvic floor physiotherapy is that it will aid in developing awareness and control of the vaginal musculature as well as restore function, improve mobility, relieve pain and overcome vaginal penetration anxiety. Physical therapists use various techniques to achieve these goals, such as breathing and relaxation, local tissue desensitization, electromyographic biofeedback (EMG), electrical stimulation, manual tissue manipulation, stretching/strengthening exercises, and vaginal dilators.

Electromyography is performed by an electromyograph, which detects the electrical potential generated by muscle cells when active and at rest to evaluate and record the activation signals of muscles.

On the other hand, in the Biofeedback technique, the woman uses electromyography, which measures muscle activation with surface electrodes on a small vaginal probe, to help her identify when she is activating the pelvic floor muscles. Physiotherapists mainly apply this technique together with pelvic floor exercises.

Psychological Managements

A variety of psychological treatment methods for vaginismus have been investigated, including marital, interactional, existential–experiential, relationship enhancement, group therapy, and hypnosis. The psychological treatments are often

Table 13.3 Management of the GPPPD

Cognition
• Verbal suggestions and encouragement
• Sexual awareness exercises
• Information about genital anatomy and physiology
• Motivational and positive thinking methods
• Information about coitus, reproduction, and contraception
Exercises
• Mirror exercises
• Breathing techniques
• Sensate focus and genital massage
• Pelvic floor muscle and Kegel exercises
• Progressive relaxation
• Progressive finger and vaginal trainer exercises
Main treatment methods
• Pelvic floor physiotherapy
• Psychological managements
• Surgical interventions
• Pharmacological agents
• Botulinum toxin injections

based on the notion that vaginismus results from marital problems, negative sexual experiences in childhood, or a lack of sexual education [39, 40].

Hypnotherapy, which can be applied in GPPPD, has benefits of muscular relaxation, reducing pain, increasing self-esteem and motivation. However, it lacks studies in larger groups.

Couples with marital problems are primarily treated with marital therapy, followed by sexual therapies. Having no pain and discomfort during complete penetration and having satisfaction during intercourse are accepted as treatment success.

Surgical Interventions

Hymenotomy (incision on hymen) and hymenectomy (removal of the hymen) operations under sedation or local anesthesia should be limited only for the patients with congenital obstructive or rigid hymen abnormalities which interfere with coitus [35]. These patients might be invited back for additional cognitive and behavioral therapy for resolving anxiety and negative conditioning. If there are concomitant male problems, consultation from a urologist is also needed. Male partners who had primary or secondary sexual dysfunctions should be treated by CBT or/and medication, and they should be advised to become more active and assertive. Sometimes they also need to get psychological support.

Partial or complete removal of vulvar mucosa (vulvar vestibulectomy operation) is a well-established treatment for PVD associated with neuroproliferation [41]. While this invasive surgical approach has high success rates, with at least partial relief of sexual pain in 88% of patients and significant relief in 78.5% of patients according to a meta-analysis of 33 previous studies, it has a risk of complications such as bleeding, infection, Bartholin cyst formation, and worsening of pain. Surgery should be the last treatment option for resistant patients [42].

Pharmacological Agents

As pharmacological treatment methods, local anesthetic creams, muscle relaxants (nitroglycerin ointment, etc.), antidepressants, and anxiolytic drugs (diazepam, etc.) were also recommended in different studies.

Topical lidocaine creams are minimally efficacious, demonstrating only a 20% improvement in pain scores which was not significantly different from placebo [43].

Examination in dyspareunia patients, firstly Q tip test should be performed to determine the signs of hyperesthesia in the vestibulum, and "pain mapping" should be done (Fig. 13.2). The first step of managing dyspareunia is educating vulvar self-care, including avoiding douches, possible irritants, and allergens. Then, the treatment should be tailored according to the underlying causative(s). In PVD patients, topical 0.03% estradiol and 0.01% testosterone creams and discontinuation of oral contraceptives were recommended [44].

Eserdağ et al. investigated histopathological results of vestibulectomy specimens in localized provoked vulvodynia of resistant PVD patients and demonstrated the comorbidity with HPV-dependent cellular abnormalities. HPV can be an important agent impairing vestibular mucosa and causing PVD [45].

Cromolyn cream (a mast cell stabilizer), enoxaparin (low molecular weight heparin), and a skin cream containing lysate of fetal fibroblasts (with anti-inflammatory cytokines) have all undergone RCTs to evaluate the efficacy of possible anti-inflammatory action, with various success. In conclusion, pharmacological treatments are limited since most studies lack placebo control groups and do not randomly assign patients to treatment, are based on small samples, or do not use standardized outcome instruments [33].

Antidepressants generally negatively affect sexuality, and they can worsen sexual functions. Thus they are limitedly used only in patients with major depression or general anxiety. However, a recent small open-label trial of SNRI seemed to reduce pain severity, coital pain, and depression symptoms [46].

Botulinum Toxin Injections

Botulinum Toxin Type A acts at nociceptors to cause local muscle paralysis of 3–6 months duration, making it an appropriate choice for women who have difficulties with pelvic floor hyperactivity causing pain. The botulinum injection to treat vaginismus was first reported by Brin and Vapnek in 1997 [37]. This reported case of secondary vaginismus was managed first with 10 units of Botox™ followed by 40 units of Botox™. The patient was able to have intercourse for the first time in 8 years. The results persisted during the 24 months of follow-up evaluation. Pacik, in his study, suggested using a total of 100 IU of botox™ and bupivacaine 0.25% with 1:400,000 epinephrine injections to the lateral walls of the vagina, triangular wedge resection of hymenal mucosa at 3 and 9 o'clock, and dilator insertion at the same session. In 1 year, 97% of the patients could achieve comfortable intercourse, or single women without partners use a large dilator. Several small studies have

Fig. 13.2 Q Tip test and pain mapping in a PVD patient

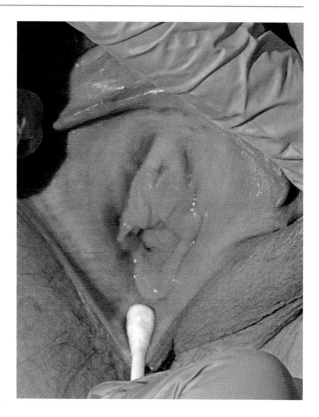

demonstrated efficacy in improving sexual pain, though larger RCTs should confirm these results before recommendation as a first-line treatment.

Although the vaginismus problem is accepted as a cause of infertility, very rarely and unexpectedly vaginismic women can get pregnant without complete penetration. It was stated in a study that vaginismic women who became pregnant in this way and whose pregnancies were at normal risk could also receive treatment during their pregnancies. Thus, with the reduction of their anxiety and involuntary pelvic contractions, it will be possible for these patients to have more comfortable pregnancy period, to have more comfortable vaginal examination, to get ability of vaginal delivery, and to solve their problems without delaying them to the intensive postpartum periods [47].

GPPPD treatments need a multidisciplinary team's multimodal approach, including gynecologist, psychiatrist, urologist, family consultant, sex therapist, psychologist, and physiotherapist. Furthermore, early management before the condition progresses into a chronic and resistant state is also important to reduce the likelihood of secondary sexual problems, such as lack of sexual desire, premature ejaculation and erectile dysfunction in men, or development of psychiatric problems, such as anxiety and depression. First, from an early age, age-appropriate sexual information should be provided to prevent the development of such problems. Second, early diagnosis and treatment should be undertaken to prevent sexual and psychiatric problems and improve marriage relationships [27].

References

1. Cherner RA, Reissing ED. A comparative study of sexual function, behavior, and cognitions of women with lifelong vaginismus. Arch Sex Behav. 2013;42:1605–14.
2. Basson R, Leiblum S, Brotto L, et al. Definitions of women's sexual dysfunction reconsidered: advocating expansion and revision. J Psychosom Obstet Gynaecol. 2003;24:221–9.
3. Ciocca G, Limoncin E, Di Tommaso S, et al. Attachment styles and sexual dysfunctions: a case-control study of female and male sexuality. Int J Impot Res. 2015;27:81–5.
4. Maseroli E, Scavello I, Cipriani S, et al. Psychobiological correlates of vaginismus: an exploratory analysis. J Sex Med. 2017;14:1392–402.
5. Ciocca G, Limoncin E, Di Tommaso S, et al. Alexithymia and vaginismus: a preliminary correlation perspective. Int J Impot Res. 2013;25:113–6.
6. American Psychiatric Association. Diagnostic and statistical manual of mental disorders. 4th ed. Text revision. Washington, DC: American Psychiatric Association; 2000.
7. American Psychiatric Association. Genito-pelvic pain/penetration disorder. In: Diagnostic and statistical manual of mental disorders. 5th ed. Arlington, VA: American Psychiatric Association; 2013. p. 437–40.
8. Lahaie MA, Boyer SC, Amsel R, et al. Vaginismus: a review of the literature on the classification/diagnosis, etiology and treatment. Womens Health (Lond). 2010;6(5):705–19.
9. Kaplan HS. The new sex therapy: active treatment of sexual dysfunctions. New York: Brunner-Mazel; 1974.
10. Mason-Hohl Trans W, editor. Trotula of Salerno: *The diseases of women*. Los Angeles, CA: The Ward Ritchie Press; 1940.
11. Butcher J. ABC of sexual health: female sexual problems II: sexual pain and sexual fears. BMJ. 1999;318(7176):110–2.
12. Sims MJ. On vaginismus. Trans Obstet Soc London. 1861;3:356–67.
13. Spector I, Carey M. Incidence and prevalence of the sexual dysfunctions: a critical review of the empirical literature. Arch Sex Behav. 1990;19:389–96.
14. Fugl-Meyer AR, Sjogren F-MK. Sexual disabilities, problems, and satisfaction in 18–74 year old Swedes. Scand J Sex. 1999;3:79–105.
15. Read S, King M, Watson J. Sexual dysfunction in primary medical care: prevalence, characteristics and detection by the general practitioner. J Public Health Med. 1997;19:387–91.
16. Oniz A, Keskinoglu P, Bezircioglu I. The prevalence and causes of sexual problems among premenopausal Turkish women. J Sex Med. 2007;4:1575–81.
17. Masters WH, Johnson VE. Human sexual inadequacy. Boston: Little, Brown; 1970.
18. Beck JG. Vaginismus. In: O'Donohue W, Greer JH, editors. Handbook of sexual dysfunctions: assessment and treatment. Boston: Allyn and Bacon Inc; 1993. p. 381–97.
19. Duddle M. Etiological factors in the unconsummated marriage. J Psychosom Res. 1977;21:157–60.
20. Reissing ED, Binik YM, Khalifé S, et al. Etiological correlates of vaginismus: sexual and physical abuse, sexual knowledge, sexual self-schemata, and relationship adjustment. J Sex Marital Ther. 2003;29:47–59.
21. Tugrul C, Kabakçi E. Vaginismus and its correlates. Sex Marital Ther. 1997;12(1):23–34.
22. Hawton K, Catalan J. Sex therapy for vaginismus: characteristics of couples and treatment outcome. Sex Marital Ther. 1990;5:39–48.
23. Biswas A, Ratnam SS. Vaginismus and outcome of treatment. Ann Acad Med. 1995;24:755–8.
24. Van de Wiel HB. Treatment of vaginismus: a review of concepts and treatment modalities. J Psychosom Obstet Gynaecol. 1990;11:1–18.
25. Eserdağ S, Kurban D, Yakut E, Mishra PC. Insights into the vaginismus treatment by cognitive behavioral therapies: correlation with sexual dysfunction identified in male spouses of the patients. J Family Reprod Health. 2021;15(1):61–9.
26. Eserdağ S, Zülfikaroğlu E, Akarsu S. Sexual dysfunction in male partners of 580 women with vaginismus: is it a result of or a reaction to vaginismus? Eur J Surg Sci. 2012;3(2):51–5.

27. Kurban D, Eserdağ S, Yakut E, et al. The treatment analysis of the patients suffering from vaginismus and the correlation with the psychological issues. Int J Reprod Contracept Obstet Gynecol. 2021;10(4):1328–36.
28. Harlow BL, Wise LA, Stewart EG. Prevalence and predictors of chronic lower genital tract discomfort. Am J Obstet Gynecol. 2001;185:545–50.
29. Friedrich EG. Vulvar vestibulitis syndrome. J Reprod Med. 1987;32:110–4.
30. Graziottin A, Gambini D. Evaluation of genito-pelvic pain/penetration disorder. In: IsHak WW, editor. The textbook of clinical sexual medicine. 1st ed. Los Angeles, CA: Springer International Publishing; 2017. p. 289–304.
31. Tympanidis P, Terenghi G, Dowd P. Increased innervation of the vulval vestibule in patients with vulvodynia. Br J Dermatol. 2003;148(5):1021–7.
32. Eserdağ S, Sevinc T, Tarlacı S. Do women with vaginismus have a lower threshold of pain? Eur J Obstet Gynecol Reprod Biol. 2021;258:189–92.
33. Conforti C. Genito-pelvic pain/penetration disorder (GPPPD): an overview of current terminology, etiology, and treatment. Univ Ottawa J Med. 2017;7(2):48–53.
34. Ramirez De Knott HM, McCormick TS, Do SO, et al. Cutaneous hypersensitivity to Candida albicans in idiopathic vulvodynia. Contact Dermatitis. 2005;53(4):214–8.
35. Eserdağ S, Dogukan AD. Importance of gynecological assessment for the treatment of vaginismus as a predictive value. J Obstet Gynaecol Res. 2021;47(7):2537–43.
36. Lamont JA. Vaginismus. Am J Obstet Gynecol. 1978;131:633–6.
37. Pacik PT. Vaginismus: review of current concepts and treatment using botox injections, bupivacaine injections, and progressive dilation with the patient under anesthesia. Aesthetic Plast Surg. 2011;35:1160–4.
38. Eserdağ S, Zülfikaroğlu E, Akarsu S, et al. Treatment outcome of 460 women with vaginismus. Eur J Surg Sci. 2011;2(3):73–9.
39. Delmonte MM. The use of relaxation and hypnotically-guided imagery as an intervention with a case of vaginismus. Aust J Clin Exp Hypn. 1988;9(1):1–7.
40. Ni C, Sinha VK. Marriage consummated after 22 years: a case report. J Sex Marital Ther. 2002;28(4):301–4.
41. Goldstein AT, Pukall CF, Brown C, et al. Vulvodynia: assessment and treatment. J Sex Med. 2016;13(4):572–90.
42. Pukall CF, Mitchell LS, Goldstein AT. Non-medical, medical, and surgical approaches for the treatment of provoked vestibulodynia. Curr Sex Health Rep. 2016;8(4):240–8.
43. Foster DC, Kotok MB, Huang L, et al. Oral desipramine and topical lidocaine for vulvodynia: a randomized controlled trial. Obstet Gynecol. 2010;116(3):583–93.
44. Burrows LJ, Goldstein AT. The treatment vestibulodynia with topical estradiol and testosterone. Sex Med. 2013;1(1):30–3.
45. Eserdağ S, Kurban D, Kiseli M, et al. The histopathological results of vestibulectomy specimens in localized provoked vulvodynia in Turkey. Pan Afr Med J. 2020;37(267):1–9.
46. Brown C, Bachmann G, Foster D, Rawlinson L, Wan J, Ling F. Milnacipran in provoked vestibulodynia: efficacy and predictors of treatment success. J Low Genit Tract Dis. 2015;19(2):140–4.
47. Eserdağ S, Akalın EA. Evaluation of characteristics and clinical outcomes of vaginismus treatment during pregnancy. South Clin Ist Euras. 2021;32(2):134–40.

Male Infertility

14

Ugo Falagario, Anna Ricapito, and Carlo Bettocchi

Abstract

One in eight couples encounter problems when attempting to conceive a first child and one in six when attempting to conceive a subsequent child. Half of the cases are linked to male infertility. The pathophysiology of male infertility is not perfectly understood. Most of infertile patients have abnormalities in the semen analysis. However, up to 30% of couples have unexplained male infertility which is defined as infertility of unknown origin with normal sperm parameters and partner evaluation.

Similarly, 30–40% of patients with impaired sperm parameters have idiopathic male infertility with no previous history of diseases affecting fertility and normal findings on physical examination as well as endocrine, genetic and biochemical laboratory testing.

Given the complexity of male infertility, accurate diagnostic evaluation is needed and it must always include physical examination, a detailed medical history, testicular ultrasound and Semen analysis. The clinical management of patients with male infertility depend indeed on the underlying etiology.

In the following paragraphs we will provide readers with a complete overview of the most clinically useful classification of male infertility with the current available evidence and recommendation on male infertility treatment.

U. Falagario · A. Ricapito · C. Bettocchi (✉)
Department of Urology and Organ Transplantation, University of Foggia, Foggia, Italy
e-mail: carlo.bettocchi@unifg.it

© The Author(s), under exclusive license to Springer Nature Switzerland AG 2022
S. Sarikaya et al. (eds.), *Andrology and Sexual Medicine*, Management of Urology,
https://doi.org/10.1007/978-3-031-12049-7_14

Epidemiology

Couple infertility is defined as the lack of conception after at least 12 months of regular unprotected sexual intercourse aimed at pregnancy and it represents a frequent clinical issue. One in eight couples encounter problems when attempting to conceive a first child and one in six when attempting to conceive a subsequent child and the half cases are linked to male infertility [1, 2]. Unexplained fertility has also to be explained: it is defined as infertility of unknown origin with normal sperm parameters and partner evaluation, and it ranges between 20% and 30% [3].

Several risk factors have been identifying, in particular age, environment, and infections. Advanced paternal age has indeed emerged as one of the main risk factors associated with the progressive increase in the prevalence of male factor infertility [4, 5].

Another important risk factor is obesity. According to the World Health Organization (WHO), obesity can be defined when BMI is higher than 30 kg/m^2 (WHO) and its prevalence has incredibly increased during last decades [6].

There is evidence of lower fertility rate in couples with an obese male partner than couples with normal-BMI male partners [7] and different mechanisms have been theorized to explain this matter [8]. Higher scrotal temperature in obese men must be considered, since spermatogenesis is process strictly linked to temperature itself. Hormonal aspect may also involve. Indeed, compared to non-obese male patients, serum levels of Sex-Hormon Binding Globulin (SHBG) have been detected higher in obese men, so inducing lower free testosterone levels [9].

Another factor altering male fertility is represented by PFAS (PerFluorinated Alkylated Substances), a class of organic molecules made of fluorinated hydrocarbon chains, hugely used in industry, and detected in human semen and testis [10, 11].

Exposure to high levels of this category of molecules is associated with reduced the concentration of normal morphology among spermatozoa in men [12, 13]. PFAS also modify spermatozoa's membrane, a crucial component for motility: this is recognized as a possible explanation of PFAS-induced sperm damage [14].

Finally HPV infection, agent of common sexually transmitted infections, plays an important role in this field [15] and it can be divided in two different groups: high-risk (HR-HPV), classified as oncogenic to humans, and low-risk (LR-HPV). Numerous studies have found a possible role of HPV in male infertility [16], due to the fact that it has been detected in sperm of men with unexplained infertility, and because it has been linked to lower sperm motility [17–21]. Additionally another connection is provided by the presence of anti-sperm antibodies (ASAs), which are higher in infected patients with fertility issues compared to non-infected ones [22].

Diagnostic Evaluation

Accurate diagnostic evaluation is needed in case of male infertility, and it must always include physical examination, detailed medical history, testicular ultrasound and Semen analysis (Fig. 14.1).

Fig. 14.1 Diagnostic
evaluation of patients with
suspected male infertility

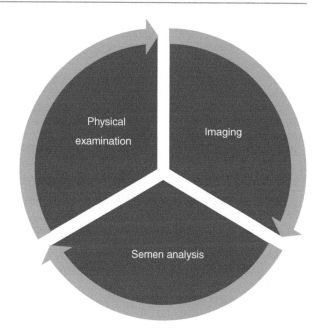

1. **Physical examination**. Accurate physical examination is mandatory, also evaluating secondary sexual characteristics. Testicular size, consistency and texture must be assessed, determining the presence of vas deferens, epididymis and eventual varicocele [23]
2. **Radiological assessment**. Testicular ultrasound provides information about testicular tissue, testicular volume, epididymal aspect, presence of varicocele or tumor. It allows the detection of obstruction when, seminal vesicle (SV) width is >1.5 cm and ejaculatory duct diameter is >2.3 mm [24]. Magnetic resonance imaging (MRI) showed to be beneficial for soft-tissue and cystic lesions, though its costs.
3. **Semen analysis** is a key step in the evaluation of the fertility of the male partner of a couple, even if it cannot precisely distinguish fertile from infertile men. Basic examination provides assessment of sperm number, which is recognized to have more diagnostic value than sperm concentration (defined as number of spermatozoa per unit volume of semen; sperm motility, divided into fast progressively motile, slow progressively motile, non-progressively motile and immotile; sperm morphology, that consists of a head and a tail connected by a midpiece [23].

   Concerning sperm number, three quantitative alterations can be distinguished (Fig. 14.2):

   • Azoospermia: absence of spermatozoa in the ejaculate and in the pellet after centrifugation.
   • Cryptozoospermia: absence of spermatozoa in the ejaculate but present in the pellet after centrifugation.

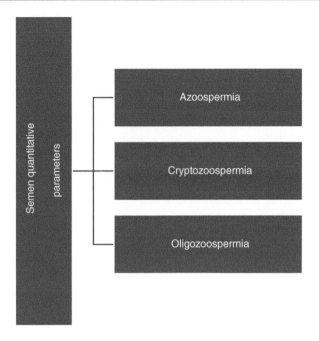

Fig. 14.2 Quantitative abnormalities in semen analysis

- Oligozoospermia: sperm concentration or TSC lower than the fifth percentile value.

The reduction in sperm motility, instead, called asthenozoospermia (total motility <42% and progressive motility <30%) can be explained with congenital or acquired factors. Especially extreme asthenozoospermia, with or without associated teratozoospermia (primary ciliary disease), is due to different genetic anomalies [25]. Table 14.1 reports the lower reference limits for semen characteristics according to the 2021 fifth edition of the WHO Manual.

Most of seminal fluids don't fulfil the WHO criteria for being considered as "normal" even when the test is performed by fertile men (WHO). In many of patients affected by teratozoospermia (normal forms <4%), head, midpiece and tail defects are mixed. So, since the overlapping values between fertile and infertile men, the application of these criteria in the clinical practice is still questionable (WHO).

Semen analysis also allows anti-sperm antibodies (ASA) detection, through evaluation of aggregation, that is the adherence of motile and immotile spermatozoa to mucus strands, and agglutinantion, that is the trend of motile spermatozoa to make clumps (WHO). The presence of ASA as an isolated abnormality is seen in less than 5% of infertile males and occurs mainly in association with normal sperm counts [26]. ASA evaluation can be requested in case of unexplained couple infertility with normozoospermic male partner [27].

Table 14.1 Lower reference limits for semen analysis according to the 2021 fifth edition of the WHO Manual

Parameter	Normal reference limit (WHO criteria, fifth edition)
Semen volume	$\geq$1.5 mL
pH	$\geq$7.2
Total sperm number	$\geq$35–40 $\times$ 10⁶/ejaculate
Sperm concentration	$\geq$16 $\times$ 10⁶/mL
Morphology	$\geq$4%
Progressive motility (PR)	$\geq$32%
Total motility (PR + NP)	$\geq$40%

4. **DNA Fragmentation Index (DFI)**. DNA fragmentation, or the accumulation of single- and double-strand DNA breaks, is a common property of sperm, and an increase in the level of sperm DNA fragmentation has been shown to reduce the chances of natural conception. Sperm DNA damage is more common in men with fertility issues and it can be increased by hormonal anomalies, varicocele and lifestyle. The suggested threshold DFI of 25% is associated with reduced natural pregnancy rates [23].

Classification and Clinical Management

Clinical management of male infertility depend on the underlying etiology and pathophysiology. In the following paragraphs we will provide readers with a complete overview of the most clinically useful classification of male infertility with the current available evidence and recommendation on male infertility treatment.

Pathophysiology of male infertility is not perfectly understood. Most of infertile patients have abnormalities in the semen analysis. However, up to 30% of couples have Unexplained male infertility which is defined as infertility of unknown origin with normal sperm parameters and partner evaluation.

Similarly, 30–40% of patients with impaired sperm parameters have idiopathic male infertility with no previous history of diseases affecting fertility and normal findings on physical examination as well as endocrine, genetic and biochemical laboratory testing.

The most frequently associated semen abnormality in infertile man is azoospermia, the absence of sperm in the ejaculate. Based on the underlining etiology, azoospermia can be categorized in:

- **Pre-testicular** abnormalities in the hypothalamic-pituitary-gonadal axis;
- **Testicular** spermatogenesis disorders occurring in the testes;
- **Post-testicular**: obstruction in the male seminal tract and ejaculatory dysfunctions.

From a clinical point of view, however, azoospermia is more commonly classified in two large groups based on the presence or absence of sperm in the testis:

- **Non-obstructive azoospermia (NOA)** or **secretory azoospermia** due to a sperm production impairment (pre-testicular and testicular etiologies);
- **Obstructive azoospermia (OA)**: the spermatogenesis is unaffected, and the complete absence of sperm in the ejaculate is due to bilateral obstruction of the passage of sperm along the seminal tract (post-testicular etiologies).

Non-obstructive Azoospermia (NOA)

NOA is defined as the absence of sperm at the semen analysis after centrifugation, with usually a normal ejaculate volume. This finding should be confirmed at least at two consecutives semen analyses [28].

Hormonal profile in these patients is mandatory even if dysfunction of the hypothalamus pituitary-gonadal (HPG) axis (pre-testicular etiology) account for less than 1% of cases of NOA.

A dysfunction of the hypothalamus or the pituitary gland led to a decreased secretion of gonadotropins with consequent HYPOGONADOTROPIC HYPOGONADISM (HH).

Congenital HH is in a third of the cases idiopathic. Remaining cases or due to genetic syndromes (Kallmann syndrome, Prader-Willi syndrome) [29]. Tumor, infections or iatrogenic injuries of the pituitary gland as well as illicit drugs intake (anabolic steroids, opiates), alcohol abuse, hyperprolactinemia, iron overload are possible etiologies of acquired HH.

The therapy is medical and depends on patient's desire for future fertility: testosterone is indicated for men who already have children or have no desire for children.

Gonadotropins with or without follicle-stimulating hormone is otherwise indicated to stimulate spermatogenesis.

The severe deficit in spermatogenesis observed in NOA patients is almost in all cases of NOA, at the gonadal level (**Testicular etiology**). These patients should undergo a comprehensive clinical assessment including a detailed history since the intrinsic disorder of spermatogenesis may derive from exposure to substances with gonadotoxic effects (chemotherapy agents, hormonal therapies, pesticides and solvents) or testicular damage due to iatrogenic causes (irradiation or previous surgery), undescended testes (cryptorchidism), varicocele-induced, testicular torsion and infections.

Genetic tests are also indicated, and sovra-numerical chromosome are the most observed abnormalities. Klinefelter syndrome (XXY) is the most common occurring in 1 out of 500 males. These patients are usually tall and with eunuchoid body proportions, and present with high levels of gonadotropins and low testosterone.

The second per frequency is the 47, XYY syndrome occurring in 1:1000 men. Patients present tall stature, azoospermia with normal serum testosterone level [29, 30]. Finally.

Y-chromosome microdeletion occurring in the AZF region (Yq) may be found. Notably, deletion of the loci AZFa and AZFb are associated with complete absence of spermatogenesis [31].

Despite definition of the exact etiology may be desirable, almost 50% of NOA are idiopatic likely determined by an unknown genetical defect or exposition to gonadotoxins.

If genetic abnormalities are found, genetic counselling is mandatory prior to any assisted reproductive technology protocols.

Treatment

Conventional medical or surgical treatments are ineffective in patients with NOA and sperm retrieval with consequent Intracytoplasmic Sperm Injection (ICSI) represents the only option.

In patients with complete AZFa and AZFb microdeletions the chance of sperm retrieval is zero and surgery is contraindicated.

Since there are no pre-operative biochemical and clinical variables predicting positive sperm retrieval at surgery, fine needle aspiration may be considered an option to evaluate the eligibility of patients for more advance techniques of sperm retrieval and to guide sampling in specific areas. Microdissection testicular sperm aspiration (microTESE) is the technique of choice for retrieving sperm in patients with NOA.

The beneficial effect of varicocele treatment in infertile patients is still debated since there is increasing evidence that the two conditions may be concomitant and not directly correlated. However, results of historical and more recent metanalysis reports improvements of the ejaculate after correction [32].

Bilateral TESE for sperm retrieval, freezing and histological evaluation may be performed in azoospermic patients simultaneously or before varicocele correction [33].

Obstructive Azoospermia (OA)

Obstruction of sperm transit at any point of the seminal tract and ejaculatory dysfunction are frequent in azoospermic or severely oligozoospermic patients, usually with normal-sized testes and normal reproductive hormones (post-Testicular etiology). Table 14.2 summarize level of obstruction and etiology of different forms of OA.

Testicular obstruction with total absence of spermatozoa in the epididymis is extremely rare. It can be found in concomitance to other congenital malformations, but it is usually associated with epididymal obstruction as a reliquate of inflammation or infection.

More commonly, **Epididymal obstruction** is found in patients with azoospermia (30–67%).

Congenital obstruction is found in up to 6% of patients with OA and manifests as bilateral agenesis of vas deferens. This condition is frequently (80% of cases) associated with mutation of the cystic fibrosis transmembrane conductance

Table 14.2 Level of obstruction and etiology of different forms of obstructive azoospermia

Location of the obstruction	Etiology
Testicles	Congenital
	Infection (acute/chronic epididymitis)
Epididymis	Infection (acute/chronic epididymitis)
	Trauma
	Post-surgical iatrogenic obstruction (i.e., MESA, hydrocelectomy or other scrotal surgery)
	Congenital epididymal obstruction (usually manifests as congenital bilateral absence of the vas deferens
	[CBAVD])
	Other congenital forms of epididymal obstruction (Young's syndrome)
Vas deferens	Vasectomy
	Vasotomy/vasography (with improper technique)
	Post-surgical iatrogenic obstruction (i.e., scrotal surgery or herniorraphy)
	Unilateral or bilateral agenesia of the vas deferens
Ejaculatory ducts	Cysts (Mullerian utricular, prostatic or seminal vesicular)
	Infection (acute/chronic epididymitis)
	Traumatic
	Postsurgical iatrogenic obstruction
Functional obstruction	Idiopathic/acquired local neurogenic dysfunction

regulator (CFTR) gene. Remaining congenital cases may be due to anormal differentiation of the mesonephric duct and may be associated with epididymal aplasia, seminal vesicle aplasia or hypospadias [34]. Patients with Congenital Epididymal obstruction presents with normal testicular volume, normal spermatogenesis and normal levels of FSH. Spermatozoa can be easily retrieved from the testis or the caput epididymis.

Sexually transmitted infections (*Chlamydia, N. Gonorreae*) and post-surgical iatrogenic lesions represents the acquired forms of epididymal obstruction.

Vas deferent obstruction etiologies include Vasectomy performed for selective sterilization, iatrogenic injuries during inguinal or scrotal surgery (surgical hernia repair and hydrocelectomy are the more common), infections and trauma can cause stop of the sperm transit at any level of the vas deferens (**Vas Deferens Obstruction**) [35].

10% of the obstructive forms of OA are due to **Ejaculatory Duct Obstruction** but this condition rarely cause male infertility [36].

The obstruction can be congenital with presence of prostatic cysts or atresia of the ejaculatory duct or acquired after catheterization, prostatic surgery or infectious diseases [24]. Patients presents with oligoasthenospermia with low-normal volume and low-normal pH (partial obstruction) or with azoospermia, low pH and absence of fructose in the ejaculate (complete obstruction).

Finally **Ejaculatory dysfunction** is an unusual cause of male infertility caused by the inability of the sperm to proceed along the seminal tract in absence of any form of obstruction. Retrograde ejaculation for example represents the abnormal backward flow of semen into the bladder with ejaculation. Prostatic surgery, abnormal contraction of the bladder neck due to neurological disorders of pharmacologic treatments (Alfa-blockers) are the most common etiologies [904].

Treatment

In the presence of OA, surgical treatment is the preferred approach and should be aimed at the relieve of the obstruction. Microsurgical vasovasostomy or epididymovasostomy should be performed for azoospermia caused by epididymal or vasal obstruction in men with female partners of good ovarian reserve.

However, the use sperm retrieval techniques, such as microsurgical epididymal sperm aspiration (MESA), testicular sperm extraction (TESE) and percutaneous techniques (PESA and TESA) to proceed with ICSI treatment is always suggested in association with reconstructive surgery and is the recommended option if surgical repair is not possible, when the ovarian reserve of the partner is limited or according to patient preferences.

Idiopathic Male Infertility and Oligo-Astheno-Terato-Zoospermia

In men with idiopathic oligo-astheno-teratozoospermia, in absence of any etiology-targeted therapy, or as adjuvant therapy in patients with NOA and OA, there is increasing evidence of the utility of non-Invasive Male Infertility Management.

Life-style changes including weight loss and increased physical activity, smoking cessation and alcohol intake reduction can improve sperm quality and the chances of conception.

International guidelines also support the use of anti-oxidants. Oxidative stress is indeed considered an important contributing factor in the pathogenesis of idiopathic infertility. Reactive oxygen species, the final products of OS, can impair sperm function acting at several levels, including plasma membrane lipid peroxidation, which can affect sperm motility, the acrosome reaction and chromatin maturation leading to increased DNA fragmentation.

Some positive results including a significant improvement in sperm and hormonal parameters and increased pregnancy rates have been reported by recent meta-nalysis on the use of selective oestrogen receptor modulators in men with idiopathic infertility [37]. However, the quality of the papers included was low and only a few studies were placebo-controlled thus no conclusive recommendations on the use of selective oestrogen receptor modulators in men with idiopathic infertility can be drawn.

Similarly, no conclusive recommendations can be drawn on the use of either steroidal (testolactone) or nonsteroidal (anastrozole and letrozole) aromatase inhibitors in men with idiopathic infertility [23].

Sperm Retrieval Techniques

Sperm retrieval and intracytoplasmic sperm injection (ICSI) is only option for patients with NOA, for patients with OA non suitable for treatment and for couples undergoing in vitro fertilization in presence of female factors.

In case of OA any sperm retrieval technique might be used with high chance of sufficient sampling for ICSI. In patients with NOA open surgical techniques are needed and the success rate are lower [38].

Several techniques have been described:

- MICROsurgical Epididymal Sperm Aspiration (MESA) with puncture of epididymis head;
- TEsticular Sperm Aspiration (TESA) and Percutaneous Epididymal Sperm Aspiration (PESA) are the simplest percutaneous techniques and consists in the percutaneous puncture of testicle or the epididymis with a butterfly 21 G needle, followed by aspiration of the testicular fluid.
- TEsticular Sperm Extraction (TESE) is slightly more invasive but allows a good amount of material to be obtained. A single surgical biopsy is performed, and the sample is microscopically examined. If no spermatozoa are found at first biopsy, multiple biopsies are taken at different testicular sites [39]. In patients with NOA the sperm recovery rate is around 50–60% [40].
- MICROsurgical Testicular Sperm Extraction (Micro-TESE). This technique has been suggested to improve outcomes of TESE and to minimize vascular damage, tissue loss, retraction of the albuginea with consequent compression of the testicular parenchyma due to multiple TESE [41]. Micro-TESE is performed under an operating microscope and single seminiferous tubules are sampled from different areas of the testicular parenchyma and sent to the laboratory for spermatozoa extraction [42]. Micro-TESE has become the gold standard procedure in men with NOA or in patients where previous techniques have been unsuccessful [31].

References

1. Greenhall E, Vessey M. The prevalence of subfertility: a review of the current confusion and a report of two new studies. Fertil Steril. 1990;54(6):978–83.
2. de Kretser DM. Male infertility. Lancet. 1997;349(9054):787–90.
3. Agarwal A, Parekh N, Panner Selvam MK, Henkel R, Shah R, Homa ST, et al. Male oxidative stress infertility (MOSI): proposed terminology and clinical practice guidelines for management of idiopathic male infertility. World J Mens Health. 2019;37(3):296–312.
4. Brandt JS, Cruz Ithier MA, Rosen T, Ashkinadze E. Advanced paternal age, infertility, and reproductive risks: a review of the literature. Prenat Diagn. 2019;39(2):81–7.
5. Jennings MO, Owen RC, Keefe D, Kim ED. Management and counseling of the male with advanced paternal age. Fertil Steril. 2017;107(2):324–8.

6. Pasquali R, Casanueva F, Haluzik M, van Hulsteijn L, Ledoux S, Monteiro MP, et al. European Society of Endocrinology Clinical Practice Guideline: endocrine work-up in obesity. Eur J Endocrinol. 2020;182(1):G1–G32.

7. Campbell JM, Lane M, Owens JA, Bakos HW. Paternal obesity negatively affects male fertility and assisted reproduction outcomes: a systematic review and meta-analysis. Reprod Biomed Online. 2015;31(5):593–604.

8. Lewin S, Williams BA. The effect of D$_2$O substitution for H$_2$O on the melting temperature of *E. coli* ribosomes. Arch Biochem Biophys. 1971;144(1):1–5.

9. Davidson LM, Millar K, Jones C, Fatum M, Coward K. Deleterious effects of obesity upon the hormonal and molecular mechanisms controlling spermatogenesis and male fertility. Hum Fertil (Camb). 2015;18(3):184–93.

10. Li N, Mruk DD, Chen H, Wong CK, Lee WM, Cheng CY. Rescue of perfluorooctanesulfonate (PFOS)-mediated sertoli cell injury by overexpression of gap junction protein connexin 43. Sci Rep. 2016;6:29667.

11. Inoue K, Okada F, Ito R, Kato S, Sasaki S, Nakajima S, et al. Perfluorooctane sulfonate (PFOS) and related perfluorinated compounds in human maternal and cord blood samples: assessment of PFOS exposure in a susceptible population during pregnancy. Environ Health Perspect. 2004;112(11):1204–7.

12. Toft G, Jonsson BA, Lindh CH, Giwercman A, Spano M, Heederik D, et al. Exposure to per-fluorinated compounds and human semen quality in Arctic and European populations. Hum Reprod. 2012;27(8):2532–40.

13. Joensen UN, Bossi R, Leffers H, Jensen AA, Skakkebaek NE, Jorgensen N. Do perfluoroalkyl compounds impair human semen quality? Environ Health Perspect. 2009;117(6):923–7.

14. Arbo MD, Altknecht LF, Cattani S, Braga WV, Peruzzi CP, Cestonaro LV, et al. In vitro cardiotoxicity evaluation of graphene oxide. Mutat Res Genet Toxicol Environ Mutagen. 2019;841:8–13.

15. Dunne EF, Nielson CM, Stone KM, Markowitz LE, Giuliano AR. Prevalence of HPV infection among men: a systematic review of the literature. J Infect Dis. 2006;194(8):1044–57.

16. Shimizu H, Ito M, Miyahara M, Ichikawa K, Okubo S, Konishi T, et al. Characterization of the myosin-binding subunit of smooth muscle myosin phosphatase. J Biol Chem. 1994;269(48):30407–11.

17. Nielson CM, Flores R, Harris RB, Abrahamsen M, Papenfuss MR, Dunne EF, et al. Human papillomavirus prevalence and type distribution in male anogenital sites and semen. Cancer Epidemiol Biomark Prev. 2007;16(6):1107–14.

18. Wahl P. Immunological factors and diabetic retinopathy. Ber Zusammenkunft Dtsch Ophthalmol Ges. 1970;70:148–52.

19. Garolla A, Pizzol D, Bertoldo A, De Toni L, Barzon L, Foresta C. Association, prevalence, and clearance of human papillomavirus and antisperm antibodies in infected semen samples from infertile patients. Fertil Steril. 2013;99(1):125–31. e2

20. Foresta C, Pizzol D, Moretti A, Barzon L, Palu G, Garolla A. Clinical and prognostic significance of human papillomavirus DNA in the sperm or exfoliated cells of infertile patients and subjects with risk factors. Fertil Steril. 2010;94(5):1723–7.

21. Foresta C, Garolla A, Zuccarello D, Pizzol D, Moretti A, Barzon L, et al. Human papillomavirus found in sperm head of young adult males affects the progressive motility. Fertil Steril. 2010;93(3):802–6.

22. Heidenreich A, Bonfig R, Wilbert DM, Strohmaier WL, Engelmann UH. Risk factors for anti-sperm antibodies in infertile men. Am J Reprod Immunol. 1994;31(2–3):69–76.

23. Salonia A, Bettocchi C, Boeri L, Capogrosso P, Carvalho J, Cilesiz NC, et al. European Association of Urology guidelines on sexual and reproductive health-2021 update: male sexual dysfunction. Eur Urol. 2021;80(3):333–57.

24. Avellino GJ, Lipshultz LI, Sigman M, Hwang K. Transurethral resection of the ejaculatory ducts: etiology of obstruction and surgical treatment options. Fertil Steril. 2019;111(3):427–43.

25. Krausz C, Riera-Escamilla A. Genetics of male infertility. Nat Rev Urol. 2018;15(6):369–84.

26. Tournaye H, Krausz C, Oates RD. Novel concepts in the aetiology of male reproductive impairment. Lancet Diabetes Endocrinol. 2017;5(7):544–53.
27. Ferlin A, Calogero AE, Krausz C, Lombardo F, Paoli D, Rago R, et al. Management of male factor infertility: position statement from the Italian Society of Andrology and Sexual Medicine (SIAMS): endorsing organization: Italian Society of Embryology, Reproduction, and Research (SIERR). J Endocrinol Investig. 2022;45(5):1085–113.
28. World Health Organization. WHO laboratory manual for the examination and processing of human semen. 5th ed. Geneva: World Health Organization; 2010.
29. Turek PJ, Pera RA. Current and future genetic screening for male infertility. Urol Clin North Am. 2002;29(4):767–92.
30. Van Assche E, Bonduelle M, Tournaye H, Joris H, Verheyen G, Devroey P, et al. Cytogenetics of infertile men. Hum Reprod. 1996;11(Suppl 4):1–24; discussion 5–6.
31. Tharakan T, Bettocchi C, Carvalho J, Corona G, Jones TH, Kadioglu A, et al. European Association of Urology guidelines panel on male sexual and reproductive health: a clinical consultation guide on the indications for performing sperm DNA fragmentation testing in men with infertility and testicular sperm extraction in nonazoospermic men. Eur Urol Focus. 2022;8(1):339–50.
32. Esteves SC, Oliveira FV, Bertolla RP. Clinical outcome of intracytoplasmic sperm injection in infertile men with treated and untreated clinical varicocele. J Urol. 2010;184(4):1442–6.
33. Salonia A, Bettocchi C, Boeri L, Capogrosso P, Carvalho J, Cilesiz NC, et al. European Association of Urology guidelines on sexual and reproductive health—2021 update: male sexual dysfunction [formula presented]. Eur Urol. 2021;80(3):333–57.
34. McCallum T, Milunsky J, Munarriz R, Carson R, Sadeghi-Nejad H, Oates R. Unilateral renal agenesis associated with congenital bilateral absence of the vas deferens: phenotypic findings and genetic considerations. Hum Reprod. 2001;16(2):282–8.
35. Costabile RA, Spevak M. Characterization of patients presenting with male factor infertility in an equal access, no cost medical system. Urology. 2001;58(6):1021–4.
36. Modgil V, Rai S, Ralph DJ, Muneer A. An update on the diagnosis and management of ejaculatory duct obstruction. Nat Rev Urol. 2016;13(1):13–20.
37. Chua ME, Escusa KG, Luna S, Tapia LC, Dofitas B, Morales M. Revisiting oestrogen antagonists (clomiphene or tamoxifen) as medical empiric therapy for idiopathic male infertility: a meta-analysis. Andrology. 2013;1(5):749–57.
38. Lee R, Li PS, Goldstein M, Schattman G, Schlegel PN. A decision analysis of treatments for nonobstructive azoospermia associated with varicocele. Fertil Steril. 2009;92(1):188–96.
39. Turunc T, Gul U, Haydardedeoglu B, Bal N, Kuzgunbay B, Peskircioglu L, et al. Conventional testicular sperm extraction combined with the microdissection technique in nonobstructive azoospermic patients: a prospective comparative study. Fertil Steril. 2010;94(6):2157–60.
40. Marconi M, Keudel A, Diemer T, Bergmann M, Steger K, Schuppe HC, et al. Combined trifocal and microsurgical testicular sperm extraction is the best technique for testicular sperm retrieval in "low-chance" nonobstructive azoospermia. Eur Urol. 2012;62(4):713–9.
41. Ramasamy R, Ricci JA, Leung RA, Schlegel PN. Successful repeat microdissection testicular sperm extraction in men with nonobstructive azoospermia. J Urol. 2011;185(3):1027–31.
42. Caroppo E, Colpi EM, Gazzano G, Vaccalluzzo L, Piatti E, D'Amato G, et al. The seminiferous tubule caliber pattern as evaluated at high magnification during microdissection testicular sperm extraction predicts sperm retrieval in patients with non-obstructive azoospermia. Andrology. 2019;7(1):8–14.

Male Contraception

15

Ioannis Sokolakis, Nikolaos Pyrgidis,
and Georgios Hatzichristodoulou

Abstract

Male Contraception is less used than female contraception and is based mainly on the use of condom and vasectomy. Recently new methods in male contraception have emerge or are under investigation. Several new pharmaceutical/hormonal applications for male contraception have been developed or are under investigation. These include testosterone monotherapy and combination of androgens with progesterone or gonadotropin releasing hormone analogues. They aim to block the hypothalamic-pituitary-testicular axis. There is a growing interest in the development of non-hormonal male contraceptives. They aim to interrupt different steps in sperm production and to block sperm transport or sperm motility. New minimal invasive methods of occlusion of vas deferens using plugs or injected polymers have also emerged. Vasectomy remains the gold standard of male contraception. It remains the safest, simplest, most highly effective, and least-expensive contraceptive method.

Introduction

Contraception, also known as anticonception, birth control or fertility control, is a method used to prevent pregnancy and regulate family planning. It has been implemented since the ancient times, but safe and effective techniques became available in the last decades. According to the World Health Organization, all people have the fundamental right to control the course of their own lives. In other words, all people can determine whether and when they may father children, how many children they want and with whom. Still, approximately 50% of the 1,000,000 daily conceptions

I. Sokolakis (✉) · N. Pyrgidis · G. Hatzichristodoulou
Department of Urology, Martha-Maria Hospital Nuremberg, Nuremberg, Germany

© The Author(s), under exclusive license to Springer Nature
Switzerland AG 2022
S. Sarikaya et al. (eds.), *Andrology and Sexual Medicine*, Management of Urology,
https://doi.org/10.1007/978-3-031-12049-7_15

worldwide remain unplanned, of which 150,000 are terminated by abortion, an intervention that, among other mental and physical complications, will lead to death for about 500 of these women [1].

To date, family planning has been anchored on female contraceptive methods. The invention of the "pill" was one of the most important milestones of the twentieth century, as it had a great impact on fertility, on sexual practices and on women's health and role in the society. Apart from oral contraceptives, a plethora of other effective contraceptive methods for females has been developed over the last years, including implants and intrauterine devices, surgical sterilization procedures, injections, transdermal patches, vaginal rings and diaphragms, as well as female condoms. Nevertheless, failure rates of these methods range from less than 1% up to more than 20%, depending on the applied contraceptive method and its correct use. Accordingly, it should be stressed that a significant proportion of women display contraindications to the available contraceptives, fear the development of adverse events or even experience devastating consequences from their use, resulting in abandoning contraception methods [2].

Therefore, the launch of a highly effective, widely available and reversible male contraceptive method is well worth considering. The ideal male contraceptive would cause azoospermia consistently and reversibly without adverse effects. To date, this contraceptive remains elusive. Nevertheless, acceptable male contraceptive methods include periodic abstinence (fertility awareness-based method), coitus interruptus (withdrawal), condoms, hormonal contraception and vasectomy. Traditional methods (periodic abstinence, coitus interruptus and male condoms) are considered as widely available and reversible contraceptive options but are associated with relatively low effectiveness. In particular, the typical first-year failure rate of traditional male contraceptive methods is approximately 20% for periodic abstinence, 19% for withdrawal and 12% for condoms. Moreover, these traditional methods can lead to a disturbance in sexual activity. It should be also highlighted that male condoms have been predominantly established as a common method for birth control due to their protective properties against sexually transmitted infections and not due to their contraceptive role [3].

Theoretically, among all available approaches for male contraception, hormonal methods hold the key, as they come closest to fulfilling the aforementioned criteria on the ideal contraceptive. More specifically, hormonal approaches display high effectiveness, wide availability and reversibility. Similar to female hormonal contraception, male hormonal contraception relies on the suppression of gonadotropins, which results to the depletion of intratesticular testosterone and, in turn, to the suppression of spermatogenesis. Importantly, the substitution of peripheral testosterone maintains androgenicity and minimizes the systematic side effects of induced contraception. To date, numerous contraceptive regimens have been implemented, including androgen monotherapy, combination therapy with androgens and gonadotropin releasing hormone (GnRH) analogues, combination therapy with androgens and progestogens, as well as other hormone-based and non-hormone-based experimental regimens. Among these options, the combination therapy with androgens and progestogens displays encouraging results, equivalent to that of female hormonal contraception methods. Still, the inconvenient administration, the restricted efficacy in some men, the safety issues raised for most regimens, the high costs of the available preparations and the lack of pharmaceutical industry support have limited the use of hormonal male contraception in everyday clinical practice [4].

Given that traditional contraceptive methods (periodic abstinence, coitus interruptus and male condoms) display relatively low effectiveness and considering that hormonal male contraception approaches are still more or less experimental, vasectomy remains the standard-of-care for male contraception. Vasectomy is a simple outpatient operation, performed under local anesthesia, in which the vas deferens is dissected bilaterally through a small scrotal incision. Even though there are significant cultural issues in the acceptability of this procedure, more than 50 million men have undergone vasectomy worldwide. Of note, vasectomy is highly effective, with a typical first-year failure rate of less than 0.5% and a low rate of complications. Nevertheless, vasectomy is mainly considered a permanent method for male contraception. Even though vasectomy reversal (vasovasostomy) restores fertility in up to 90% of the cases, its success depends on the time elapsed between the vasectomy and the vasovasostomy procedure, as well as on the type of preferred technique for both procedures. Based on the previous notion, given that about 3% of men with vasectomy request reversal, semen cryopreservation may be recommended before the initial procedure. Therefore, vasectomy is predominantly reserved for men who do not desire any future fertility.

Male contraception is essential for the further reduction of unintended pregnancies and for the fair distribution of the risks of contraception between women and men. To date, only 30% of couples rely on male contraceptive methods, i.e., condoms and vasectomy. The aforementioned shortcomings of these methods have sparked the interest in new types of male contraceptives. In this chapter, we described the principles of male reproductive physiology and we explored the role of current pharmaceutical and surgical approaches for male contraception.

Principles of the Male Reproductive Physiology

The spermatogenesis is regulated by the hypothalamic-pituitary-testicular axis, which works as a classic negative-feedback hormonal loop. Under normal circumstances, the hypothalamus releases GnRH, which further stimulates the anterior pituitary gland to release gonadotropins (LH and FSH). Consequently, LH stimulates the Leydig cells of the testes to produce testosterone in large concentrations, which is, in turn, mandatory for the activation of the Sertoli cells and for the maintenance of spermatogenesis. Concurrently, FSH directly stimulates the Sertoli cells of the testes, which act supportively to the maturation of the spermatozoa. Accordingly, testosterone binds to androgen receptors located in the hypothalamus and in the anterior pituitary gland and regulates the release of GnRH and gonadotropins, closing the negative-feedback hormonal loop. Similarly, testosterone binds to androgen receptors throughout the whole body to exert its normal central and peripheral androgenic effects.

The existing non-hormonal approaches for male contraception focus on interrupting different steps in sperm production, on blocking sperm transport during ejaculation and on impairing the ability of the spermatocytes to gain motility after ejaculation. On the contrary, the existing hormonal approaches for male contraception target the negative-feedback hormonal loop of the hypothalamic-pituitary-testicular axis. All available hormonal regimens rely on the administration of exogenous androgens, which bind to androgen receptors located in the hypothalamus and in the anterior pituitary gland and inhibit the release of GnRH, LH and FSH. This gonadotropin inhibition depletion spermatogenesis in most men by depleting the production of testosterone from the Leydig cells and by leading to Sertoli cell dysfunction. Concurrently, the exogenously administered androgens bind to the androgen receptors located in other tissues, maintaining the androgenic action of testosterone and preventing the development of male hypogonadism [5]. The normal function of the hypothalamic-pituitary-testicular axis, as well as the effects of male hormonal contraceptive regimens on the axis are presented in Fig. 15.1.

The available clinical trials on hormonal male contraceptive regimens have showcased that combination therapy with androgens and progestogens provides a firm suppression of the hypothalamic-pituitary-testicular axis. Therefore, it is currently considered the most effective type of male hormonal contraception compared to other regimens. The goal of suppressing the hypothalamic-pituitary-testicular axis is to reduce sperm concentrations to levels low enough for contraceptive

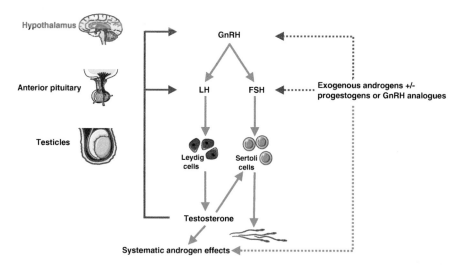

Fig. 15.1 The normal hypothalamic-pituitary-testicular axis physiology and the effects of male hormonal contraceptive regimens on the axis. FSH follicle-stimulating hormone, GnRH gonadotropin-releasing hormone, LH luteinizing hormone. All images have been drawn from Servier Medical Art, licensed under Creative Commons Attribution 3.0 unported License

protection (lower than 10^6 spermatozoa/mL of ejaculate) or, ideally, to azoospermic levels. A complete circle for the production of mature sperm in the human testes lasts approximately 72 days. Therefore, all available male contraceptives that inhibit sperm production display a delay in the onset of efficacy of more than 2 months. Based on the previous notion, sperm production is only restored several months after discontinuation of a male contraceptive method.

Spermatogenesis begins at puberty and is categorized in four distinct phases: (1) spermatocytogenesis; (2) spermatidogenesis; (3) spermiogenesis and; (4) spermiation. Spermatogenesis starts with proliferation of the spermatogonial stem cells. These cells are located in a basal niche in the epithelial wall of the seminiferous tubules, next to the basement membrane and are closely associated with the Sertoli cells. Spermatogonia initially undergo a mitotic phase, also known as spermatocytogenesis, in which they give rise to the diploid, primary spermatocytes. This mitotic phase is followed by a meiotic phase, also known as spermatidogenesis, in which these spermatocytes double their chromosome complement and undergo two consecutive meiotic cell divisions, resulting in haploid spermatids. Accordingly, the spermatids are transformed into spermatozoa by the process of spermiogenesis. Spermiogenesis involves spermatid nuclear condensation and flagellum formation. Spermatogenesis ends with the spermiation, which comprises the maturation of the spermatozoa and their release into the tubular lumen [6]. The steps of the spermatogenesis in the seminiferous tubules are depicted in Fig. 15.2. The storage and further maturation of spermatocytes until ejaculation occur in the epididymis. Finally, spermatocytes gain their full motility and fertilizing capacity once being in the female genital tract.

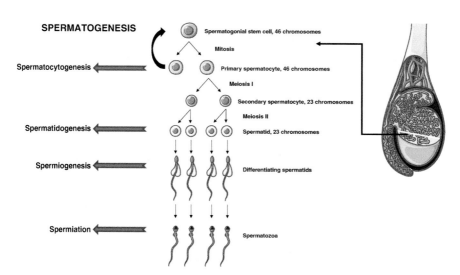

Fig. 15.2 The normal steps of the spermatogenesis in the seminiferous tubules. All images have been drawn from Servier Medical Art, licensed under Creative Commons Attribution 3.0 unported License

Current Pharmaceutical Approaches for Male Contraception

Testosterone Monotherapy

The administration of testosterone orally or topically was initially considered ineffective, as it is quickly degraded by the liver. As a result, most trials on male hormonal contraceptive regimens were conducted with testosterone injections or implants. In the early clinical trials, sperm parameters were used as a surrogate marker for efficacy. Therefore, two multicenter, pivotal trials on testosterone-based hormonal male contraception were conducted by the World Health Organization to assess, based on pregnancy rates, the efficacy of testosterone enanthate administered as weekly intramuscular injections. In the first study, 60% of men displayed azoospermia, while an additional 30% presented severe oligospermia. In the second study, testosterone enanthate demonstrated an overall contraceptive efficacy of 96.6%. Even though these landmark studies showcased the feasibility of a hormonal approach to attain male contraception, they did not offer a practical method. More specifically, the androgenic adverse events (mood and libido changes, acne, polycythemia, weight gain, hypertension and abnormal liver function tests), the dissatisfaction with the weekly injection schedule, the long duration of onset of and recovery from azoospermia, as well as the racial differences in the efficacy of testosterone monotherapy limited its implementation [7, 8].

Given that longer-acting testosterone preparations seemed more promising regarding practicability and acceptability, efforts were made to evaluate other androgen compounds. Among the available compounds, testosterone undecanoate was considered the most promising, as it required monthly intramuscular administration. In a phase II clinical trial, Chinese investigators demonstrated an overall efficacy rate of 94.8% on sperm suppression with testosterone undecanoate injections [9]. Based on these encouraging findings, the investigators conducted a phase III multicenter, clinical trial in 1045 men in China. Testosterone undecanoate 500 mg was administered as monthly injections after an initial loading dose of 1000 mg. Overall, the efficacy of testosterone undecanoate on sperm suppression was 93.9%. A total of nine pregnancies in 1554.1 person-years of exposure were reported. This corresponded to a cumulative contraceptive failure rate of 1.1 per 100 men [10]. These studies provided substantial evidence that testosterone undecanoate monotherapy may be a safe, effective and reversible contraceptive method for Asian men. However, the androgenic adverse events, the long duration of onset of and recovery from azoospermia and the lack of high efficacy in Caucasian males were still considered major concerns.

Other testosterone monotherapies were also evaluated in some relatively small clinical trials, demonstrating limited efficacy. The role of testosterone implants on male hormonal contraception was also explored as a surrogate to avoid regular intramuscular injections. The relatively low proportion of men attaining sperm suppression thresholds, as well as the intervention required for its implantation have restricted the use of testosterone implants in clinical practice [11]. The landmark efficacy trials exploring the role of testosterone monotherapy as male hormonal contraception are summarized in Table 15.1.

Combination of Androgens with GnRH Analogues

In an attempt to increase the efficacy of androgens on suppression of spermatogenesis, a combination therapeutic approach with androgens and GnRH analogues has been evaluated in some clinical trials. The potency of GnRH analogues on the suppression of the male hypothalamus-pituitary-testicular axis is well-established from studies on prostate cancer. GnRH agonists suppress gonadotropins and, in turn, intratesticular testosterone by GnRH receptor downregulation, after an initial phase of stimulation. However, their efficacy when combined with testosterone was not superior compared to testosterone monotherapy. On the contrary, GnRH agonists combined with testosterone seemed to be more effective compared to testosterone monotherapy. Still, despite these encouraging findings, the need for regular injections and the high costs of the existing regimens pose a barrier on this male contraception approach and have also discouraged the pharmaceutical industry from implementing high-quality trials on the matter. Oral GnRH antagonists may be the future of male contraception, but they have not yet been available for testing as a contraceptive method [12].

Combination of Androgens with Progestogens

The potency of progestogens on the suppression of gonadotropins as an effective supplement to estrogens is well-established from studies on female contraceptives. Similarly, multiple studies combining androgens (mainly testosterone) with different progestogens have been performed to identify a suitable regimen for male contraception. Most studies demonstrated high efficacy in terms of spermatogenesis suppression. Nevertheless, they suffered from methodological flaws as they did not follow internationally accepted guidelines on their conduction and did not have a randomized controlled design. Accordingly, it should be noted that most of these trials were investigator-initiated and were not performed as trials for approval from the regulatory authorities. Motivated by the growing interest, the pharmaceutical industry finally performed two high-quality trials. Even though these studies confirmed the high efficacy of combination treatment with androgens and progestogens, their findings were not corroborated by further studies on the field. It even seems that the pharmaceutical industry was discouraged from the conduction of additional clinical trials about novel hormonal male contraceptives [13].

In the first industry-sponsored, double-blind, randomized, placebo-controlled clinical trial, testosterone undecanoate injections were evaluated in combination with etonogestrel implants in different regimens. This clinical trial involved 354 volunteers randomized into seven groups. Participants received a low- or high-release etonogestrel implant combined with intramuscular testosterone undecanoate

I. Sokolakis et al.

Table 15.1 Pivotal high-volume, multicenter studies on testosterone monotherapy and on combination therapy with testosterone and progestogens for male hormonal contraception

Study	Sperm concentration threshold (10^6/mL)	Contraception regimen	Participants, n	Ethnicity	Participants completing suppression phase, n (%)	Participants reaching sperm threshold, n (%)	Participants entering efficacy phase, n	Participants completing efficacy phase, n	Participants with sperm rebound, n (%)	Person-years for pregnancy rate	Number of pregnancies, n
WHO (1990)	Azoospermia	TE im 200 mg/week	271	Mixed	225 (83%)	157 (70%)	157	119	21 (1.4%)	123.8	1
WHO (1996)	<3	TE im 200 mg/week	399	Mixed	357 (89%)	349 (97.8%)	268	209	4 (0.2%)	279.9	4
Gu et al. (2003)	<3	TU im 1000 mg load +500 mg/month	308	Asian	308 (100%)	299 (97.1%)	296	280	6 (2.3%)	143	0
Gu et al. (2009)	<1	TU im 1000 mg load +500 mg/month	1045	Asian	898 (86%)	855 (95.2%)	855	733	10 (1.3%)	1554.1	9
Mommers et al. (2008)	<1	TU im 750 mg/10 weeks or 12 weeks or TU im 1000 mg/12 weeks + Etonogestrel implants low/high dose or Placebo	354	Caucasian	No suppression phase	293 (89%)	349	324	17 (5.2%)	Not assessed	Not assessed
Behre et al. (2016)	<1	TU im 1000 mg + Norethisterone enanthate 200 mg/8 weeks	320	Caucasian	283 (88%)	274 (95.9%)	266	111	6	NA	4

im intramuscular, *NA* not available, *TE* testosterone enanthate, *TU* testosterone undecanoate injections (750 mg every 10 weeks, 750 mg every 12 weeks or 1000 mg every 12 weeks) or placebo implant and injections. Across all treatment groups, the efficacy of combination therapy was approximately 90% on sperm suppression. Unfortunately, the pharmaceutical companies sponsoring this trial did not further pursue this work due to changes in their policy and due to the inconvenient administration of both implants and injections [14].

In the second pivotal high-volume, multicenter phase II clinical trial, testosterone undecanoate injections were evaluated in combination with intramuscular norethisterone enanthate every 8 weeks. A total of 320 males were recruited in this prospective, single-arm trial across 10 participating centers. Four pregnancies occurred resulting in a failure rate of 2.2 per 100 person-years. Importantly, 96% of the participants achieved the sperm suppression threshold. However, an external safety review committee issued the early termination of this trial due to concerns regarding mood changes (including a suicide), depression, pain at the injection site and increased libido. Despite its early termination, this study may serve as a valuable reference for the design and implementation of further high-quality trials on male contraceptives. Additionally, it provided robust evidence regarding the high efficacy of combination treatment with androgens and progestogens. Of note, more than 85% of the participating couples stated that they would have used this method of contraception if it were made commercially available, despite its safety concerns [15]. The landmark efficacy trials exploring the role of combination therapy with testosterone and progestogens as male hormonal contraception can be seen in Table 15.1.

Several small-scale clinical studies have been performed with various schemata of testosterone and progestogens. Depot medoxyprogesterone acetate was the first progestogen that was evaluated in the context of clinical trials for male contraception. However, it was associated with high discontinuation rates and a long duration of onset of and recovery from azoospermia. Similar to etonogestrel, desogestrel has also shown good suppression levels of spermatogenesis. Levonorgestrel has been also evaluated in multiple clinical studies. Although levonorgestrel seems to be effective for the suppression of spermatogenesis, its drawbacks include greater weight gain and reduction in HDL cholesterol, compared to testosterone monotherapy. Furthermore, cyproterone acetate has also been studied in small clinical trials, demonstrating high efficacy when combined with testosterone injections [16].

Hormone-Based and Non-hormonal Experimental Regimens

Most available clinical trials on male hormonal contraceptives have implemented regular injections or short-lasting implants. To date, oral hormonal regimens were not adequately studied due to concerns about hepatotoxicity or due to the need for multiple daily doses. Accordingly, topical regimens were not frequently studied due to their restricted efficacy. Similar to the female oral pill, research is now focusing on oral and topical male contraceptive methods to increase their convenience of administration, to maximize their efficacy and to minimize their adverse events. To date, several oral and topical hormonal regimens have been launched in the setting of a clinical trial. Both progestogens such as segesterone acetate and androgens such as dimethandrolone or 11β-19-nortestosterone have been evaluated with promising findings. Still, even though these agents have the potential for clinical utility, their efficacy and safety in large clinical trials remain to be determined [17].

There is a growing interest in the development of non-hormonal male contraceptives. Non-hormonal male contraceptive approaches do not utilize compounds that block the hypothalamic-pituitary-testicular axis. On the contrary, they aim to interrupt different steps in sperm production and to block sperm transport or sperm motility. Even though non-hormonal contraceptive regimens do not have any impact on testosterone and thus, may not cause testosterone-related adverse events, their lack of efficacy has limited so far their use.

Current Surgical Approaches for Male Contraception

Vas-Occlusive Methods

Vas-occlusive methods are alternatives to vasectomy. They also aim at blocking and preventing the passage of sperm to the ejaculate, but with higher, faster and easier reversibility. Over five decades, many attempts at vas-occlusive contraception have been made using various devices such as injectable intra-vas plugs and in situ forming polymers. In situ forming polymers are injected as a liquid and form the gel or implant within the lumen of vas deferens. To date, no vas-occlusive method has successfully gained regulatory approval [18].

Vas-occlusion, a concept initially introduced in the late 1960s, describes a method for inducing infertility in the male by implanting a device (plug) into the vas deferens to block sperm transport. Five decades of research on vas-occlusion has shown that the ideal vas-occlusive contraceptive should have the following properties: (a) should be easily administered by a single physician, (b) should form instantaneously within the lumen without subsequent migration, (c) should effectively block the passage of sperm, (d) should be easily reversible by dissolution or via minor procedure, and (e) should have no significant permanent histological effects on the vas deferens, sperm, or genitourinary tissues. If these criteria are fulfilled, vas-occlusive methods have great potential to become the first class of long-lasting, nonhormonal, and reversible male contraception [19].

Reversible Inhibition of Sperm Under Guidance (RISUG) and Vasalgel

There are mainly two in situ forming polymers, which have been widely studied in the literature. The first one is RISUG (Reversible Inhibition of Sperm Under Guidance). It was developed and first tested in Indian population. RISUG is a formulation containing 60 mg of the crystal-clear polymer styrene maleic anhydride (SMA) dissolved in 120 μL of the organic solvent dimethyl sulfoxide (DMSO). When the solution is injected into an aqueous environment, such as the lumen of the vas deferens, the SMA polymer precipitates to form a partial or complete occlusion.

At the same time, it develops morphological aberrations of the sperm that manage to pass through. This could be attributed to SMA pH lowering effects, which result in sperm to undergo degeneration and morphological changes upon contact with the polymer [20].

Clinical trials investigating the effectiveness and safety of RISUG have successfully demonstrated no reported pregnancies within a 1-year follow-up period, after a single application. A recent phase III clinical trial in 139 young males showed that 95% achieved after a single injection either severe oligozoospermia or azoospermia at the first sperm examination 1 month following the treatment. 83% of the participants had continued azoospermia in the following month and the rest 17% manifested azoospermia within 3–6 months [21]. However, the surgical approach requires exteriorization of the vas deferens. The vas deferens is elevated using sutures and blunt instruments for stabilization during the injection. Once isolated, the vas was injected with 120 μL of RISUG using a 22-gauge needle in the cranial direction [18].

A single application seems to be effective, has few adverse effects and is easily reversible by injecting 200–500 μL of DMSO or 5% $NaHCO_3$ into the vas deferens, causing the extrusion of RISUG from the urethra. Adverse effects include slight testicular swelling without associated pain, which is self-limited within 15 days. In contrast to vasectomy, it does not cause granulomas or an autoimmune response. There are concerns with respect to the potential toxic effects and teratogenicity of the material, also regarding adverse effects on male reproductive organs. Ongoing studies are needed to prove the efficacy and long-term safety of the method [20].

A similar in situ polymer-based product being developed in the United States is Vasalgel, which comprises the polymer styrene maleic acid dissolved in DMSO rather than the anhydride form used in RISUG. Compared to RISUG, Vasalgel claims no spermicidal effects and it is rather described as a plug impenetrable to sperm. As with RISUG, the high viscosity of the Vasalgel solution requires a significant amount of pressure to instil the material in the narrow lumen of the vas deferens with the potential for damage associated with infiltration of Vasalgel into the wall of the vas deferens. It could be reversed by injection of $NaHCO_3$. No follow-up studies have been conducted to date assessing fertility and pregnancy rates after Vasalgel of RISUG reversal [18].

Percutaneous Intra-Vas Plugs

Two different types of injectable intraluminal plugs have been tested: medical polyurethane (MPU) and medical silicone resin (MSR) plugs. These plugs are usually inserted through a percutaneous delivery approach. The percutaneous method is less invasive and may offer fewer complications such as swelling, hematomas, and infection. Furthermore, given the non-surgical approach, men may also be more willing to undergo the procedure and thus, acceptability and usage of the contraceptive could be higher. The MPU plugs have been tested mainly in China in large-scale clinical trials, with the largest group including 12,000 men. Almost 98% of men achieved azoospermia. However, 18–24 months were required to achieve this level of efficiency. Furthermore, following the study, there were significant uncertainties about the safety of the MPU material, including potential carcinogenic effects of the aromatic amines contained in MPU. So far, the experience of many years of use in China has been free of incidents of toxicity [18].

The results for the MSR plugs were not particularly promising as azoospermia rates did not exceed 80%. On the other hand, their placement is easier. One concern for using plugs such as polyurethane and silicone are that large hand-pumps or applicators are required to inject the material. The complication rate is low, while plug removal is performed under local anesthesia on an outpatient basis and restores fertility in approximately 85% of men. The reversal of the contraceptive action is slow but steady and may be achieved in 2–4 years. Moreover, it has the theoretical advantage of repeatability, since removing and replacing can be performed without substantial damage. However, in the Dutch study, it was determined that the silicone plugs caused extensive fibrosis and tissue reaction around the occlusion site. This suggests simple plug removal for reversal could be difficult, most likely requiring excision and re-anastomosis of the vas deferens [20].

Recently an image-guided percutaneous delivery of a propriety vas-occlusive hydrogel has been evolved. Unlike plugs, hydrogels may be injected in aqueous solvents. Once formed, they are semi-open network systems joined by cross-links, and as such, they can entrap a large fraction of solvent such as biological fluid within the pores or interstitial space. The ability to swell and absorb fluid may allow for vas-occlusive hydrogels to alleviate hydrostatic pressure within the vas deferens or epididymis, resulting in occlusion and contraception, although this property requires further investigation [5].

Vasectomy

Vasectomy is safer, simpler, less expensive, and equally as effective as female sterilization. However, it remains one of the least known and least used methods of contraception. Female sterilization is used about three times as often. Vasectomy often is ignored, despite its being one of the safest, simplest, most highly effective, and least-expensive contraceptive method. Vasectomy remains the family planning method that is least known, understood, or used, a fact confirmed in Demographic and Health Survey studies conducted in 21 countries over the past 5 years [22].

Worldwide, an estimated 33 million of married women aged 15–49 (less than 3%) rely on their partner's vasectomy for contraception. Vasectomy is more common than female sterilization in only five countries: Bhutan, Canada, the Netherlands, New Zealand, and the Great Britain. Globally, after steadily increasing in the 1990s, the number of couples relying on vasectomy has dropped back to a level seen in the early 1980s. According to data from the National Study of Family Growth, approximately 17% of women between the ages of 15 and 44 years have had tubal sterilization, while only 6% rely on male sterilization for contraception. Vasectomy is utilized by 6–13% of American couples for their form of contraception and more than 75% of vasectomies are performed by urologists [23].

The benefits of vasectomy over tubal ligation include faster recovery and return to work, local rather than general anesthesia, and ability to perform the procedure in the office rather than in the operating suite. Complications are rare for both procedures. Men in every part of the world and every cultural, religious, or socioeconomic setting have demonstrated interest in or acceptance of vasectomy despite commonly held assumptions about negative male attitudes or societal prohibitions. Because men lack full access to information and services, however, they cannot make informed decisions or take an active part in family planning.

Preoperative Counselling

Preoperative counselling of the patient is extremely important, and may prevent postoperative patient dissatisfaction or even litigation. Preoperative consultation should inform and prepare the patients for the potential risks, benefits and alternatives prior to committing to a procedure. A face-to-face consultation with the patient is recommended before planning the vasectomy and it is sometimes beneficial for the patient's partner to be present. Patients should be counselled that vasectomy should be considered a permanent and irreversible form of contraception. Although options for fertility after vasectomy are possible (vasectomy reversal or sperm retrieval with in vitro fertilization), these are expensive and not 100% successful. The European guidelines on vasectomy note young age and absence of a relationship as relative contraindications to vasectomy [24].

During consultation the patient should be counselled that vasectomy is not immediately effective for sterility, and another form of birth control should be used until successful vas occlusion is confirmed by post-vasectomy semen analysis. The time from vasectomy to azoospermia or rare non-motile sperm can vary from weeks to months, depending on frequency of ejaculation, patient age and anatomical variation. Post-vasectomy semen analyses are necessary to demonstrate success of the procedure. Patients who fail to achieve azoospermia may require repeat vasectomy. Once the post-vasectomy spermiogram demonstrates sterility, a very small risk of future pregnancy remains (around 1 in 2000) [22].

Most vasectomies can be performed in the clinician's office, utilizing local anesthesia. Preoperative consultation should involve an examination of the scrotal contents, including mobilization of vas, to identify whether a patient may require sedation during vasectomy. If the patient is unable to tolerate this examination while isolating the vas deferens, he may not be a good candidate for local anesthesia [24]. The most important points to be addressed at the preoperative visit are shown in Table 15.2.

Techniques

There is a myriad of vasal isolation and occlusion techniques. Generally, prophylactic antimicrobials are not indicated at the time of vasectomy unless the patient is at high risk for infection. Scrotal skin should be shaved, and the patient prepped with antimicrobial solution and draped in a standard sterile fashion. The procedure may be noticeably easier if the Dartos smooth muscle is relaxed, so using warm preparation solution and avoiding cold room temperatures may be beneficial [24].

Table 15.2 The most important points to be addressed at the preoperative visit before vasectomy

Important points to be addressed at preoperative visit
• Alternatives to vasectomy
• Risk of infection or hematoma (1–2%)
• Risk of chronic scrotal pain (1–3%)
• Refrain from ejaculation for 1 week after the procedure
• Vasectomy is considered permanent
• Vasectomy does not produce immediate sterility; another form of contraception is required after the procedure until vasectomy success is confirmed by semen analysis
• Early vasectomy failure: risk of needing repeat vasectomy (<1%)
• Late vasectomy failure: after vasectomy success is confirmed by semen analysis, there is still a small chance of pregnancy (approximately 1 in 2000)

The target site for the vasectomy should be the straight portion of the vas deferens using a scrotal approach. There is no clear advantage of using one midline incision rather than bilateral incisions, and this should be decided upon based on surgeon preference and comfort. The bilateral incision approach may decrease the chance of cutting the same vas. if a single scrotal incision is made, the surgeon should confirm that the bilateral vasa deferentia have been occluded.

Vasectomy is performed in two distinct steps: delivering and exposing the vas deferens out of the scrotum (vas isolation), and occluding the vas. The no-scalpel technique in comparison to the classic technique refers to vas isolation only and does not denote a method of vas occlusion. The no-scalpel technique has been found to have shorter operative times and to decrease the rate of hematomas, infections, and pain during the procedure. Today the standard of care is to perform a no-scalpel technique or a modified variation of it that remains minimally invasive. Once a loop of bare vas deferens is outside of the wound (regardless the isolation technique), it is then divided with scissors. The American and European guidelines agree that routine histologic examination of the vas deferens is not required [25, 26]. Therefore, a segment of the vas should not be routinely excised. If a segment of vas is excised, it should not exceed 1–2 cm in length [27].

In terms of achieving vasectomy success, the most important step comes after division of the vas and it is the vasal occlusion. There are several vasal occlusion techniques. They include intraluminal cautery of one or both ends, ligation with suture, occlusion with clips, fascial interposition, and any combination of these. Review of the literature reveals many studies examining each of these techniques, yet it is difficult to conclude which occlusion method is superior, owing to study flaws and lack of uniformity in terms of patient follow-up and measurement of success. Intraluminal cautery, or mucosal cautery, is performed by applying thermal cautery or low-voltage electrical cautery with a needle tip within the lumen of the vas. Fascial interposition has become a commonly used technique, because when used with other methods of occlusion it decreases vasectomy failure rates. The goal is to separate the two newly divided ends of the vas to reduce the chance of recanalization [28]. Another commonly used method of vas occlusion is suture ligation or clip occlusion of the vas. Because of the higher rates of failure, ligation of the vas without fascial interposition is not recommended. In an attempt to decrease the risk of post-vasectomy chronic pain, some have advocated using a variation of an open-ended vasectomy whereby the testicular end of the vas is left open, the abdominal end is occluded with mucosal cautery, and fascial interposition is then performed. Leaving the testicular end open is proposed to decrease back pressure on the epididymis and decrease the risk of chronic pain, although this has not yet been proved in clinical studies. Finally, there is the Marie Stopes International technique, where the vas is not divided. Instead, occlusion of the vas occurs after cauterization of the outside of the vas, creating a full-thickness injury on one side and a partial thickness injury on the other [22].

The skin opening can be closed with suture or left open, depending on surgeon preference. Strictly speaking, to be called a no-scalpel vasectomy the skin is not sutured.

Postoperative Care and Follow-Up

Typically, patients are recommended to apply intermittent ice applications to the scrotum for 8–12 h after the procedure to minimize swelling. Athletic support devices may be worn for scrotal support for 48 h after the surgery. Postoperative pain is a common concern of vasectomy patients. Paracetamol alone often provides adequate analgesia. Patients are usually instructed to avoid strenuous activity for 1 week after the procedure. After vasectomy, alternative methods of contraception should be used for 12 weeks as patients are considered fertile until sterility is documented by post-vasectomy semen analysis [24].

Although no standard protocol for determining sterility exists, semen analysis generally is performed 2–3 months after vasectomy. The issue of azoospermia as a required endpoint is controversial. Many investigators advocate performing post-vasectomy spermiogram after a minimum of 20 ejaculations. If the postoperative spermiogram demonstrates azoospermia, patients require no further testing and can be considered sterile. If it shows nonmotile sperm at this time, further testing on a monthly basis is required until azoospermia is documented. For men with persistent sperm concentrations >100,000/mL of ejaculate, serial semen analyses may be performed until 6 months after vasectomy, at which time a repeat vasectomy should be offered [29].

Complications

The frequency of complications of vasectomy is low, ranging from below 1% and up to 3%. Complications of vasectomy described in the literature include hematoma formation, infection, sterilization failure, sperm granulomas, short-term postoperative pain (nodal pain, scrotal pain, and ejaculation pain), and chronic pain syndrome [30]. The long-term safety of vasectomy is mainly threatened by cardiovascular disease, testicular or prostate cancer, long-term loss of sexual function after the operation, and the formation of antisperm antibodies. All possible complications of vasectomy with their incidence rate are shown in Table 15.3. There is no increased risk with vasectomy and autoimmune disease, cardiovascular disease, prostate cancer and sexual dysfunction. But long-term observation is still needed to obtain more

Table 15.3 Possible vasectomy complications

Vasectomy complications	Incidence rate
• Infection and hematoma	1–2% in minimal invasive techniques, hematoma up to 20% with the classic technique
• Chronic scrotal pain/post-vasectomy pain syndrome	Usually 1–3%, up to 14% in some series
• Early or late vasectomy failure	Usually <1%
• Sperm granulomas	Up to 40%
• Antisperm antibodies	No increased risk after vasectomy
• Sexual dysfunction[a]	No increased risk after vasectomy
• Cardiovascular disease[a]	No increased risk after vasectomy
• Changes in reproductive hormones[a]	No increased risk after vasectomy
• Prostate and testicular cancer[a]	No increased risk after vasectomy

[a]These possible complications of vasectomy are uncertain or proven wrong, but they are listed here because they can be found in the literature

evidence. Numerous reports have confirmed that vasectomy is a safe, reliable, and low-complication method for male birth control [31].

Vasectomy Reversal

A small proportion of patients after vasectomy (3–6%) will undergo vasectomy reversal operation. Desire for fertility and relief from post-vasectomy pain syndrome are the most frequent reasons. For patients desiring fertility, their options include undergoing either a vasectomy reversal operation or in vitro fertilization with intracytoplasmic sperm injection (IVF/ICSI). Several factors should be considered by the couple when choosing between these two options, such as time to pregnancy, number of desired children, time commitment, cost, and maternal age. Vasectomy reversal is typically more cost-effective and is the favored approach for patients desiring multiple pregnancies with unimpaired female partner fertility. Sperm extraction and cryopreservation at the time of vasectomy reversal should be discussed preoperatively. It should be offered as an option for patients who want to avoid a future sperm extraction in the event of persistent oligospermia or azoospermia following reversal [32].

Vasectomy reversal is accomplished by one of two techniques: vasovasostomy (VV) or vasoepididymostomy (VE). After identifying the two occluded ends of vas deferens, the first step is to reverse the occlusion technique usually by removing the damaged/occluded end. The most important step before proceeding to re-anastomosis is the macroscopic and microscopic evaluation of the vasal fluid. The macro- and microscopic appearance of the vasal efflux will inform the surgeon if secondary epididymal obstruction has ensued. In that case a VE is required. As can be expected, the finding of motile sperm within the vas deferens eliminates the possibility of epididymal obstruction, with post-VV patency rates approaching 96% for some series. Macroscopic the presence of "toothpaste"-like fluid is a product of the vasal epithelium, and in the absence of sperm, necessitates VE. However, clear fluid in large amounts after transection of the vas deferens generally indicate a patent epididymis, even in the absence of sperm [33].

The vasectomy reversal operation should be performed in experience high-volume centers. The vasovasostomy or vasoepididymostomy anastomosis is usually performed using a surgical microscope and 9-0 Nylon sutures (8-0 to 10-0) [34]. Recently some case series reported the efficacy of robotic assisted vasectomy reversal procedures with high success rates [35]. The complications rate is low. Return of sperm to the ejaculate occurred between a mean range of 1.7–4.3 months for VV and up to 6.6 months for VE. Late failures, defined as a return to seminal azoospermia, happened in up to 12% and 50% for VV and VE, respectively [36].

References

1. Planning F. A global handbook for providers. Geneva: WHO; 2007.
2. Guideline F. Correction: FSRH guideline (January 2019) combined hormonal contraception. Reprod Health. 2019;45:1–93.
3. Minhas S, Bettocchi C, Boeri L, Capogrosso P, Carvalho J, Cilesiz NC, et al. European Association of Urology guidelines on male sexual and reproductive health: 2021 update on male infertility. Eur Urol. 2021;80(5):603–20.
4. Thirumalai A, Page ST. Male hormonal contraception. Annu Rev Med. 2020;71:17–31.
5. Amory JK. Male contraception. Fertil Steril. 2016;106(6):1303–9.
6. de Kretser DM, Loveland KL, Meinhardt A, Simorangkir D, Wreford N. Spermatogenesis. Hum Reprod. 1998;13(Suppl_1):1–8.
7. World Health Organization Task Force on Methods for the Regulation of Male Fertility. Contraceptive efficacy of testosterone-induced azoospermia and oligozoospermia in normal men. Fertil Steril. 1996;65(4):821–9.
8. Contraceptive efficacy of testosterone-induced azoospermia in normal men. World Health Organization Task Force on methods for the regulation of male fertility. Lancet. 1990;336(8721):955–9.
9. Gu Y-Q, Wang X-H, Xu D, Peng L, Cheng L-F, Huang M-K, et al. A multicenter contraceptive efficacy study of injectable testosterone undecanoate in healthy Chinese men. J Clin Endocrinol Metab. 2003;88(2):562–8.
10. Gu Y, Liang X, Wu W, Liu M, Song S, Cheng L, et al. Multicenter contraceptive efficacy trial of injectable testosterone undecanoate in Chinese men. J Clin Endocrinol Metab. 2009;94(6):1910–5.
11. Chao JH, Page ST. The current state of male hormonal contraception. Pharmacol Ther. 2016;163:109–17.
12. Wang C, Festin MPR, Swerdloff RS. Male hormonal contraception: where are we now? Curr Obstet Gynecol Rep. 2016;5:38–47.
13. Nieschlag E. Clinical trials in male hormonal contraception. Contraception. 2010;82(5):457–70.
14. Mommers E, Kersemaekers WM, Elliesen J, Kepers M, Apter D, Behre HM, et al. Male hormonal contraception: a double-blind, placebo-controlled study. J Clin Endocrinol Metab. 2008;93(7):2572–80.
15. Behre HM, Zitzmann M, Anderson RA, Handelsman DJ, Lestari SW, McLachlan RI, et al. Efficacy and safety of an injectable combination hormonal contraceptive for men. J Clin Endocrinol Metab. 2016;101(12):4779–88.
16. Grimes DA, Lopez LM, Gallo MF, Halpern V, Nanda K, Schulz KF. Steroid hormones for contraception in men. Cochrane Database Syst Rev. 2012;3:CD004316.
17. Thirumalai A, Amory JK. Emerging approaches to male contraception. Fertil Steril. 2021;115(6):1369–76.

18. Khourdaji I, Zillioux J, Eisenfrats K, et al. The future of male contraception: a fertile ground. Transl Androl Urol. 2018;7:S220–35.

19. Cook LA, Van Vliet HA, Lopez LM, et al. Vasectomy occlusion techniques for male sterilization. Cochrane Database Syst Rev. 2014;2014:CD003991.

20. Kanakis GA, Goulis DG. Male contraception: a clinically-oriented review. Hormones (Athens). 2015;14:598–614.

21. Sharma RS, Mathur AK, Singh R, et al. Safety & efficacy of an intravasal, one-time injectable & non-hormonal male contraceptive (RISUG): a clinical experience. Indian J Med Res. 2019;150:81–6.

22. Rogers MD, Kolettis PN. Vasectomy. Urol Clin North Am. 2013;40:559–68.

23. Pile JM, Barone MA. Demographics of vasectomy—USA and International. Urol Clin North Am. 2009;36:295–305.

24. Johnson D, Sandlow JI. Vasectomy: tips and tricks. Transl Androl Urol. 2017;6:704–9.

25. Dohle GR, Diemer T, Kopa Z, et al. European Association of Urology guidelines on vasectomy. Eur Urol. 2012;61:159–63.

26. Velez D, Pagani R, Mima M, et al. Vasectomy: a guidelines-based approach to male surgical contraception. Fertil Steril. 2021;115:1365–8.

27. Art KS, Nangia AK. Techniques of vasectomy. Urol Clin North Am. 2009;36:307–16.

28. Dassow P, Bennett JM. Vasectomy: an update. Am Fam Physician. 2006;74:2069–74.

29. Sokal DC, Labrecque M. Effectiveness of vasectomy techniques. Urol Clin North Am. 2009;36:317–29.

30. Yang F, Li J, Dong L, et al. Review of vasectomy complications and safety concerns. World J Mens Health. 2021;39:406–18.

31. Adams CE, Wald M. Risks and complications of vasectomy. Urol Clin North Am. 2009;36:331–6.

32. Kirby EW, Hockenberry M, Lipshultz LI. Vasectomy reversal: decision making and technical innovations. Transl Androl Urol. 2017;6:753–60.

33. Patel AP, Smith RP. Vasectomy reversal: a clinical update. Asian J Androl. 2016;18:365–71.

34. Lipshultz LI, Rumohr JA, Bennett RC. Techniques for vasectomy reversal. Urol Clin North Am. 2009;36:375–82.

35. Gözen AS, Tokas T, Tawfick A, et al. Robot-assisted vasovasostomy and vasoepididymostomy: current status and review of the literature. Turk J Urol. 2020;46:329–34.

36. Namekawa T, Imamoto T, Kato M, et al. Vasovasostomy and vasoepididymostomy: review of the procedures, outcomes, and predictors of patency and pregnancy over the last decade. Reprod Med Biol. 2018;17:343–55.

Male Hypogonadism

16

Z. Kopa, F. St. Laurent, and N. Szücs

Abstract

In this chapter, the reader will get acquainted with the andrological importance, clinical features, diagnosis and treatment of Male hypogonadism. Primary-, secondary- and Late-onset hypogonadism are discussed in the aspect of andrology, sexual health and fertility.

Testosterone

Testosterone in the Male Development

The male embryo is already determined genetically by the time of fertilization, the SRY (Sex-determining region on Y chromosome) gene will stimulate testicular- and suppress ovarian development, by activation of downstream genes including SOX9 and steroidogenesis factor 1 (SF1), which lead to the differentiation of primordial germ cells into Sertoli and Leydig cells [1, 2]. At the seventh week of gestation, foetal Testosterone (T) levels will start to rise and will peak at week 12–18 of gestation, then rapidly decline. This T peak is essential for the development of male external genitalia. The second peak of T occurs in the second to third month after birth (mini-puberty) due to the activation of the Hypothalamo-Pituitary-Testicular Axis (HPTA). The activation HPTA will lead to high gonadotropin and sex steroid levels, which then decline to prepubertal levels by 6–9 months of age [3]. This T rise

Z. Kopa (✉) · F. St. Laurent
Andrology Centre, Department of Urology, Semmelweis University, Budapest, Hungary

N. Szücs
2nd Department of Internal Medicine, Faculty of Medicine, Semmelweis University, Budapest, Hungary

289

is responsible for the development of Ad spermatogonia, masculine sexual behaviour and penile growth. The third rise of T occurs at puberty (approximately 12–17 years of age), when the release of hypothalamic GnRH (Gonadotropin-releasing hormone) leads to the stimulation of sex-steroid synthesis and spermatogenesis due to LH (Luteinizing hormone) and FSH (Follicle stimulating hormone). In men, LH stimulates the secretion of testosterone from Leydig cells and FSH stimulates spermatogenesis and tubular growth. In a normally functioning HPT axis, the arcuate nucleus of the hypothalamus generates a pulsating release of gonadotropin-releasing hormone (GnRH) into the hypothalamic-pituitary portal system [4]. This results in the secretion of FSH and LH. In turn, these gonadal hormones decrease FSH and LH production, resulting in a negative feedback loop. FSH also stimulates the release of inhibin B from Sertoli cells, as such, both FSH and inhibin B are markers of spermatogenesis and Sertoli cell functions. FSH levels correlate with the number of spermatogonia, while low inhibin B levels indicate a stronger correlation with spermatogenic damage [5, 6]. FSH levels may be in the normal range when the number of spermatogonia is adequate, but there is a complete blockage of the spermatocyte or spermatid. Leydig cell function can be deduced from testosterone and insulin-like factor 3 levels (INSL3). INSL3 is secreted by both foetal and fully differentiated Leydig cells. Prepubertal immature Leydig cells and transformed cells only weakly express INSL3. As a result, INSL3 is thought to be more sensitive than testosterone in determining Leydig cell function. Please note, that not only the actions of T are responsible for the pubertal development but also its active metabolites dihydrotestosterone (DHT) and estradiol, metabolized by the target tissues [7].

Testosterone and its active form, DHT is responsible for a wide range of male characteristics and functions. DHT is linked to the development of the urogenital tract, genital skin, hair follicles, and liver. Furthermore, it is responsible for the masculine development of the external genitalia, the growth of the prostate gland and the penis, pubertal changes, darkening and folding of the scrotum, growth of pubic hair, and increase muscle mass. DHT is associated with acnes in the skin due to the activation of the sebaceous glands. Actions of T include the stimulation of Sertoli cells (spermatogenesis), increasing very low and low lipoprotein levels while decreasing high density lipoproteins, promoting the deposition of abdominal adipose tissue, increasing erythropoiesis, deepening the voice, stimulating bone growth, and it also has anabolic effects on the muscles resulting in a male physique. Male behaviour, emotional stability and sexual drive are also T linked [8].

Testosterone in Adulthood

T exhibits diurnal fluctuations in cyclic rises and falls during the day, higher morning levels can be measured, peaking between 05.30 and 08.00 (assuming an 8 hour-long sleep at night) and it falls over the next 12 hours, resulting in lower levels in the evening. Unfortunately, these high human T levels do not stay constant forever, several studies have shown that in men over the age of 35 there is an age related decline. The European Male Aging study showed that men in the age group of 40–70 years had a serum total T declined of 0.4% per year, bear in mind that obesity and lifestyle factors influenced this decline of T [9].

Hypogonadism

Hypogonadism is a condition with low or total absence of androgen secretion due to impaired physiologic functioning of the testicles. The signs and symptoms present-ing will be those linked to a lacking or low circulating T levels, and can affect all previously listed testosterone-dependent characteristics and functions, according to the onset of the dysfunction.

Developmental abnormalities, phenotypic alterations of the male body, loss of muscle mass, virilisation defects, and absence of sexual maturation, altered second-ary male sexual characteristics can be observed. Altered erythropoiesis (mild anae-mia), decreased bone density, increased BMI (Body Mass Index), poor concentration and memory, fatigue, decreased motivation and energy, diminished performance, sleep disturbances, hot flushes and depression are all common signs of male hypo-gonadism. Spermatogenic failure, male infertility is also a highly important conse-quence of the hypogonadal state. Sexual symptoms, the loss of libido, erectile dysfunction and delayed ejaculation are also characteristic of the condition. Type 2 diabetes mellitus, metabolic syndrome (MS), chronic obstructive lung disease (COPD), obstructive sleep apnoea syndrome (OSAS), renal failure, osteoporosis are conditions commonly associated with low testosterone levels. All of the above symp-toms will result in a significant reduction of the quality of life. Moreover, several studies proved, that hypogonadal males will have a shorter life span and will develop more comorbidities [10].

The origin of hypogonadism might be due to damages or defects on one of three levels: Testicular (primary), or Hypothalamo-pituitary (secondary), and a special form is linked to the aging process (late-onset).

Primary (Hypergonadotropic) Hypogonadism

Primary hypogonadism (PH) is more common than secondary, it results from a testicular failure, and can be classified as congenital or acquired. Maldescended or ectopic testicles, congenital anorchia, Klinefelter syndrome, disorders of sexual development (DSD), gonadal dysgenesis, 46,XX male syndrome, Noonan syn-drome and LH receptor mutations are congenital forms. Most common acquired causes of PH are testicular cancer, orchitis, testicular injuries, chemo- and radio-therapy, and acquired anorchia [11].

In PH the HPT axis is disrupted at the level of the testes, resulting in normal or low testosterone-, normal or elevated estradiol levels, elevated concentrations of sex-hormone-binding-globulin (SHBG) and increased FSH and LH levels. SHBG binds free testosterone, resulting in a further decrease in free testosterone levels. FSH levels correlate negatively with spermatogenesis; when spermatogonia are diminished or absent, FSH levels are generally elevated. Biochemically PH is characterized by low levels of T, as the total serum testosterone concentration is below the normal range: <12 nmol/L (350 ng/dL), with elevated gonadotropins (FSH and LH), accompanied by testosterone deficiency symptoms. In general, a testicular damage or malfunction caused Leydig- and/or Sertoli cell dysfunction will lead to a decreased or absent T production, where as a consequence of the lack of the negative feedback inhibition in the hypothalamus and pituitary gland elevated levels of GnRH, FSH and LH will arise. Impaired spermatogenesis is also a consequence, as these hormones will no longer exert their physiological function on the testicular cells.

Diagnosis

The diagnosis of primary hypogonadism is based on the presence of the symptoms of low or absent T, AND the biochemical evaluation of hypogonadism. Physical examination focuses on phenotype, secondary sexual characteristics, gynecomastia, testicular volume, testis consistency, and penile length. The clinical onset of pubertal changes can be followed using the "Tanner stages", which assess the secondary sexual characteristics in terms of genital and pubic hair changes [12]. Scrotal ultrasound is recommended, as it yields more information about testicular structure. Low tT (total Testosterone) levels mean values below the optimal range: <12 nmol/L (350 ng/dL). SHBG and calculated free testosterone level can add relevant information. The physician should take into account the diurnal fluctuations of T, with serum T peaking in the morning hours (08.00) and declining towards the evening (20.00) [13]. Elevated gonadotropins FSH over 6.9 IU/L, and LH over 8.0 IU/L are classical alterations. Laboratory measurement of prolactin levels is also recommended. In case of fertility issues, Inhibin B can provide more relevant information. For men of reproductive ages, semen analysis is essential for fertility evaluation [14].

Treatment

Hormone replacement (Testosterone Replacement Therapy—TRT) is the standard treatment for Hypergonadotropic hypogonadism. Lifelong testosterone supplementation is usually initiated when the patient's testosterone levels fall below the normal range and these laboratory findings are accompanied by the symptoms and features of hypogonadism. The treatment guidelines include oral testosterone undecanoate capsules, subdermal implants, pellets, transdermal gels or intramuscular testosterone ester preparations. The oral forms are eliminated through the liver, thus even larger doses might not be sufficient to reach normal levels of T, thus the desired effects, therefore, their use has recently decreased. Transdermal preparations should be rubbed into the skin early in the morning, the dose can be personally tailored, adjusted to individual needs. Gels are generally well tolerated, caution is needed to avoid the transfer of the gel onto another person. Parenteral injections (i.m.) have a long-term and consistent effect with mostly good compliance from the patient. Regular follow-up is needed, prostate-specific antigen (PSA), haemoglobin, haematocrit and liver functions should be controlled.

Testosterone supplementation clearly improves quality of life, it has been shown to increase libido, erectile function, body hair, and it reduces fatigue and irritability. It also improves symptomps of depression, social maladjustment, and intellectual and neuro-motor functions. Bone mineral density and erythropoiesis are also positively affected, as well as cardiovascular health, improving angina threshold and lowering vascular reactivity in hypogonadal men. Although, Testosterone substitution does correct most of the symptoms of androgen deficiency, but it has a clear negative effect on fertility.

Improving the chances for fathering a child in PH, endocrine interventions focus on improving testosterone without the use of TRT. Therapeutic protocol for hypogonadism using gonadotropins, selective estrogenic receptor modulators (SERMS), and aromatase inhibitors seeks to increase intratesticular testosterone levels and improve quality and quantity of sperm. Gonadotropins, such as human chorionic gonadotropin (hCG) or human menopausal gonadotropin (hMG), act by mimicking LH and FSH, respectively. These then stimulate Sertoli cells and increase intratesticular testosterone levels. SERMS function by blocking the negative feedback mechanism of testosterone on the HPA axis, decreasing their sensitivity to testosterone and increasing endogenous FSH and LH levels. Aromatase inhibitors block the conversion of androgens to estradiol, decreasing the level of circulating estrogens and re-equilibrating the testosterone/estrogen balance. The use of these pharmaceutical agents changes the intratesticular environment and supports remaining spermatogenic foci found in the testis of patients with Klinefelter syndrome (KS).

In the case of non-obstructive azoospermia (NOA), these therapies are usually initiated 3 months prior to surgical interventions. These therapies are not found to be beneficial in improving sperm retrieval rates (SRR) in normal karyotype NOA men. NOA patients can have residual foci of spermatogenesis (approx. 50% of the cases); so spermatozoa can be found in the testicular tissue. These foci of spermatogenesis can be found and sperm cells can be retrieved via surgical sperm retrieval techniques with a convenient safety profile: conventional or multifocal, random testicular sperm extraction (TESE) or microsurgical dissection (mTESE) and used for assisted reproduction, intracytoplasmic sperm injection (ICSI) treatments [15, 16].

Congenital Forms

Congenital Anorchia
It is a rare condition, testicles temporarily begin their development in utero, but a disruption of blood supply (intrauterine infections or testicular torsion) may lead to the atrophy of the testicles. Postnatally testes cannot be found neither via imaging nor with laparoscopy and the hCG evoked T rise is absent. Puberty will not be achieved and the phenotype becomes eunuchoid. After the expected time of puberty, testosterone replacement therapy is recommended, in case of intersex external genitalia, corrective plastic surgery is possible. Infertility cannot be treated.

Cryptorchidism
Cryptorchidism literally means hidden or obscure testis, it is the failure of the testicular descent into the scrotum; a congenital abnormality affecting about 1–3% of term infants, but more frequent in preterm boys (30–45%). The testes may descend into the scrotum in 75% of full-term neonates and in 90% of premature new-born boys by

the age of 1 year. The explanation can be the LH and FSH rise during the mini puberty. The diagnosis based on palpation and imaging techniques (ultrasonography and MRI) is insufficient, as non-palpable testicles cannot be accurately detected, so most recently laparoscopic surgery is recommended in the diagnosis and immediate treatment of non-palpable undescended testicles. Endocrinological and genetic examinations are required in cases of bilateral testicular maldescent. Anorchia can be diagnosed in cases of non-palpable testicles, when hCG evoked T response (hCG test) is lacking at postnatal ages of over 3 months. Inhibin B and AMH tests are useful tools in the diagnosis of bilateral agenesia of the testes [17, 18].

Cryptorchidism poses a higher risk for infertility, 10% of infertile males have a history of testicular maldescent, azoospermia occurs in 13% and 89% in men with unilateral and bilateral cryptorchidism, respectively. The risk for testicular cancer is 35–48 fold higher in cryptorchid patients, 10% of testicular cancer patients have a history of testicular maldescent. In adult patients there is a higher risk reported for testicular torsion [19].

It has been shown that the longer the time the testes spend undescended, the higher the degree of damage to germinal cells and Leydig cells [20]. Treatment should be initiated at the age of 6 months and is recommended to be completed by the age of 12 months. Hormonal treatment (testosterone, hCG, GnRH, hMG, hCG + FSH) has lower success rate (19–25%) and has recently become controversial [21]. Surgical corrections with orchiopexy or laparoscopic surgery have a higher success rates (90%), recently it has become the first line treatment modality. Despite the surgical treatment the risk for infertility still remains a question. Infertility amongst surgically treated patients was reported to be 54% in bilateral- and 9% in unilateral cases, 35% of early orchiopexy-treated patients were also found to be infertile. Malignancy risk was reported in several studies not be influenced by early orchiopexy, but a six fold increase was published in non-treated patient populations.

Noonan-Syndrome (Ullrich-Noonan Syndrome)
An autosomal dominant disorder associated with varying degrees of testicular hypogonadism and often uni- or bilateral cryptorchidism. It can occur in either sexes with an incidence of 1 in 1000–2500 new-borns. Noonan syndrome is associated with characteristic somatic stigmas, such as low stature, webbed neck (pterygium colli), cardiac malformations (atrial septal defects, hypertrophic cardiomyopathy, pulmonary stenosis), learning difficulties and coagulation disorders of varying severity. Testosterone replacement is usually required from puberty.

Androgen Insensitivity Syndrome
Androgen-insensitivity (AIS) is a result of a loss-of-function mutation of the androgen receptor encoding gene in persons with a karyotype of 46,XY. It is characterized by functioning testicles and sustained testosterone production. The clinical presentation greatly varies according to the severity of androgen resistance. In case of complete androgen resistance (CAIS) a female phenotype is observed, in moderate forms, partial androgen resistance (PAIS) ambiguous genitalia are present, and in mild cases, partial resistance (MAIS) leads to a male phenotype with varying degrees of hypogonadism or solely infertility.

Klinefelter Syndrome (KS)

The majority of KS patients (80–90%) have a 47,XXY karyotype, the remaining patients have a higher-grade aneuploidy (48,XXXY, 49,XXXXY), or possess fragments of supranumeral X chromosomes, or mosaicism (46,XY/47,XXY). The true number of mosaic KS patients may be under-identified as chromosomal mosaicism can be tissue-specific to the testes, with a normal karyotype in peripheral lymphocytes. Some mosaic KS men have less severe forms of infertility and can present with oligozoospermia [22].

The exact mechanism of androgen deficiency in KS is largely unknown, there is thought to be a correlation between the androgen receptor CAG repeat length and the variability in KS patient phenotype. An androgen receptor polymorphic trinucleotide repeat (three DNA building blocks (cytosine, adenine, and guanine) appear multiple times in a row—CAGn) located on the X-chromosome is in correlation with the phenotypic differences seen in KS. Normally, these repeats are 9 to 37 trinucleotides long, and the polyglutamine repeat length is correlated with physiological androgen effects [23].

Klinefelter's syndrome presents as a constellation of endocrine, metabolic, neurologic and psychosocial symptoms that vary in degree, and is also associated with a wide range of comorbidities.

The 'prototypic' features of KS include tall stature, gynecomastia, small but firm testicles, Hypergonadotropic hypogonadism, sub/infertility. Presenting symptoms of androgen deficiency in KS are largely age-dependent and range from severe signs of hypogonadism, such as testicular hypotrophy, infertility, decreased libido, erectile dysfunction, increased stature, reduced male-pattern body and facial hair, eunuchoid body habitus and gynecomastia, to the normally virilised male phenotype. Hormonal changes are especially age related. Prepubescent patients have normal plasma gonadotropin levels and a normal response to GnRH. Several studies showed that serum levels of FSH, LH, Testosterone, Inhibin B and AMH levels can be normal in prepubertal boys. During puberty, there is an increased concentration of plasma gonadotropin levels and an exaggerated response to GnRH. In pubertal patients, FSH and LH are elevated, a clear negative correlation can be seen between age and gonadotropins (FSH and LH). These observations are pivotal in the infertility treatment of KS patients. Regarding Leydig cell function, INSL3 plasma concentrations in prepubescent KS patients show no significant difference when compared to healthy boys, however, during mid-puberty, INSL3 levels decrease despite high levels of LH. By adulthood, INSL3 levels in KS patients are well below normal. Testosterone levels are normal or subnormal until puberty when, relative to the surge in normal males, they are substantially reduced. Testosterone levels are below normal in 65–85% of adult KS patients, but some patients may show concentrations within the normal range [24, 25].

Testicular hypotrophy in KS begins during early foetal life and progresses with age. Testicular degeneration has been observed in 47,XXY foetuses at gestational ages of 18–22 weeks. Histological changes include a decrease in the number of germ cells and a proportional increase in tubules devoid of germ cells. In prepubertal patients, testicular degeneration is already evident and shows accelerated degeneration during puberty. The regression of Sertoli cell function is supported by the observed decrease in inhibin B serum concentrations after early puberty. With age, KS presents histologically with abnormal seminiferous tubules that have extensive fibrosis and are entirely hyalinised. An absence of spermatogenesis, and interstitial hyperplastic Leydig cell nodules can be observed. Physically, testicular hypotrophy manifests as small, but firm testes [26].

The wide variety of phenotypes makes the clinical recognition of KS difficult and is still often diagnosed only upon treatment for infertility or endocrine function abnormalities later in life. It is estimated that as few as 25% of all males carrying the 47,XXY genotype are ever diagnosed. A phenotypic clinical presentation and higher physician awareness can lead to earlier suspected diagnosis. Testicular biopsy showing Leydig-cell hyperplasia and seminiferous tubule fibrosis is diagnostic after puberty. Definitive diagnosis is made by karyotype analysis.

Hormone replacement (Testosterone Replacement Therapy—TRT) is the standard treatment also for KS. Lifelong testosterone supplementation is usually initiated when the patient's testosterone levels fall below the normal range, which generally occurs in the middle of the third decade of life, however, TRT should be started as early as possible to avoid symptoms and features of hypogonadism. Early diagnosis and treatment of KS can profoundly improve the patient's quality of life and lower the risk for many of the comorbidities associated with the syndrome.

The age for the initiation of testosterone supplementation is frequently debated. Early observations showed that KS boys started on testosterone from early puberty were better adjusted and had improved cognitive abilities. Recent studies show that supplementation as early as infancy, also has an effect. Despite such evidence, there is still disagreement if testosterone therapy should be clinically indicated in the absence of Hypergonadotropic hypogonadism, as in KS infants and boys prior to puberty.

Since KS was first described, testosterone substitution has been the standard of treatment, despite there having been no controlled clinical studies aimed at determining appropriate dosing or optimal route of treatment. During the last decades, there have been more controlled studies and it is becoming acutely apparent that, although the positive effect of testosterone supplementation on the androgen deficiency aspect of KS is known, KS is associated with a variety of other social and health-related challenges that require more than what testosterone substitution can provide the patients with [27].

Regarding fertility aspects, KS is the most common genetic aetiology of infertility seen in 11% of azoospermic men. 47,XXY men are usually azoospermic (nonobstructive azoospermia) while mosaic XXY/XY men show varying rates of spermatogenesis from oligozoospermia to normozoospermia. Progressively degenerating testicular function ultimately leads to tubular atrophy, maturation arrest, fibrosis or hyalinization. In addition, KS is commonly associated with cryptorchidism resulting in further augmentation of testicular deficit [28].

Aromatase inhibitors are recommended for endocrinological treatment of KS patients with low tT levels. They block the conversion of androgens to estradiol, and improve testosterone levels. The use of these pharmaceutical agents changes the intratesticular environment and supports remaining spermatogenic foci found in the testis of KS patients. Most commonly, they are initiated 3 months prior to surgical interventions. KS patients generally start showing signs of hypergonadotropic hypogonadism at younger ages, thus requiring life-long androgen replacement therapy. Though this treatment does help with the various symptoms of hypogonadism and can lower the risk of developing significant comorbidities, the excess of exogenous androgens further suppresses remaining testicular functions and spermatogenesis. In adolescent KS patients aged 20 years or below, 70% had sperm in the ejaculated semen samples. It is therefore important to investigate the ability and willingness of the patient to provide sperm or testicular sperm for cryopreservation prior to the initiation of testosterone substitution. In the case of azoospermia surgical sperm retrieval and cryopreservation is the method of choice. Successful sperm retrieval is defined as the retrieval of an adequate number and quality of sperm for the use in subsequent ICSI. Conventional TESE and mTESE frequently show similar SRR and a younger patient age at the time of TESE is associated with more positive SRR, though thresholds have yet to be determined [29]. BMI was recently found to be significantly associated with SRR. The significance of the effect of serum testosterone level on SRR has been inconsistent, though higher levels have been found to be associated with positive SRR. The European Association of Urology (EAU) reports SRR in KS men to be 50%. However, infertility literature reporting SRRs in KS men continues to show inconsistency in the data. In the US, SRR in a population of KS men was reported as 72% in 2005 by Schiff et al. and 66% in 2009 by Schlegel et al. Multinational meta-analysis from Plotton et al. in 2014 and Corona et al. in 2017 report SRRs of approximately 50%. These rates are similar to the SRRs found in men with NOA not associated with chromosomal abnormalities [30–35]. Most recently however, several studies ran in Europe, Iran, Turkey and the UK have demonstrated significantly lower SRR varying between 20% and 35%. The cause of these lower retrieval rates has not been determined; however, demographics, real-life settings, and pharmacological stimulation have been considered as confounding factors attributing to lower reported SRR [36, 37].

Although this allows for the possibility of previously infertile KS men to become biological parents, KS patients are still found to have a lower quality of life compared to the general population. The most frequently cited causes of dissatisfaction are infertility and psychological challenges. There are still no universally implemented guidelines for KS treatment and it is critical that attention continues to be paid to the clinical outcome of testosterone substitution, optimizing treatment regimens and implementing comprehensive KS care [20, 38].

The 46,XX Males

It is the translocation of the SRY gene onto the X chromosome (or onto one of the autosomes), which is rare, occurring in 1 out of every 20,000 male new-borns with a varying degree of HG. Patients are short in stature, hypospadias is often observed and testosterone replacement may be necessary, but infertility is definitive [2].

Acquired Forms

Surgical Castration

This bilateral testicular dysfunction is caused by the loss of the testicles due to an accident, severe infection, torsion or surgical removal (testicular tumor). In long-term aspects, hypogonadism can be treated with testosterone replacement, but not infertility.

In the case of an accident or disease affecting both testicles, semen can be stored or sperm can still be surgically retrieved. Cryopreservation is strongly recommended for fertility preservation.

Infections

Viral mumps orchitis is the infection irreversibly affecting testicular function. It occurs more commonly in adults and in 80% of cases, only one testicle is affected. In children, mumps usually resolves without a trace, but if it occurs after puberty, it can damage seminiferous tubules. Testicular pain, scrotal swelling and fever are the leading symptoms, in adulthood testicular atrophy and abnormal semen analysis can be seen, mostly in bilateral cases. Today the incidence of mumps orchitis has decreased due to the compulsory vaccination protocol [39, 40].

Chemo and Radiotherapy

Chemotherapy has gonadotoxic effects, due to targeting rapidly proliferating cells. The severity of the harmful effect depends on the type of the agent, dosage and effect's location. Spermatogenic defect and disruption, moreover hyalinisation and fibrosis can be the consequence of drugs crossing the blood-testis barrier. Chemotherapy with alkylating agents are the most harmful in terms of spermatogenesis and hormonal balance. Leydig cells have a lower turnover and are therefore more resistant, but a dose-dependent Leydig cell dysfunction after chemotherapy is proven.

Radiotherapy affects testicular function depending on the gonadal dosage and delivery method. Irreversible damage occurs to spermatogenesis at 4 Gy dose. The more resistant Leydig cells can withstand a dose of up to 30 Gy. Recovery of spermatogenesis may start as late as 9 years post treatment, more accurate and gonad-protective deliveries allow for earlier recoveries, with doses of up to 1 Gy, recovery may start between 9–18 months, with 2–3 Gy, after 30 months and with 4 Gy, after 5 years if it even occurs. Irradiation causes sperm functional alteration in the form of increased sperm DNA fragmentation, which may continue for up to 2 years after treatment.

Combination of radio- and chemotherapy is more harmful than either treatment alone.

Hypogonadisms Associated with Systemic Diseases

Consecutive, i.e., Hypergonadotropic hypogonadisms associated with systemic diseases are a very heterogeneous entity in which primary testicular damage is dominant. In hemochromatosis, iron is deposited in the testes and in 1/3 of the patients it can lead to a varying degree of hypogonadism. The pituitary gland may also be affected, if so, hypogonadotropic hypogonadism develops. Excessive alcohol consumption decreases testosterone production by causing toxin-mediated hepatic cirrhosis and also, by the accumulation of SHBG, binding more free testosterone leading to hypogonadism. The inflammatory bowel disease—Crohn's disease itself, leads to primary hypogonadism by damaging the testicle, but also, sulphasalazin used in its treatment results in reversible germ cell damage. In case of severe chronic renal insufficiency a varying degree of hypogonadism can also be observed.

Secondary (Hypogonadotropic) Hypogonadism

Secondary hypogonadism is caused by hypothalamic or pituitary malfunctions, therefore gonadotropin levels are low, which result in the lack of stimulation of Leydig and Sertoli cells in the testes, resulting in a low or completely absent testosterone production and the lack of spermatogenesis (hypogonadotropic hypogonadism). Hypothalamic or pituitary damages can be classified as congenital or acquired. Amongst conditions of congenital origin, Kallmann syndrome has the highest impact, but Leptin receptor mutations, Prader-Willi syndrome and idiopathic isolated gonadotropin deficiencies should also be mentioned. Hyperprolactinaemia, drug induced gonadotropin suppression, diabetes mellitus and anabolic steroid use are acquired suppressive factors, whereas tumors, cysts, infiltrative diseases, infections, traumas and iatrogenic factors can be mentioned as other acquired causes that damage gonadotropic cells [41, 42].

Diagnosis

Biochemically, since GnRH cannot be measured, LH, FSH, testosterone serum concentration and calculated free testosterone are used instead for the diagnosis, with diagnostic criteria being: LH < 1.7 IU/L, FSH < 2.0 IU/L, and tT < 12.0 nmol/L (350 ng/dL). In secondary hypogonadism the measurement of prolactin levels is essential, since hyperprolactinaemia is one of the most common acquired causes of the disease. In secondary hypogonadism, pituitary imaging (MRI) is highly recommended to exclude pituitary and/or hypothalamic tumors or infiltrative diseases, especially when panhypopituitarism, persistent hyperprolactinemia, symptoms or signs of a tumor's mass effect, such as headache, visual impairment, or visual field defect, are present.

Treatment

In prepubertal and adolescent boys the aim of the treatment is to induce puberty and the development of the secondary sexual characteristics. In adults, the therapy should focus on maintaining normal sexual hormone levels, returning serum testosterone levels into the physiological range, improving the symptoms of hypogonadism, and avoiding secondary male characteristics. TRT usually means a life-long hormone replacement treatment. In the case of appropriate treatment and follow-up, secondary hypogonadism is not associated with decreased life expectancy, but can be accompanied by osteopenia or osteoporosis.

Testosterone replacement therapy was already discussed in the Primary hypogonadism chapter.

Fertility can be restored through the use of GnRH or gonadotropins, depending on the level of defect (hypothalamic or pituitary). GnRH can be given, if the pituitary gland is functioning normally. GnRH is usually given episodically by a pump mimicking its physiological release [43].

Gonadotropins can be given both to patients having dysfunctions in the hypothalamus or in the pituitary. For gonadotropin replacement, human chorionic gonadotropin (hCG) is usually given instead of LH. hMG (human menopausal gonadotropin) can also be used, it consists of both FSH and LH at a ratio of 1:1 and thus has the biological properties of both gonadotropins [44, 45].

The use of gonadotropin therapy (hCG + hMG or recombinant FSH) for fertility issues is the recommended way of treatment [46].

Hyperprolactinaemia

Causes of hyperprolactinemia include prolactin secreting tumors (prolactinomas) and medications, like phenothiazine and tricyclic antidepressants.

Hyperprolactinemia leads to the inhibition of GnRH secretion from the hypothalamus and subsequently, a decrease of FSH and LH, which in turn leads to a drop in T levels and alteration of spermatogenesis.

Kallmann Syndrome

A rare form of congenital isolated GnRH deficiency (10 in 100,000 boys) characterized by low serum gonadotropin (FSH and LH) levels and by consequent signs of hypogonadism. The lack of sexual maturity and absence of secondary male characteristics are accompanied by hyposmia or anosmia (decreased or absent smell) which is caused by failed migration of GnRH neurons from the olfactory placode into the hypothalamus during the embryonal stage of life.

Clinical, hormonal, genetic and imaging diagnostic work-up is required. Lack of puberty and hypogonadal features with hyposmia/anosmia can raise the suspicion. Typical features on the body observed are the absence of facial and pubic hair, small testicular volumes, shorter penile length, eunuchoid phenotype, long arms, decreased muscle mass and renal agenesis.

As a cause of this disease, more than 20 gene mutations have been detected. KAL1 was the first responsible gene associated with an X linked pattern of inheritance. These mutations occur especially in men with unilateral renal agenesis and mirror movements-bimanual synkinesis. FGR1 (KAL2) mutations are inherited as autosomal dominant traits associated with midline facial abnormalities, dental agenesis and short metacarpals. Although in most of the cases radiographic appearance of the hypothalamic-pituitary region is normal, MRI can be recommended to rule out any anatomical structural abnormalities (e.g., absence of olfactory structures).

Other forms of congenital isolated hypogonadotropic hypogonadism are also known without smell dysfunction. These congenital forms can be associated with mutations in the following genes: *GNRH1, KISS1, KISS1R (GPR54), TAC3, TACR3*, etc.

Therapy is the classical treatment recommended for secondary hypogonadism (TRT), in terms of fertility aspects, the above listed management strategy (hCG + gonadotropins) should be followed. At present, no treatment is available for the lack of smell and mirror-movements of the hands.

Anabolic Steroid Use

Androgenic-steroid use leads to hypogonadotropic hypogonadism, through the negative feedback loop of the hypothalamus and pituitary gland. This leads to the suppression of GnRH and a subsequent decrease of LH and FSH, resulting in the termination of endogenous testosterone synthesis and sperm production. The chronic use of exogenous androgens leads to decreased testicular volume, later in time, to testicular atrophy, decreased spermatogenesis and infertility. Once exogenous androgens are discontinued, symptoms of hypogonadism also arise. Other common side effects are gynecomastia, sexual dysfunction and polycythaemia. The prevalence of hypogonadism due to exogenous androgen use is not known, but shows an increasing tendency. This finding raises the importance of obtaining a detailed drug history, before prescribing testosterone to men with apparent hypogonadism.

Late-Onset Hypogonadism

Serum testosterone levels decrease with age. As they reach the subnormal levels, late-onset hypogonadism (LOH) occurs. LOH affects one in four men in the 65-year-old population, and its incidence has recently risen from 12% to 49% for the age group of 50–80 years old [5]. LOH is characterized by a co-occurrence of decreased testosterone levels and associated sexual, physical, and psychological symptoms. In the majority of men with LOH, co-morbidities are present, metabolic syndrome being the most common amongst them.

Diagnosis is based on the symptoms and laboratory findings (lower testosterone levels). The most common symptoms of LOH are decreased sexual desire and activity, erectile dysfunction, lack of morning erections, impaired physical fitness, and mood swings. Testosterone has no age-related normal value. Based on a summary of the literature, the cut-off level for optimal total testosterone is 12.1 nmol/L (351.0 ng/dL) [47].

Appropriate examinations are needed to exclude other organic factors, and to evaluate all possible functional alterations caused by the low testosterone level.

The first and most important step in treating LOH is lifestyle change, in many cases, this is already an effective treatment. If treatment for underlying conditions and lifestyle changes are not sufficient, testosterone replacement therapy is required. In LOH the topical (gel) treatment seems to be the first choice, intermittent therapy is recommended with careful follow-up of the patients.

Over the past decade, the number of testosterone medications prescribed to middle-aged or older men has increased exponentially. In addition to the many beneficial effects, the risk of testosterone supplementation has sparked serious professional debates. Also, some retrospective and prospective randomized studies have suggested that testosterone supplementation increases the incidence of cardiovascular diseases. In 2014, the FDA (U.S. Food and Drug Administration) issued a safety warning about the possibility of potential cardiovascular side effects. Low serum levels of endogenous testosterone alone are associated with increased cardiovascular risks, and this association has been shown in several cohort studies. A substantial association between hypogonadism and cardiovascular mortality and mortality from other causes has also been demonstrated in middle-aged and aging men [48]. Regarding the link between hormone replacement and cardiovascular disease, the findings are contradictory: some retrospective studies based on a prescription database have shown an increased incidence of cardiovascular events in TRT, while other studies have found a neutral or beneficial effect. Thus, the safe use of testosterone supplementation from a cardiovascular perspective is still under discussion. Regarding mortality, most studies have shown a protective effect of testosterone, although results have been reported where no such association has been found.

References

1. Coerdt W, Rehder H, Gausmann I, Johannisson R, Gropp A. Quantitative histology of human fetal testes in chromosomal disease. Pediatr Pathol. 1985;3:245–59.
2. Kashimada K, Koopman P. Sry: the master switch in mammalian sex determination. Development. 2010;137(23):3921–30.
3. Sadler TW. Langman's medical embryology. Philadelphia: Lippincott Williams & Wilkins; 2011.
4. Handelsman DJ, et al. Age-specific population centiles for androgen status in men. Eur J Endocrinol. 2015;173(6):809–17.
5. Anawalt BD, Bebb RA, Matsumoto AM, Groome NP, Illingworth PJ, McNeilly AS, Bremner WJ. Serum inhibin B levels reflect Sertoli cell function in normal men and men with testicular dysfunction. J Clin Endocrinol Metab. 1996;81(9):3341–5. https://doi.org/10.1210/jcem.81.9.8784094.
6. Kumanov P, Nandipati K, Tomova A, Agarwal A. Inhibin B is a better marker of spermatogenesis than other hormones in the evaluation of male factor infertility. Fertil Steril. 2006;86(2):332–8. https://doi.org/10.1016/j.fertnstert.2006.01.022.
7. Foresta C, Bettella A, Vinanzi C, Dabrilli P, Meriggiola MC, Garolla A, Ferlin A. Insulin-like factor 3: a novel circulating hormone of testis origin in humans. J Clin Endocrinol Metab. 2004;89(12):5952–8.
8. Stanton BA, Koeppen BM, Berne RM. Berne & Levy physiology, updated edition e-book. 6th ed., updated ed. Philadelphia: Mosby; 2010.
9. Harman SM, Metter EJ, Tobin JD, Pearson J, Blackman MR, et al. Longitudinal effects of aging on serum total and free testosterone levels in healthy men. Baltimore Longitudinal Study of Aging. J Clin Endocrinol Metab. 2001;86:724–31.
10. Kumar P, et al. Male hypogonadism: symptoms and treatment. J Adv Pharm Technol Res. 2010;1(3):297–301.
11. Vakalopoulos I, Dimou P, Anagnostou I, Zeginiadou T. Impact of cancer and cancer treatment on male fertility. Hormones (Athens). 2015;14(4):579–89. https://doi.org/10.14310/horm.2002.1620.
12. Marshall WA, Tanner JM. Variations in the pattern of pubertal changes in boys. Arch Dis Child. 1970;45(239):13–23.
13. Brambilla DJ, et al. The effect of diurnal variation on clinical measurement of serum testosterone and other sex hormone levels in men. J Clin Endocrinol Metab. 2009;94(3):907–13.
14. Travison TG, et al. Harmonized reference ranges for circulating testosterone levels in men of four cohort studies in the United States and Europe. J Clin Endocrinol Metab. 2017;102(4):1161–73.
15. Raheem AA, Ralph D. Complications of male fertility surgery for sperm retrieval in the azoospermic male. In: Rizk B, Gerris J, editors. Complications and outcomes of assisted reproduction. Cambridge: Cambridge University Press; 2017. p. 186–94. https://doi.org/10.1017/9781107295391.018.
16. Schlegel PN. Non-obstructive azoospermia: a revolutionary surgical approach and results. Semin Reprod Med. 2009;27:165–70. https://doi.org/10.1055/s-0029-1202305.

17. Josso N, Rey R, Picard J-Y. Testicular anti-Müllerian hormone: clinical applications in DSD. Semin Reprod Med. 2012;30(5):364–73.
18. Rodprasert W, Virtanen HE, Mäkelä J-A, Toppari J. Hypogonadism and cryptorchidism. Front Endocrinol. 2020;10:906. https://doi.org/10.3389/fendo.2019.00906.
19. Sabanegh ES. Male infertility. New York: Springer; 2011.
20. Vloeberghs V, Verheyen G, Santos-Ribeiro S, Staessen C, Verpoest W, Gies I, Tournaye H. Is genetic fatherhood within reach for all azoospermic Klinefelter men? PLoS One. 2018;13(7):e0200300. https://doi.org/10.1371/journal.pone.0200300.
21. Abacı A, Çatlı G, Anık A, Böber E. Epidemiology, classification and management of undescended testes: does medication have value in its treatment? J Clin Res Pediatr Endocrinol. 2013;5(2):65–72. https://doi.org/10.4274/Jcrpe.883.
22. Bojesen A, Juul S, Gravholt CH. Prenatal and postnatal prevalence of Klinefelter syndrome: a national registry study. J Clin Endocrinol Metab. 2003;88(2):622–6. https://doi.org/10.1210/jc.2002-021491.
23. Murken JD, Stengel-Rutkowski S, Walther JU, Westenfelder SR, Remberger KH, Zimmer F. Klinefelter's syndrome in a fetus (letter). Lancet. 1974;2(7873):171.
24. Lanfranco F, Kamischke A, Zitzmann M, Nieschlag E. Klinefelter's syndrome. Lancet. 2004;364:272–83.
25. Nieschlag E, Werler S, Wistuba J, Zitzmann M. New approaches to the Klinefelter syndrome. Ann Endocrinol (Paris). 2014;75(2):88–97. https://doi.org/10.1016/j.ando.2014.03.007.
26. Aksglaede L, Wikström AM, Rajpert-De Meyts E, Dunkel L, Skakkebaek NE, Juul A. Natural history of seminiferous tubule degeneration in Klinefelter syndrome. Hum Reprod Update. 2006;12(1):39–48. https://doi.org/10.1093/humupd/dmi039.
27. Chang S, Skakkebaek A, Davis SM, Gravholt CH. Morbidity in Klinefelter syndrome and the effect of testosterone treatment. Am J Med Genet C Semin Med Genet. 2020;184(2):344–55. https://doi.org/10.1002/ajmg.c.31798.
28. Wikström AM, Dunkel L. Testicular function in Klinefelter syndrome. Horm Res. 2008;69(6):317–26. https://doi.org/10.1159/000117387.
29. Hawksworth DJ, Szafran AA, Jordan PW, Dobs AS, Herati AS. Infertility in patients with Klinefelter syndrome: optimal timing for sperm and testicular tissue cryopreservation. Rev Urol. 2018;20(2):56–62. https://doi.org/10.3909/riu0790.
30. Corona G, Minhas S, Giwercman A, Bettocchi C, Dinkelman-Smit M, Dohle G, Fusco F, Kadioglou A, Kliesch S, Kopa Z, Krausz C, Pelliccione F, Pizzocaro A, Rassweiler J, Verze P, Vignozzi L, Weidner W, Maggi M, Sofikitis N. Sperm recovery and ICSI outcomes in men with non-obstructive azoospermia: a systematic review and meta-analysis. Hum Reprod Update. 2019;25(6):733–57. https://doi.org/10.1093/humupd/dmz028.
31. Johnson M, Sangster P, Raheem A, Zainal Y, Poselay S, Hallerstrom M, Johnson TF, Mohammadi B, Hafez K, Bhandari C, Vincens A, Yap T, Shabbir M, Minhas S, Ralph D. 040 A UK multicentre study analysing the surgical sperm retrieval rates in men with non-mosaic Klinefelter's syndrome undergoing mTESE. J Sex Med. 2018;15:S141. https://doi.org/10.1016/j.jsxm.2018.04.044.
32. Ozer C, Caglar Aytac P, Goren MR, Toksoz S, Gul U, Turunc T. Sperm retrieval by microdissection testicular sperm extraction and intracytoplasmic sperm injection outcomes in non-obstructive azoospermic patients with Klinefelter syndrome. Andrologia. 2018; https://doi.org/10.1111/and.12983.
33. Plotton I, Brosse A, Cuzin B, Lejeune H. Klinefelter syndrome and TESE-ICSI. Ann Endocrinol (Paris). 2014;75(2):118–25. https://doi.org/10.1016/j.ando.2014.04.004.
34. Rohayem J, Fricke R, Czeloth K, Mallidis C, Wistuba J, Krallmann C, Zitzmann M, Kliesch S. Age and markers of Leydig cell function, but not of Sertoli cell function predict the success of sperm retrieval in adolescents and adults with Klinefelter's syndrome. Andrology. 2015;3(5):868–75. https://doi.org/10.1111/andr.12067.
35. Schiff JD, Palermo GD, Veeck LL, Goldstein M, Rosenwaks Z, Schlegel PN. Success of testicular sperm extraction [corrected] and intracytoplasmic sperm injection in men with

Klinefelter syndrome. J Clin Endocrinol Metab. 2005;90(11):6263–7. https://doi.org/10.1210/jc.2004-2322.

36. Boeri L, Palmisano F, Preto M, Sibona M, Capogrosso P, Franceschelli A, Ruiz-Castañé E, Sarquella-Geli J, Bassas-Arnau L, Scroppo FI, Saccà A, Gentile G, Falcone M, Timpano M, Ceruti C, Gadda F, Trost L, Colombo F, Rolle L, Gontero P, Montorsi F, Sánchez-Curbelo J, Salonia A, Montanari E. Sperm retrieval rates in non-mosaic Klinefelter patients undergoing testicular sperm extraction: What expectations do we have in the real-life setting? Andrology. 2020;8(3):680–7. https://doi.org/10.1111/andr.12767.

37. Chehrazi M, Rahimiforoushani A, Sabbaghian M, Nourijelyani K, Sadighi Gilani MA, Hoseini M, Vesali S, Yaseri M, Alizadeh A, Mohammad K, Samani RO. Sperm retrieval in patients with Klinefelter syndrome: a skewed regression model analysis. Int J Fertil Steril. 2017;11(2):117–22. https://doi.org/10.22074/ijfs.2017.4702.

38. Turriff A, Macnamara E, Levy HP, Biesecker B. The impact of living with Klinefelter syndrome: a qualitative exploration of adolescents and adults. J Genet Couns. 2017;26(4):728–37. https://doi.org/10.1007/s10897-016-0041-z.

39. Centers for Disease Control and Prevention. Mumps: for healthcare providers. 2019. https://www.cdc.gov/mumps/hcp.html.

40. Hviid A, Rubin S, Mühlemann K. Mumps. Lancet. 2008;371(9616):932–44.

41. Stamou MI. Georgopoulos: Kallmann syndrome: phenotype and genotype of hypogonadotropic hypogonadism. Metabolism. 2018;86:124–34. https://doi.org/10.1016/j.metabol.2017.10.012.

42. UpToDate. Hypothalamic-pituitary-testicular axis. 2019. https://www.uptodate.com/contents/image?imageKey=ENDO%2F97670&topicKey=ENDO%2F7462&search=semen%20analysis&source=outline_link&selectedTitle=2~45

43. Boehm U, Bouloux PM, Dattani MT, de Roux N, Dodé C, Dunkel L, Dwyer AA, Giacobini P, Hardelin JP, Juul A, Maghnie M, Pitteloud N, Prevot V, Raivio T, Tena-Sempere M, Quinton R, Young J. European Consensus Statement on congenital hypogonadotropic hypogonadism—pathogenesis, diagnosis and treatment. Nat Rev Endocrinol. 2015;11:547–64. https://doi.org/10.1038/nrendo.2015.112.

44. Agarwal A, et al. A unique view on male infertility around the globe. Reprod Biol Endocrinol. 2015;13(1):37.

45. Raivio T, Falardeau J, Dwyer A, Quinton R, Hayes FJ, Hughes VA, Cole LW, Pearce SH, Lee H, Boepple P, Crowley WF, Pitteloud N. Reversal of idiopathic hypogonadotropic hypogonadism. N Engl J Med. 2007;357:863–73. https://doi.org/10.1056/NEJMoa066494.

46. Young J, Xu C, Papadakis GE, Acierno JS, Maione L, Hietamäki J, Raivio T, Pitteloud N. Clinical management of congenital hypogonadotropic hypogonadism. Endocr Rev. 2019;1(40):669–710. https://doi.org/10.1210/er.2018-00116.

47. Bhasin S, Pencina M, Jasuja GK, Travison TG, Coviello A, Orwoll E, et al. Reference ranges for testosterone in men generated using liquid chromatography tandem mass spectrometry in a community- based sample of healthy nonobese young men in the Framingham Heart Study and applied to three geographically distinct cohorts. J Clin Endocrinol Metab. 2011;96:2430–9.

48. Baillargeon J, Kuo YF, Westra JR, Urban RJ, Goodwin JS. Testosterone prescribing in the United States, 2002–2016. JAMA. 2018;320:200–2.

Sexually Transmitted Diseases (STDs)

17

Andrea Cocci and Andrea Romano

Abstract

The term "sexually transmitted infection" (STI) refers to a pathogen that causes infection through sexual contact, whereas the term "sexually transmitted disease" (STD) refers to a recognizable disease state that has developed from an infection. Physicians and other health care providers have a crucial role in preventing and treating STIs.

Learning Objectives
- To define sexually transmitted diseases (STDs)
- To describe the etiopathogenesis of STDs
- To indicate the appropriate STDs diagnostic and therapeutic flow-chart
- To describe the characteristics of each type of infections and skin lesion

Introduction

The term "sexually transmitted infection" (STI) refers to a pathogen that causes infection through sexual contact, whereas the term "sexually transmitted disease" (STD) refers to a recognizable disease state that has developed from an infection. Physicians and other health care providers have a crucial role in preventing and treating STIs.

A. Cocci (✉) · A. Romano
Department of Urology, Careggi Hospital, University of Florence, Florence, Italy

Epidemiology

Prevention and control of STIs are based on the following five major strategies:

- Accurate risk assessment and education and counseling of persons at risk regarding ways to avoid STIs through changes in sexual behaviors and use of recommended prevention services
- Pre-exposure vaccination for vaccine-preventable STIs
- Identification of persons with an asymptomatic infection and persons with symptoms associated with an STI
- Effective diagnosis, treatment, counseling, and follow-up of persons who are infected with an STI
- Evaluation, treatment, and counseling of sex partners of persons who are infected with an STI.

Primary Prevention

Pre-exposure vaccination represents the most effective way for preventing transmission of STIs as HPV, HBV, HAV and others. Using external condoms (known as male condoms) correctly is the best way to prevent HIV and other STIs, not only for occasional intercourses but also to avoid relapsing and chronic re-infection due to partner undiagnosed and asymptomatic conditions. Although limited data, also internal condoms (known as female condoms) use is recommended, despite these are more costly than external ones. Cervical diaphragms has been demonstrated to protect against cervical infections (e.g., gonorrhoea, chlamydia and trichomoniasis). Unprotected intercourse exposes women to risks for STIs and unplanned pregnancy. Providers should offer counseling about the option of emergency contraception if pregnancy is not desired. Male circumcision reduces risk for HPV, HIV and certain STIs.

Secondary Prevention

Viral STI's may expose patients to risk of cancer if they are not screened and checked with accuracy. Great example is represented by cervix cancer related to HPV infection; in female patients this condition may be diagnosed with Pap-test in young women and HPV test in older ones.

Bacterial Infections

Syphilis

Pathology
Syphilis is a systemic disease caused by a bacterial agent called Treponema Pallidum.

Treponema Pallidum is a thin, tightly spiralized spirochaete with straight, pointed ends.

Traditional diagnostic tests are of little value because spirochaetes are too thin to visualize microscopically in Gram-stained specimens and do not grow in vitro cultures.

In addition, spirochaetes are anaerobic and microaerobic and are extremely sensitive to oxygen, in line with the finding that bacteria lack the genes for catalepsy or superoxide necessary for protection from oxygen toxicity.

Epidemiology

Syphilis is a disease widespread throughout the world and represents the third sexually transmitted disease in the United States, after the infections with Chlamydia trachomatis and Neisseria Gonorrhoeae.

The incidence of this pathology decreased dramatically after the discovery of penicillin.

At present, an increase in incidence has been observed year after year since 2000.

This probably reflects the wrong condition that sexually transmitted diseases, including HIV, can be controlled with antibiotics. This leads individuals to consider unprotected sexual intercourse as low-risk events for contracting sexually transmitted diseases.

In fact, for this reason, patients infected with syphilis presented an increased risk of acquiring an HIV infection when genital lesions are present.

Syphilis has man as its only known reservoir.

Treponema Pallidum is very labile and is unable to survive contact with disinfectants or drying. For this reason, its diffusion by contact with objects (e.g., toilet tablet) is not possible.

In fact, the most common way of transmission is direct sexual contact, but it can be acquired by congenital infection or as a result of transfusion with infected blood.

Nevertheless, Syphilis is not very contagious.

The probability of contracting this infection following sexual intercourse with an infected subject is equal to 30%. Its contagiousness depends on the stage at which the disease occurs in the patient.

T. Pallidum is transmitted mainly during the early stages of the disease, that is, when many microorganisms are present on the newly formed lesions both on the skin and on the mucous membranes.

Clinical Manifestations

This disease has been divided into stages on the basis of clinical findings: primary, secondary and tertiary syphilis.

Primary syphilis classically presents as a single painless ulcer or chancre at the site of infection but can also present with multiple, atypical, or painful lesions [1].

After a period ranging from 10 to 90 days, we have the onset of primary syphilis, characterized by syphiloma, the specific elementary lesion. Syphiloma is represented by an inflammatory nodule that derives from the immunocytic infiltration of the dermis and subcutaneous tissue and has the characteristic of being eroded in the central part, from which a liquid rich in Treponemas leaks out, giving it a great contagiousness (Figs. 17.1 and 17.2).

Usually the syphiloma is a single lesion, but it is also possible to find more than one.

The syphiloma undergoes a spontaneous healing process through the action of cell-mediated immunity.

After a second incubation period of 3–6 weeks, secondary syphilis begins.

By this time, T. Pallidum gains access to lymphatic system arriving in few time to the blood, causing a true treponemic septicemia.

Treponema reaches virtually all organs but can survive only at the level of the skin. Specific pathological phenomena may virtually occur in each organ it can localize in: periostitis, meningoencephalitis, hepatitis, nephritis. All these phenomena, however, are temporary and of little clinical relevance.

The interaction between Treponema and the cell-mediated response in the skin determines the clinical manifestation of secondary syphilis: the roseola (erythematous syphiloderma) and papules (papular syphiloderma). These clinical manifestations last a few days, can recur within a few months and are increasingly attenuated

Fig. 17.1 Penile mutiple Syphiloma; non-painful ulcers with indurated borders. (*Lee V, Kinghorn G: Syphilis: an update, Clin Med* 8:330–333, 2008-https://clinicalgate.com/syphilis-3/)

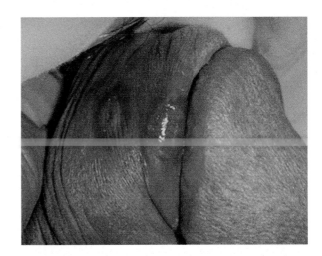

Fig. 17.2 Penile mutiple Syphiloma; inflammatory, very contagious ulcers with fluids rich in bacteria (*International Journal of Dermatology, Volume 55, Issue 7*-https://onlinelibrary.wiley.com/journal/13654632)

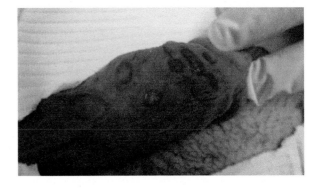

with each recurrence, until they disappear completely. From this moment, begins a long period of clinical silence of the disease: early latent syphilis and late latent syphilis.

In the first case, when the syphilis forms, the body is not yet able to produce antibodies in sufficient quantity to defend itself and we are not able, with the tests available, to serologically detect the presence of the disease.

These antibodies become quantitatively sufficient to be detected only after 10 days from the appearance of the syphiloma.

From this moment onwards, antibodies become detectable. Initially, during the syphiloma phase, the antibody titer is low; it rises significantly during treponemic septicaemia and then falls again, to remain constant during early and late latent syphilis.

Tertiary syphilis can present with cardiac involvement (e.g., lieti aortitits) and lesions in centrale nervous system (CNS) as gummatous lesions, tabes dorsalis, and general paresis.

Latent infections are diagnosed by seriologic testing.

Latent syphilis acquired within the preceding year is referred to as early latent syphilis; all other cases of latent syphilis are classified as late latent syphilis or latent syphilis of unknown duration.

Treponema pallidum can cause infections to CNS, which can occur at any stage of syphilis and result in neurosyphilis.

Early neurologic clinical manifestations or syphilitic meningitis (e.g., cranial nerve dysfunction, meningitis, meningovascular syphilis, stroke, and acute altered mental status) are usually present within the first few months or years of infection.

Late neurologic manifestations (e.g., tabes dorsalis and general paresis) occur after a long period of time by primary infection as 10 to >30 years. Infection of the visual system (ocular syphilis) or auditory system (otosyphilis) can occur at any stage of syphilis but is commonly identified during the early stages and can present with or without additional CNS involvement.

Ocular syphilis often presents as panuveitis but can involve structures in both the anterior and posterior segment of the eye, including conjunctivitis, anterior uveitis, posterior interstitial keratitis, optic neuropathy, and retinal vasculitis. Ocular syphilis can result in permanent vision loss.

Otosyphilis typically presents with cochleo-vestibular symptoms, including tinnitus, vertigo, and sensorineural hearing loss. Hearing loss can be unilateral or bilateral, have a sudden onset, and progress rapidly. This condition can result in permanent hearing loss.

Darkfield examinations and molecular tests for detecting T. Pallidum directly from lesion exudate or tissue are the definitive methods for diagnosing early syphilis and congenital syphilis.

Diagnosis

Although no T. pallidum direct-detection molecular NAATs are commercially available, certain laboratories provide locally developed and validated PCR tests for detecting T. pallidum DNA.

A presumptive diagnosis of syphilis requires use of two laboratory serologic tests:

- Non Treponemal test (i.e., Venereal Disease Research Laboratory—VDRL—or rapid plasma reagin—RPR—test)
- Treponemal test (i.e., the T. Pallidum passive particle agglutination—TP-PA—assay, various EIAs, chemiluminescence immunoassays—CIAs—and immunoblots, or rapid Treponemal assays.

Use of only one type of serologic test (Non Treponemal or Treponemal) is insufficient for diagnosis and can result in false-negative results among persons tested during primary syphilis and false-positive results among persons without syphilis or previously treated syphilis.

False-positive Non Treponemal test results can be associated with multiple medical conditions and factors unrelated to syphilis, including other infections (e.g., HIV), autoimmune conditions, vaccinations, injecting drug use, pregnancy, and older age.

Therefore, persons with a reactive Non treponemal test should always receive a Treponemal test to confirm the syphilis diagnosis.

Non treponemal test antibody titers might correlate with disease activity and are used for monitoring treatment response. Serum should be diluted to identify the highest titer, and results should be reported quantitatively. Sequential serologic tests for a patient should be performed using the same testing method (Veneral Disease Research Laboratory-VDRL or Rapid Plasmatic Reagent-RPR), preferably by the same laboratory. VDRL and RPR are equally valid assays; however, quantitative results from the two tests cannot be compared directly with each other because the methods are different, and RPR titers frequently are slightly higher than VDRL titers.

Atypical non-treponemal serologic test results (e.g., unusually high, unusually low, or fluctuating titers) might occur regardless of HIV status. When serologic tests do not correspond with clinical findings indicative of primary, secondary, or latent syphilis, presumptive treatment is recommended for persons with risk factors for syphilis, and use of other tests (e.g., biopsy for histology and immunostaining and PCR of lesion) should be considered.

For the majority of persons with HIV infection, serologic tests are accurate and reliable for diagnosing syphilis and evaluating response to treatment.

Treatment and Prevention

Penicillin G, administered parenterally, is the preferred drug for treating patients in all stages of syphilis. The preparation used (i.e., benzathine, aqueous procaine, or aqueous crystalline), dosage, and length of treatment depend on the stage and clinical manifestations of the disease (Table 17.1).

Available data demonstrate that use of additional doses of benzathine penicillin G, amoxicillin, or other antibiotics do not enhance efficacy of this recommended regimen when used to treat primary and secondary syphilis, regardless of HIV status [2–4].

Table 17.1 Primary and Secondary Syphilis recommended treatment among adults and Children. (Sexually Transmitted Infections Treatment Guidelines, 2021-Centers for disease control and prevention-Recommendations and reports/Vol. 70, N.4)

Recommended regimen for primary and secondary syphilis among adults
Benzathine penicillin G 2.4 million units IM in a single dose
Recommended regimen for syphilis among infants and children
Benzathine penicillin G 50,000 units/kg body weight IM, up to the adult dose of 2.4 million units in a single dose

Table 17.2 Latent and Tertiary Syphilis recommended treatment among adults. (Sexually Transmitted Infections Treatment Guidelines, 2021-Centers for disease control and prevention-Recommendations and reports/Vol. 70, N.4)

Recommended regimens for latent syphilis* among adults
Early latent syphilis: Benzathine penicillin G 2.4 million units IM in a single dose
Late latent syphilis: Benzathine penicillin G 7.2 million units total, administered as 3 doses of 2.4 million units IM each at 1-week intervals
* Recommendations for treating syphilis in persons with HIV and pregnant women are discussed elsewhere in this report (see Syphilis Among Persons with HIV Infection; Syphilis During Pregnancy).
Recommended regimen for tertiary syphilis among adults
Tertiary syphilis with normal CSF examination: Benzathine penicillin G 7.2 million units total, administered as 3 doses of 2.4 million units IM each at 1-week intervals

Selection of the appropriate penicillin preparation is important because T. Pallidum can reside in sequestered sites (e.g., the CNS and aqueous humor) that are poorly accessed by certain forms of penicillin.

Treatment for late latent syphilis (>1 years' duration) and tertiary syphilis requires a longer duration of therapy because organisms might be dividing more slowly but the validity of this therapeutic approach has not been assessed. Longer treatment duration is required for persons with latent syphilis of unknown duration to ensure that those who did not acquire syphilis within the preceding year are adequately treated (Table 17.2).

Persons who have syphilis and symptoms or signs indicating neurologic disease (e.g., cranial nerve dysfunction, meningitis, stroke, or altered mental state) should have an evaluation that includes CSF analysis. Persons with syphilis who have symptoms or signs of ocular syphilis (e.g., uveitis, iritis, neuroretinitis, or optic neuritis) should have a thorough cranial nerve examination and ocular slit-lamp and ophthalmologic examinations.

Invasion of cerebra-spinal fluid (CSF) by T. pallidum accompanied by CSF laboratory abnormalities is common among adults who have primary or secondary syphilis but has unknown medical significance [5].

Combinations of Benzathine penicillin, Procaine penicillin, and oral penicillin preparations are not considered appropriate for syphilis treatment.

After about 4 years represented by the early and late latent phase, three things can happen:

- Spontaneous healing
- Asymptomatic condition with a positive antibody titer
- Evolution to tertiary and quaternary syphilis; almost 5 years after infection, syphilitic gums begin to appear in skin and bone tissue. This particular name is due to syphilitic nodules' morphology that are colliquate in the central part becoming soft as a gum.

The so-called quaternary syphilis, i.e., the cardiovascular and neurological form, may also develop 10–15 years after the infection. Neurosyphilis is characterized by the presence of granulomas in the central nervous system; the lesion becomes symptomatic when it localizes in specific functional areas. In cardiovascular syphilis, granulomas typically affect the thoracic aorta, the aortic arch and the abdominal aorta.

The lesions are perivascular and the artery wall undergoes severe damage caused mainly by obliteration of the vasa vasorum.

Bacterial Vaginosis (BV)

Pathology
BV is a vaginal dysbiosis resulting from replacement of normal hydrogen peroxide and lactic-acid-producing *Lactobacillus* species in the vagina with high concentrations of anaerobic bacteria, including *G. vaginalis*, *Prevotella* species, *Mobiluncus* species, *A. vaginae*, and other BV-associated bacteria. A notable feature is the appearance of a polymicrobial biofilm on vaginal epithelial cells [6] (Fig. 17.3).

Epidemiology
BV is a highly prevalent condition and the most common cause of vaginal discharge worldwide [7]. However, in a nationally representative survey, the majority of women with BV were asymptomatic [8].

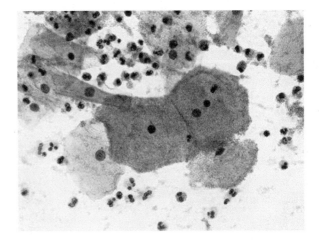

Fig. 17.3 Microscopic picture of vaginal epithelial clue cells coated by Gardnerella Vaginalis (https://www.researchgate.net/figure/Vaginal epithelial cells are coated by Gardnerella vaginalis-fig14 276290839)

BV is associated with having multiple male sex partners, female partners, sexual relationships with more than one person [9], a new sex partner, lack of condom use [10], douching [11, 12], and HSV-2 seropositivity [13]. Male circumcision reduces the risk for BV among women [14]. In addition, BV prevalence increases during menses [15, 16]. Women who have never been sexually active are rarely affected [17]. The cause of the microbial alteration that precipitates BV is not fully understood, and whether BV results from acquisition of a single sexually transmitted pathogen is unknown. BV prevalence has been reported to increase among women with copper-containing IUDs [7, 18]. Hormonal contraception does not increase risk for BV (983) and might protect against BV development [19, 20]. Vitamin D deficiency has not been reported to be a risk factor for BV [21].

Women with BV are at increased risk for STI acquisition, such as HIV, *N. gonorrhoeae*, *C. trachomatis*, *T. vaginalis* [13], *M. genitalium* [22], HPV [23], and HSV-2 [24]; complications after gynecologic surgery; complications of pregnancy; and recurrence of BV [25–28]. BV also increases HIV infection acquisition [29] because specific BV-associated bacteria can increase susceptibility to HIV [30, 31] and the risk for HIV transmission to male sex partners [32]. Evaluation of short-term valacyclovir suppression among women with HSV-2 did not decrease the risk for BV, despite effective suppression of HSV-2 [33].

Although BV-associated bacteria can be identified on male genitalia [34, 35], treatment of male sex partners has not been beneficial in preventing the recurrence of BV [36]. Among WSW, a high level of BV concordance occurs between sex partners [37]; however, no studies have evaluated treatment of female sex partners of WSW to prevent BV recurrence.

Clinical Manifestations

With bacterial vaginosis, the discharge is usually thin, homogenous, gray or off-white, and has a foul smell, which typically worsens after unprotected sexual intercourse (Fig. 17.4).

The vulva is not affected, and there are usually no other symptoms—and if there are, that suggests a mixed infection.

Fig. 17.4 Greyish discharge with fishy smell is commonly seen in bacterial vaginosis (https://screening.iarc.fr/atlascolpodetail.php?Index=31&e=)

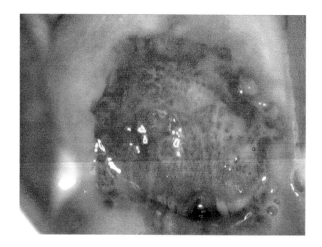

Diagnosis

BV can be diagnosed by using clinical criteria (i.e., Amsel's diagnostic criteria) [38] or by determining the Nugent score from a vaginal Gram stain [39]. Vaginal Gram stain, considered the reference standard laboratory method for diagnosing BV, is used to determine the relative concentration of lactobacilli (i.e., long gram-positive rods), small gram-negative and gram-variable rods (i.e., *G. vaginalis* or *Bacteroides*), and curved gram-negative rods (i.e., *Mobiluncus*) characteristic of BV. A Nugent score of 0–3 is consistent with a *Lactobacillus*-predominant vaginal microbiota, 4–6 with intermediate microbiota (emergence of *G. vaginalis*), and 7–10 with BV.

Clinical diagnosis of BV by Amsel's criteria requires at least three of the following four symptoms or signs:

- Homogeneous, thin discharge (Milk-like consistency) that smoothly coats the vaginal walls
- Clue cells (e.g., vaginal epithelial cells studded with adherent bacteria) on microscopic examination
- pH of vaginal fluid >4.5
- A fishy odor of vaginal discharge before or after addition of 10% KOH (i.e., the whiff test)

Detection of at least three Amsel criteria has been correlated with results by Gram stain [40]. The sensitivity and specificity of the Amsel criteria are 37–70% and 94–99%, respectively, compared with the Nugent score [41].

In addition to the Amsel criteria, multiple POC tests are available for BV diagnosis. The Osom BV Blue test (Sekisui Diagnostics) detects vaginal sialidase activity [42, 43]. The Affirm VP III (Becton Dickinson) is an oligonucleotide probe test that detects high concentrations of *G. vaginalis* nucleic acids ($>5 \times 10^5$ CFU of *G. vaginalis*/mL of vaginal fluid) for diagnosing BV, *Candida* species, and *T. vaginalis*. This test has been reported to be most useful for symptomatic women in conjunction with vaginal pH measurement and presence of amine odor (sensitivity of 97%); specificity is 81% compared with Nugent.

Multiple BV NAATs are available for BV diagnosis among symptomatic women [42].

BV NAATs should be used among symptomatic women only (e.g., women with vaginal discharge, odor, or itch) because their accuracy is not well defined for asymptomatic women.

Despite the availability of BV NAATs, traditional methods of BV diagnosis, including the Amsel criteria, Nugent score, and the Affirm VP III assay, remain useful for diagnosing symptomatic BV because of their lower cost and ability to provide a rapid diagnosis. Culture of *G. vaginalis* is not recommended as a diagnostic tool because it is not specific. Cervical Pap tests have no clinical utility for diagnosing BV because of their low sensitivity and specificity.

Treatment and Prevention

Treatment for BV is recommended for women with symptoms. Established benefits of therapy among non-pregnant women are to relieve vaginal symptoms and signs of infection. Other potential benefits of treatment include reduction in the risk for acquiring *C. trachomatis, N. gonorrhoeae, T. vaginalis, M. genitalium,* HIV, HPV, and HSV-2 [22–25, 27, 44]. No data are available that directly compare the efficacy of oral and topical medications for treating BV.

Women should be advised to refrain from sexual activity or to use condoms consistently and correctly during the BV treatment regimen. Douching might increase the risk for relapse, and no data support use of douching for treatment or symptom relief.

Alternative regimens include secnidazole oral granules [45–47], multiple oral tinidazole regimens [48], or clindamycin (oral or intravaginal) [49]. Secnidazole is listed as an alternative regimen, due to its higher cost and lack of long-term outcomes compared with recommended BV treatments (Tables 17.3 and 17.4).

Neisseria Gonorrhoeae

Pathology

Neisseria gonorrhoeae, the gonococcus, is a non-spore-forming, nonmotile bacterium that appears under the microscope as a Gram-negative coccus occurring in

Table 17.3 Bacterial Vaginosis recommended therapy. (Sexually Transmitted Infections Treatment Guidelines, 2021-Centers for disease control and prevention-Recommendations and reports/Vol. 70, N.4)

Recommended regimens for bacterial vaginosis
Metronidazole 500 mg orally 2 times/day for 7 days
or
Metronidazole gel 0.75% one full applicator (5 g) intravaginally, once daily for 5 days
or
Clindamycin cream 2% one full applicator (5 g) intravaginally at bedtime for 7 days

Table 17.4 Bacterial Vaginosis alternative therapy. (Sexually Transmitted Infections Treatment Guidelines, 2021-Centers for disease control and prevention-Recommendations and reports/Vol. 70, N.4)

Alternative regimens
Clindamycin 300 mg orally 2 times/day for 7 days
or
Clindamycin ovules 100 mg intravaginally once at bedtime for 3 days
or
Secnidazole 2 g oral granules in a single dose
or
Tinidazole 2 g orally once daily for 2 days
or
Tinidazole 1 g orally once daily for 5 days

Fig. 17.5 Microscopic picture of Neisseria Gonorrhoeae, Gram-negative coccus occurring in pairs (diplococci) with flattening of the adjacent sides (https://en. wikipedia.org/wiki/ Neisseria_gonorrhoeae)

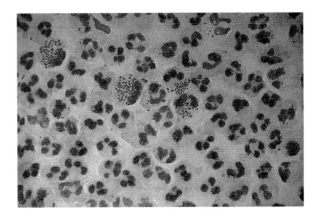

pairs (diplococci) with flattening of the adjacent sides. Gonococci are adapted to growth on mucous membranes and cannot tolerate drying (Fig. 17.5).

N. Gonorrohoeae grows only on enriched agar-chocolate medium and other supplementary media.

It requires a humid atmosphere supplemented with 5% carbon dioxide and temperature between 35 °C and 37 °C.

Epidemiology

Gonorrhea is one of the most common sexually transmitted diseases.

Its incidence has greatly increased in Eastern European and Baltic countries: immigration from these countries to Western Europe has led to an increase in incidence in these areas as well.

Man is the only reservoir for gonorrhea. This pathology is second only to Chlamydia infections in the United States.

The infection rate is the same for both men and women with higher prevalence in African-Americans than in Asians and Caucasians and with a peak incidence between 15 and 24 years.

However, the true incidence of the pathology is underestimated like other sexually transmitted infections due to the lack of diagnosis or reporting.

N. Gonorrhoeae is transmitted mainly by sexual contact. Women have a 50% risk of acquiring the infection following a single exposure to an infected male subject, while for men the risk of becoming infected with the contact of an infected woman is equal to 20%.

Clearly the risk increases if the subject has numerous intercourses with infected partners.

The largest reservoir for gonococci are asymptomatic infected individuals.

The probability of being an asymptomatic carrier is higher for men than for women.

Infected women have asymptomatic or mild infections. In contrast, most men show symptoms already at the beginning of the infection.

Generally the symptoms disappear after a few weeks in subjects with untreated pathology, determining the status of chronic carrier.

Clinical Manifestations

Clinical presentation depends on sex and it's different in male and female patients.

Incubation lasts from 1 to 7 days. In men, Gonorrhea occurs after an incubation period ranging from 1 to 7 days (average 3 days) and then appears itching, burning and redness of the urinary tract, sided by dysuria (i.e., difficult emission of urine) and pollakiuria (i.e., frequent emission of urine).

These symptoms are accompanied by an abundant urethral discharge that presents as a thick, creamy, purulent, yellowish color fluid. Symptoms, without therapy, are maintained for about 2 months with gradual involvement of the entire urethra up to the bladder.

Most frequent manifestations are: anterior urethritis, posterior urethritis, pharyngitis, ano-proctitis, vulvovaginitis in the girl (usually due to sexual abuse) and conjunctivitis in the newborn due to passage through an infected birth canal.

Other less frequent manifestations and complications, due to antibiotics therapy, concern the male genital tracts such as prostatitis and epididymitis, but also the female ones such as pelvic inflammatory disease(PID), salpingitis and endocervicitis.

Neglected gonococcal infections can lead to infection's dissemination and gonococcal bacteremia with septic shock, if untreated.

Diagnosis

In male subjects with purulent urethritis, Gram staining has high sensitivity (90%) and specificity (98%) in detecting Gonococcal infection.

In case of asymptomatic infection, Sensitivity does not exceed 60%.

This test also has problems in the diagnosis of gonococcal cervicitis in asymptomatic and symptomatic women.

Therefore all negative results to Gram staining in asymptomatic women and men must be confirmed.

The anti-hygienic test for N. Gonorrhoeae is less sensitive than culture and nucleic acid amplification tests (NAATs) and is not recommended unless confirmatory tests are performed on negative samples.

For the detection of the pathogen directly from clinical samples, Nucleic Acid Amplification (NAA) assays have been developed.

The tests using these assays are rapid, sensitive and specific although a confirmatory text for non-genital material is required.

N. Gonorrhoeae can also be isolated by cultural examinations. To prevent the sample from being contaminated with commensal pathogens that normally colonize the mucous membranes, all genital, rectal and pharyngeal samples should be analyzed on both non-selective (e.g., chocolate agar-blood) and selective (e.g., modified Thayer-Martin) solis.

Treatment and Prevention

Treating this condition may be achieved and requires a third generation cephalosporin such as Ceftriaxone intramuscularly associated with a macrolide such as Azithromycin; this one has to be used if the co-presence of Chlamydia cannot be excluded (Tables 17.5 and 17.6).

Treatment of the partner is also essential to avoid re-infection.

Table 17.5 Gonococcal infection recommended and alternative therapeutic regimens. (Sexually Transmitted Infections Treatment Guidelines, 2021-Centers for disease control and prevention-Recommendations and reports/Vol. 70, N.4)

Recommended regimen for uncomplicated gonococcal infection of the cervix, urethra, or rectum among adults and adolescents
Ceftriaxone 500 mg IM in a single dose for persons weighing <150 kg. For persons weighing ≥150 kg, 1 g ceftriaxone should be administered.
If chlamydial infection has not been excluded, treat for chlamydia with doxycycline 100 mg orally 2 times/day for 7 days.

Table 17.6 Gonococcal infection alternative therapeutic regimen. (Sexually Transmitted Infections Treatment Guidelines, 2021-Centers for disease control and prevention-Recommendations and reports/Vol. 70, N.4)

Alternative regimen if ceftriaxone is not available
Gentamicin 240 mg IM in a single dose
plus
Azithromycin 2 g orally in a single dose or **Cefixime*** 800 mg orally in a single dose
* If chlamydial infection has not been excluded, providers should treat for chlamydia with doxycycline 100 mg orally 2 times/day for 7 days.

Chancroid

Pathology

Chancroid or soft ulcer is a sexually transmitted disease, characterized by a painful papilla with an erythematous basis that progresses to a painful ulceration associated to lymphadenopathy.

This pathology is caused by a Haemophilus Ducreyi, a gram negative pleomorphic bacterium.

Unlike the other species of Haemophilus, which constitute the oropharyngeal bacterial flora of man, H. Ducreyi causes exogenous infections transmitted by sexual contact.

Epidemiology

Chancroid is a very frequent pathology in developing countries and less frequent in the West, although in recent years its incidence has gradually increased. An important problem is that its presence facilitates HIV infection: therefore, from the medical point of view, it is a very important pathology.

H. Ducreyi is a major cause of genital ulcers in Africa and Asia, but is less common in Europe and North America. The incidence of the disease in the United States is cyclical. A peak incidence of over 5000 cases was, for example, reported in 1988, to decrease to 8 cases in 2011.

Despite this favorable trend, the centers for control and prevention of infective diseases have documented that this pathology is reported in a lower share than its real incidence, who therefore remains unknown.

Clinical Manifestations

This infection is acquired through a wound of genital epithelium due, for example, to a trauma during an sexual intercourse. After an incubation period of 4–7 days, an initial lesion starts to appear, i.e., a papule surrounded by an eritematous halo.

In few days, this papule evolves into a pustule and the pustule spontaneously ruptures, resulting in the formation of a sharply demarcated and sparsely infiltrated ulcer (Fig. 17.6).

The ulcer is painful, tender and nonindurating; it bleeds easily, while the surrounding skin is normal or only slightly inflamed.

The lymphnodes are very painful and swollen; outward fistulisation is a very frequent event (Fig. 17.7).

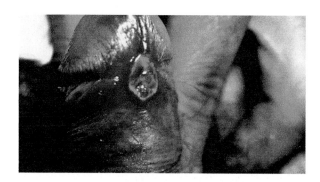

Fig. 17.6 Penile Chancroid; painful, tender, non indurated and necrotizing genital ulcer localized on frenulum (Chaux A, Cubilla AL. Chancroid-https://www.pathologyoutlines.com/topic/penscrotumchancroid.html)

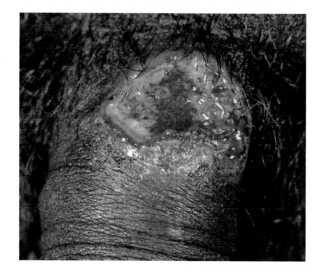

Fig. 17.7 Penile Ulcer in Chancroid infection; presence of necrotizing and bleeding ulcer at the base of penis, with surrounding normal or slightly inflamed skin. (Morrone A. (2020) Donovanosis, Chancroid, and Endemic Treponematoses: Clinical Features and Control. In: Cristaudo A., Giuliani M. (eds) Sexually Transmitted Infections. Springer, Cham. https://doi.org/10.1007/978-3-030-02200-6_16)

Table 17.7 Chancroid/Soft ulcer recommended therapy. (Sexually Transmitted Infections Treatment Guidelines, 2021-Centers for disease control and prevention-Recommendations and reports/Vol. 70, N.4)

Recommended regimens for chancroid
Azithromycin 1 g orally in a single dose
or
Ceftriaxone 250 mg IM in a single dose
or
Ciprofloxacin 500 mg orally 2 times/day for 3 days
or
Erythromycin base 500 mg orally 3 times/day for 7 days

Diagnosis

Samples for the detection of H. Ducreyi should be taken with a swab moistened from the base or margin of the ulcer. It is possible to perform cultures of purulent material taken from the aspiration of an enlarged lymphnode, but generally the sensitivity of this diagnostic exam is inferior to cultural examination of the ulcer. The laboratory must also be informed as H. Ducreyi needs specific culture media [50].

In fact, less than 85% of the culture tests are positive for this microorganism.

Sensitivity increases by using gonococcal agar (GC) supplemented with 1–2% haemoglobin, 5% fetal bovine serum, IsoVitaleX and Vancomycin (3 mcg/mL) as a culture medium. Crops should be brought to a temperature of 33 °C in 5–10% carbon dioxide for more than 7 days [51].

Treatment and Prevention

Azithromycin and Erythromycin represent the therapy of choice for this pathological condition [52] (Table 17.7).

Lymphogranuloma Venereum (LGV)

Pathology

Lymphogranuloma Veneruem (LGV) is caused by *C. trachomatis* serovars L1, L2, or L3 [53–55]. LGV can cause severe inflammation and invasive pathology, in contrast with *C. trachomatis* serovars A–K that cause mild or asymptomatic infection. Clinical manifestations of LGV can include genito-urinary discharge (GUD), lymphadenopathy, or proctocolitis. Rectal exposure among men who have sex with men (MSM) or women can result in proctocolitis, which is the most common presentation of LGV infection [56], and can mimic inflammatory bowel disease with clinical findings of mucoid or hemorrhagic rectal discharge, anal pain, constipation, fever, or tenesmus [57–63]. LGV proctocolitis can be an invasive, systemic infection and, if it is not treated early, can lead to chronic colorectal fistulas and strictures; reactive arthropathy has also been reported. However, reports indicate that rectal LGV can also be asymptomatic.

Epidemiology

C. Trachomatis has a ubiquitous distribution and causes trachoma (chronic kerato-conjunctivitis), oculomotor-genital infections, atypical pneumonia and lympho-granuloma venero (LGV).

While trachoma, the first cause of preventable blindness in the world, and interstitial pneumonia are more frequent infectious phenomena in children, lymphogranuloma venereum concerns adults.

C. trachomatis is believed to be the most frequent sexually transmitted infectious disease of bacterial origin in the United States. Nevertheless, LGV is sporadic in the United States but very frequent and widespread in Africa, Asia, and South America.

However, the estimate is believed to be underestimated because most infected patients do not require medical treatment or are treated without a specific diagnosis.

Most genital tract infections are caused by D to K types.

Clinical Manifestations

A common clinical manifestation of LGV among heterosexuals is tender inguinal or femoral lymphadenopathy that is typically unilateral. A self-limited genital ulcer or papule sometimes occurs at the site of inoculation; from painless papules, there is a transition to papulovesicle or papulopustule, which ulcerates flat and drains serous secretion. Then it results in a flat and greasy ulcer (Fig. 17.8).

The second stage of infection consists of inflammation and swelling of the lymph nodes draining the site of the initial infection. Inguinal lymph nodes are the most commonly involved; they may undergo colliquation and fistula formation (Fig. 17.9).

Proctitis is a more common clinical picture in women with LGV, as a result of spread from the vagina and cervix. In men, proctitis develops following anal intercourse or as a result of urethral infection.

Fig. 17.8 Penile flat and greasy ulcer in LGV infection. (https://www.altmeyers.org/en/dermatology/venereal-lymphogranuloma-121803)

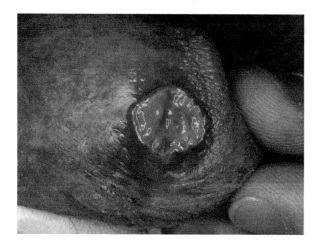

Fig. 17.9 Inguinal Lymphoadenopathy in LGV infection; swelling lymph nodes in the first phase of infection (https://www.altmeyers.org/en/dermatology/venereal-lymphogranuloma-121803)

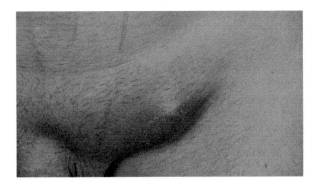

At this point, untreated LGV may regress or evolve into a chronic ulcerative phase with formation of ulcers, fistulas, stenosis or elephantiasis of the genitals.

However, by the time persons seek care, the lesions have often disappeared.

LGV-associated lymphadenopathy can be severe, with bubo formation from fluctuant or suppurative inguinal or femoral lymphadenopathy.

Oral ulceration can occur and might be associated with cervical adenopathy [64, 65].

Diagnosis

A definitive LGV diagnosis can be made only with LGV-specific molecular testing (e.g., PCR-based genotyping). These tests can differentiate LGV from non–LGV *C. trachomatis* in rectal specimens.

However, these tests are not widely available, and results are not typically available in a time frame that would influence clinical management. Therefore, diagnosis is based on clinical suspicion, epidemiologic information, and a *C. trachomatis* NAAT at the symptomatic anatomic site, along with exclusion of other etiologies for proctocolitis, inguinal lymphadenopathy, or genital, oral, or rectal ulcers [65, 66].

Genital or oral lesions, rectal specimens, and lymph node specimens (i.e., lesion swab or bubo aspirate) can be tested for *C. trachomatis* by NAAT or culture. NAAT is the preferred approach for testing because it can detect both LGV strains and non–LGV *C. trachomatis* strains [67]. Therefore, all persons presenting with proctocolitis should be tested for chlamydia with a NAAT performed on rectal specimens. Severe symptoms of proctocolitis (e.g., bloody discharge, tenesmus, and rectal ulcers) indicate LGV. A rectal Gram stain with >10 white blood cells (WBCs) has also been associated with rectal LGV [59, 68, 69].

Chlamydia serology (complement fixation or micro-immunofluorescence) should not be used routinely as a diagnostic tool for LGV because the utility of these serologic methods has not been established, interpretation has not been standardized, and validation for clinical proctitis presentation has not been done. It might support an LGV diagnosis in cases of isolated inguinal or femoral lymphadenopathy for which diagnostic material for *C. trachomatis* NAAT cannot be obtained.

Table 17.8 Lymphogranuloma Venereum recommended and alternative therapy. (Sexually Transmitted Infections Treatment Guidelines, 2021-Centers for disease control and prevention-Recommendations and reports/Vol. 70, N.4)

Recommended regimen for lymphogranuloma venereum
Doxycycline 100 mg orally 2 times/day for 21 days
Alternative regimens
Azithromycin 1 g orally once weekly for 3 weeks *or* **Erythromycin** base 500 mg orally 4 times/day for 21 days

Treatment and Prevention

Any patients with suspect symptoms for LGV infection or signs of proctocolitis as bloody discharge, tenesmus, or ulceration should undergo empirical antibiotic therapy, especially in cases of severe inguinal lymphadenopathy with buboes and a recent history of a genital ulcer.

Doxycicline represent the gold standard therapy (Table 17.8).

Treating the infection and preventing tissue damages are the principal goals to achieve; nevertheless, infection can result in tissutal reactions as scarring.

To prevent formation of femoral and inguinal ulcers, buboes should be aspired through skin or drained through an incision.

Donovanosis

Pathology

Calymmatobacterium or Klebsiella granulomatis is a pleoiomorphic gram-negative intracellular pathogen responsible for Donovanosis, a chronic infection with destructive behavior. The disease is endemic in some populations, such as the aborigines of central Australia, or the inhabitants of southeastern India and Papua New Guinea [70].

Epidemiology

In the United States, Donovanosis was endemic in some areas, and some small outbreaks may still occur. In the US, however, there are about 20 cases each year, partly because early diagnosis has greatly limited the spread of the disease.

Clinical Manifestations

After an incubation period of about 1–4 weeks, one or more nodules appear and subsequently ulcerate, forming painless, well cleansed ulcers with clear margins (Figs. 17.10 and 17.11).

Fig. 17.10 Major labia ulcer in female patients with Donovanosis; bumps in inguinal region. (https://phil.cdc.gov//PHIL_Images/20041119/adf42721ff9746838da4aa36adddde5f/6431_lores.jpg)

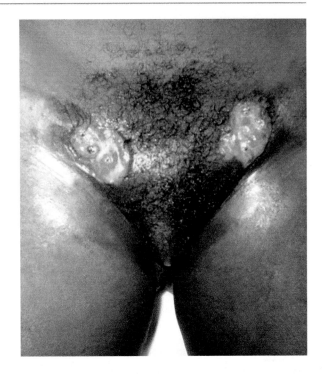

Fig. 17.11 Penile ulcerogranulomatous lesione in male patient with Donovanosis; painless and destructive lump on preputial groove that slowly spreads to glans and penile body. (https://www.msdmanuals.com/professional/infectious-diseases/sexually-transmitted-diseases-stds/granuloma-inguinale)

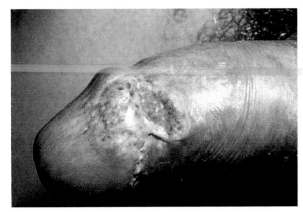

There are four types of Donovanosis:

- Ulcerogranulomatous (most frequent typology);
- Hypertrophic (or verrocous);
- Necrotic;
- Fibrous.

The types are characterized by lesions appearance. Most commonly, the ulcer becomes ulcerogranulomatous, with a beefy-red appearance and granulation tissue that is highly vascular (i.e., containing many blood vessels). For this reason, these ulcers bleed easily despite being painless. Hypertrophic, or verrucous, ulcers have an irregular edge and can be completely dry, while necrotic ulcers are deeper, foul-smelling, and often painful to the touch. Lastly, fibrous ulcers resemble painless scar tissue.

These lesions tend to expand slowly but may become extremely penetrating and destructive. Frequently the lesions cause lymphedema. Phimosis may be a result of scarring.

Other rare localizations include the oral cavity and bone tissue.

Diagnosis

Clinical suspicion especially in patients with a sexual history suggestive of exposure and presenting with genital ulceration.

Donovanosis can be diagnosed by taking a culture of the ulcer using a cotton swab. The swab is then rolled across a slide and stained using Giemsa stain, a common microscopic stain used for diagnosis.

Electron microscopy can then be used to look for Donovan bodies, which are clusters of dark-staining bacteria seen within large, mononuclear cells. These are microscopic features specific to the bacteria that cause donovanosis.

Other techniques that can be used for diagnosis include polymerase chain reaction (PCR), which allows clinicians to identify the specific bacteria in the ulcer based on its DNA, as well as blood tests and biopsies. Biopsies taken from the infected area would show changes in the cell types that indicate inflammation and can confirm diagnosis of Donovanosis.

Treatment and Prevention

Donovanosis can be treated with Azithromycin or Doxycycline (Tables 17.9 and 17.10).

Table 17.9 Donovanosis recommended therapy. (Sexually Transmitted Infections Treatment Guidelines, 2021-Centers for disease control and prevention-Recommendations and reports/Vol. 70, N.4)

Recommended regimen for granuloma inguinale (donovanosis)
Azithromycin 1 g orally once/week or 500 mg daily for >3 weeks and until all lesions have completely healed

Table 17.10 Donovanosis alternative therapy. (Sexually Transmitted Infections Treatment Guidelines, 2021-Centers for disease control and prevention-Recommendations and reports/Vol. 70, N.4)

Alternative regimens
Doxycycline 100 mg orally 2 times/day for at least 3 weeks and until all lesions have completely healed
or
Erythromycin base 500 mg orally 4 times/day for >3 weeks and until all lesions have completely healed
or
Trimethoprim-sulfamethoxazole one double-strength (160/800 mg) tablet orally 2 time/day for >3 weeks and until all lesions have completely healed

Pelvic Inflammatory Disease (PID)

Pathology
PID comprises a spectrum of inflammatory disorders of the upper female genital tract, including any combination of endometritis, salpingitis, tubo-ovarian abscess, and pelvic peritonitis [71–73].

Sexually transmitted organisms, especially N. gonorrhoeae and C. trachomatis, often are implicated.

PID cases attributable to *N. gonorrhoeae* or *C. trachomatis* is decreasing; of women who received a diagnosis of acute PID, approximately 50% have a positive test for either of those organisms [74, 75].

Micro-organisms that comprise the vaginal flora, such as strict and facultative anaerobes and G. vaginalis, H. influenzae, enteric gram-negative rods, and Streptococcus agalactiae, have been associated with PID.

Indeed Cytomegalovirus (CMV), T. vaginalis, M. hominis, and U. urealyticum might be associated with certain PID cases.

Screening and treating sexually active women for chlamydia and gonorrhea reduces their risk for PID [76, 77].

Epidemiology
Risk factors for pelvic inflammatory disease include:

- IUD (or IUD Intra Uterin Device), an intrauterine device for contraception with efficacy equal to hormonal contraception. The disadvantage of this device is that it goes up the vagina through the cervical canal, facilitating the ascent of microorganisms.
- Pregnant episodes of PID
- Invasive diagnostic procedures (e.g., hysterosalpingography, hysteroscopy, endometrial biopsy).

Clinical Manifestations
The diagnosis of pelvic inflammatory disease is very difficult and is based primarily on the presence of signs and symptoms that may indicate the presence of an infection. This is a condition whose diagnosis is clinical.

It is necessary to think about the presence of PID in the event that the following symptoms are present:

- Abdomino-pelvic pain (symptom, however, very specific)
- Uterine mobilization pain (also present in case of endometriosis)
- Dyspareunia (pain during sexual intercourse)
- Irritated urinary symptoms (e.g., dysuria, stranguria)
- Fever, even above 38 °C (not necessary for diagnosis)

Diagnosis
Acute PID is difficult to diagnose because of the considerable variation in symptoms and signs associated with this condition. Women with PID often have subtle or

nonspecific symptoms or are asymptomatic. Delay in diagnosis and treatment probably contributes to inflammatory sequelae in the upper genital tract. Laparoscopy can be used to obtain a more accurate diagnosis of salpingitis and a more complete bacteriologic diagnosis.

However, this diagnostic tool frequently is not readily available, and its use is not easily justifiable when symptoms are mild or vague. Moreover, laparoscopy will not detect endometritis and might not detect subtle inflammation of the fallopian tubes. Consequently, a PID diagnosis usually is based on imprecise clinical findings. Episodes of PID often go unrecognized. Although certain cases are asymptomatic, others are not diagnosed because the patient or the health care provider do not recognize the implications of mild or nonspecific symptoms or signs (e.g., abnormal bleeding, dyspareunia, and vaginal discharge) (Fig. 17.12).

Even women with mild or asymptomatic PID might be at risk for infertility.

Because of the difficulty of diagnosis and the potential for damage to the reproductive health of women, health care providers should maintain a low threshold for the clinical diagnosis of PID.

The recommendations for diagnosing PID are intended to assist health care providers to recognize when PID should be suspected and when additional information should be obtained to increase diagnostic certainty. Diagnosis and management of other causes of lower abdominal pain (e.g., ectopic pregnancy, acute appendicitis, ovarian cyst, ovarian torsion, or functional pain) are unlikely to be impaired by initiating antimicrobial therapy for PID. Presumptive treatment for PID should be initiated for sexually active young women and other women at risk for STIs if they are experiencing pelvic or lower abdominal pain, if no cause for the illness other than PID can be identified, or if one or more of the following three minimum clinical

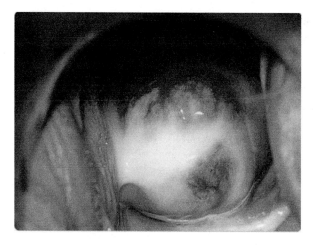

Fig. 17.12 Vaginal discharge in Pelvic inflammatory disease; an inflamed, beefy-red and swollen cervix with pus coming out of the external os. The columnar epithelium becomes oedematous and friable. Visualization of the endocervical canal becomes difficult because of profuse purulent discharge. (https://screening.iarc.fr/atlascolpodetail.php?Index=31&e=)

criteria are present on pelvic examination: cervical motion tenderness, uterine tenderness, or adnexal tenderness.

More specific criteria for diagnosing PID include:

- endometrial biopsy with histopathologic evidence of endometritis;
- transvaginal sonography or magnetic resonance imaging techniques demonstrating thickened, fluid-filled tubes with or without free pelvic fluid or tubo-ovarian complex, or Doppler studies indicating pelvic infection (e.g., tubal hyperemia);
- laparoscopic findings consistent with PID (e.g., peri-hepatic adherences, as Fitz-Hugh-Curtis Syndrome) (Figs. 17.13 and 17.14). The major symptom and signs include an acute onset of right upper quadrant (RUQ) abdominal pain worsened by coughing, laughing or breathing. These symptoms may be referred to the right shoulder. There is usually also tenderness on palpation of the RUQ and tenderness to percussion of the lower ribs which protect the liver.

Requiring that all three minimum criteria be present before the initiation of empiric treatment can result in insufficient sensitivity for a PID diagnosis. After

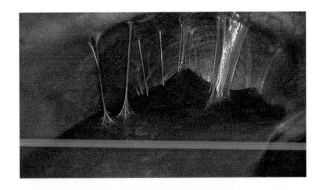

Fig. 17.13 Peri hepatic fibrotic adherences in Fitz-Hugh-Curtis Syndrome; liver capsule inflammation leading to the creation of adhesion. (https://en.wikipedia.org/wiki/Fitz-Hugh–Curtis_syndrome#/media/File:Perihepatic_adhesions_2.jpg)

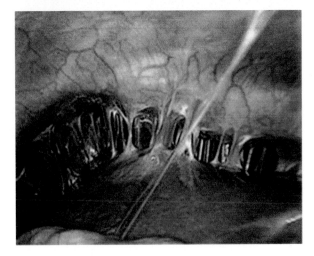

Fig. 17.14 Peri hepatic fibrotic adherences in Fitz-Hugh-Curtis Syndrome. (Theofanakis, C.P., Kyriakidis, A.V. Fitz-Hugh–Curtis syndrome. *Gynecol Surg* **8,** 129–134 (2011)-https://doi.org/10.1007/s10397-010-0642-8)

deciding whether to initiate empiric treatment, clinicians should also consider the risk profile for STIs. More elaborate diagnostic evaluation frequently is needed because incorrect diagnosis and management of PID might cause unnecessary morbidity. For example, the presence of signs of lower genital tract inflammation (predominance of leukocytes in vaginal secretions, cervical discharge, or cervical friability), in addition to one of the three minimum criteria, increases the specificity of the diagnosis.

One or more of the following additional criteria can be used to enhance the specificity of the minimum clinical criteria and support a PID diagnosis:

- Oral temperature > 38.3 °C (>101 °F)
- Abnormal cervical mucopurulent discharge or cervical friability
- Presence of abundant numbers of WBCs on saline microscopy of vaginal fluid
- Elevated erythrocyte sedimentation rate
- Elevated C-reactive protein
- Laboratory documentation of cervical infection with N. gonorrhoeae or C. trachomatis

The majority of women with PID have either mucopurulent cervical discharge or evidence of WBCs on a microscopic evaluation of a saline preparation of vaginal fluid (i.e., wet prep). If the cervical discharge appears normal and no WBCs are observed on the wet prep of vaginal fluid, a PID diagnosis is unlikely, and alternative causes of pain should be considered. A wet prep of vaginal fluid also can detect the presence of concomitant infections (e.g., Bacterial Vaginosis or trichomoniasis).

Treatment and Prevention

Treatment PID treatment regimens should provide empiric, broadspectrum coverage of likely pathogens. Multiple parenteral and oral antimicrobial regimens have been effective in achieving clinical and microbiologic cure in randomized clinical trials with short-term follow-up.

The optimal treatment regimen and long-term outcome of early treatment of women with subclinical PID are unknown.

All regimens used to treat PID should also be effective against N. gonorrhoeae and C. trachomatis because negative endocervical screening for these organisms does not rule out upper genital tract infection. Anaerobic bacteria have been isolated from the upper genital tract of women who have PID, and data from in vitro studies have revealed that some anaerobes (e.g., Bacteroides fragilis) can cause tubal and epithelial destruction. BV is often present among women who have PID [75, 78–80].

Until treatment regimens that do not cover anaerobic microbes have been demonstrated to prevent long-term sequelae (e.g., infertility and ectopic pregnancy) as successfully as the regimens that are effective against these microbes, using regimens with anaerobic activity should be considered. Treatment should be initiated as soon as the presumptive diagnosis has been made because prevention of long-term sequelae is dependent on early administration of recommended antimicrobials.

IM or oral therapy can be considered for women with mild-to-moderate acute PID because the clinical outcomes among women treated with these regimens are similar to those treated with IV therapy [30].

The decision of whether hospitalization is necessary should be based on provider judgment and whether the woman meets any of the following criteria:

- Surgical emergencies (e.g., appendicitis) cannot be excluded
- Tubo-ovarian abscess
- Pregnancy
- Severe illness, nausea and vomiting, or oral temperature > 38.5 °C (101 °F)
- Unable to follow or tolerate an outpatient oral regimen
- No clinical response to oral antimicrobial therapy No evidence is available to indicate that adolescents have improved outcomes from hospitalization for treatment of PID, and the clinical response to outpatient treatment is similar among younger and older women. The decision to hospitalize adolescents with acute PID should be based on the same criteria used for older women.

Because of the pain associated with IV infusion, doxycycline should be administered orally when possible. Oral and IV administration of doxycycline and metronidazole provide similar bioavailability. Oral metronidazole is well absorbed and can be considered instead of IV for women without severe illness or tubo-ovarian abscess when possible. After clinical improvement with parenteral therapy, transition to oral therapy with doxycycline 100 mg 2 times/day and metronidazole 500 mg 2 times/day is recommended to complete 14 days of antimicrobial therapy (Tables 17.11, 17.12, and 17.13).

Table 17.11 Pelvic inflammatory disease recommended parenteral regimen. (Sexually Transmitted Infections Treatment Guidelines, 2021-Centers for disease control and prevention-Recommendations and reports/Vol. 70, N.4)

Recommended parenteral regimens for pelvic inflammatory disease
Ceftriaxone 1 g by every 24 h + **Doxycycline** 100 mg orally or IV every 12 h + **Metronidazole** 500 mg orally or IV every 12 h
or
Cefotetan 2 g IV every 12 h + **Doxycycline** 100 mg orally or IV every 12 h
or
Cefoxitin 2 g IV every 6 h + **Doxycycline** 100 mg orally or IV every 12 h

Table 17.12 Pelvic inflammatory disease alternative parenteral regimen. (Sexually Transmitted Infections Treatment Guidelines, 2021-Centers for disease control and prevention-Recommendations and reports/Vol. 70, N.4)

Alternative parenteral regimens
Ampicillin-sulbactam 3 g IV every 6 h + **Doxycycline 100 mg orally or IV every 12 h**
or
Clindamycin 900 mg IV every 8 h + **Gentamicin** loading dose IV or IM (2 mg/kg body weight), followed by a maintenance dose (1.5 mg/kg body weight) every 8 h; single daily dosing (3–5 mg/kg body weight) can be substituted

Table 17.13 Pelvic inflammatory disease recommended intramuscolar-oral regimen. (Sexually Transmitted Infections Treatment Guidelines, 2021-Centers for disease control and prevention-Recommendations and reports/Vol. 70, N.4)

Recommended intramuscular or oral regimens for pelvic inflammatory disease
Ceftriaxone 500 mg* IM in a single dose + **Doxycycline** 100 mg orally 2 times/day for 14 days with **metronidazole** 500 mg orally 2 times/day for 14 days
or
Cefoxitin 2 g IM in a single dose and **probenecid** 1 g orally administered concurrently in a single dose + **Doxycycline** 100 mg orally 2 times/day for 14 days with **metronidazole** 500 mg orally 2 times/day for 14 days
or
Other parenteral third-generation cephalosporin (e.g., ceftizoxime or cefotaxime) + **Doxycycline 100 mg orally 2 times/day for 14 days with metronidazole 500 mg orally 2 times/day for 14 days**

Viral Infections

Human Papilloma Virus (HPV)

Pathology
HPV is a circular double-stranded DNA virus with no pericapside (Fig. 17.15).

The replication cycle of HPV is related to the life cycle of the keratinocyte and skin and mucosal epithelial cells. The virus accesses the cells of the basal layer through small continuous solutions of the skin. With its early genes, the virus stimulates cell growth, facilitating the replication of the viral genome by the DNA polymerase of the host cell when the cells divide themselves.

The increase in cells, induced by the virus, makes the basal and spinous layer thicker, leading to the formation of condyloma.

While the cells of the basal layer differentiate nuclear factors expressed in the different layers favor transcription of different viral genes. Instead, thanks to late genes, structural proteins are encoded.

These are necessary for the assembly of the viral capsid that occurs in the most superficial and most differentiated layer of the skin.

Epidemiology
Approximately 150 types of HPV have been identified, at least 40 of which infect the genital area [81].

HPV is resistant to inactivation and can be transmitted following contact with contaminated objects. Asymptomatic elimination of the virus can promote transmission.

HPV infections are transmitted by:

- Direct contact;
- Sexual contact;
- During passage of a newborn through the infected birth canal.

Fig. 17.15 Electron microscopy visione of Human Papilloma Virus (HPV). (https://en. wikipedia.org/wiki/ Papillomaviridae)

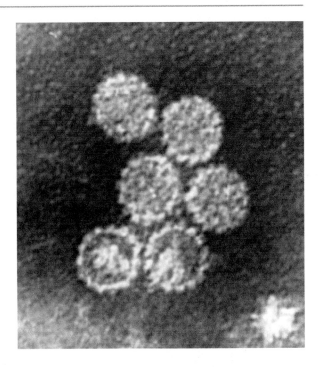

HPV is probably the most common sexually transmitted infection in the world; some types of HPV are very common among sexually active men and women.

In addition, HPV is present in more than 99.7% of all cervical cancers and HPV-16 and 18 make up 70% of detections. Other high-risk genotypes have higher prevalence in certain ethnic groups such as types 33, 35, 58 and 68 in African Americans.

High-risk HPV types are also present in oropharyngeal, anal, and penile cancers.

In contrast, HPV-6 and 11 are low-risk HPV types for cervical cancer but cause condylomata acuminata and oro-pharyngeal papillons.

Clinical Manifestations

The majority of HPV infections are self-limited and are asymptomatic or unrecognized.

Sexually active persons are usually exposed to HPV during their lifetime [82–84].

Oncogenic, high-risk HPV infection (e.g., HPV types 16 and 18) causes the majority of cervical, penile, vulvar, vaginal, anal, and oropharyngeal cancers and precancerous lesions, whereas other HPV infection (e.g., HPV types 6 and 11) causes genital warts (Figs. 17.16, 17.17, and 17.18) and recurrent respiratory papillomatosis [85].

Persistent oncogenic HPV infection is the strongest risk factor for development of HPV-attributable precancerous lesions and cancers (Fig. 17.19). A substantial proportion of cancers and anogenital warts are attributable to HPV in the United

Fig. 17.16 Penile warts
due to HPV genital
infection; the warts appear
as a small bump or group
of bumps. They are
flesh-colored and can be
flat or look bumpy like
cauliflower. (https://
dermnetnz.org/cme/
viral-infections/
viral-warts-cme)

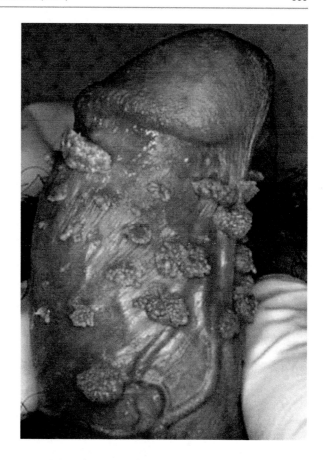

Fig. 17.17 Penile warts
due to HPV genital
infection; small flat warts
on the foreskin. (https://
commons.wikimedia.org/
wiki/File:Penile_warts.jpg)

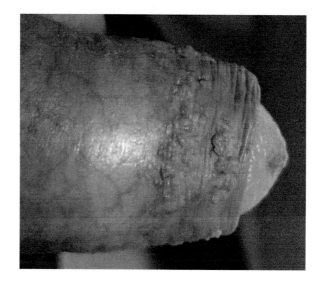

Fig. 17.18 Vaginal warts caused by HPV female infection; presence of multiple warts (Dexeus S., Cararach M., Dexeus D. (2012) Colposcopic Appearance of HPV Infection. In: Borruto F., De Ridder M. (eds) HPV and Cervical Cancer. Springer, New York, NY. https://doi.org/10.1007/978-1-4614-1988-4_7)

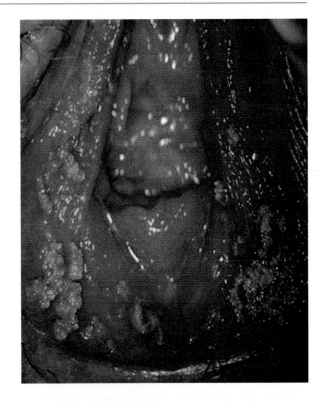

Fig. 17.19 Colposcopic vision of squamocellular cervical cancer induced by HPV (https://screening.iarc.fr/atlascolpodetail.php?Index=31&e=)

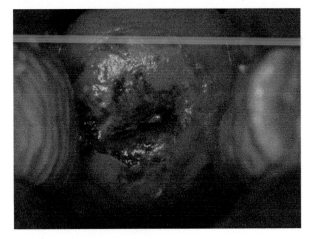

States. An estimated 34,800 new HPV-attributable cancers occurred every year during 2012–2016. Before HPV vaccines were introduced, approximately 355,000 new cases of anogenital warts occurred every year.

HPV Prevention is based on three HPV vaccines:

- Cervarix, a 2-valent vaccine that targets HPV types 16 and 18;
- Gardasil, a 4-valent vaccine that targets HPV types 6, 11, 16, and 18;
- Gardasil 9, a 9-valent vaccine that targets HPV types 6, 11, 16, 18, 31, 33, 45, 52, and 58. Types 16 and 18 account for 66% of all cervical cancers, whereas the five additional types targeted by the 9-valent vaccine account for 15%. Types 6 and 11 cause >90% of genital warts.

HPV Vaccines

- Routine HPV vaccination for all adolescents at age 11 or 12 years.
- Administering vaccine starting at age 9 years.
- Catch-up vaccination through age 26 years for those not vaccinated previously.
- Not using HPV vaccination for all adults aged >26 years. Instead, shared clinical decision-making between a patient and a provider regarding HPV vaccination is recommended for certain adults aged 27–45 years not vaccinated previously.
- A 2-dose vaccine schedule (at 0- and 6–12-month intervals) is recommended for persons who initiate vaccination before their 15th birthday.
- A 3-dose vaccine schedule (at 0-, 1–2-, and 6-month intervals) for immunocompromised persons regardless of age of initiation. HPV vaccines are not recommended for use in pregnant women. HPV vaccines can be administered regardless of history of anogenital warts, abnormal Pap test or HPV test, or anogenital precancer. Women who have received HPV vaccine should continue routine cervical cancer screening.

Abstaining from sexual activity is the most reliable method for preventing genital HPV infection. Persons can decrease their chances of infection by practicing consistent and correct condom use and limiting their number of sex partners. Although these interventions might not fully protect against HPV, they can decrease the chances of HPV acquisition and transmission.

Diagnosis

HPV tests are available for detecting oncogenic types of HPV infection. They are also available for cervical cancer screening and management or follow-up of abnormal cervical cytology or histology.

These tests should not be used for male partners of women with HPV or women aged <25 years, for diagnosis of genital warts, or as a general STI test.

Treatment and Prevention

Treatment is directed to the macroscopic (e.g., genital warts) or pathologic precancerous lesions caused by HPV.

Imiquimod is a patient-applied, topically active immune enhancer that stimulates production of interferon and other cytokines. Imiquimod 5% cream should be applied once at bedtime, 3 times/week for <16 weeks [86]. Similarly, imiquimod

3.75% cream should be applied once at bedtime every night for <8 weeks [87]. With either formulation, the treatment area should be washed with soap and water 6–10 h after the application. Local inflammatory reactions, including redness, irritation, induration, ulceration or erosion, and vesicles might occur with using imiquimod, and hypopigmentation has also been described [88] (Table 17.14).

After medical therapy, these lesions can be removed with surgery or alternative methods as criotherapy, electro-cautery (Table 17.14).

Subclinical genital HPV infection typically clears spontaneously; therefore, specific antiviral therapy is not recommended to eradicate HPV infection. Precancerous lesions are detected through cervical cancer screening.

When counseling persons with anogenital HPV infection, the provider should discuss the following:

- Anogenital HPV infection is common. It usually infects the anogenital area but can infect other areas, including the mouth and throat. The majority of sexually active persons get HPV at some time during their lifetime, although most never know it.
- Partners tend to share HPV, and it is not possible to determine which partner transmitted the original infection. HPV infection is in many cases undetected and its healing process spontaneous.
- If HPV infection persists, it may hide an undiagnosed immunodepression condition and this situation can lead to genital or head and neck tumors.
- Tobacco suspension is recommended and should be encouraged.
- The types of HPV that cause genital warts are different from the types that can cause cancer.
- Many types of HPV are sexually transmitted through anogenital contact, mainly during vaginal and anal sex. HPV also might be transmitted during oral sex and

Table 17.14 Available recommended regimens for HPV infection. (Sexually Transmitted Infections Treatment Guidelines, 2021-Centers for disease control and prevention-Recommendations and reports/Vol. 70, N.4)

Recommended regimens for external anogenital warts (i.e., penis, groin, scrotum, vulva, perineum, external anus, or perianus)
Patient-applied: Imiquimod 3.75% or 5% cream
or
Podofilox 0.5% solution or gel
or
Sinecatechins 15% ointment[†]
Provider-administered: Cryotherapy with liquid nitrogen or cryoprobe
or
Surgical removal by tangential scissor excision, tangential shave excision, curettage, laser, or electrosurgery
or
Trichloroacetic acid (TCA) or bichloroacetic acid (BCA) 80%–90% solution

genital-to-genital contact without penetration. In rare cases, a pregnant woman can transmit HPV to an infant during delivery.

- Treatments are available for the conditions caused by HPV but not for the virus itself.
- No HPV test can determine which HPV infection will become undetectable and which will persist or progress to disease. However, in certain circumstances, HPV tests can determine whether a woman is at increased risk for cervical cancer.

Herpes Simplex Virus (HSV)

Pathology

Genital herpes is caused by HSV-2, a virus of the herpes simplex family (Fig. 17.20).

Herpes viruses have a large capsid with a lipoprotein envelope containing a circular double-stranded DNA genome.

They are capable of producing many proteins that affect the host cell and immune response. In addition, they encode enzymes (e.g., DNA polymerase) that promote viral DNA replication and are a target for available antiviral drugs.

DNA replication and assembly of the capsid take place in the nucleus. Subsequently, the virus is released by mechanisms of exocytosis, cell lysis and through cell-cell bridges.

Herpes viruses are ubiquitous and produce mythic, persistent, latent and, in the case of Epstein-Barr Virus (EBV), immortalizing infections.

Cell-mediated immunity is essential for the control of infection.

HSV initially infects the mucous membranes or penetrates through skin lesions. Subsequently, the virus reproduces in the cells at the base of the lesion and infects the innervating neurons, reaching the ganglion by a retrograde pathway (e.g., the trigeminal nerve ganglion for oro-labial HSV and the sacral ganglion for genital HSV).

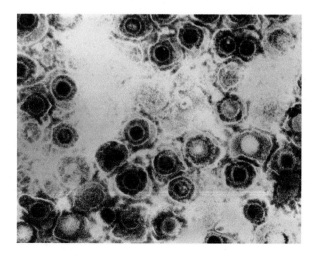

Fig. 17.20 Electron microscopy vision of Herpes Simplex Virus (HSV). (https://en.wikipedia.org/wiki/Herpes simplex virus)

CD8+ T lymphocytes and interferon gamma (IFN-gamma) keep HSV in a latent state.

After reactivation, the virus returns to the site of primary infection, resulting in re-infection that may be inapparent or may manifest as vesicular lesions, riches in virions.

Tissue damage is caused by viral pathology and immune damage. However, the lesions disappear without scarring.

Herpes viruses are numerous, you can remember:

- HSV-1, cold sore virus
- VZV, chickenpox and shingles viruses
- CMV, responsible for several diseases of the immunocompromised host and a form of mononucleosis
- EBV, infectious mononucleosis virus, as well as associated with some neoplastic diseases
- HHV-6
- HHV-7, pityriasis rosea of Gibert virus
- HHV-8, Kaposi's Sarcoma virus

Therefore, the herpetic pathology enjoys a wide spread, always increasing at the global level.

Epidemiology

The person infected with HSV represents a lifelong source of infection since HSV can establish latent infections with even asymptomatic recurrent episodes.

The virus is transmitted via secretions in close contact. Because it has a pericapsid, HSV is extremely sensitive and is quickly inactivated by drying, the gastrointestinal tract and cleaning agents.

Furthermore, HSV infection is exclusively human. HSV is transmitted by vesicle fluid, saliva, and vaginal secretions, and the site of infection is determined by which mucous membranes come into contact with each other.

Both HSV-1 and HSV-2 can cause oral and genital lesions.

While HSV-1 is predominantly spread by oral contact, HSV-2 is primarily transmitted by sexual contact, by autoinoculation or transmitted to the child during childbirth by the infected mother (by secretion of HSV-2 from the cervix during vaginal passage).

Depending on sexual practices and hygiene, HSV-2 can infect genitalia such as the oro-pharynx.

The incidence of HSV-1 in causing genital infections is increasingly similar to that of HSV-2.

However, primary HSV-2 infection is statistically more prevalent in adulthood and more advanced than HSV-1 infection because it correlates with increased sexual activity.

Clinical Manifestations

From a clinical point of view, genital herpes is classified into:

Primary Genital Herpes

First manifestation of genital herpes in subject naive to both HSV-1 and HSV-2 viruses.

Initial Genital Herpes

First manifestation of HSV-2 infection in an individual who has already encountered HSV-1 and therefore has antibodies to it.

Relapsing Genital Herpes

When the virus penetrates the body it localizes as a pro-virus in a nerve cell of a sensory ganglion and when it reactivates it causes recurrent genital herpes. The reactivation occurs in conjunction with transient immunodepression: a flu, a tiring trip, a very tense mood, heavy menstruation, excessive sun exposure.

Atypical Genital Herpes

Atypical genital herpes is a relapsing form of herpes, so defined because it is characterized by clinical manifestations that cannot be traced back to genital herpes.

Asymptomatic Genital Herpes

Also this is a form of relapsing genital herpes: in this case, however, we have no obvious clinical manifestations, but we have a reactivation with viral shedding from the skin and mucosal surface. This is a highly infectious condition that accounts for the uncontrollable spread of herpes infection.

After 2–3 days after sexual intercourse, the subject begins to have an erythematous lesion in the area of infection and cluster vesicles appear on edematous and erythematous skin or mucosa (Figs. 17.21, 17.22, and 17.23).

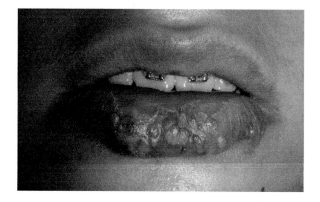

Fig. 17.21 Oral herpetic blisters in HSV infection; presence of multiple groups of blisters surrounded by erythematous halo. When the wabs break, crusts may become infected (e.g., Staphylococci and other gram + bacteria), leading to impetigo. (*Reactivation of herpes simplex*-http://www.researchgate.net/figure-virus)

Fig. 17.22 Genital herpetical blisters; multiple lesions (blisters) located on whole glans and distal part of penile body. (https://www.dermatologo-torino.it/herpes-genitale)

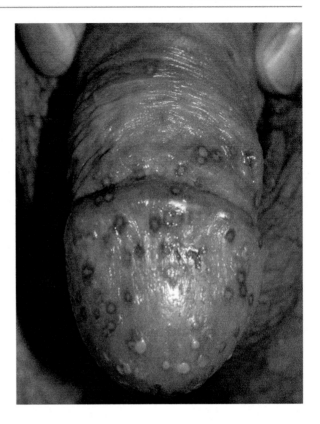

The vesicles then come to break at the apex of the disease with the formation of post-vesicular erosions; from the erosions grows liquid that congeals to form crusts that will then fall off. The duration of the lesions is about 3 weeks and the subject is contagious in the first 10–12 days, that is until the crusts appear [89, 90].

At the time of contagion, the virus goes up through the sensory endings and localizes itself at the level of a sensory ganglion and there it installs itself as a pro-virus in the cellular genome. If at this point the virus is able to give rise to an immediate productive infection, the new viral copies retrace the path of the nerve ending and only in this case we will have the clinical manifestation of the primary infection. Otherwise, the virus remains at the ganglion level and maintains a very low level of replication: this occurs in 80% of cases, so a subject can become infected without realizing it. The genital manifestation can sometimes be associated with a sacral radiculitis that can also cause intestinal symptoms such as transient ileus and brachial paresthesias.

In severe immunodepression (e.g., HIV co-infection), the most feared complication is represented by the dissemination of the disease and neurological forms such as meningoencephalitis with involvement of the temporal lobes [91].

Diagnosis
Diagnosis is based on direct detection by PCR detection of viral DNA and indirect detection by detection of IgM and IgG-anti HSV-2.

Fig. 17.23 Vulvar
herpetic blisters; blisters
and deroofed cold sores
located on major and
minor labia. (https://www.
dermatologo-torino.it/
herpes-genitale)

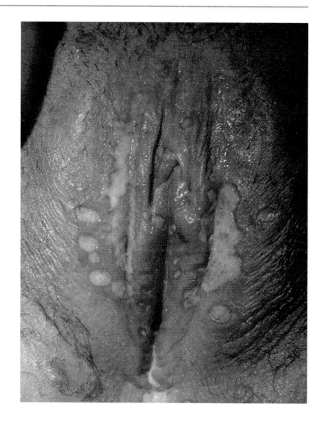

Table 17.15 Genital Herpes recommended therapy for first episode. (Sexually Transmitted Infections Treatment Guidelines, 2021-Centers for disease control and prevention-Recommendations and reports/Vol. 70, N.4)

Recommended regimens for first clinical episode of genital herpes
Acyclovir[†] 400 mg orally 3 times/day for 7–10 days
or
Famciclovir 250 mg orally 3 times/day for 7–10 days
or
Valacyclovir 1 g orally 2 times/day for 7–10 days

Treatment and Prevention

The therapy of the primary infection is based on Acyclovir and propharmaceuticals such as Famciclovir and Valacyclovir, taken systemically (Tables 17.15, 17.16, and 17.17).

Table 17.16 Genital Herpes recommended therapy for suppression of recurrent infections (Sexually Transmitted Infections Treatment Guidelines, 2021-Centers for disease control and prevention-Recommendations and reports/Vol. 70, N.4)

Recommended regimens for suppression of recurrent HSV-2 genital herpes
Acyclovir 400 mg orally 2 times/day
or
Valacyclovir 500 mg orally once a day
or
Valacyclovir 1 g orally once a day
or
Famciclovir 250 mg orally 2 times/day

Table 17.17 Genital herpes recommended therapy for episodic therapy of recurrent infections. (Sexually Transmitted Infections Treatment Guidelines, 2021-Centers for disease control and prevention-Recommendations and reports/Vol. 70, N.4)

Recommended regimens for episodic therapy for recurrent HSV-2 genital herpes
Acyclovir 800 mg orally 2 times/day for 5 days
or
Acyclovir 800 mg orally 3 times/day for 2 days
or
Famciclovir 1 g orally 2 times/day for 1 day
or
Famciclovir 500 mg orally once, followed by 250 mg 2 times/day for 2 days
or
Famciclovir 125 mg orally 2 times/day for 5 days
or
Valacyclovir 500 mg orally 2 times/day for 3 days *or* **Valacyclovir** 1 g orally once daily for 5 days

Human Immunodeficiency Virus (HIV)

Pathology

There are four main genotypes of HIV-1 called M (main), N, O, P. The main ones are of the M subtype which is divided into 11 subtypes or clades, called A-K (for HIV-2, A-F). The designations are based on differences in their genetic sequences regarding the env and gag genes, thus on their antigenicity and recognition by the immune system of Gp-120 and capsidic proteins of these viruses (Figs. 17.24 and 17.25).

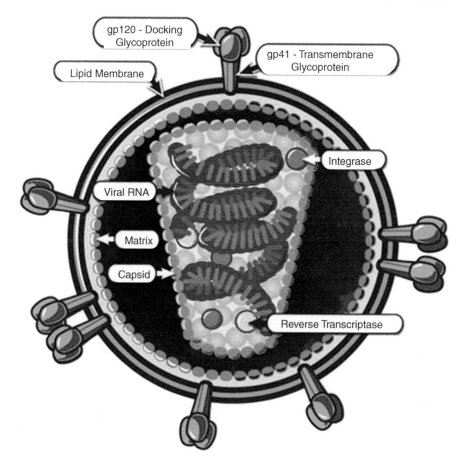

Fig. 17.24 HIV structure's representation (https://microbeonline.com/describe-structure-of-hiv-virus-t-u-2058)

Epidemiology

AIDS was first detected in male homosexuals in the United States, but has spread with epidemic proportions throughout the population. Although the prevalence has been increasing for several years in drug users and heterosexual partners, since 2014 the rate of increase has stabilized due to prevention campaigns.

HIV-1 infections are spreading worldwide, with the highest number of AIDS cases in Sub-Saharan Africa.

HIV-2 has the highest prevalence in Africa and causes a disease similar to AIDS but of lesser severity. The presence of HIV in the blood, seminal fluid and vaginal secretions of those infected and the long asymptomatic period of infection have favored the spread of the disease through sexual contact and exposure.

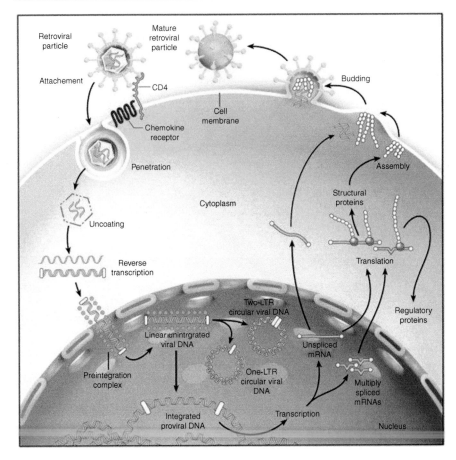

Fig. 17.25 HIV replication process (*Cell-associated HIV RNA: A dynamic biomarker of viral persistence*-http://www.researchgate.net/publication/236183663)

Clinical Manifestations

The course of HIV disease runs parallel to the reduction in the number of CD4+ T lymphocytes and in the amount of virions in the blood. HIV infects and destroys CD4+ lymphocytes presenting the CCR5 gene immediately after the onset of the infectious process.

T lymphocytes begin to proliferate following antigen presentation by infecting macrophage, dendritic cells and also CD4 T lymphocytes. This causes the onset of a mononucleosis-like syndrome. CD8+ T lymphocytes kill many virus-infected cells, limiting their replication.

Virus levels in the blood decrease and the individual is asymptomatic, i.e., in the latent period. Viral replication continues in the lymph nodes, causing damage to the CD4+ T lymphocytes which continue to decrease.

In the late phase of the disease, CD4+ lymphocytes decrease so much that the anti-viral activity carried out by CD8+ lymphocytes fails to keep up that the level of virus in the blood increases.

Infection with HIV causes an acute but brief and nonspecific influenza-like retroviral syndrome that can include fever, malaise, lymphadenopathy, pharyngitis, arthritis, or skin rash. Most persons experience at least one symptom; however, some might be asymptomatic or have no recognition of illness (406–409). Acute infection transitions to a multiyear, chronic illness that progressively depletes CD4+ T lymphocytes crucial for maintenance of effective immune function. Ultimately, persons with untreated HIV infection experience symptomatic, life-threatening immunodeficiency (i.e., AIDS).

The fundamental role played by CD4+ lymphocytes in the control of innate and adaptive responses is demonstrated by the occurrence of opportunistic infections after HIV infection.

CD4+ Th17-mediated responses that activate neutrophils protect the mucoepithelium are the first to be diminished (CD4+ <500/mcL). Thus fungal and bacterial infections increase.

When CD4+ drop below 200/mcL, CD4+ Th1 also lose function causing further bacterial and viral infections.

In addition to causing immunodepression, HIV infection damages microglia cells, causing neurological disorders. These infected cells are able to release neurotoxic substances and chemotactic factors that promote inflammation and neuronal death.

The HIV virus is able to evade the immune system in several ways, the main one being to undergo mutations. These alter its immunogenicity and thus allow it to evade the action of antibody removal. By persistently infecting macrophages and CD4+ lymphocytes, the virus has the ability to maintain itself in immunologically privileged tissues.

HIV infection may progress from an aspecific and asymptomatic infection to important immunodepression (AIDS). Linfoadenopathy and fever appear insidiously and may be accompanied by weight loss.

Commun benign infections often are responsible of serious pathologies.

Pneumocystis jirovecii induced pneumonia represents the principal sign of AIDS.

Depending on CD4+ count, different opportunistic infection can occur:

- CD4+ <500/mcL: HAART beginning
- CD4+ <200/mcL: Multifocal progressive leucoencephalopathy, Pneumocystosis, hystoplasmosis
- CD4+ <100/mcL: Esophageal candidiasis, Cryptococcosis, Cryptosporidiosis, Cerebral Toxoplasmosis, HSV relapsing, Bacillar angiomatosis
- CD4+ <50/mcL: CMV, DLBCL CNS, M.avium complex

Also tumors leads the way in this infection as Kaposi's sarcom, related to HHSV-8.

This rare skin tumor spreads in infected patients' body through different organs. Unfortunately, EBV-related lymphomas are very common in this kind of patients.

Neurological symptoms may present too due to microglia-cells damages and can be worsened by CNS opportunistic infections.

Diagnosis

HIV infection can be diagnosed by HIV 1/2 Ag/Ab combination immunoassays. Available serologic tests can detect all known subtypes of HIV-1. The majority also detect HIV-2 and uncommon variants of HIV-1 (e.g., group O and group N).

According to an algorithm for HIV diagnosis, CDC recommends that HIV testing begin with a laboratory- based HIV-1/HIV-2 Ag/Ab combination assay, which, if repeatedly reactive, is followed by a laboratory-based assay with a supplemental HIV-1/HIV-2 antibody differentiation assay.

This algorithm confers an additional advantage because it can detect HIV-2 antibodies after the initial immunoassay.

RNA testing should be performed on all specimens with reactive immunoassay but negative supplemental antibody test results to determine whether the discordance represents acute HIV infection.

When providers test by using the CDC algorithm, specimens collected during acute infection might give indeterminate or negative results because insufficient anti-HIV antibodies and potentially insufficient antigen are present to be reactive on Ag/Ab combination assays and supplemental HIV-1/HIV-2 antibody differentiation assays. Whenever acute HIV infection is suspected, additional testing for HIV RNA is recommended. If this additional testing for HIV RNA is also negative, repeat testing in a few weeks is recommended to rule out very early acute infection when HIV RNA might not be detectable.

Detecting HIV is very important for four reasons:

- Identifying infected patients to start anti-retroviral therapy (ART)
- Discovering healthy carrier able to spread infection to other persons
- Monitoring illness history and confirming diagnosis

Treatment and Prevention

Providers serving persons at risk for STIs are in a position to diagnose HIV infection during its acute phase. Diagnosing HIV infection during the acute phase is particularly important because persons with acute HIV have highly infectious disease due to the concentration of virus in plasma and genital secretions, which is extremely elevated during that stage of infection [92, 93].

ART during acute HIV infection is recommended because it substantially reduces infection transmission to others, improves laboratory markers of disease, might decrease severity of acute disease, lowers viral setpoint, reduces the size of the viral reservoir, decreases the rate of viral mutation by suppressing replication, and preserves immune function.

Persons who receive an acute HIV diagnosis should be referred immediately to an HIV clinical care provider, provided prevention counseling (e.g., advised to reduce the number of partners and to use condoms correctly and consistently), and screened for STIs.

Effective ART that suppresses HIV replication to undetectable levels reduces morbidity, provides a near-normal lifespan, and prevents sexual transmission of HIV to others [94–99]. Early diagnosis of HIV and rapid linkage to care are essential for achieving these goals.

Principal drugs for HIV therapy can be classified by:

- Nucleosidic reverse transcriptase inhibitors (NRTI): Zidovudina, Didanosina, Stavudina, Lamivudina, Abacavir, Emtricitabina
- Non-nucleosidic reverse transcriptase inhibitors (NNRTI): Nevirapina, Delavirdina, Efavirenz, Etravirena, Rilpivirina
- Protease inhibitors (PI): Indinavir, Nelfinavir, Atazanavir, Fosamprenavir, Ritonavir, Darunavir, Tipranavir
- Fusion inhibitors: Enfuvirtide (T-20), Maraviroc (CCR5-inhibitor)
- Integrase inhibitors: altegravir

HIV testing should be recommended to all patients with STI's evaluation who are not already known to have HIV infection.

Persons at higher risk for HIV acquisition, including sexually active gay, bisexual, and other MSM, should be screened for HIV at least annually. Providers can consider the benefits of offering more frequent screening (e.g., every 3–6 months) among MSM at increased risk for acquiring HIV [100, 101].

All pregnant women should be tested for HIV during the first prenatal visit. A second test during the third trimester, preferably at <36 weeks' gestation, should be considered and is recommended for women who are at high risk for acquiring HIV infection, women who receive health care in jurisdictions with high rates of HIV, and women examined in clinical settings in which HIV incidence is ≥1 per 1000 women screened per year [102–104].

HIV screening requires an informed consent, a general one is sufficient without any kind of specific consent. This type of screening should be voluntary and free from coercion and, of course, patients should not be tested without their knowledge.

Providers should use a laboratory-based antigen/antibody (Ag/Ab) combination assay as the first test for HIV, unless persons are unlikely to follow up with a provider to receive their HIV test results; in those cases screening with a rapid POC test can be useful.

Preliminary positive screening tests for HIV should be followed by supplemental testing to establish the diagnosis.

Persons with HIV infection who achieve and maintain a viral load suppressed to <200 copies/mL with ART have effectively no risk for sexually transmitting HIV [97–99].

Early HIV diagnosis and treatment is thus not only vital for individual health but also as a public health intervention to prevent new infections. Knowledge of the prevention benefit of treatment can help reduce stigma and increase the person's commitment to start and remain adherent to ART [105].

The importance of adherence should be stressed as well as the fact that ART does not protect against other STIs that can be prevented by using condoms.

Interventions to assist persons to remain adherent to their prescribed HIV treatment, to otherwise reduce the possibility of transmission to others, and to protect themselves against STIs, have been developed for diverse populations at risk [106].

Behavioral and psychosocial services are integral to caring for persons with HIV infection. Providers should expect persons to be distressed when first informed that they have HIV. They face multiple adaptive challenges, including coping with the reactions of others to a stigmatizing illness, developing and adopting strategies to maintain physical and emotional health, initiating changes in behavior to prevent HIV transmission to others, and reducing the risk for acquiring additional STIs. Many persons will require assistance gaining access to health care and other support services and coping with changes in personal relationships.

Persons with HIV infection might have additional needs (e.g., referral for substance use or mental health disorders). Others require assistance to secure and maintain employment and housing. Persons capable of reproduction might require family planning counseling, information about reproductive health choices, and referral for reproductive health care.

The following recommendations apply to managing persons with diagnosed HIV infection:

- Link persons with HIV infection to care and start them on ART as soon as possible.
- Report cases (in accordance with local requirements) to public health and initiate partner services.
- Provide prevention counseling to persons with diagnosed HIV infection.
- Ensure all persons with HIV infection are informed that if they achieve and maintain a suppressed viral load, they have effectively no risk for transmitting HIV. Stress that a suppressed viral load is not a substitute for condoms and behavioral modifications because ART does not protect persons with HIV against other STIs.
- Provide additional counseling, either on-site or through referral, about the psychosocial and medical implications of having HIV infection.
- Assess the need for immediate medical care and psychosocial support.
- Link persons with diagnosed HIV infection to services provided by health care personnel experienced in managing HIV infection. Additional services that might be needed include substance misuse counseling and treatment, treatment for mental health disorders or emotional distress, reproductive counseling, risk-reduction counseling, and case management. Providers should follow up to ensure that patients have received services for any identified needs.
- Persons with HIV infection should be educated about the importance of ongoing medical care and what to expect from these services.

Hepatitis B Virus (HBV)

Pathology

HBV is the principal member of the Hepadnaviruses.

This virus has a very limited tissue tropism and host spectrum; HBV infects the liver and, to a lesser extent kidneys and pancreas.

The virus has pericapsid virions containing a circular, partially double-stranded DNA genome.

Replication occurs through a circular overlapping RNA intermediate. The virus encodes and carries a reverse transcriptase (Fig. 17.26).

HBV encodes a series of proteins (HBsAg L-M-S; HBe-HBc antigens) that share gene sequences but with different initial condones. The virus has a narrow tissue tropism for the liver.

HBV-infected cells produce and release a large amount of DNA-free HBsAg particles.

Its genome can integrate into the chromosome of the host cell.

Epidemiology

In the United States, more than 12 million people are infected with HBV. Worldwide, approximately one in three people are infected with HBV, with 1 million deaths per year and more than 350 million worldwide have chronic HBV infection.

Seroprevalence is high in Italy, Greece, Africa, and Southeast Asia.

In some areas of the world, such as South Africa and Southeast Asia, the degree of seroconversion is 50%. In these areas of the world, PHC is endemic and a long-term consequence of infection.

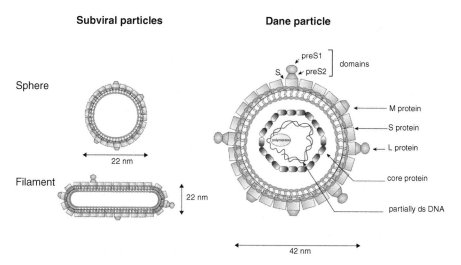

Fig. 17.26 Hepatitis B Virus (HBV) structure; representation of hepatitis B virus particles (Dane particles) and hepatitis B surface antigen (HBsAg). (*Hepatits B Virus entry into cells*-https://doi.org/10.3390/cells9061486)

The virus is primarily transmitted perinatally, parenterally, and sexually.

The highest concentrations of HBV are located in blood, with lower concentrations in other body fluids including wound exudates, semen, vaginal secretions, and saliva [107, 108].

Transmission occurs via blood or blood components during transfusion, exchange of syringes, tattoos, piercings, acupuncture or close contacts involving seminal fluid, saliva and vaginal secretions (e.g., sexual intercourse and childbirth).

Healthcare workers are at risk from accidents involving syringes or sharp instruments.

The main risk factors for HBV infection are sexual promiscuity and drug abuse.

HBV can be transmitted to infants through contact with maternal blood at birth and through the mother's milk. In fact, infants born to HBV-positive mothers with chronic infection are at high risk for infection.

Serologic screening of the blood unit and precautions against sexual intercourse have helped to decrease the incidence and transmission of both HIV and HBV.

However, the major problem associated with HBV infection is PHC.

Clinical Manifestations

The clinical manifestation of HBV in children is less severe than in adults, and infection may also be asymptomatic. The disease is clinically evident in 25% of infected individuals.

The incubation period for HBV infection from time of exposure to symptom onset ranges from 6 weeks to 6 months. The highest concentrations of HBV are located in blood, with lower concentrations in other body fluids including wound exudates, semen, vaginal secretions, and saliva. HBV is more infectious and more stable in the environment than other bloodborne pathogens (e.g., HCV or HIV). HBV infection can be either self-limited or chronic. Among adults, approximately half of newly acquired HBV infections are symptomatic, and approximately 1% of reported cases result in acute liver failure and death. Risk for chronic infection is inversely related to age at acquisition; approximately 90% of infected infants and 30% of infected children aged.

Symptoms during the prodromal period may include fever, malaise followed by nausea, vomiting, and abdominal pain. After a short time, typical signs and symptoms of liver damage such as jaundice, hypocolic stools and hyperchromic urine appear.

The recovery is manifested by a decrease in fever and reappearance of appetite.

Fulminant hepatitis occurs in 15 patients and can be fatal, presenting with symptoms and signs of severe liver damage, such as ascites and hemorrhage.

In addition, HBV infection can trigger hypersensitivity reactions from immune complexes consisting of HBsAg and antibodies. Possible manifestations are polyarthritis, rash, fever, glomerulonephritis and necrotizing vasculitis.

Chronic hepatitis occurs in 5–10% of HBV-infected individuals, usually after a mild or asymptomatic onset of the disease. Approximately 1/3 of these individuals present with chronic active hepatitis with ongoing liver damage leading to liver fibrosis, cirrhosis, and liver failure. The other 2/3 of patients present with non-active chronic hepatitis and are less likely to experience such consequences.

Patients with chronic infection represent the main source of virus spread and are at risk of fulminant hepatitis in case of co-infection with HDV.

Diagnosis

While the initial diagnosis of hepatitis can be made on the basis of clinical findings and elevation of liver enzymes in the blood, a serological investigation can accurately describe the course and nature of the liver disease.

Because HBsAg is present in both acute and chronic infection, presence of IgM antibody to hepatitis B core antigen (IgM anti-HBc) is diagnostic of acute or recently acquired HBV infection. Antibody to HBsAg (anti-HBs) is produced after a resolved infection and is the only HBV antibody marker present after vaccination. The presence of HBsAg and anti-HBc, with a negative test for IgM anti-HBc, indicates chronic HBV infection. The presence of total anti-HBc alone might indicate acute, resolved, or chronic infection or a false-positive result (Fig. 17.27).

Quantification of virus in the blood by quantitative genomic analysis is useful in determining the efficacy of antiviral therapy.

Treatment and Prevention

No specific therapy is available for persons with acute HBV infection; treatment is supportive. Persons with chronic HBV infection should be referred for evaluation to a provider experienced in managing such infections. Therapeutic agents approved by FDA for treatment of chronic HBV infection can achieve sustained suppression of HBV replication and remission of liver disease [109].

Hepatitis B immunoglobulins can be administered within 1 week of exposure and to children born to HBsAg positive mothers for prevention and improvement of the disease course.

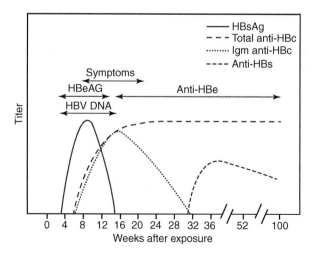

Fig. 17.27 Antigen response to HBV during and after infection (*Anti-HBc*, antibodies to hepatitis B core antigen [HBcAg]; *Anti-HBe*, antibodies to hepatitis B "e" antigen [HBeAg]; *Anti-HBs*, antibodies to HBsAg). (*Prevention of Hepatitis B Virus Infection in the United States: Recommendations of the Advisory Committee on Immunization Practices*-https://www.research-gate.net/figure/Acute-hepatitis-B-virus-infection-with-recovery_fig2_322439363)

In case of chronic infection, antiviral drugs targeting polymerase (e.g., Lamivudine, Entecavir, Telbivudine or Tenofovir, i.e., reverse transcriptase inhibitors) or nucleoside analogs (e.g., Adefovir dipivoxil and Famciclovir) are used.

Pegylated interferon-alpha is effective and can be administered for 4 months.

Transmission of HBV occurs through blood or blood products; it has been greatly reduced by screening of blood donors and by numerous prevention campaigns based on safe sex, a healthy lifestyle that avoids practices that facilitate the spread of the virus such as intravenous drug use.

Vaccination against HBV is recommended for infants, children and high-risk persons; it is also useful after infection, for those born to HBsAg positive mothers and for those accidentally infected through percutaneous contact or mucous membrane contact.

HBV vaccines contain virus-like particles.

The vaccination cycle consists of a series of three injections, with the second and third given 1 and 6 months after the first. The single serotype and limited host spectrum (human) facilitate the success of an immunization program.

Hepatitis C Virus (HCV)

Pathology
HCV is the only member of the genus Hepacvirus, belonging to the Flaviviridae family. There are six genotypes of HCV (called clades) and within each genotype there is great antigenic and genetic variability.

This virus has a positive-stranded RNA genome and is equipped with a pericapside.

HCV also possesses an RNA-dependent RNA polymer that is particularly prone to make errors and determine mutations in its genes. Because of these phenomena, it is characterized by antigenic variability that makes the development of a vaccine very difficult (Fig. 17.28).

Humans and chimpanzees constitute the only reservoirs for HCV.

The ability of the virus to remain associated with the host cell and to avoid death promotes persistent infection, which is subsequently the cause of hepatopathy.

As with HBV, chronic infection results in the depletion of CD8+ lymphocytes, thus preventing resolution of the infection.

Continuous repair processes, inflammatory cytokines, and induction of cell growth during the chronic phase of infection are responsible for the predisposition to the development of PHC.

Epidemiology
HCV is most prevalent in southern Italy, Spain, central Europe, Japan and parts of the Middle East. The high incidence of asymptomatic chronic infections promotes the spread of the virus in the population.

HCV infection is the most common chronic blood-borne infection in the United States, with an estimated 2.4 million persons living with chronic infection.

HCV is not efficiently transmitted through sex [110–112]. Studies of HCV transmission between heterosexual couples and MSM have yielded mixed results;

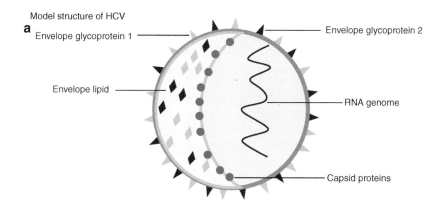

Fig. 17.28 Hepatits C Virus (HCV) model structure and genome organization; Notes: (**a**) Model structure of HCV. (**b**) Proteins encoded by the HCV genome. Expert review in Molecular Medicine © 2003 Cambridge University Press. (https://www.researchgate.net/figure/HCV model structure and genome organization-Notes: A Model structure of HCV-B_fig1_311784847/actions#reference)

however, studies have reported either no or minimally increased rates of HCV infection among partners of persons with HCV infection compared with partners of those without HCV [111, 113–115].

HCV is mainly transmitted with infected blood. Intravenous drug addicts individuals who undergo tattoos are at increased risk of HCV infection. Screening procedures have resulted in reduced levels of blood transfusion transmission by organ donation point.

Over 90% of individuals with HIV infections and natural history or previous drug addiction are also infected with HCV.

Studies of HCV transmission between heterosexual couples and MSM have yielded mixed results; however, studies have reported either no or minimally increased rates of HCV infection among partners of persons with HCV infection compared with partners of those without HCV.

However, data indicate that sexual transmission of HCV can occur, especially among persons with HIV infection. Increasing incidence of acute HCV infection among MSM with HIV infection has been reported in multiple U.S. and European cities.

A recent systematic review reported an HCV incidence of 6.35 per 1000 person years among MSM with HIV infection. An association exists with high-risk and traumatic sexual practices (e.g., condom-less receptive anal intercourse or receptive fisting) and concurrent genital ulcerative disease or STI-related proctitis. HCV transmission among MSM with HIV infection has also been associated with group sex and chem-sex (i.e., using recreational drugs in a sexual context).

Shedding of HCV in the semen and in the rectum of men with HIV infection has been documented.

Certain studies have revealed that risk increases commensurate with increasing numbers of sex partners among heterosexual persons and MSM with HIV infection, especially if their partners are also co-infected with HIV.

More recently, acute HCV infections have been reported among MSM on PrEP, increasing concerns that certain MSM might be at increased risk for incident HCV infection through condom-less sexual intercourse with MSM with HCV infection.

However, infected persons are a source of transmission to others and are at risk for cirrhosis and hepatocellular carcinoma decades after infection. HCV is primarily transmitted parenterally, usually through shared drug-injecting needles and paraphernalia. HCV also can be transmitted through exposures in health care settings as a consequence of inadequate infection control practices.

HCV causes three types of diseases:

- acute hepatitis with resolution of the infection healing in 15% of cases;
- chronic persistent infection with possible disease progression much later in life in 70% of infected people;
- rapid and severe cirrhosis progressions in 15% of patients.

Clinical Manifestations

Persons newly infected with HCV typically are either asymptomatic or have a mild clinical illness. HCV RNA can be detected in blood within 1–3 weeks after exposure. The average time from exposure to antibody to HCV (anti-HCV) seroconversion is 4–10 weeks, and anti-HCV can be detected among approximately 97% of persons by 6 months after exposure. Chronic HCV infection develops among 75–85% of persons with HCV infection, and 10–20% of persons with chronic infection develop cirrhosis in 20–30 years of active liver disease. The majority of infected persons remain unaware of their infection because they are not clinically significant.

Viraemias can be detected within 1–3 weeks of a transfusion of HCV-contaminated blood.

In the acute comma form, HCV infection is similar to acute HIV and HBV infection, but the inflammatory response is less intense and symptoms are usually milder.

Most commonly (>70% of cases), the initial disease is asymptomatic but evolves into the chronic persistent form (Fig. 17.29).

The predominant symptom is chronic fatigue.

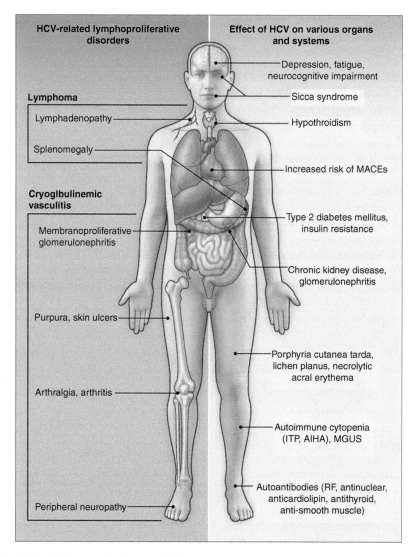

Fig. 17.29 HCV systemic effects on different organs; These can be present long before the stage of advanced liver disease and include non-specific symptoms such as fatigue, nausea, abdominal or musculoskeletal pain, loss of weight, and neuropsychiatric symptoms including depression, fatigue and neurocognitive impairment. Other specific extra-hepatic manifestations are cryoglobulinaemia vasculitis, lymphoproliferative disorders (e.g., B-cell non-Hodgkin lymphoma), renal disease, type II diabetes mellitus, cerebrovascular and cardiovascular events, porphyria cutanea tarda and lichen planus. (*Extrahepatic manifestations of chronic HCV infection*-https://www.nejm.org/doi/full/10.1056/NEJMra2033539)

Persistent chronic disease often degenerates into active chronic hepatitis in about 10–15 years and into cirrhosis (20% of chronic cases) and liver failure (20% of cirrhosis cases) after about 20 years.

HCV-induced liver damage can be worsened by alcohol, certain medications, and other hepatitis viruses, thus favoring evolution into cirrhosis. HCV promotes the development of hepatocellular carcinoma over years in 5% of patients with infection chronic.

Diagnosis

Diagnosis of infection is based on finding anti-HCV antibodies by ELISA or detection of the RNA genome. Seroconversion usually occurs within 7–31 weeks of infection. However, the gold standard for confirming infection by HCV consists of the detection and quantification of the viral genome by RT-PCR, branched DNA technology and related techniques.

Treatment and Prevention

For a long time, interferon-alpha was the only treatment available for HCV until the introduction of prosthetic specific inhibitors such as Boceprevir, Telaprevir and Ledipasvir more recently.

A polymerase inhibitor, Sofosfbuvir, is also available.

The introduction of these new HCV-specific drugs, as happened for HIV, has limited the evolution of drug resistance and determined a great difference in the level of therapeutic efficacy.

Obviously, the precautions to avoid HCV transmission are similar to those taken with HBV and various blood-borne pathogens, including practicing safe sex, avoiding sharing personal care accessories or syringe needles and limiting, in this case, excessive alcohol consumption.

Funginal Infections

Candida Albicans

Pathology

Approximately 95% of all Candida bloodstream infections are associated with four species: C. albican, C. Glabrata, C parapsilosis, C tropicalis.

Among these common species, only C. GLabrata can be narrowly defined as an emerging cause of bloodstream infections, in part because of its intrinsic and acquired resistance to atolls and other commonly used antifungal agents.

All Candida species are yeast-like organisms that produce budding or blastoconidia. Candidate species except C. glabrata, also produce pseudohyphae and true hyphae.

In addition, C. albicans has thick-walled terminal germ tubes and clamidioconidia. C slabbrata, the second most frequent species in several clinical settings, is unable to form pseudohyphae, germ tubes, or true hyphae under most conditions.

Most Candida colonies form smooth, white, creamy, domed colonies. C albicans and other species can undergo phenotypic switching, in which a single Candida strain can reversibly switch between different morphotypes. These can range from the classic smooth, white colony with lievitiform elements to very "wrinkled" and "hairy" colonies composed of hyphal and pseudohyphal forms.

It has been hypothesized that this process makes it possible for Candida to adapt to the various environmental micronuclei within the human host.

Epidemiology

Candida species are known colonizing species of humans and other warm-blooded animals. So they are ubiquitous in humans and in nature. The primary site of colonization is the castro-intestinal tract, although they are present at the cutaneous and genital level.

C. albicans is the most common causative agent of disease in humans and can also be found at an environmental level.

Colonization rates increase especially in hospitalized patients, diabetic patients, immunosuppressed patients for HIV, antiblastic chemotherapy or chronic corticosteroid use.

The main source of Candida infection is the patient; most candidiasis consists of endogenous infections.

In these cases, the host's resident microbial population takes advantage of the momentary drop in immune defenses to cause an infection.

Exogenous transmission of Candida may also contribute in part to certain types of candidiasis. Examples may be irrigation solutions, parenteral nutrition fluids, heart valves, infected corneas, central or peripheral venous catheters, and pressure transducers.

C. Albicans is predominant among the various species of Candida capable of causing infection in humans and is also responsible for infections affecting the genital areas.

Differences in the number and species of Candida that cause infections can be influenced by numerous factors, including patient age, increased immunosuppression, exposure to antifungal drugs, or differences in infection control practices. Each of these farms alone or in combination, can influence the prevalence of different Candida species in any situation.

Clinical Manifestations

A diagnosis of *Candida* vaginitis is clinically indicated by the presence of external dysuria and vulvar pruritus, pain, swelling, and redness. Signs include vulvar edema, fissures, excoriations associated to thick, curdy and milky vaginal discharge. Most healthy women with uncomplicated vulvovaginal candidiasis (VVC) have no identifiable precipitating factors (Figs. 17.30, 17.31, 17.32, and 17.33).

Under the right conditions, Candida can potentially cause infections in any organ. Infections can range from superficial cutaneous and mucosal candidiasis to diffuse blood spread and septicemia. This clinical picture can lead to the involvement of important organs such as heart, brain, kidney, spleen and liver.

Fig. 17.30 Genital candidiasis infection in male patient (lateral view of glans); multiple erythematous spots often associated with itching. (https://www.altmeyers. org/en/dermatology/ candida-balanitis-118722)

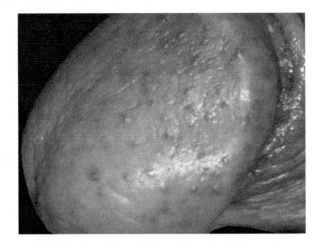

Fig. 17.31 Genital candidiasis infection in male patient (frontal view of glans); presence of a thick cheesy white discharge under the retracted foreskin and over the glans. (https:// sidriinternational.in/ penis-male-yeast-infection- candidiasis-symptoms- causes-complications- treatment)

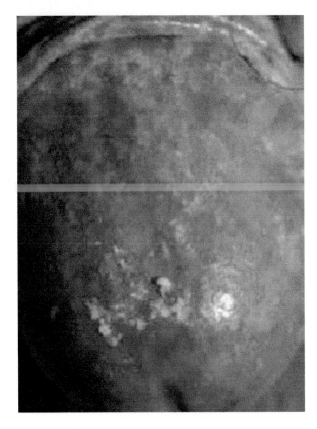

In case of encephalic involvement, the mortality rate attributable to the infection reaches 50%.

Mucosal infections due to Candida species may be limited to the oropharynx or extend to the esophagus and entire gastrointestinal tract. In women, the vaginal

Fig. 17.32 Vulvar and cervical Candidiasis infection; this condition is characterized by curdy or cheesy and often sticky white discharge. Discharge and secretions may be visible on the vulvar region and on minor labia if neglected. (https://en.wikipedia.org/wiki/Vaginal_yeast_infection)

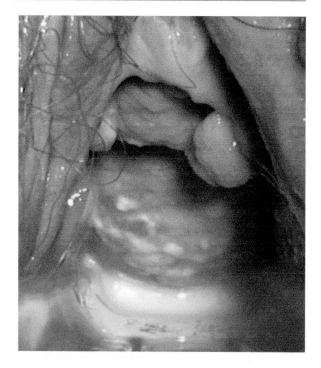

Fig. 17.33 Cervical candidiasis; presence of white milky discharge from cervical canal associated with itching. (https://screening.iarc.fr/atlascolpodetail.php?Index=31&e=)

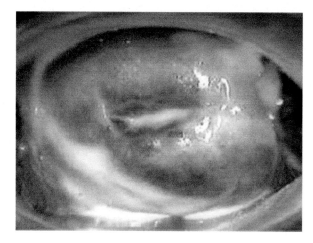

mucosa is also a common site of infection. These infections are generally observed in individuals with local or generalized immunosuppression.

The infections present as white patches on the mucosal surface with the appearance of an itchy rash and erythematous vesicular-papular lesions.

Diagnosis

Laboratory diagnosis of candidiasis involves the search for clinical material followed by microscopic examination and culture.

Budding yeast forms and pseudo-hyphae are easily detected by fluorescent microscopic examination and this finding is sufficient for the diagnosis of candidiasis. However, blood cultures, tissue cultures and normally sterile body fluids can be performed.

Identification of the Candida species is necessary for therapy setting because of the different responses to various antifungal agents. This can be accomplished by testing for germ tubes (C. Albicans), tests on cromogenic essays, PNA-FISH (peptide nucleic acid-fluorescence in situ hybridization) and with sugars assimilation pannels.

Treatment and Prevention

Mucosal and cutaneous infections can be treated with topically applied creams and lotions containing azoic antifungal agents. Systemic oral therapy of these infections can be performed with Fluconazole or Itraconazole (Table 17.18).

Short-course topical formulations (i.e., single dose and regimens of 1–3 days) effectively treat uncomplicated VVC. Treatment with azoles results in relief of symptoms and negative cultures in 80–90% of patients who complete therapy.

Table 17.18 Vulvovaginal candidiasis recommended therapy. (Sexually Transmitted Infections Treatment Guidelines, 2021-Centers for disease control and prevention-Recommendations and reports/Vol. 70, N.4)

Recommended regimens for vulvovaginal candidiasis
Over-the-counter intravaginal agents
Clotrimazole 1% cream 5 g intravaginally daily for 7–14 days
or
Clotrimazole 2% cream 5 g intravaginally daily for 3 days
or
Miconazole 2% cream 5 g intravaginally daily for 7 days
or
Miconazole 4% cream 5 g intravaginally daily for 3 days
or
Miconazole 100 mg vaginal suppository one suppository daily for 7 days
or
Miconazole 200 mg vaginal suppository one suppository for 3 days
or
Miconazole 1200 mg vaginal suppository one suppository for 1 day
or
Tioconazole 6.5% ointment 5 g intravaginally in a single application
Prescription intravaginal agents
Butoconazole 2% cream (single-dose bioadhesive product) 5 g intravaginally in a single application
or
Terconazole 0.4% cream 5 g intravaginally daily for 7 days
or
Terconazole 0.8% cream 5 g intravaginally daily for 3 days
or
Terconazole 80 mg vaginal suppository one suppository daily for 3 days
Oral agent
Fluconazole 150 mg orally in a single dose

Deeper infections require systemic therapy, the choice of which depends on the type of infection, the infecting species, and the status of the host.

In many cases, oral fluconazole can be quite effective in treating candidiasis.

As with many infectious diseases, prevention is clearly preferable to treatment for Candida infection. The use of broad-spectrum antimicrobial agents should be avoided at all costs, catheter cleaning should be ensured, and infection control precautions should be followed carefully.

Follow-up typically is not required. Only women with persistent or recurrent symptoms after treatment should be return to follow-up visit.

Uncomplicated VVC is not usually acquired through sexual intercourse, and data do not support treatment of sex partners. A minority of male sex partners have balanitis, characterized by erythematous areas on the glans of the penis and thick cheesy white discharge in conjunction with pruritus or irritation. These men benefit from treatment with topical antifungal agents to relieve symptoms.

Ectoparasitic Infections

Trichomoniasis

Pathology
Trichomonas Vaginalis is a protozoan that causes urogenital infections; its movement is ensured by four flagella and a shrewd undulating membrane (Fig. 17.34). This parasite exists only as a trophozoite, can infect both men and women and is localized in the urethra, vagina and prostate glands.

Epidemiology
Trichomoniasis is estimated to be the most prevalent non-viral STI worldwide. Trichomoniasis has not a general screening for his ectoparasite, *T. Vaginalis;* indeed, the epidemiology of trichomoniasis has largely come from population-based and clinic-based surveillance studies.

Trichomoniasis prevalence is as high among women aged >24 years as they are for women aged <24 years.

Clinical Manifestations
The majority of cases about trichomoniasis (70–85%) have minimal or no genital symptoms; untreated infections might last from months to years.

Men with trichomoniasis may report mild symptoms of urethritis, epididymitis, or prostatitis, and women with trichomoniasis sometimes have vaginal discharge, which can be diffuse, malodorous, or yellow-green with or without vulvar irritation, and might have a characteristic strawberry-appearing cervix, which is observed more often on colposcopy than on physical examination (Fig. 17.35).

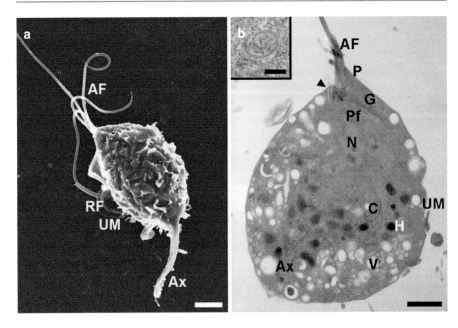

Fig. 17.34 Trichomonas Vaginalis biological structure; Trichomonads have four flagella that project from the organism's anterior and one flagellum that extends backward across the middle of the organism, forming an undulating membrane. (**a**) Scanning electron microscopy image of T. vaginalis. AF, anterior flagella; Ax, axostyle; RF, recurrent flagellum; UM, undulating membrane. (**b**) TEM image of T. vaginalis. C, costa; G, Golgi complex; H, hydrogenosome; N, nucleus; P, pelta; Pf, parabasal filament; V, vacuole. (*Three dimensional structure of the cytoskeleton in Trichomonas vaginalis revealed new features*-http://www.researchgate.net/publication/24350321)

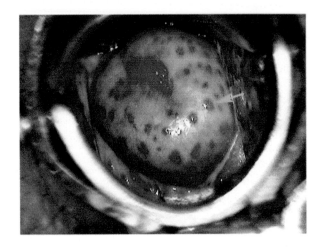

Fig. 17.35 Strawberry cervix in Trichomonas Vaginalis infection; this condition is associated with multiple erythematous spots that recall a strawberry's appearance and a rothy greenish or yellowish foul-smelling discharge (https://screening.iarc.fr/atlascolpodetail.php?Index=31&e=)

Among sexually active persons, use of condoms represents the best way to prevent genital trichomoniasis. Reduced risk for T. Vaginalis is described in partner whose men have been circumcised.

Table 17.19 Trichomoniasis regimen for men and women. (Sexually Transmitted Infections Treatment Guidelines, 2021-Centers for disease control and prevention-Recommendations and reports/Vol. 70, N.4)

Recommended regimen for trichomoniasis among women and men
Metronidazole 500 mg orally 2 times/day for 7 days
Metronidazole 2 g orally in a single dose

T. vaginalis causes reproductive morbidity and has been reported to be associated with a 1.4-times greater likelihood of preterm birth, premature rupture of membranes, and infants who are small for gestational age. A meta-analysis demonstrated an association between *T. vaginalis* and a 2.1-fold increased risk for cervical cancer.

Another meta-analysis reported a slightly elevated but not statistically significant association between *T. vaginalis* and prostate cancer.

Diagnosis

The method of choice for diagnosis of Trichomoniasis is microscopic examination of vaginal or urethral secretions for trophozoites.

Diagnostic accuracy can be increased by culture examination of the organism or by using fluorescent monoclonal antibody staining.

Treatment and Prevention

Treatment reduces symptoms and signs of *T. vaginalis* infection and might reduce transmission. Treatment recommendations for women are based on a meta-analysis [116] and a multicenter, randomized trial of mostly symptomatic women without HIV infection [117]. The study demonstrated that multidose metronidazole (500 mg orally 2 times/day for 7 days) reduced the proportion of women retesting positive at a 1-month test of cure visit by half, compared with women who received the 2-g single dose (Table 17.19).

No published randomized trials are available that compare these doses among men.

Pediculosis Pubis

Pathology

Different species of lice infest humans as hematological parasites. Only the body louse plays an important role in medicine as a vector of typhoid rickettsias and trench fever. The body louse, Pedicures humans, and the head louse, Pediculus capiti, are morphologically identical. They have an elongated body, flat back-ventrally, they are wingless and have three pairs of legs; the mouth appendages are adapted for piercing the meat and sucking blood. The pubic louse or flat, Phtirus pubis, has a short abdomen, similar to that of a crab and the second and third pair of legs equipped with claws (Fig. 17.36).

Pediculosis pubis is caused by the parasite *Phthirus pubis* and is usually transmitted by sexual contact [118].

Fig. 17.36 Microscopic vison of Phtirus pubis. (https://it.wikipedia.org/wiki/Pthirus_pubis)

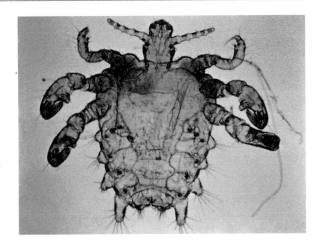

Epidemiology

Outbreaks of pediculosis of the head are very frequent, particularly among school-age children.

Head lice live and reproduce in the hair and are transmitted by direct physical contact or by sharing brushes and hair.

Pubic lice are usually localized on the hair of the pubic and perinatal areas, but the spread can affect all hairy areas of the body such as eyelashes, armpits and eyebrows with the exception of hair. All lice during the meal inject saliva which determines in humans varying degrees of sensitization.

Clinical Manifestations

Pediculosis are itchy infestations caused by Pedicules, small arthropods without wings, order-specific parasites of the mammals.

Pedicules that are relevant to humans are: Pediculus humanus capitis and Phtirus pubis (crab).

These creatures lay their eggs (nits) on the hair shafts and hairs. In addition to affecting the hair, pediculosis can also affect the hair (especially pubic) and eyebrows. Malathion and Permethrin have proved to be the most effective drugs. It is advisable to use a thick comb and warm vinegar to remove the eggs.

Diagnosis

The clinical diagnosis is based on typical symptoms of itching in the pubic region.

Lice and nits can be observed on pubic hair (Figs. 17.37 and 17.38).

Treatment and Prevention

Permethrin 1% cream rinse or Pyrethrin with piperonyl butoxide applied to affected areas and washed off after 10 min represents the best treatment option (Table 17.20).

Reported resistance to pediculcides (permethrin and pyrethrin) has been increasing and is widespread [119, 120].

Fig. 17.37 Direct observation of Phtirus pubis on pubic hair. (Phthirus pubis alive and his lendine.jpg-http:// commons.wikimedia.org/ wiki)

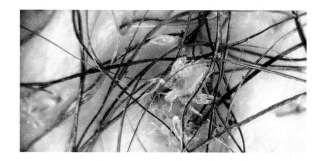

Fig. 17.38 Evidence of several Pedicules on pubic hair. (https://www.std-gov. org/std_picture/crabs_std_ pubic_lice_pictures.htm)

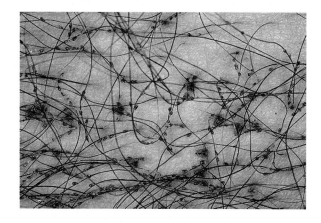

Table 17.20 Pediculosis pubis recommended therapy. (Sexually Transmitted Infections Treatment Guidelines, 2021-Centers for disease control and prevention-Recommendations and reports/Vol. 70, N.4)

Recommended regimens for pediculosis pubis
Permethrin 1% cream rinse applied to affected areas and washed off after 10 min
or
Pyrethrin with piperonyl butoxide applied to the affected area and washed off after 10 min

Alternative Regimens may be Malathion 0.5% lotion applied to affected areas and washed off after 8–12 h or Ivermectin 250 μg/kg body weight orally, repeated in 7–14 days (Table 17.21).

Malathion can be used when treatment failure is believed to have occurred as a result of resistance. The odor and longer duration of application associated with malathion therapy make it a less attractive alternative compared with the recommended pediculicides.

Ivermectin has limited ovicidal activity [121]; so it might not prevent recurrences from eggs at the time of treatment, and therefore treatment should be repeated in 7–14 days [122, 123].

Table 17.21 Pediculosis pubis recommended therapy. (Sexually Transmitted Infections Treatment Guidelines, 2021-Centers for disease control and prevention-Recommendations and reports/Vol. 70, N.4)

Alternative regimens
Malathion 0.5% lotion applied to affected areas and washed off after 8–12 h
or
Ivermectin 250 μg/kg body weight orally, repeated in 7–14 days

Ivermectin should be taken with food because bioavailability is increased, thus increasing penetration of the drug into the epidermis. Adjustment of ivermectin dosage is not required for persons with renal impairment; however, the safety of multiple doses among persons with severe liver disease is unknown. Lindane is not recommended for treatment of pediculosis because of toxicity, contraindications for certain populations (pregnant and breastfeeding women, children aged).

Scabies

Pathology

Human scabies is an ectoparasitosis that is characterized by very typical lesions-the pearly vesicle and the burrowing-as well as by particularly intense itching (especially at night) and great contagiousness.

The etiological agent is the mite Sarcoptes Scabiei Hominis, a mite that lives in the human skin as an obliged parasite, spending there all its life cycle.

Adult mites average 300–400 μm in length, have an oval-shaped body with four pairs of legs.

The first and second pairs are separated by the third and fourth.

The body of this parasite is equipped with bristles, spines and transverse and parallel ridges. The eggs measure 100–150 μm in size (Fig. 17.39).

The pregnant females penetrate the skin, digging in the stratum corneum of the epidermis burrows where they lay their eggs. From the eggs develop the larvae that emerge from the burrow, take shelter in the hair follicles or in small skin craters specially dug, in which they mature in nymphs and, then, in adults.

Females lay eggs and feces in the burrows for about 2 months, after which they die.

Usually, the mites are localized where the skin is thinner, that is the popliteal folds, interdigital, the wrist, the inguinal region and the mammary folds.

The presence of the mite and its secretions causes intense itching, especially at night.

Sarcoptes Scabiei is an obligate parasite and can perpetuate itself in a single host indefinitely.

Scabies among adults frequently is sexually acquired, although scabies among children usually is not [124, 125].

Fig. 17.39 Direct observation of Sarcoptes scabiei hominis. (https://it.wikipedia.org/wiki/Sarcoptes_scabiei)

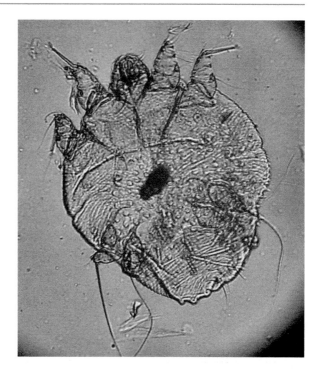

This creature, once pregnant with eggs, digs in the lower part of the stratum corneum of the human epidermis, using mandibles together proteolytic thus realizes the burrow, from 3 to 20 mm long, inside which is able to lay 2–3 eggs per day.

Epidemiology

Scabies is widespread worldwide, with an estimated global prevalence of about 300 million cases.

Sarcoptes spp. is an obligate and permanent parasite of pets and humans. In fact, it is able to survive for some time away from the host, thus facilitating its spread.

Transmission occurs by direct contact with a parasitic individual or with his clothing and personal effects such as sheets, towels. Sexual transmission has been well documented.

Diffusion to other areas of the body occurs with treatment and subsequent manual transfer.

Scabies can occur in an epidemic manner in conditions of particular crowding such as in prisons, military bases, nurseries and nursing homes.

Clinical Manifestations

After 7 days, hexapod larvae emerge from the eggs and in 16 days become octapod nymphs. After 28 days, the nymphs mutate into adult mites that mate. The male mite dies after mating and the female lives in the burrow for 30–40 days. The larvae, nymphs and adult males live under the scales of the stratum corneum. Transmission modality is essentially through prolonged contact with the skin. Scabies can therefore be considered a sexually transmitted disease. The mite can survive on bedding and clothing for about 7 days; for this reason, indirect contagion is also possible (Figs. 17.40 and 17.41).

Incubation period is about 16 weeks. Scabies lesions are most frequently seen on the hands, on the volar surface of the wrists, on the skin of the penis shaft and, in children, on the soles of the feet. When the disease becomes established, scratching lesions and sensitization lesions from inflammatory response, such as papules and inflammatory nodules, are also present (Figs. 17.42 and 17.43).

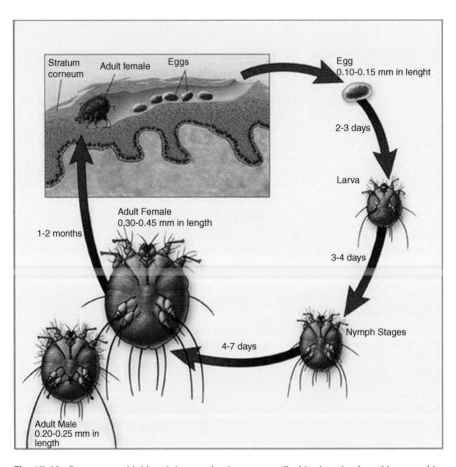

Fig. 17.40 Sarcoptes scabiei hominis reproductive process (Scabies in animals and humans: history, evolutionary perspectives and modern clinical management-https://www.researchgate.net/publication/221894813)

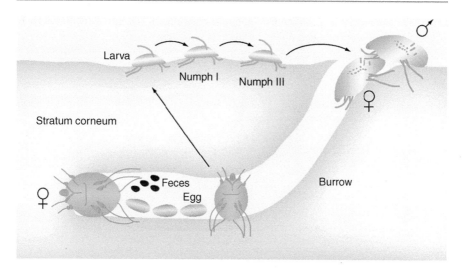

Fig. 17.41 Sarcoptes scabiei hominis vital cycle; the pregnant females penetrate the skin, digging in the stratum corneum of the epidermis burrows where they lay their eggs. From the eggs develop the larvae that emerge from the burrow, take shelter in the hair follicles or in small skin craters specially dug, in which they mature in nymphs and, then, in adults. (https://www.researchgate.net/figure/Life-cycle-of-the-scabies-mite-Only-the-female-mite-creates-a-burrow-in-the-skin-Larvae_fig9_233628791)

Fig. 17.42 Cunicles and itchy papules on dorsal hand. (https://www.healthline.com/health/scabies-vs-eczema)

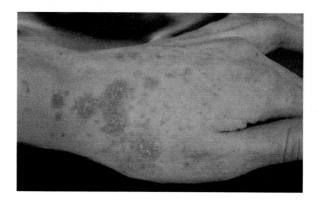

Itching is very intense especially during the night due to both the mechanical action of the mite but also to the immune response of the host directed towards the antigens of the mite, mainly consisting of chitin of the exoskeleton of its excrements. The hypersensitivity that develops thus scabies both type 1 and type 4.

Fig. 17.43 Diffuse Abdominal papules and cunicles. (https://www.frontiersin.org/articles/10.3389/fmed.2021.628392/full)

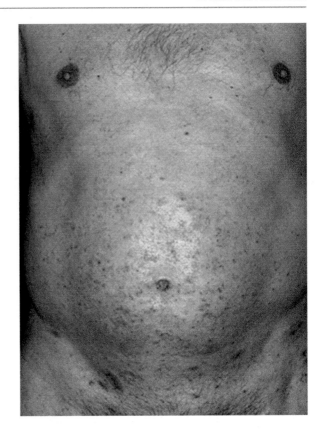

Diagnosis

The clinical diagnosis of Scabies is made on the basis of characteristic lesions and their distribution on the patient's body.

However, definitive diagnosis requires direct identification of the mite from skin scarifications. Usually the female is found in the terminal portion of a fresh burrow.

Mites can also be identified in sections of skin biopsies.

Treatment and Prevention

This pathology is treated by topical application of drugs such as Benzylbenzoate 25–30% and especially Permethrin 5%, the most widely used presidium (Table 17.22).

As hygienic precautions it is necessary to change the personal linen and disinfect the clothes that have come into contact with the patient.

Table 17.22 Scabies recommended regimens. (Sexually Transmitted Infections Treatment Guidelines, 2021-Centers for disease control and prevention-Recommendations and reports/Vol. 70, N.4)

Recommended regimens for scabies
Permethrin 5% cream applied to all areas of the body from the neck down and washed off after 8–14 h
or
Ivermectin 200 ug/kg body weight orally, repeated in 14 days
or
Ivermectin 1% lotion applied to all areas of the body from the neck down and washed off after 8–14 h; repeat treatment in 1 week if symptoms persist

References

1. Towns JM, Leslie DE, Denham I, Azzato F, Fairley CK, Chen M. Painful and multiple ano-genital lesions are common in men with Treponema pallidum PCR-positive primary syphilis without herpes simplex virus coinfection: a cross-sectional clinic-based study. Sex Transm Infect. 2016;92:110–5. https://doi.org/10.1136/sextrans-2015-052219.
2. Rolfs RT, Joesoef MR, Hendershot EF, et al. A randomized trial of enhanced therapy for early syphilis in patients with and without human immunodeficiency virus infection. N Engl J Med. 1997;337:307–14. https://doi.org/10.1056/NEJM199707313370504.
3. Yang CJ, Lee NY, Chen TC, et al. One dose versus three weekly doses of benzathine penicillin G for patients co-infected with HIV and early syphilis: a multicenter, prospective observational study. PLoS One. 2014;9:e109667. https://doi.org/10.1371/journal.pone.0109667.
4. Ganesan A, Mesner O, Okulicz JF, et al. A single dose of benzathine penicillin G is as effective as multiple doses of benzathine penicillin G for the treatment of HIV-infected persons with early syphilis. Clin Infect Dis. 2015;60:653–60. https://doi.org/10.1093/cid/ciu888.
5. Lukehart SA, Hook EW 3rd, Baker-Zander SA, Collier AC, Critchlow CW, Handsfield HH. Invasion of the central nervous system by Treponema pallidum: implications for diagnosis and treatment. Ann Intern Med. 1988;109:855–62. https://doi.org/10.7326/0003-4819-109-11-855.
6. Swidsinski A, Mendling W, Loening-Baucke V, et al. Adherent biofilms in bacterial vaginosis. Obstet Gynecol. 2005;106:1013–23. https://doi.org/10.1097/01.AOG.0000183594.45524.d2.
7. Peebles K, Velloza J, Balkus JE, McClelland RS, Barnabas RV. High global burden and costs of bacterial vaginosis: a systematic review and meta-analysis. Sex Transm Dis. 2019;46:304–11. https://doi.org/10.1097/OLQ.0000000000000972.
8. Koumans EH, Sternberg M, Bruce C, et al. The prevalence of bacterial vaginosis in the United States, 2001–2004; associations with symptoms, sexual behaviors, and reproductive health. Sex Transm Dis. 2007;34:864–9. https://doi.org/10.1097/OLQ.0b013e318074e565.
9. Kenyon CR, Buyze J, Klebanoff M, Brotman RM. Association between bacterial vaginosis and partner concurrency: a longitudinal study. Sex Transm Infect. 2018;94:75–7. https://doi.org/10.1136/sextrans-2016-052652.
10. Sanchez S, Garcia PJ, Thomas KK, Catlin M, Holmes KK. Intravaginal metronidazole gel versus metronidazole plus nystatin ovules for bacterial vaginosis: a randomized controlled trial. Am J Obstet Gynecol. 2004;191:1898–906. https://doi.org/10.1016/j.ajog.2004.06.089.
11. Ness RB, Soper DE, Holley RL, et al. Douching and endometritis: results from the PID evaluation and clinical health (PEACH) study. Sex Transm Dis. 2001;28:240–5. https://doi.org/10.1097/00007435-200104000-00010.

12. Gondwe T, Ness R, Totten PA, et al. Novel bacterial vaginosis-associated organisms mediate the relationship between vaginal douching and pelvic inflammatory disease. Sex Transm Infect. 2020;96:439–44. https://doi.org/10.1136/sextrans-2019-054191.

13. Abbai NS, Reddy T, Ramjee G. Prevalent bacterial vaginosis infection—a risk factor for incident sexually transmitted infections in women in Durban, South Africa. Int J STD AIDS. 2016;27:1283–8. https://doi.org/10.1177/0956462415616038.

14. Morris BJ, Hankins CA, Banerjee J, et al. Does male circumcision reduce women's risk of sexually transmitted infections, cervical cancer, and associated conditions? Front Public Health. 2019;7:4. https://doi.org/10.3389/fpubh.2019.00004.

15. Srinivasan S, Liu C, Mitchell CM, et al. Temporal variability of human vaginal bacteria and relationship with bacterial vaginosis. PLoS One. 2010;5:e10197. https://doi.org/10.1371/journal.pone.0010197.

16. Gajer P, Brotman RM, Bai G, et al. Temporal dynamics of the human vaginal microbiota. Sci Transl Med. 2012;4:132ra52. https://doi.org/10.1126/scitranslmed.3003605.

17. Fethers KA, Fairley CK, Morton A, et al. Early sexual experiences and risk factors for bacterial vaginosis. J Infect Dis. 2009;200:1662–70. https://doi.org/10.1086/648092.

18. Achilles SL, Austin MN, Meyn LA, Mhlanga F, Chirenje ZM, Hillier SL. Impact of contraceptive initiation on vaginal microbiota. Am J Obstet Gynecol. 2018;218:622.e1–622.e10. https://doi.org/10.1016/j.ajog.2018.02.017.

19. Vodstrcil LA, Plummer ME, Fairley CK, et al. Combined oral contraceptive pill-exposure alone does not reduce the risk of bacterial vaginosis recurrence in a pilot randomised controlled trial. Sci Rep. 2019;9:3555. https://doi.org/10.1038/s41598-019-39879-8.

20. Brooks JP, Edwards DJ, Blithe DL, et al. Effects of combined oral contraceptives, depot medroxyprogesterone acetate and the levonorgestrel-releasing intrauterine system on the vaginal microbiome. Contraception. 2017;95:405–13. https://doi.org/10.1016/j.contraception.2016.11.006.

21. Moore KR, Harmon QE, Baird DD. Serum 25-hydroxyvitamin D and risk of self-reported bacterial vaginosis in a prospective cohort study of young African American women. J Womens Health (Larchmt). 2018;27:1278–84. https://doi.org/10.1089/jwh.2017.6804.

22. Lokken EM, Balkus JE, Kiarie J, et al. Association of recent bacterial vaginosis with acquisition of Mycoplasma genitalium. Am J Epidemiol. 2017;186:194–201. https://doi.org/10.1093/aje/kwx043.

23. Brusselaers N, Shrestha S, van de Wijgert J, Verstraelen H. Vaginal dysbiosis and the risk of human papillomavirus and cervical cancer: systematic review and meta-analysis. Am J Obstet Gynecol. 2019;221:9–18.e8. https://doi.org/10.1016/j.ajog.2018.12.011.

24. Abbai NS, Nyirenda M, Naidoo S, Ramjee G. Prevalent herpes simplex virus-2 increases the risk of incident bacterial vaginosis in women from South Africa. AIDS Behav. 2018;22:2172–80. https://doi.org/10.1007/s10461-017-1924-1.

25. Brotman RM, Klebanoff MA, Nansel TR, et al. Bacterial vaginosis assessed by Gram stain and diminished colonization resistance to incident gonococcal, chlamydial, and trichomonal genital infection. J Infect Dis. 2010;202:1907–15. https://doi.org/10.1086/657320.

26. Laxmi U, Agrawal S, Raghunandan C, Randhawa VS, Saili A. Association of bacterial vaginosis with adverse fetomaternal outcome in women with spontaneous preterm labor: a prospective cohort study. J Matern Fetal Neonatal Med. 2012;25:64–7. https://doi.org/10.3109/14767058.2011.565390.

27. Cherpes TL, Wiesenfeld HC, Melan MA, et al. The associations between pelvic inflammatory disease, trichomonas vaginalis infection, and positive herpes simplex virus type 2 serology. Sex Transm Dis. 2006;33:747–52. https://doi.org/10.1097/01.olq.0000218869.52753.c7.

28. Nelson DB, Hanlon A, Hassan S, et al. Preterm labor and bacterial vaginosis-associated bacteria among urban women. J Perinat Med. 2009;37:130–4. https://doi.org/10.1515/JPM.2009.026.

29. Atashili J, Poole C, Ndumbe PM, Adimora AA, Smith JS. Bacterial vaginosis and HIV acquisition: a meta-analysis of published studies. AIDS. 2008;22:1493–501. https://doi.org/10.1097/QAD.0b013e3283021a37.

30. Gosmann C, Anahtar MN, Handley SA, et al. Lactobacillus-deficient cervicovaginal bacterial communities are associated with increased HIV acquisition in young South African women. Immunity. 2017;46:29–37. https://doi.org/10.1016/j.immuni.2016.12.013.
31. McClelland RS, Lingappa JR, Srinivasan S, et al. Evaluation of the association between the concentrations of key vaginal bacteria and the increased risk of HIV acquisition in African women from five cohorts: a nested case-control study. Lancet Infect Dis. 2018;18:554–64. https://doi.org/10.1016/S1473-3099(18)30058-6.
32. Cohen SE, Chew Ng RA, Katz KA, et al. Repeat syphilis among men who have sex with men in California, 2002–2006: implications for syphilis elimination efforts. Am J Public Health. 2012;102:e1–8. https://doi.org/10.2105/AJPH.2011.300383.
33. Johnston C, Magaret A, Srinivasan S, et al. P239 Genital HSV-2 suppression is not associated with alterations in the vaginal microbiome: a one-way, cross-over study. Sex Transm Infect. 2019;95(Suppl 1):A148.
34. Zozaya M, Ferris MJ, Siren JD, et al. Bacterial communities in penile skin, male urethra, and vaginas of heterosexual couples with and without bacterial vaginosis. Microbiome. 2016;4:16. https://doi.org/10.1186/s40168-016-0161-6.
35. Liu CM, Hungate BA, Tobian AA, et al. Penile microbiota and female partner bacterial vaginosis in Rakai, Uganda. mBio. 2015;6:e00589. https://doi.org/10.1128/mBio.00589-15.
36. Mehta SD. Systematic review of randomized trials of treatment of male sexual partners for improved bacteria vaginosis outcomes in women. Sex Transm Dis. 2012;39:822–30. https://doi.org/10.1097/OLQ.0b013e3182631d89.
37. Marrazzo JM, Koutsky LA, Eschenbach DA, Agnew K, Stine K, Hillier SL. Characterization of vaginal flora and bacterial vaginosis in women who have sex with women. J Infect Dis. 2002;185:1307–13. https://doi.org/10.1086/339884.
38. Amsel R, Totten PA, Spiegel CA, Chen KC, Eschenbach D, Holmes KK. Nonspecific vaginitis. Diagnostic criteria and microbial and epidemiologic associations. Am J Med. 1983;74:14–22. https://doi.org/10.1016/0002-9343(83)91112-9.
39. Nugent RP, Krohn MA, Hillier SL. Reliability of diagnosing bacterial vaginosis is improved by a standardized method of Gram stain interpretation. J Clin Microbiol. 1991;29:297–301. https://doi.org/10.1128/JCM.29.2.297-301.1991.
40. Schwebke JR, Hillier SL, Sobel JD, McGregor JA, Sweet RL. Validity of the vaginal gram stain for the diagnosis of bacterial vaginosis. Obstet Gynecol. 1996;88:573–6. https://doi.org/10.1016/0029-7844(96)00233-5.
41. Coleman JS, Gaydos CA. Molecular diagnosis of bacterial vaginosis: an update. J Clin Microbiol. 2018;56:e00342–18. https://doi.org/10.1128/JCM.00342-18.
42. Myziuk L, Romanowski B, Johnson SC. BVBlue test for diagnosis of bacterial vaginosis. J Clin Microbiol. 2003;41:1925–8. https://doi.org/10.1128/JCM.41.5.1925-1928.2003.
43. Bradshaw CS, Morton AN, Garland SM, Horvath LB, Kuzevska I, Fairley CK. Evaluation of a point-of-care test, BVBlue, and clinical and laboratory criteria for diagnosis of bacterial vaginosis. J Clin Microbiol. 2005;43:1304–8. https://doi.org/10.1128/JCM.43.3.1304-1308.2005.
44. Schwebke JR, Desmond R. A randomized trial of metronidazole in asymptomatic bacterial vaginosis to prevent the acquisition of sexually transmitted diseases. Am J Obstet Gynecol. 2007;196:517.e1–6. https://doi.org/10.1016/j.ajog.2007.02.048.
45. Hillier SL, Nyirjesy P, Waldbaum AS, et al. Secnidazole treatment of bacterial vaginosis: a randomized controlled trial. Obstet Gynecol. 2017;130:379–86. https://doi.org/10.1097/AOG.0000000000002135.
46. Schwebke JR, Morgan FG Jr, Koltun W, Nyirjesy P. A phase-3, double-blind, placebo-controlled study of the effectiveness and safety of single oral doses of secnidazole 2 g for the treatment of women with bacterial vaginosis. Am J Obstet Gynecol. 2017;217:678.e1–9. Erratum in: Am J Obstet Gynecol 2018;219;110. https://doi.org/10.1016/j.ajog.2017.08.017.
47. Chavoustie SE, Gersten JK, Samuel MJ, Schwebke JR. A phase 3, multicenter, prospective, open-label study to evaluate the safety of a single dose of secnidazole 2 g for the treatment of women and postmenarchal adolescent girls with bacterial vaginosis. J Womens Health (Larchmt). 2018;27:492–7. https://doi.org/10.1089/jwh.2017.6500.

48. Livengood CH 3rd, Ferris DG, Wiesenfeld HC, et al. Effectiveness of two tinidazole regimens in treatment of bacterial vaginosis: a randomized controlled trial. Obstet Gynecol. 2007;110:302–9. https://doi.org/10.1097/01.AOG.0000275282.60506.3d.

49. Sobel JD, Nyirjesy P, Brown W. Tinidazole therapy for metronidazole- resistant vaginal trichomoniasis. Clin Infect Dis. 2001;33:1341–6. https://doi.org/10.1086/323034.

50. Lewis DA, Mitjà O. Haemophilus ducreyi: from sexually transmitted infection to skin ulcer pathogen. Curr Opin Infect Dis. 2016;29:52–7. https://doi.org/10.1097/QCO.0000000000000226.

51. Lockett AE, Dance DA, Mabey DC, Drasar BS. Serum-free media for isolation of Haemophilus ducreyi. Lancet. 1991;338:326. https://doi.org/10.1016/0140-6736(91)90473-3.

52. Romero L, Huerfano C, Grillo-Ardila CF. Macrolides for treatment of Haemophilus ducreyi infection in sexually active adults. Cochrane Database Syst Rev. 2017;12:CD012492. https://doi.org/10.1002/14651858.CD012492.pub2.

53. Mabey D, Peeling RW. Lymphogranuloma venereum. Sex Transm Infect. 2002;78:90–2. https://doi.org/10.1136/sti.78.2.90.

54. White JA. Manifestations and management of lymphogranuloma venereum. Curr Opin Infect Dis. 2009;22:57–66. https://doi.org/10.1097/QCO.0b013e328320a8ae.

55. de Vries HJ, Zingoni A, White JA, Ross JD, Kreuter A. 2013 European Guideline on the management of proctitis, proctocolitis and enteritis caused by sexually transmissible pathogens. Int J STD AIDS. 2014;25:465–74. https://doi.org/10.1177/0956462413516100.

56. Ward H, Martin I, Macdonald N, et al. Lymphogranuloma venereum in the United kingdom. Clin Infect Dis. 2007;44:26–32. https://doi.org/10.1086/509922.

57. Martin-Iguacel R, Llibre JM, Nielsen H, et al. Lymphogranuloma venereum proctocolitis: a silent endemic disease in men who have sex with men in industrialised countries. Eur J Clin Microbiol Infect Dis. 2010;29:917–25. https://doi.org/10.1007/s10096-010-0959-2.

58. De Voux A, Kent JB, Macomber K, et al. Notes from the field: cluster of lymphogranuloma venereum cases among men who have sex with men—Michigan, August 2015–April 2016. MMWR Morb Mortal Wkly Rep. 2016;65:920–1. https://doi.org/10.15585/mmwr.mm6534a6.

59. Pallawela SN, Sullivan AK, Macdonald N, et al. Clinical predictors of rectal lymphogranuloma venereum infection: results from a multicentre case-control study in the U.K. Sex Transm Infect. 2014;90:269–74. https://doi.org/10.1136/sextrans-2013-051401.

60. De Vrieze NH, de Vries HJ. Lymphogranuloma venereum among men who have sex with men. An epidemiological and clinical review. Expert Rev Anti Infect Ther. 2014;12:697–704. https://doi.org/10.1586/14787210.2014.901169.

61. Koper NE, van der Sande MA, Gotz HM, Koedijk FD, Dutch STI Clinics. Lymphogranuloma venereum among men who have sex with men in the Netherlands: regional differences in testing rates lead to underestimation of the incidence, 2006–2012. Euro Surveill. 2013;18:20561. https://doi.org/10.2807/1560-7917.ES2013.18.34.20561.

62. Haar K, Dudareva-Vizule S, Wisplinghoff H, et al. Lymphogranuloma venereum in men screened for pharyngeal and rectal infection, Germany. Emerg Infect Dis. 2013;19:488–92. https://doi.org/10.3201/eid1903.121028.

63. Riera-Monroig J, Fuertes de Vega I. Lymphogranuloma venereum presenting as an ulcer on the tongue. Sex Transm Infect. 2019;95:169–70. https://doi.org/10.1136/sextrans-2018-053787.

64. Andrada MT, Dhar JK, Wilde H. Oral lymphogranuloma venereum and cervical lymphadenopathy. Case report. Mil Med. 1974;139:99–101. https://doi.org/10.1093/milmed/139.2.99.

65. Ilyas S, Richmond D, Burns G, et al. Orolabial lymphogranuloma venereum, Michigan, USA. Emerg Infect Dis. 2019;25:2112–4. https://doi.org/10.3201/eid2511.190819.

66. Kersh EN, Pillay A, de Voux A, Chen C. Laboratory processes for confirmation of lymphogranuloma venereum infection during a 2015 investigation of a cluster of cases in the United States. Sex Transm Dis. 2017;44:691–4. https://doi.org/10.1097/OLQ.0000000000000667.

67. CDC. Recommendations for the laboratory-based detection of Chlamydia trachomatis and Neisseria gonorrhoeae—2014. MMWR Recomm Rep. 2014;63(RR-2):1–19.

68. Pathela P, Jamison K, Kornblum J, Quinlan T, Halse TA, Schillinger JA. Lymphogranuloma venereum: an increasingly common anorectal infection among men who have sex with men attending New York City sexualhealthclinics. Sex Transm Dis. 2019;46:e14–7. https://doi.org/10.1097/OLQ.0000000000000921.

69. Cohen S, Brosnan H, Kohn R, et al. P494 Diagnosis and management of lymphogranuloma venereum (LGV) in a municipal STD clinic, San Francisco, 2016–18. Sex Transm Infect. 2019;95(Suppl 1):A229.

70. O'Farrell N. Donovanosis. Sex Transm Infect. 2002;78:452–7. https://doi.org/10.1136/sti.78.6.452.

71. Darville T, Pelvic Inflammatory Disease Workshop Proceedings Committee. Pelvic inflammatory disease: identifying research gaps—proceedings of a workshop sponsored by Department of Health and Human Services/National Institutes of Health/National Institute of Allergy and Infectious Diseases, November 3–4, 2011. Sex Transm Dis. 2013;40:761–7. https://doi.org/10.1097/OLQ.0000000000000028.

72. Wiesenfeld HC, Sweet RL, Ness RB, Krohn MA, Amortegui AJ, Hillier SL. Comparison of acute and subclinical pelvic inflammatory disease. Sex Transm Dis. 2005;32:400–5. https://doi.org/10.1097/01.olq.0000154508.26532.6a.

73. Wiesenfeld HC, Hillier SL, Meyn LA, Amortegui AJ, Sweet RL. Subclinical pelvic inflammatory disease and infertility. Obstet Gynecol. 2012;120:37–43. https://doi.org/10.1097/AOG.0b013e31825a6bc9.

74. Ness RB, Soper DE, Holley RL, et al. Effectiveness of inpatient and outpatient treatment strategies for women with pelvic inflammatory disease: results from the Pelvic Inflammatory Disease Evaluation and Clinical Health (PEACH) Randomized Trial. Am J Obstet Gynecol. 2002;186:929–37. https://doi.org/10.1067/mob.2002.121625.

75. Wiesenfeld HC, Meyn LA, Darville T, Macio IS, Hillier SL. A randomized controlled trial of ceftriaxone and doxycycline, with or without metronidazole, for the treatment of acute pelvic inflammatory disease. Clin Infect Dis. 2021;72:1181–9. https://doi.org/10.1093/cid/ciaa101.

76. Scholes D, Stergachis A, Heidrich FE, Andrilla H, Holmes KK, Stamm WE. Prevention of pelvic inflammatory disease by screening for cervical chlamydial infection. N Engl J Med. 1996;334:1362–6. https://doi.org/10.1056/NEJM199605233342103.

77. Oakeshott P, Kerry S, Aghaizu A, et al. Randomised controlled trial of screening for Chlamydia trachomatis to prevent pelvic inflammatory disease: the POPI (Prevention of Pelvic Infection) trial. BMJ. 2010;340:c1642. https://doi.org/10.1136/bmj.c1642.

78. Ness RB, Hillier SL, Kip KE, et al. Bacterial vaginosis and risk of pelvic inflammatory disease. Obstet Gynecol. 2004;104:761–9. https://doi.org/10.1097/01.AOG.0000139512.37582.17.

79. Ness RB, Kip KE, Hillier SL, et al. A cluster analysis of bacterial vaginosis-associated microflora and pelvic inflammatory disease. Am J Epidemiol. 2005;162:585–90. https://doi.org/10.1093/aje/kwi243.

80. Haggerty CL, Totten PA, Tang G, et al. Identification of novel microbes associated with pelvic inflammatory disease and infertility. Sex Transm Infect. 2016;92:441–6. https://doi.org/10.1136/sextrans-2015-052285.

81. De Villiers EM, Fauquet C, Broker TR, Bernard HU, zur Hausen H. Classification of papillomaviruses. Virology. 2004;324:17–27. https://doi.org/10.1016/j.virol.2004.03.033.

82. Kreisel KM, Spicknall IH, Gargano JW, et al. Sexually transmitted infections among US women and men: prevalence and incidence estimates, 2018. Sex Transm Dis. 2021;48:208–14. https://doi.org/10.1097/OLQ.0000000000001355.

83. Myers ER, McCrory DC, Nanda K, Bastian L, Matchar DB. Mathematical model for the natural history of human papillomavirus infection and cervical carcinogenesis. Am J Epidemiol. 2000;151:1158–71. https://doi.org/10.1093/oxfordjournals.aje.a010166.

84. Chesson HW, Dunne EF, Hariri S, Markowitz LE. The estimated lifetime probability of acquiring human papillomavirus in the United States. Sex Transm Dis. 2014;41:660–4. https://doi.org/10.1097/OLQ.0000000000000193.

85. Cogliano V, Baan R, Straif K, Grosse Y, Secretan B, El Ghissassi F, WHO International Agency for Research on Cancer. Carcinogenicity of human papillomaviruses. Lancet Oncol. 2005;6:204. https://doi.org/10.1016/S1470-2045(05)70086-3.
86. Gotovtseva EP, Kapadia AS, Smolensky MH, Lairson DR. Optimal frequency of imiquimod (aldara) 5% cream for the treatment of external genital warts in immunocompetent adults: a meta-analysis. Sex Transm Dis. 2008;35:346–51. https://doi.org/10.1097/OLQ.0b013e31815ea8d1.
87. Baker DA, Ferris DG, Martens MG, et al. Imiquimod 3.75% cream applied daily to treat anogenital warts: combined results from women in two randomized, placebo-controlled studies. Infect Dis Obstet Gynecol. 2011;2011:806105. https://doi.org/10.1155/2011/806105.
88. Mashiah J, Brenner S. Possible mechanisms in the induction of vitiligo- like hypopigmentation by topical imiquimod. Clin Exp Dermatol. 2008;33:74–6.
89. Benedetti J, Corey L, Ashley R. Recurrence rates in genital herpes after symptomatic first-episode infection. Ann Intern Med. 1994;121:847–54. https://doi.org/10.7326/0003-4819-121-11-199412010-00004.
90. Engelberg R, Carrell D, Krantz E, Corey L, Wald A. Natural history of genital herpes simplex virus type 1 infection. Sex Transm Dis. 2003;30:174–7. https://doi.org/10.1097/00007435-200302000-00015.
91. Masese L, Baeten JM, Richardson BA, et al. Changes in the contribution of genital tract infections to HIV acquisition among Kenyan high-risk women from 1993 to 2012. AIDS. 2015;29:1077–85. https://doi.org/10.1097/QAD.0000000000000646.
92. Wawer MJ, Gray RH, Sewankambo NK, et al. Rates of HIV-1 transmission per coital act, by stage of HIV-1 infection, in Rakai, Uganda. J Infect Dis. 2005;191:1403–9. https://doi.org/10.1086/429411.
93. Pilcher CD, Eron JJ Jr, Vemazza PL, et al. Sexual transmission during the incubation period of primary HIV infection. JAMA. 2001;286:1713–4. https://doi.org/10.1001/jama.286.14.1713.
94. Legarth RA, Ahlström MG, Kronborg G, et al. Long-term mortality in HIV-infected individuals 50 years or older: a nationwide, population-based cohort study. J Acquir Immune Defic Syndr. 2016;71:213–8. https://doi.org/10.1097/QAI.0000000000000825.
95. Marcus JL, Chao CR, Leyden WA, et al. Narrowing the gap in life expectancy between HIV-infected and HIV-uninfected individuals with access to care. J Acquir Immune Defic Syndr. 2016;73:39–46. https://doi.org/10.1097/QAI.0000000000001014.
96. Cohen MS, Chen YQ, McCauley M, et al. Antiretroviral therapy for the prevention of HIV-1 transmission. N Engl J Med. 2016;375:830–9. https://doi.org/10.1056/NEJMoa1600693.
97. Rodger AJ, Cambiano V, Bruun T, et al. Sexual activity without condoms and risk of HIV transmission in serodifferent couples when the HIV-positive partner is using suppressive antiretroviral therapy. JAMA. 2016;316:171–81. https://doi.org/10.1001/jama.2016.5148.
98. Bavinton BR, Pinto AN, Phanuphak N, et al. Viral suppression and HIV transmission in sero-discordant male couples: an international, prospective, observational, cohort study. Lancet HIV. 2018;5:e438–47. https://doi.org/10.1016/S2352-3018(18)30132-2.
99. Rodger AJ, Cambiano V, Bruun T, et al. Risk of HIV transmission through condomless sex in serodifferent gay couples with the HIV-positive partner taking suppressive antiretroviral therapy (PARTNER): final results of a multicentre, prospective, observational study. Lancet. 2019;393:2428–38. https://doi.org/10.1016/S0140-6736(19)30418-0.
100. Branson BM, Handsfield HH, Lampe MA, et al. Revised recommendations for HIV testing of adults, adolescents, and pregnant women in health-care settings. MMWR Recomm Rep. 2006;55(RR-14):1–17.
101. DiNenno EA, Prejean J, Irwin K, et al. Recommendations for HIV screening of gay, bisexual, and other men who have sex with men—United States, 2017. MMWR Morb Mortal Wkly Rep. 2017;66:830–2. https://doi.org/10.15585/mmwr.mm6631a3.
102. Owens DK, Davidson KW, Krist AH, et al. Screening for HIV infection: US Preventive Services Task Force recommendation statement. JAMA. 2019;321:2326–36. https://doi.org/10.1001/jama.2019.6587.

103. Centers for Disease Control and Prevention. Health and Human Services Panel on Treatment of HIV-Infected Pregnant Women and Prevention of Perinatal Transmission. Recommendations for use of antiretroviral drugs in pregnant HIV-1- infected women for maternal health and interventions to reduce perinatal HIV transmission in the United States. Bethesda, MD: US Department of Health and Human Services, National Institutes of Health, AIDSinfo; 2014. https://npin.cdc.gov/publication/recommendations-use-antiretroviral-drugs-pregnant-hiv-1-infected-women-maternal-health.

104. Committee on Obstetric Practice HIV Expert Work Group. ACOG Committee opinion no. 752: prenatal and perinatal human immunodeficiency virus testing. Obstet Gynecol. 2018;132:e138–42. https://doi.org/10.1097/AOG.0000000000002825.

105. Calabrese SK, Mayer KH. Providers should discuss U=U with all patients living with HIV. Lancet HIV. 2019;6:e211–3. https://doi.org/10.1016/S2352-3018(19)30030-X.

106. Gilbert P, Ciccarone D, Gansky SA, et al. Interactive "Video Doctor" counseling reduces drug and sexual risk behaviors among HIV-positive patients in diverse outpatient settings. PLoS One. 2008;3:e1988. https://doi.org/10.1371/journal.pone.0001988.

107. Alter HJ, Purcell RH, Gerin JL, et al. Transmission of hepatitis B to chimpanzees by hepatitis B surface antigen-positive saliva and semen. Infect Immun. 1977;16:928–33. https://doi.org/10.1128/IAI.16.3.928-933.1977.

108. Villarejos VM, Visoná KA, Gutiérrez A, Rodríguez A. Role of saliva, urine and feces in the transmission of type B hepatitis. N Engl J Med. 1974;291:1375–8. https://doi.org/10.1056/NEJM197412262912602.

109. Terrault NA, Lok ASF, McMahon BJ, et al. Update on prevention, diagnosis, and treatment of chronic hepatitis B: AASLD 2018 hepatitis B guidance. Hepatology. 2018;67:1560–99. https://doi.org/10.1002/hep.29800.

110. Lockart I, Matthews GV, Danta M. Sexually transmitted hepatitis C infection: the evolving epidemic in HIV-positive and HIV-negative MSM. Curr Opin Infect Dis. 2019;32:31–7. https://doi.org/10.1097/QCO.0000000000000515.

111. Terrault NA, Dodge JL, Murphy EL, et al. Sexual transmission of hepatitis C virus among monogamous heterosexual couples: the HCV partners study. Hepatology. 2013;57:881–9. https://doi.org/10.1002/hep.26164.

112. Price JC, McKinney JE, Crouch PC, et al. Sexually acquired hepatitis C infection in HIV-uninfected men who have sex with men using preexposure prophylaxis against HIV. J Infect Dis. 2019;219:1373–6. https://doi.org/10.1093/infdis/jiy670.

113. Tohme RA, Holmberg SD. Transmission of hepatitis C virus infection through tattooing and piercing: a critical review. Clin Infect Dis. 2012;54:1167–78. https://doi.org/10.1093/cid/cir991.

114. Brettler DB, Mannucci PM, Gringeri A, et al. The low risk of hepatitis C virus transmission among sexual partners of hepatitis C-infected hemophilic males: an international, multicenter study. Blood. 1992;80:540–3. https://doi.org/10.1182/blood.V80.2.540.540.

115. Kao JH, Hwang YT, Chen PJ, et al. Transmission of hepatitis C virus between spouses: the important role of exposure duration. Am J Gastroenterol. 1996;91:2087–90.

116. Loo SK, Tang WY, Lo KK. Clinical significance of Trichomonas vaginalis detected in Papanicolaou smear: a survey in female Social Hygiene Clinic. Hong Kong Med J. 2009;15:90–3.

117. Howe K, Kissinger PJ. Single-dose compared with multidose metronidazole for the treatment of trichomoniasis in women: a meta- analysis. Sex Transm Dis. 2017;44:29–34. https://doi.org/10.1097/OLQ.0000000000000537.

118. Galiczynski EM Jr, Elston DM. What's eating you? Pubic lice (Pthirus pubis). Cutis. 2008;81:109–14.

119. Meinking TL, Serrano L, Hard B, et al. Comparative in vitro pediculicidal efficacy of treatments in a resistant head lice population in the United States. Arch Dermatol. 2002;138:220–4. https://doi.org/10.1001/archderm.138.2.220.

120. Yoon KS, Gao JR, Lee SH, Clark JM, Brown L, Taplin D. Permethrin- resistant human head lice, Pediculus capitis, and their treatment. Arch Dermatol. 2003;139:994–1000. https://doi.org/10.1001/archderm.139.8.994.

121. Burkhart CG, Burkhart CN. Oral ivermectin for Phthirus pubis. J Am Acad Dermatol. 2004;51:1037–8. https://doi.org/10.1016/j.jaad.2004.04.041.

122. Scott GR, Chosidow O, IUSTI/WHO. European guideline for the management of pediculosis pubis, 2010. Int J STD AIDS. 2011;22:304–5. https://doi.org/10.1258/ijsa.2011.011114.

123. Goldust M, Rezaee E, Raghifar R, Hemayat S. Comparing the efficacy of oral ivermectin vs malathion 0.5% lotion for the treatment of scabies. Skinmed. 2014;12:284–7.

124. Leung AKC, Lam JM, Leong KF. Scabies: a neglected global disease. Curr Pediatr Rev. 2020;16:33–42. https://doi.org/10.2174/1573396315666190717114131.

125. Shimose L, Munoz-Price LS. Diagnosis, prevention, and treatment of scabies. Curr Infect Dis Rep. 2013;15:426–31. https://doi.org/10.1007/s11908-013-0354-0.

Penile Cancer

18

Laura Elst, Federica Peretti, Esther Lee, Arie Parnham, Marco Falcone, and Maarten Albersen

Abstract

Penile cancer (PC) is a rare disease with a prevalence of 0.1–1 in 100,000 men in Western countries. However, risk factors such as phimosis, low socioeconomic status, smoking and human papillomavirus (HPV) affect prevalence rates. Different histological subtypes of PC have been described and moreover, since 2016 the World Health Organization has stratified PC by HPV status as pathways of carcinogenesis strongly differ.

Primary treatment of PC includes topical therapy, radiotherapy, laser therapy and surgical approaches. Historically, radical excision of localized disease with a 2 cm margin was the gold standard. Since radical surgery affects the ability to void in the upright position, sexual function and psychological wellbeing, a paradigm shift has occurred towards penile-sparing approaches. Organ-sparing surgery aims to minimize loss of penile function and to preserve patients' quality of life, without compromising oncological outcome. Since PC is characterized by early lymphatic spread and as lymph node involvement is known as the most important predictor of survival in PC, in-depth and upfront lymph node staging is required. In advanced stages of disease, a multimodal approach is needed, including inguinopelvic lymphadenectomy followed by adjuvant chemotherapy.

L. Elst · M. Albersen (✉)
Department of Urology, University Hospitals Leuven, Leuven, Belgium
e-mail: maarten.albersen@uzleuven.be

F. Peretti · M. Falcone
Urology Department, "Città della Salute e della Scienza", Molinette Hospital, University of Turin, Turin, Italy
e-mail: marco.falcone@unito.it

E. Lee · A. Parnham
Department of Urology, University College London Hospital, London, UK

© The Author(s), under exclusive license to Springer Nature Switzerland AG 2022
S. Sarikaya et al. (eds.), *Andrology and Sexual Medicine*, Management of Urology,
https://doi.org/10.1007/978-3-031-12049-7_18

To date, Platinum- and Taxane-based chemotherapy is mainstay of systemic therapy, however burdened by poor response rates and early therapy resistance.

Dealing with the diagnosis of PC and their appropriate treatments can have a substantial impact on psychological and physical wellbeing, by affecting sexual, esthetical, and urinary penile function.

Introduction

Laura Elst and Maarten Albersen

Penile cancer (PC) is a rare disease with a prevalence of 0.1–1 in 100,000 men in Western countries [1]. However, the prevalence is dependent on the country and the exposure to risk factors, such as phimosis, lack of circumcision, low socioeconomic status, smoking, lichen sclerosus et atrophicans and Human Papilloma Virus (HPV) [2]. As a result, the incidence of PC is negligible in countries with religious circumcision in children and can be up to 6.8 in 100,000 men in low-income countries such as Brazil [3, 4]. Currently, a rise in incidence rates is observed in developed countries, which may be explained due to a higher exposure to HPV [5]. Ninety-five percent of penile cancers are penile squamous cell carcinomas (pSCC), originating in the squamous epithelial cells of the glans and the prepuce [1]. These pSCC could be divided into various histological subgroups, characterized by HPV status, aggressiveness and growth patterns [1]. Most common histological subtypes are usual squamous cell carcinoma (SCC), papillary carcinoma, basaloid carcinoma, warty carcinoma, mixed warty-basaloid carcinoma, verrucous carcinoma and mixed carcinomas [1]. Since 2016 the WHO has recognized two different pathways of carcinogenesis: non-HPV related pSCC and HPV-related pSCC, in which the latter is considered responsible for 50.8% of cases worldwide [6, 7].

Since pSCC is characterized by an aggressive clinical course with early lymphatic and metastatic dissemination, the treatment of PC is strongly depending on the pathological staging and grading of the tumor, which is currently defined by the American Joint Committee on Cancer (AJCC) and the Union Internationale Contre le Cancer (UICC) TNM clinical classification system (8th edition) [3, 8]. This universal classification systems should assist healthcare providers to predict the prognosis and to choose an appropriate treatment.

Primary treatment of PC can be divided into non-surgical and surgical approaches, including organ-sparing surgery (OSS) or more radical surgery. Primary PC spreads into the superficial and deep inguinal lymph nodes followed by the pelvic lymph nodes and finally to retroperitoneal lymph nodes, resulting in systemic metastases. Since lymph node involvement is known as the most important predictor of survival in PC, in-depth lymph node staging is required.

In addition to primary tumor treatment, when lymph nodes are involved, they should be accurately treated with inguinal or pelvic lymph node dissection (ILND or PLND), depending on the TNM classification. In cases of advanced disease (pN2 or pN3) adjuvant chemotherapy after ILND is the mainstay of therapy, however response rates are poor [1]. Despite a low quality of evidence, the European Association of Urology guidelines recommend neo-adjuvant chemotherapy if patients have fixed, unresectable nodal disease (cN3) [3]. Hithertho, there is no evidence on the role of radiotherapy in advanced PC, so it's use is not recommended except for clinical trials [1].

The diagnosis of PC and its related treatments can have a devastating impact on the patients' psychological well-being and its quality of life. Current treatment strategies aim to preserve as much as possible penile length and penile function to keep the ability to void in the upright position and the penile sexual function, however tumor stage and grade should be taken into account and as a result a complete excision of tumor tissue is sometimes required [9].

Primary Tumor Management

Laura Elst and Maarten Albersen

Penile Sparing Non-surgical Treatment

5-Fluoroacil (5-FU)

Five-fluoroacil is a topical treatment which can be used in superficial penile intraepithelial neoplasia (PeIN). Five-fluoroacil is the first line treatment for PeIN. After topical application of 5-FU and topical application of 5-FU with circumcision, complete response rates of 50% to 74% respectively, have been described [10, 11]. However, small multicenter studies reported recurrence rates of 20–25% after complete response [10, 11]. Since recurrence rates are high, a long-term surveillance is required. Moreover, the threshold to take biopsy should be low as persistence and recurrence of lesions is high and non-responsiveness could imply underlying invasive disease [1]. Inflammatory responses may occur which can be treated with topical steroids [9].

Imiquimod

Imiquimod is an immunotherapeutic local treatment, which can be used in PeIN. Imiquimod contains Toll-like seven receptor agonists which stimulate the immune response against malignant cells in the penile skin. A systematic review by Deen et al. demonstrated a complete response rate in PeIN after Imiquimod therapy of 63% [12]. However, few studies are investigating the use of Imiquimod monotherapy. No evidence-based data on dose and application protocol are available, however in our center we advise to apply Imiquimod 5% 3 times a week for 12 weeks. Inflammation of tissue is a common complication through activation of the immune system.

Radiotherapy: External Beam Radiotherapy (EBRT), Surface Mold Brachytherapy and Interstitial Brachytherapy

Radiotherapy is an organ-sparing treatment which is indicated in case of Ta, T1 and T2 tumors <4 cm in diameter and can be an option in T3 tumors smaller than 4 cm in diameter [1]. Radiotherapy is a well examined treatment in other squamous cell tumors such as vulva, cervix, head and neck and anal cancer. However, there is limited evidence in PC. The type of radiotherapy should be chosen depending on tumor extent and patient characteristics. EBRT is widely available, surface mold brachytherapy is a good option in superficial lesions and interstitial brachytherapy in more invasive lesions [13]. Surface mold brachytherapy is a relatively new option in PC in which the patient selection is really important as it is only appropriate for superficial stage Tis and T1a tumors less than 3 mm thick [13]. EBRT has higher recurrence rates than brachytherapy, 38–43% versus 13–20%, respectively [9, 14]. Moreover, penile preservation rates are higher in brachytherapy (high dose and low dose) compared to EBRT, 60% versus 80–86% respectively [13].

Before radiotherapy, patients need a circumcision in order to exactly visualize the lesion and in addition to avoid a paraphimosis due to swelling of the foreskin. Most common complications after EBRT and brachytherapy are radiation necrosis, urethral strictures and meatal stenosis. Cordoba et al. reported 6.8% of patients requiring penile amputation due to high necrosis rates [15].

Lasertherapy

Lasertherapy, with Neodymium: yttrium-aluminium-garnet (Nd:YAG) or Carbon dioxide (CO_2) lasers, is an appropriate treatment for PeIN and T1 penile cancers [1]. Potassium titanyl phosphate (KTP) lasers are used less frequently. Lasertherapy is mostly combined with circumcision for oncological improvement, however combination therapies of laserexcision and local chemotherapy or radiotherapy have also been described [16]. Evidence on lasertherapy is low and studies are demonstrating heterogeneous data. Application of acetic acid 5% is adviced to accurately define the area of interest, which should be marked before starting lasertherapy, though lesions are difficult to delineate [17]. A retrospective study on 224 PeIN and T1 patients treated by CO_2 lasertherapy demonstrated a 10-year recurrence rate of 17.5% [17]. Another study on Nd:YAG lasertherapy in 54 patients, including PeIN, T1 and 4 patients suffering T2 pSCC, demonstrated a higher recurrence rate of 42% during 11 years [18]. Care should be taken to counsel patients for strict follow-up protocols as lasertherapy damages tissue and as a result pathological staging may be compromised. Despite high local recurrence rates, lasertherapy portrays excellent esthetic and functional outcomes without chances in erection capability [17].

Penile Sparing Surgical Treatment

Historically, aggressive treatment of PC through surgical excision with 2-cm margins was the standard of care [19, 20]. However, partial and total penectomy result in the inability to void in the upright position, compromise masculinity and reduce penile sexual function and appearance [9]. During the last decennium, the treatment of PC has shifted to less aggressive and penile-sparing approaches. Nowadays, OSS is the mainstay of therapy, aiming to minimize loss of penile function and preservation of patients' quality of life, while not compromising oncological results [21]. Different studies have demonstrated a higher rate of local recurrence after OSS, though not influencing overall survival (OS) [22, 23]. As long as resection margins are clear, margins as small as 1 mm seem to be oncollogically safe and do not influence overall survival [23, 24]. Nonetheless, a recent study demonstrated that local recurrence after upfront glansectomy was associated with worse OS and cancer specific survival (CSS), particularly in high-grade tumors, thereby challenging the use of OSS [25]. Since most recurrences (92%) are observed during the first 5 years after surgery, clinical examination is advised every 3 months during the first 2 years, every 6 months in the third, fourth and fifth year and afterwards annually [1, 19]. A careful patient selection is crucial in OSS, as patients must be compliant to strict follow-up appointments. The National Comprehensive Cancer Network (NCCN) advocates the use of OSS only in lower grade and stage tumors, whereas the European Association of Urology (EAU) recommends to implement OSS whenever possible, indicating that further research is required [1, 26]. In this section, we aim to give a brief overview of organ-sparing surgical techniques.

Wide Local Excision and Circumcision

Based on location and tumor invasiveness a circumcision or a wide local excision (WLE) can be indicated for local disease. PeIN and pT1 tumors, which are limited to the prepuce only, can be treated by a radical circumcision in which negative radical margins should be achieved [27]. If the tumor invades the glans, a circumcision combined with a WLE can be an appropriate treatment. Although circumcision is one of the most common urological procedures, almost 30% of men globally underwent a circumcision for several purposes, the procedure results in sensation changes of the glans [28, 29]. Circumcision could cause lower sexual sensations and higher levels of discomfort and pain [28]. However, circumcision is an imperative part of PC surgery because of two main reasons. Firstly, it can remove the chronic inflammatory stimulus of PC and thereby minimizing progression of malignant cells [9]. Secondly, it facilitates clinical examination and critical follow-up, which is of the utmost importance to early recognize local recurrence in OSS.

Glans Resurfacing and Split-Thickness Skin Graft (STSG)

Glans resurfacing is a surgical technique used for localized and superficial tumors of the glans. It can be performed in PeIN and pT1a tumors in patients with failure of topical therapies and who are not eligible for rigorous follow-up protocols. Glans resurfacing includes removal of the glandular epithelium and subepithelium. Since the whole glandular skin is excised, glans resurfacing has the advantage of obtaining a complete histopathological report, which optimizes staging of primary lesions. If less than 50% of glandular tissue is involved, a partial glans resurfacing can be performed in order to preserve the penile corona to maintain penile sensitivity [30]. Partial glans resurfacing has a higher risk of local recurrence as an incomplete resection occurs, however local recurrence does not compromise patients' OS [22, 23]. Total glans resurfacing excises the complete glandular epithelium resulting in lower recurrence rates [31, 32].

The surgical procedure starts with a circumcision in uncircumcised patients. Afterwards, a tourniquet is applied at the glans penis. The glans epithelium and subepithelium are incised, starting at the meatus, which is marked in four quadrants, and terminating at the coronal sulcus. The tip of each quadrant of glandular skin is lifted and dissected from the meatus to the coronal sulcus (Fig. 18.1). After complete removal of glandular epithelial and subepithelial tissue, the tourniquet should be removed to identify and control excessive bleeding by bipolar energy.

A split-thickness skin graft (STSG), which is harvested preferably from the thigh using a dermatome, can be used to cover the spongious tissue of the glans. In our center we use a graft thickness of 0.018 inches to optimize graft taking rates. However, the use of STSG should be discouraged in patients who suffer severe vascular disease, diabetes or who refuse to stop smoking as this can compromise graft taking rates. The graft is quilted with absorbable sutures monofilament poliglecaprone 5.0 (Fig. 18.2). Small cuts with a nr. 15 blade are made though the graft

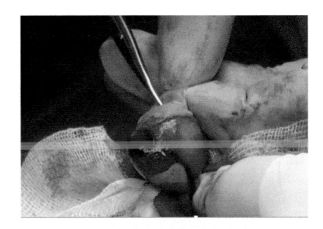

Fig. 18.1 The glans is marked in four quadrants and then the glandular epithelium and subepithelium are incised, starting at the meatus and terminating at the coronal sulcus. The tip of each quadrant of glandular skin is lifted and dissected from the meatus to the coronal sulcus

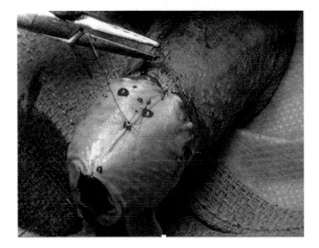

Fig. 18.2 An extragenital STSG, preferably harvested from the thigh, is applied over the corpora and the neoglans is quilted with absorbable monofilament 5.0 sutures to compress the graft to its bed

Fig. 18.3 A paraffin soaked tie-over dressing is applied and sutured, as described by Malone and colleagues [34]

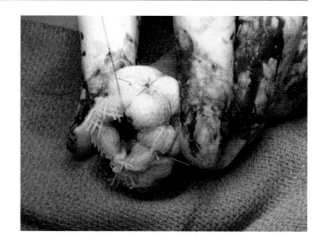

to prevent hematoma formation underneath. The graft donor site is infiltrated with 1% lidocaine and 1:200000 adrenaline to optimize hemostasis and afterwards an alginate dressing is applied [33]. After the surgical procedure, a urinary catheter is applied and a paraffin soaked dressing is sutured as described by Malone et al. (Fig. 18.3) [34]. This dressing, consisting of silicone gauze and several layers of paraffin gauze, is applied to provide compression of the graft against the graft bed and to reduce sheer, allowing the patient to early mobilize [33, 34]. The dressing and catheter are left in place for 5–10 days postoperative.

The glans resurfacing with STSG surgical procedure provides acceptable esthetic outcomes and preservation of penile function. However, a reduced glandular sensation has been described [35]. Most frequent complications are graft failure and infection, though since the graft bed is thoroughly perfused, these complications are still very uncommon [9]. Local recurrence is described in between 0–6% of patients [19, 36].

Glansectomy

A glansectomy is a surgical procedure indicated for high grade pT1 and T2 tumors. Austoni et al. firstly described the corpora cavernosa as a well-defined anatomical structure, not contiguous with the corpus spongiosum [37]. In case of locally advanced disease, the removal of the glans spongiosum from the corpora cavernosa, is an appropriate surgical treatment. However, a good clinical examination of the penile tumor is required to provide optimal staging. In case of suspected invasion into the corpora cavernosa (cT3), preoperative imaging through ultrasound or MRI, can help to stratify and choose the appropriate treatment [33]. Depending on the extent of tumor invasion, the surgical procedure should be performed over versus under Buck's fascia.

Dissection over Buck's fascia is sufficient if tumor invasion is confined to the glans, without invasion into the corporal tips (Fig. 18.5). This approach provides the advantage of protecting the dorsal neurovascular bundle and preserving a well vascularized graft bed to enhance graft taking rates. However, dissection over Buck's fascia could jeopardize the oncological resection margins.

In cases of high-risk tumors where corporal tip involvement is suspected, a dissection under Buck's fascia is advised. In addition, a corporal tip excision can be considered to provide wider resection margins [27]. However, dissection under Buck's fascia poses two risks. Firstly to damage the neurovascular bundle and secondly to have worse graft healing as the tunica albuginea is avascular, compromising graft taking rates.

When the tumor invades less than 50% of the glans, a partial glansectomy or a WLE should be considered. The glans can be primarily closed or in case of larger lesions covered by STSG or buccal mucosa grafts (BMG) [27].

The surgical procedure starts with a subcoronal skin incision (Fig. 18.4). The continuation of the procedure is depending on the grade of invasiveness.

1. If dissection over Buck's fascia is sufficient, the plane between the glans and Buck's fascia is approached and dissected (Fig. 18.5). Dissection is continued until the glans is separated from the corporal heads and only the urethra remains intact (Fig. 18.6). Finally, the urethra is transected below the tumor lesion and splayed in between the cavernosal tips. Care should be taken to provide a thor-

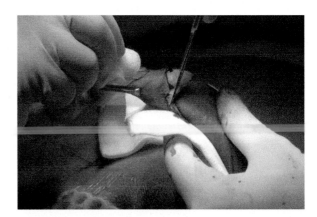

Fig. 18.4 A subcoronal skin incision is made

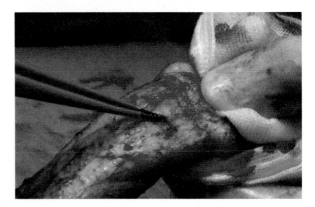

Fig. 18.5 Dissection over Buck's fascia. A thorough hemostasis is provided by bipolar diathermy to prevent for hematoma formation

Fig. 18.6 Dissection continues until the glans is separated from the corporal heads and only the urethra remains intact. Finally, the urethra is transected below the tumor lesion and placed in between the cavernosal tips

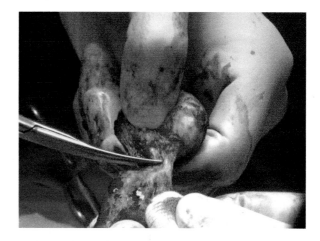

Fig. 18.7 Dissection under Buck's fascia and identification of the neurovascular bundle

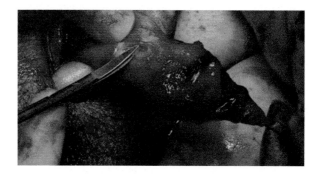

ough hemostasis to prevent hematoma formation. Afterwards, the penile shaft skin is sutured to the corporal bodies and a neoglans is created through preservation of a 2.5 cm gap [33]. When the patient is fit, a STSG could be harvested from the thigh to cover the neoglans to the Buck's fascia, with a technique analogous to the glans resurfacing technique. Neovascularization of the graft takes 5–7 days, entailing a risk of infection and graft failure [33].

2. If, because of suspicious corporal tip involvement, dissection under Buck's fascia is required, the procedure starts with a subcoronal incision. Afterwards, the plane between the glans and Buck's fascia is dissected longitudinally until Buck's fascia is circumferentially excised. The neurovascular bundle should be approached and ligated from the tunica albuginea (Fig. 18.7). Finally, Buck's fascia is dissected of the corporal heads and the urethra is divided under the tumor lesion. The continuation is equal to dissection over Buck's fascia, apart from the STSG which should be placed to the tunica albuginea.

A glansectomy provides satisfactory oncological and functional outcomes. Sexual penile functions are mostly maintained, though a reduction in glans sensitivity is described [38, 39]. Further research on functional and sexual outcomes is required.

Complications of glansectomy are graft failure, infection and meatal stenosis. Parnham et al. demonstrated partial graft loss and total graft loss rates of 20% and 3.4%, respectively [33]. Local recurrences rates are strictly depending on tumor stage and grade, however studies described recurrence rates in between 4–9.3% [33, 40].

Non-penile Sparing Surgical Treatment

Partial Penectomy

Partial penectomy is a radical, non-organ sparing treatment, which is indicated for extensive disease with invasion into the corpora cavernosa (cT3). This procedure has the main purpose to provide oncological control, with as a secondary aim to maintain penile function [41]. Therefore, urologists should carefully reflect upon the remaining penile length before performing surgery [27]. A penile stump of sufficient length is required to preserve the ability to void in the upright position and to maintain sexual activity [27]. If the tumor invades the corpora cavernosa to a large extent and the maintenance of genitourinary function could not be guaranteed, a total penectomy with perineal urethrostomy should be considered.

The surgical procedure starts with a circumferential incision proximal of the tumor. Historically, surgical margins of 2 cm were advised, however currently there is a shift towards smaller margins if oncollogically feasible and with the aim to optimize genitourinary function. Though OSS contains a higher risk of local recurrence, while not affecting OS, recent studies have stated that in higher risk lesions, local recurrence is predictive for disease specific survival, as a result broader margins should be envisaged as well [22, 23, 25, 42]. Afterwards, Buck's fascia should be carefully dissected and the neurovascular bundle ligated [41]. As a next step, a tourniquet is applied and the corpus cavernosum is transected. Before transecting the corpus spongiosum, the urethra is identified and transected, thereby preserving an urethral stump of 1–1.5 cm in order to spatulate this stump to the ventral penile shaft skin [20]. Finally, the tourniquet is released and bleeding vessels are identified and coagulated. This technique has some drawbacks. Firstly, a ventrally located urethra causes a poor esthetic result, leading to psychological morbidity. Secondly, meatal stenosis can occur. A number of alternative techniques have been described, e.g., the formation of a neoglans by using a STSG or the urethral centralization after partial penectomy (UCAPP) technique, which was first performed by Kranz et al. [43]. These techniques are aiming to provide a higher satisfaction of cosmetic results and to minimize psychological burden [20, 41]. Seven to ten days post-operative, the applied dressings and catheter could be removed [20, 43]. Recurrence rates are strongly dependent of tumor stage, however local recurrence rates of 18% and 20% have been described in T2 and T3, respectively [21]. A study of Korets et al. demonstrated a 3-year OS rate of 56% [44].

Fig. 18.8 Total penectomy. The urethra is brought through the inverted Y-incision posterior of the scrotum in the perineum. A catheter is placed in the neomeatus. The catheter can be removed 5–7 days post-operative

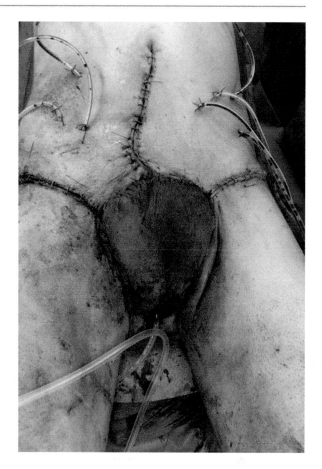

Total Penectomy With Perineal Urethrostomy

In patients with locally advanced disease (pT4) and where partial penectomy cannot achieve negative surgical margins or cannot preserve a penile length sufficient to provide the genitourinary function, a total penectomy is indicated [45]. Since advanced penile cancers have a higher risk of secondary infection, broad spectrum antibiotics are administered preoperatively.

A lithotomy position is advised for this surgical procedure. After marking a rhombic incision around the penis, the penis should be mobilized proximally and dissection through the skin can be performed. The suspensory ligament is divided in order to continue dissection until the neurovascular bundle is reached and can be ligated. Posterior of the scrotum, an inverted Y-incision is made to form the urinary outlet. The urethra is fixed to the inverted Y-incision in the perineum without angulation and with ventral spatulation in order to prevent stenosis of the perineal urethrostomy (Fig. 18.8), which is a complication possibly requiring revision surgery [20, 46].

Lymph Node Staging and Groin Management

Federica Peretti and Marco Falcone

Lymphatic drainage of the penis is based on two lymphatic networks:

- a superficial one, represented by the satellite circle of the superficial dorsal vein of the penis, that drains into the superficial inguinal lymph nodes
- a deep one, satellite of the deep dorsal vein of the penis, that includes the lymph nodes draining the glans, corpora cavernosa, and urethra

The two networks are interconnected at the level of the glans and the foreskin [47].

Considering the aforementioned lymphatic anatomy, it becomes clear how the loco-regional extension of a PC primarily involves the inguinal lymph nodes, both in superficial and deep stations, and secondary the pelvic ones.

Additionally, the current scientific evidence has shown that, if a loco-regional extension of the tumor occurs, it primarily involves the supero-medial inguinal lymph nodes and only then the central and distal ones [48]. There have been no cases in which neoplastic cells have involved lymph nodes located more distally in the drainage chain without involving proximal ones, nor have there been cases of infiltration of pelvic or retroperitoneal abdominal (para-aortic and/or para-caval) lymph nodes without the primary involvement of inguinal lymph nodes. These evidence comes from the results of studies performed using the dynamic sentinel lymph node biopsy (DSNB), in which a specific nanocolloid (Technetium-99m) is injected in the proximity if the tumor. The nanocolloid rapidly spreads in the lymphatic network reaching the sentinel lymph node, which is the first lymph node in the lymphatic chain and therefore the first to be affected by any possible tumor metastasis. The sentinel lymph node is than identified by a lymphoscintigraphy associated to an intraoperative use of a gamma probe.

In most case the lymph node metastatic spread in PC seems to follow an orderly and predictable pattern. Considering the rich lymphatic network of the penis and its structures, the study of inguinal and pelvic lymph nodes and the consequent treatment decision is a fundamental step in the management of the disease.

The correct lymph node management has a decisive influence on the outcomes of recurrence-free survival (RFS) and overall CSS.

Objective Examination: Clinical Staging at Lymph Node Palpation

Clinical examination based on palpation of bilateral groin lymph nodes is a key element in the staging pathway of PC and guides its subsequent diagnostic-therapeutic course. Indeed, therapeutic strategies and follow-up depend on risk stratification.

Based on the objective examination, two main types of scenarios are defined:

1. *Clinically negative inguinal lymph node palpation*: no pathologically enlarged or suspicious lymph nodes are detected on palpation. These patients are defined as cN0.

2. *Clinically positive inguinal lymph node palpation:* on palpation, one or more
   pathologically enlarged lymph nodes are detected, monolaterally or bilaterally.
   These patients are defined as cN1 (monoliteral pattern) and cN2 (bilateral
   pattern).

In addition, patients with positive inguinal palpation include those with pathologically severely enlarged, fixed lymph nodes with possible areas of ulceration and/or
suppuration, monolaterally or bilaterally. These patients are defined as cN3.

Role of Imaging in Nodal Staging

In case of a clinically negative inguinal lymph node palpation imaging studies do
not play a detrimental role in staging the disease. Indeed neither inguinal ultrasound
(US), computed tomography (CT) or MRI are able to detect micrometastases.

   Groin US is suggested in obese patients where a clinical evaluation is deemed
not reliable due to the excessive of adipose tissue.

   On the contrary, in case of a positive inguinal lymph node palpation, pelvic CT
is suggested to stage pelvic nodal status.

Management in Case of Negative Inguinal Palpation (cN0)

In patients who are clinically negative at the inguinal physical examination (cN0), a
risk-stratified invasive nodal staging should be proposed. Indeed, recent evidence
has highlighted that up to 25% of cN0 patients may have a micrometastasis not
detectable neither by clinical examination or imaging techniques.

   In the problem handling, we are aided by risk stratification of primary disease
based on stage, grade and the lymphovascular involvement status on histologic
examination of the penile lesion [23]. Following these issues we may classify PC as:

– **Low risk of lymphatic involvement:** superficial tumors such as carcinoma in
  situ (pTis) or (pTa); tumors infiltrating the submucosal layer (pT1) but of a low
  histopathological grade (G1).
– **Medium risk of lymphatic involvement:** moderately differentiated tumors of
  intermediate grade (G2) localized to the submucosal layer (pT1).
– **High risk of lymphatic involvement:** tumors localized in the submucosa (pT1)
  but of high grade and poorly differentiated (G3) and all tumors infiltrating
  deeper layers.

Based on risk stratification, three different diagnostic-therapeutic pathways with
increasing invasivity can be proposed to cN0 patients [49]:

Active Surveillance
Active surveillance is the most conservative option, consisting in a strict clinical and
radiological follow-up aimed at detecting early signs and symptoms of a loco-
regional lymph node recurrence, in order to guarantee an early and curative surgical

approach. On the one hand, this approach has the advantage of avoiding a surgery, with all the related risks, that could be unnecessary from the point of view of onco- logical radicality. This approach requires compliance. Additionally, it is necessary to counsel the patient about possible risk related to a deferred node disease. In fact, there are cases of loco-regional lymph node recurrence not detectable by imaging techniques and then misrecognized up to more advanced stages in which it was then necessary to perform an invasive approach with outcomes, in terms of survival, less satisfactory than the same surgery performed early.

In 2007, Meijer et al. conducted a study showing that early lymphadenectomy in cN0 patients is associated with a survival rate of about 90%, while the same surgery performed in later settings, practiced only when there are clinical and radiological signs of recurrence, correlates with survival rates of 40% [50].

To summarize, the conservative approach offered by surveillance is a strategy that should be applied only in selected cases of cN0 patients who satisfy certain requirements:

- Low risk PC
- Elderly pluricomorbid patients in whom surgery is charged with multiple risks
- Strict adherence to cadenced follow-up

Invasive Lymph Node Staging

Invasive lymph node staging involves the use of invasive surgical techniques to study the loco-regional inguinal lymph nodes.

There are two lymph node staging techniques:

- *The dynamic sentinel lymph node biopsy (DSNB) technique* uses Technetium-99m (TC99-m), which is injected the previous day in the site adjacent to the area of malignancy; subsequently, any lymph node uptake is searched for, as a sign of regional disease involvement. The procedure can be made more effective, in terms of sensitivity and specificity, if the use of TC-99m is associated also to the blue-patent according to the latest EAU Guidelines [1]. Recent evidences sup- port the use of intraoperative indocyanine green (ICG) fluorescence to optimize outcomes of DSNB.
- The *modified inguinal lymph node dissection (mILND)* consists in the surgical removal, laparoscopic or with open technique, of the first lymph nodes of the penile drainage chain, specifically the supero-medial and central inguinal lymph nodes bilaterally.

Even in pursuing these more invasive staging pathways it is necessary to carefully evaluate the patients to whom they are proposed, it is essential to examine the clini- cal scenario an overall and the risks and benefits of the individual case.

Several authors in the past have conducted studies aimed at measuring the sensi- tivity and specificity as well as reliability and reproducibility of mILND and DSNB: according to the study conducted by Rothenberg K.H et al. in 1994 and then con- firmed by the subsequent work in 2007 by Meijer et al. in the case of DSNB the rate of false negatives (FN) is around 12–15%, even in referral centers [49, 51].

It should be kept in mind that neither of the two techniques on which the proposed invasive staging is based guarantees 100% detection of lymph node micrometastases in cN0 patients [17, 52]. If inguinal lymph nodes analyzed by invasive staging techniques are positive for malignancy, radical inguinal lymphadenectomy (ILND) becomes imperative.

Management in Case of Doubtful or Positive Inguinal Palpation (cN1 and cN2)

In patients with positive mono or bilateral inguinal lymph node palpation—cN1 and cN2, respectively—the therapeutic pathway should include first of all the radiological study of the pelvis, in fact CT with contrast or MRI allow a better local characterization of the regional lymph node status than the clinical examination alone as recommended by the EAU Guidelines [1].

Because, in case of positive lymph node palpation, the hypothesis of metastatic disease is highly probable, staging must be aimed at excluding metastatic spread.

In doubtful cases a *cytologic examination by ultrasound-guided needle aspiration (FNA)* is a viable option. According to the 2006 study by Sairson et al. conducted on 16 patients with pSCC and positive lymph node palpation, the FNA technique has good sensitivity, specificity and accuracy and allows an early ILND even in cases that are not clinically exhaustive [53]. Otherwise, the gold standard approach is represented by *surgical excision of palpable inguinal lymph nodes* with intraoperative histologic evaluation by frozen section followed by a ILND if positive.

If local staging is positive for metastatic disease to the inguinal lymph nodes the use of 18F-FDGPET/CT may be appropriate with the intent of detecting other metastatic locations, while it should not be interpreted as an alternative option to invasive techniques in the staging procedure, as the risk of false negatives is high as demonstrated by the study of Rosevear et al. in 2012 [54].

Radical Inguinal Lymphadenectomy (ILND)

After positive local staging in cN1 or cN2 patients, surgical removal of inguinal lymph nodes is indicated: bilateral ILND can be performed with traditional open technique or by minimally invasive techniques such as laparoscopy (Video endoscopic inguinal lymphadenectomy: VEIL) or robot-assisted laparoscopy (R-VEIL).

ILND Step by Step Technique

A transversal inguinal incision of approximately 7 cm in length 1 cm below the inguinal ligament was performed (Figs. 18.9 and 18.10: right side). The Camper's fascia was incised. The dissection of superficial nodal stations between Camper's and lata fascia was performed. The saphenous veins was isolated and spared if not involved in nodal disease. A progressive ligation of the pudendal, epigastric, and

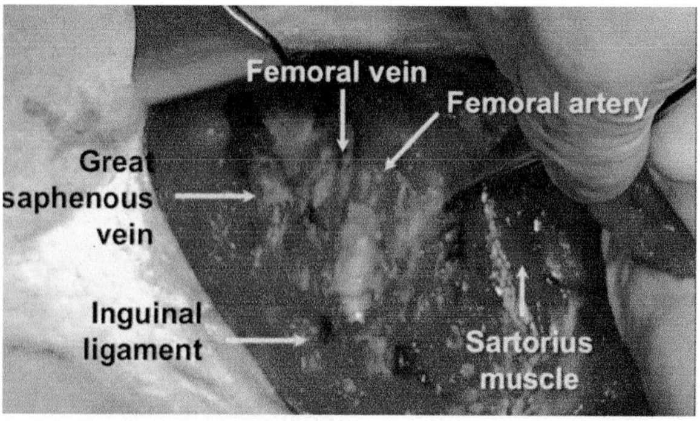

Fig. 18.9 Open ILND. Scarpa's Triangle: the upper the inguinal ligament, the lateral the sartorius muscle and the medial the adductor muscle. Excision of the lymph nodes along the course of the femoral vessels and the saphenous vein, which is spared if possible

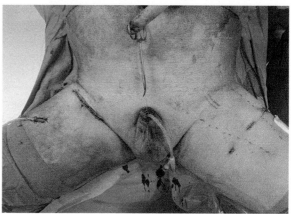

Fig. 18.10 Open ILND at the right groin versus VEIL at the left groin

circumflex vascular pedicles was performed. Superficial lymph node packages were isolated. Lymphostasis was obtained with selective use of metallic ligaclips or with application of automatic sealing systems. Fascia lata was incised longitudinally at the level of ovalis fossa. Deep nodal packages were isolated and excised. Hemostasis was achieved. Tubular drainage was left in place.

Video Endoscopic Inguinal Lymphadenectomy (VEIL) Step by Step Technique

An Hasson's trocar was inserted at the apex of Scarpa's triangle. A digital development of a working space below Camper's fascia was obtained. Two 5 mm trocars were placed 5 cm laterally to the Hasson in a triangle fashion (Fig. 18.10: left side, Figs. 18.11 and 18.12). Insufflation with CO_2 at 10 mmHg. Progressive development of working space. Progressive isolation and selective ligation of the pudendal, epigastric and circumflex pedicles with the use of ligaclips or automatic sealing systems. Isolation and sparing of the saphenous vein (Fig. 18.13). Progressive excision of the superficial lymph node packages. Incision of the fascia lata at the level of the ovalis fossa. Excision of the deep lymph node packages. Hemostasis was obtained. Tubular drainage was left in place.

Fig. 18.11 Laparoscopic dissection goes up to the inguinal ligament

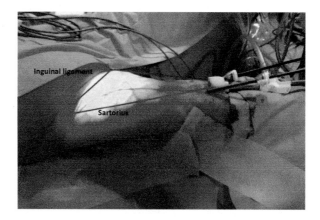

Fig. 18.12 VEIL: Two 5 mm trocars were placed 5 cm laterally to the Hasson in a triangle fashion

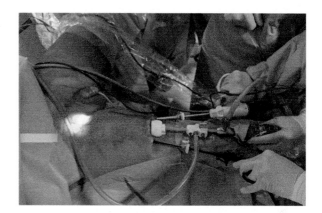

Fig. 18.13 VEIL: Isolation and sparing of the saphenous vein. Haemostasis and lymphostasis by Thunderbeat

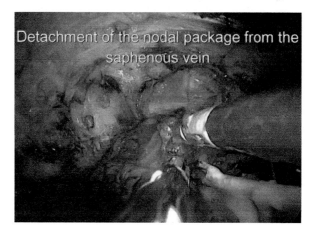

Focusing on the surgical technique, in order to be as minimally invasive as possible, preservation of the saphenous vein is recommended, if surgically feasible, as it reduces morbidity. On the other hand, the use of a pedicled sartorius muscle flap to cover the dissected inguinal area is not recommended, as it does not improve the outcomes of oncological radicality, but worsens morbidity [1].

The surgical removal of all inguinal lymph nodes provides an excellent oncological radicality of the disease and in cases of exclusive involvement of inguinal lymph nodes is considered as curative treatment [55].

While ILND play an essential role in the treatment of PC, it is also burden by important morbidities [56]. In fact, according to the main reports by Koifman in 2013 and Yao in 2010, in addition to the classic complications related to any surgery, as the surgical site infection, bleeding and hematoma formation, specific complications as skin necrosis, lymphedema and lymphoceles formations are frequently described [57, 58].

Therefore an accurate selection of the type of patient to submit to ILND must be considered, resulting in precise balance between risks and benefits.

Overall, in order to reduce the morbidity of the procedure, some postoperative precautions are recommended, such as the use of suction drainage techniques, elastic compression medications, elastocompression socks and prolonged antibiotic therapy in accordance with the findings of y by La-Touche et al. [1, 59].

Pelvic Lymphadenectomy (PLND)

Ipsilateral pelvic lymphadenectomy (PLND) is demanded in high-risk patients with:

- Two or more ipsilateral inguinal lymph nodes positive for disease at inguinal staging
- Inguinal lymph node diameter more than 3 cm
- Extracapsular lymph node extension of disease to the explored inguinal lymph nodes

The aforementioned features are associated with increased risk of pelvic lymph node involvement as already anticipated by the study conducted by Graafland et al. in 2010 [60] and confirmed by the conclusions of the study conducted by Lunghezzani et al. in 2014 where among 142 patients analyzed (with histological diagnosis of PC) the finding of these three features at the staging of inguinal lymph nodes was associated in 57% of cases with pelvic lymph node metastases compared with no cases in patients who did not have these features [61].

The choice of performing PLND at the same surgical time as the ILND or at a later time will depend on the individual case (Fig. 18.14).

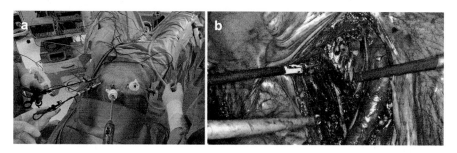

Fig. 18.14 (**a**) Videolaparoscopic pelvic lymphadenectomy: open-laparoscopy placement of supra-umbilical Hasson and four other trocars according to classical scheme. (**b**) Excision of lymph node envelopes along the axis of the iliac vessels. (**a**, **b**) Pelvic laparoscopic lymphadenectomy

Management in Case of Clearly Positive Inguinal Palpation With Voluminous Fixed Lymphadenopathies (cN3)

cN3 patients are defined as those who present at clinical diagnosis a severe inguinal lymph node disease characterized by very bulky, bilateral, fixed, and often ulcerated lymphadenopathies. The locally advanced stage requires a more complete radiological staging aimed to the inguinal-pelvic study of the disease and also to a total-body evaluation in order to confirm or exclude the presence of distant metastatic disease. Therefore, in these patients the staging procedure is based on thoracic-abdominal and pelvic contrast CT scans. The indication for histological staging of inguinal lymph nodes, which consists exclusively on surgical removal of suspicious lymph nodes, may not be systematic, in fact, in those cases in which the clinic is unequivocal, this step can be bypassed and proceed directly to bilateral and inguinal lymphadenectomy and then pelvic necessary.

In literature and also according to what reported in the EAU Guidelines, between the end of the 90s and the first decade of the 2000s a therapeutic scheme based on neoadjuvant chemotherapy (CT) in cN3 patients followed by surgery only in cases of good clinical and radiological response has been proposed, so currently this represents the standard of care [1, 62–66]. All authors currently agree on the poor prognosis that characterizes this class of patients.

Adjuvant Chemotherapy

According to EAU Guidelines 2021 treatment scheme based on lymphadenectomy followed by adjuvant chemotherapy (CT) in pN2 and/or pN3 patients seems to significantly increase the disease free-survival (DSF) rate [1, 67–70]. There is no evidence in the literature currently regarding adjuvant radiation therapy.

Nodal Recurrence

In case of lymph node recurrence, the EAU Guidelines [6] recommend surgical treatment. However, as always, it is necessary to adapt the treatment based on the individual case, because if the regional recurrence occurs in subjects who have already undergone to invasive staging techniques, the diffusion of lymph node metastases will be subverted and will no longer follow the classic linear model mentioned at the beginning of this chapter.

The alteration of the original anatomy of the inguinal and pelvic lymphatic drainage pathway will make the scheme of disease spread disorderly and unpredictable. Recently, DSNB has been described as effective in salvage settings, with a nodal recurrence after a previous invasive nodal staging.

According to current knowledge, the EAU guidelines propose a multimodal approach for these patients based on different personalized chemotherapy regimens. The prognosis of this group of patients is extremely poor [63, 71].

Advanced Disease

Esther Lee and Arie Parnham

Introduction

Most penile cancers are confined to the glans and prepuce, a significant number of patients will present late with locally advanced disease associated with inguinal metastases. This may be due to a combination of patient, healthcare, and disease factors. Many patients cite embarrassment, guilt, and fear as explanations for ignoring symptomatic and in some circumstances clearly abnormal fungating infiltrative lesions on the penis or in the groin [72]. The rarity of the disease also means that the awareness of healthcare professionals both in primary and secondary care is limited, often leading to misdiagnosis and false reassurance. Finally, its presentation can be covert with the disease developing unchecked under a phimotic foreskin or an inguinal node being passed off as a small hernia left on surveillance, leading to delays in diagnosis and definitive management [73].

The management of advanced tumors as with many cancers, benefits from being placed within an extended multidisciplinary team including oncologists, surgeons, radiologists, specialist nursing, and palliative care physicians. The patient and family, however, should rightly be placed in the center of decision making where possible. It is worth recognizing that many interventions for advanced disease in PC have a limited evidence base which makes the already complex interplay between preserving quality of life versus extending life even harder.

The presentation of men with advanced PC is varied and can be because of local effects from the primary or inguinal/pelvic lymphadenopathy, and metastatic disease.

Locally Advanced Primary

Local effects from an advanced primary can include (although not limited to) bleeding, pain, discharge, and a distinctive foul odor. An advanced tumor can have a profound influence on urinary function depending on its location with dribbling incontinence and urinary retention being a feature of those with distal tumors, and urinary incontinence with more proximal membranous urethral involvement [74]. These can usually be temporized or palliated with the provision of a urethral or suprapubic catheter until a definitive management strategy is established. Where a primary tumor extends into the anorectal area it may result in lower gastrointestinal problems such as pain, rectal bleeding, tenesmus, and bowel obstruction. In such cases a palliative diversion using a colostomy may be used.

Management of a locally advanced PC should always be taken in context of lymphatic, and metastatic burden, as well as patient factors such as pre-existing morbidity predicted survival and patient's preferences. The aim of intervention should always be explicit whether it is for palliation or curative intent. Where there is uncertainty regarding the extent of infiltration, pre-operative MRI can be used to identify the extent of proximal invasion and the presence of skip lesions [75]. This can facilitate pre-operative planning including liaising with plastic surgical colleagues for the use of flaps to cover defects, pelvic surgeons for urinary and bowel diversion etc. and other surgical disciplines. It also allows for adequate counselling and consent of the patient.

In rare cases of verrucous carcinomas or giant condyloma accuminatum (Buschke–Löwenstein tumour), where the primary can be large and locally infiltrative but does not metastasize, the decision making is relatively straight forward and can be excised surgically based on clinical and radiological imaging to guide extent of resection [76–79].

Further details on Partial penectomy, and radical penectomy are discussed earlier in this chapter.

In cases that are deemed inoperable, data extrapolated from trials in oropharynx, vulval, cervix and anal cancers have demonstrated the radiosensitive nature of squamous cell carcinomas [80]. In combination with chemotherapy there have been some reports reporting success in treatment, however this is limited by small sample sizes [81, 82].

Advanced Inguinal Disease and Pelvic Disease

As discussed earlier in the chapter most penile cancers disseminate in a step wise manner spreading from the primary along lymphatic channels to the superficial and then deep inguinal lymph nodes, before passing through the femoral canal to the pelvic nodes. In cases of advanced inguinal disease, patients may present with bulky disease, which may be adherent or erode through the skin, causing pain, discharge, bleeding, lymphoedema and a foul odor.

In such cases imaging with CT of the thorax, abdomen and pelvis is essential so that an assessment of resectability can be made. Further, as per managing the primary, it is important to consider the context of the disease in terms of pelvic nodal involvement and metastasis. Most will demonstrate extracapsular spread indicating a higher risk of pelvic involvement and metastasis which may preclude early resection and justify neoadjuvant or palliative chemoradiotherapy. Finally, a small proportion of patients presenting with locally advanced inguinal disease will involve the femoral vein or artery and as such represent a risk for catastrophic haemorrhage. This is invariably a terminal event for which patients, carers, family members and staff should be made aware of, and advice/protocols given on how to manage appropriately and sensitively.

In those patients with bulky nodes but not fixed (N1/2) radical ILND as previously described is appropriate. Where significant defects are created from the excision of disease such that tension free closure is not possible, mobilization of the flaps can be performed along with Sartorius transposition to protect the vessels. Early engagement with plastic surgical services can be critical for larger defects requiring coverage with pedicled grafts such as rectus femoris pedicled flap, vertical rectus abdo-minis myocutaneous (VRAM), anterolateral thigh (ALT), and tensor fascia lata (TFL) [83, 84].

In patients with fixed inguinal nodal disease, it is important to recognise that in such cases the evidence for intervention is far from mature and doubt still exists regarding the optimal strategy and outcomes remain universally poor. In such circumstances the importance of multidisciplinary decision making with patient involvement is critical.

Surgical excision of disease is feasible using the principles set out in brief above and can be employed in the palliative setting, although it is important to recognize that the risk of complications in such cases are increased and a careful assessment of risks versus perceived benefits should be made.

It is recognized that in the curative setting however the chances of positive margins and residual disease are too high to provide conclusive benefit and ignores the risk of systemic malignancy. Many patients may find that subsequent complications of surgery (which are increased in these cases) prevent patients ever receiving adjuvant systemic therapy, or patients' disease progresses during the time of recovery.

In cases where a curative intent is deemed suitable, neoadjuvant chemotherapy with cisplatin and taxane based regimens have been used with some effect to help downstage disease locally and allow treatment of systemic disease early on. In those patients that respond they can then go onto have completion ILND with long term survival in 37% of cases [62, 66]. This has been supported by further studies showing similar outcomes although, it is worth recognizing that that triple regimen chemotherapy is associated with significant toxicity and as such many patients are ineligible for treatment who present with cN3 disease due to reduction in their performance status and existing co-morbidity [63]. The most used regimens are paclitaxel, ifosfamide, and cisplatin (TIP) and docetaxel, 5-fluorouracil and cisplatin (TPF) with pathological response rates of 15% and an objective response rate of 50% [66, 68, 84–88].

The use of radiotherapy in the management of advanced inguinal and pelvic disease remains unclear. Data from other squamous cell cancer sites including oropharynx, vulval, cervix and anal cancer, have demonstrated benefit, however this has not been conclusively replicated in PC with a systematic review of seven studies in 2018 failing to identify a positive benefit [89].

Metastatic Disease

Although metastatic disease can appear throughout the body, the most common sites are lung, liver, retroperitoneum and bone [90].

It is worth recognizing that the prognosis for metastatic PC is extremely poor and many patients will endure a significant reduction in their quality of life consequently. Involvement of palliative care physicians and allied teams is essential.

Patients with PC may present with paraneoplastic hypercalcaemia even without evidence of bone metastasis because of release of parathyroid hormone protein analogues [91, 92]. Symptoms include thirst, lethargy, and confusion are all potentially reversible with bisphosphonates and fluid resuscitation which may improve performance status and allow subsequent palliative intervention, i.e., surgery, radiotherapy, systemic therapy.

Skin metastases can be devastating and multiple, causing pain, bleeding, and mal odor. Although they can be excised, they invariably appear elsewhere.

Depending on the patient's co-morbidity and performance status they can be offered systemic therapy usually TIP or TPF, recognizing however the severe toxicity associated with such regimens may limit their utility in the palliative setting. More tolerable regimens have been investigated including vinflunine, cisplatin and irinotecan, which demonstrated a clinical benefit rate of 45.5% (n-25), although no standard first line option exists [93]. More recently new trials have opened exploring the use of immunotherapy and basket trials.

Quality of Life

Esther Lee and Arie Parnham

The investigation and management of PC holds many challenges for patients. Dealing with the diagnosis of a cancer many will not have had a prior knowledge of, makes managing the inevitable uncertainties and effects of investigations and treatments all the harder patients. It is well understood and documented that the penis holds enormous psychological importance for men as well and so it is little surprise to find that PC can be a devastating disease with a considerable effect on quality of life [94]. What is surprising however is despite the implicit effects of the disease on patients there is little good quality evidence available to inform us.

Psychological

The psychological effect of PC treatment can be profound. In a systematic review by Maddineni et al. it was found that 40% of patients had impaired wellbeing (General Health Questionnaire), 31% had pathological anxiety (HADS) and 53% exhibited signs of mental illness (DSM 3R) [95]. Many of the themes around mental health identified in patients having undergone treatment for PC relate to a loss of masculinity and concerns regarding the appearance of the penis. Many patients express reticence in showing the penis to partners or its appearance as a barrier to engaging in relationships. The value of the clinical nurse specialist (CNS) role in improving the experiences of those diagnosed with cancer cannot be underestimated and patients should have access to psychological and psychosexual support. Many men also find benefit in support groups. In a qualitative study the authors reported that meeting men with a similar condition and sharing experiences of living with the disease were important to them [96].

Relaxing attitudes towards safe margins for surgery and regarding local recurrence on the penis, has meant that the paradigm has shifted from oncological control with cursory attention to function to one that considers form, function as well [22, 23, 97–99]. There have been numerous studies published examining penile preserving techniques both surgically and using brachytherapy/radiotherapy with many showing improved satisfaction.

Voiding

The effect of PC management on voiding is poorly documented. Many men following penile preserving surgery will be able to void, however may find that they spray when passing urine and require a funnel. In those men undergoing total penectomy and perineal urethrostomy and depending on preserved length those post partial penectomy will find that they must sit to void. The impact on the male psyche of these changes to perceived 'normal' male behaviors is yet not well documented.

Sexual Dysfunction

Several studies have examined the effects of PC management on sexual function.

Much of the evidence confirms what could be assumed, the more aggressive the surgery the larger the effect on sexual function. In a study from Norway, patients that underwent radical penectomy and partial penectomy were more likely to have reduced sexual interest, severely limited sexual ability, markedly reduced sexual enjoyment and frequency [100]. This was in sharp contrast to those men undergoing penile preserving forms of management (glansectomy, local excision, radiotherapy), who still had effects on function but to a lesser degree [100]. The relationship between extent of penile resection to sexual function has been confirmed in similar studies and cemented the role of penile preserving surgery [38, 101]. The importance of a psychosexual counsellor and attention to penile preservation should always therefore be considered in those men wanting to preserve sexual function. In addition, for those men who have had more aggressive forms of surgery clear referral pathways should be in place to allow consideration for genital reconstruction such as phalloplasty.

Lymphoedema

One of the main concerns of PC patients is lymphoedema, which can affect the lower limbs and genitals following groin node surgery. Both DSNB and ILND carry a risk of complications of 3.4% and 42–57% respectively [102, 103]. Without doubt the use of DSNB has reduced the number of patients requiring ILND. For those undergoing groin node dissection, the issue persists however. Modifications in technique, including adoption of laparoscopic and robotic approaches, have demonstrated reduced rates of lymphoedema, and hospital stay with comparable oncological outcomes [104].

With no clear solution to the issue, it is important to have clear information regarding care for patients and well-defined pathways for lymphoedema support services co-located where possible.

References

1. Hakenberg OW, Compérat E, Minhas S, Necchi A, Protzel C, Watkin N. Guidelines on penile cancer 2018. https://uroweb.org/wp-content/uploads/EAU-Guidelines-Penile-Cancer-2018.pdf.
2. Douglawi A, Masterson TA. Penile cancer epidemiology and risk factors: a contemporary review. Curr Opin Urol. 2019;29(2):145–9.
3. Thomas A, Necchi A, Muneer A, Tobias-Machado M, Tran ATH, Van Rompuy A-S, et al. Penile cancer. Nat Rev Dis Primers. 2021;7(1):11.
4. Favorito LA, et al. Epidemiologic study on penile cancer in Brazil. Int Braz J Urol. 2008;34(5):587–91; discussion 591–3
5. Hansen BT, Orumaa M, Lie AK, Brennhovd B, Nygård M. Trends in incidence, mortality and survival of penile squamous cell carcinoma in Norway 1956–2015. Int J Cancer. 2018;142(8):1586–93.
6. Moch H, Cubilla AL, Humphrey PA, Reuter VE, Ulbright TM. The 2016 WHO classification of tumours of the urinary system and male genital organs—part A: renal, penile, and testicular tumours. Eur Urol. 2016;70(1):93–105.
7. Olesen TB, Sand FL, Rasmussen CL, Albieri V, Toft BG, Norrild B, et al. Prevalence of human papillomavirus DNA and p16INK4a in penile cancer and penile intraepithelial neoplasia: a systematic review and meta-analysis. Lancet Oncol. 2019;20(1):145–58.
8. Amin MB, Edge SB, Greene FL, et al. AJCC cancer staging manual. 8th ed. New York: Springer; 2017.
9. Skrodzka M, Ayres B, Watkin N. Penile-sparing surgical and non-surgical approaches. In: Spiess PE, Necchi A, editors. Penile carcinoma: therapeutic principles and advances. Cham: Springer; 2021. p. 59–73.
10. Alnajjar HM, Lam W, Bolgeri M, Rees RW, Perry MJ, Watkin NA. Treatment of carcinoma in situ of the glans penis with topical chemotherapy agents. Eur Urol. 2012;62(5):923–8.

11. Lucky M, Murthy KV, Rogers B, Jones S, Lau MW, Sangar VK, et al. The treatment of penile carcinoma in situ (CIS) within a UK supra-regional network. BJU Int. 2015;115(4):595–8.
12. Deen K, Burdon-Jones D. Imiquimod in the treatment of penile intraepithelial neoplasia: an update. Australas J Dermatol. 2017;58(2):86–92.
13. Crook J. Organ preserving radiation strategies for penile cancer. Urol Oncol. 2022;40(5):184–90.
14. de Crevoisier R, Slimane K, Sanfilippo N, Bossi A, Albano M, Dumas I, et al. Long-term results of brachytherapy for carcinoma of the penis confined to the glans (N- or NX). Int J Radiat Oncol Biol Phys. 2009;74(4):1150–6.
15. Cordoba A, Escande A, Lopez S, Mortier L, Mirabel X, Coche-Dequeant B, et al. Low-dose brachytherapy for early stage penile cancer: a 20-year single-institution study (73 patients). Radiat Oncol. 2016;11:96.
16. Piva LNN, Di Palo A, et al. Alternative terapeutiche nel trattamento del carcinoma spinocellulare del pene di categoria T1N0: indicazioni e limiti [Therapeutic alternatives in the treatment of class T1N0 squamous cell carcinoma of the penis: indications and limitations]. Arch Ital Urol Androl. 1996;68(3):157–61.
17. Bandieramonte G, Colecchia M, Mariani L, Lo Vullo S, Pizzocaro G, Piva L, et al. Peniscopically controlled CO2 laser excision for conservative treatment of in situ and T1 penile carcinoma: report on 224 patients. Eur Urol. 2008;54(4):875–82.
18. Schlenker B, Tilki D, Seitz M, Bader MJ, Reich O, Schneede P, et al. Organ-preserving neodymium-yttrium-aluminium-garnet laser therapy for penile carcinoma: a long-term follow-up. BJU Int. 2010;106(6):786–90.
19. Alnajjar HM, Randhawa K, Muneer A. Localized disease: types of reconstruction/plastic surgery techniques after glans resurfacing/glansectomy/partial/total penectomy. Curr Opin Urol. 2020;30(2):213–7.
20. Pang KH, Alnajjar HM, Muneer A. Management of primary penile tumours: partial and total penectomy. In: Spiess PE, Necchi A, editors. Penile carcinoma: therapeutic principles and advances. Cham: Springer; 2021. p. 75–84.
21. Raskin Y, Vanthoor J, Milenkovic U, Muneer A, Albersen M. Organ-sparing surgical and nonsurgical modalities in primary penile cancer treatment. Curr Opin Urol. 2019;29(2):156–64.
22. Leijte JA, Kirrander P, Antonini N, Windahl T, Horenblas S. Recurrence patterns of squamous cell carcinoma of the penis: recommendations for follow-up based on a two-centre analysis of 700 patients. Eur Urol. 2008;54(1):161–8.
23. Philippou P, Shabbir M, Malone P, Nigam R, Muneer A, Ralph DJ, et al. Conservative surgery for squamous cell carcinoma of the penis: resection margins and long-term oncological control. J Urol. 2012;188(3):803–8.
24. Sri D, Sujenthiran A, Lam W, Minter J, Tinwell BE, Corbishley CM, et al. A study into the association between local recurrence rates and surgical resection margins in organ-sparing surgery for penile squamous cell cancer. BJU Int. 2018;122(4):576–82.
25. Roussel E, Peeters E, Vanthoor J, Bozzini G, Muneer A, Ayres B, et al. Predictors of local recurrence and its impact on survival after glansectomy for penile cancer: time to challenge the dogma? BJU Int. 2021;127(5):606–13.
26. Thomas W, Flaig PES, et al. National Comprehensive Cancer Network. Guidelines on penile cancer 2021. https://www.nccn.org/professionals/physician_gls/pdf/penile.pdf
27. Burnett AL. Penile preserving and reconstructive surgery in the management of penile cancer. Nat Rev Urol. 2016;13(5):249–57.
28. Bronselaer GA, Schober JM, Meyer-Bahlburg HFL, T'Sjoen G, Vlietinck R, Hoebeke PB. Male circumcision decreases penile sensitivity as measured in a large cohort. BJU Int. 2013;111(5):820–7.
29. World Health Organization and UNAIDS. Male circumcision: global trends and determinants of prevalence, safety and acceptability. Geneva: World Health Organization; 2007.

30. Cakir OO, Schifano N, Venturino L, Pozzi E, Castiglione F, Alnajjar HM, et al. Surgical technique and outcomes following coronal-sparing glans resurfacing for benign and malignant penile lesions. Int J Impot Res. 2022;34(5):495–500.
31. Shabbir M, Muneer A, Kalsi J, Shukla CJ, Zacharakis E, Garaffa G, et al. Glans resurfacing for the treatment of carcinoma in situ of the penis: surgical technique and outcomes. Eur Urol. 2011;59(1):142–7.
32. Issa A, Sebro K, Kwok A, Janisch F, Grossmann NC, Lee E, et al. Treatment options and outcomes for men with penile intraepithelial neoplasia: a systematic review. Eur Urol Focus. 2021; https://doi.org/10.1016/j.euf.2021.04.026.
33. Parnham AS, Albersen M, Sahdev V, Christodoulidou M, Nigam R, Malone P, et al. Glansectomy and split-thickness skin graft for penile cancer. Eur Urol. 2018;73(2):284–9.
34. Malone PR, Thomas JS, Blick C. A tie-over dressing for graft application in distal penectomy and glans resurfacing: the TODGA technique. BJU Int. 2011;107(5):836–40.
35. Pappas A, Katafigiotis I, Waterloos M, Spinoit AF, Ploumidis A. Glans resurfacing with skin graft for penile cancer: a step-by-step video presentation of the technique and review of the literature. Biomed Res Int. 2019;2019:5219048.
36. Hadway P, Corbishley CM, Watkin NA. Total glans resurfacing for premalignant lesions of the penis: initial outcome data. BJU Int. 2006;98(3):532–6.
37. Austoni E, Fenice O, Kartalas Goumas Y, Colombo F, Mantovani F, Pisani E. New trends in the surgical treatment of penile carcinoma. Arch Ital Urol Androl. 1996;68(3):163–8.
38. Gulino G, Sasso F, Falabella R, Bassi PF. Distal urethral reconstruction of the glans for penile carcinoma: results of a novel technique at 1-year of followup. J Urol. 2007;178(3 Pt 1):941–4.
39. Morelli G, Pagni R, Mariani C, Campo G, Menchini-Fabris F, Minervini R, et al. Glansectomy with split-thickness skin graft for the treatment of penile carcinoma. Int J Impot Res. 2009;21(5):311–4.
40. Smith Y, Hadway P, Biedrzycki O, Perry MJ, Corbishley C, Watkin NA. Reconstructive surgery for invasive squamous carcinoma of the glans penis. Eur Urol. 2007;52(4):1179–85.
41. Horenblas S, Malone P, Muneer A. Surgical treatment of penile cancer. In: Muneer A, Jordan GH, Arya M, editors. Atlas of male genitourethral surgery: the illustrated guide. Weinheim: Wiley; 2013. p. 134–50.
42. Rosa S, Djajadiningrat EVW, Meinhardt W, van Rhijn BWG, Bex A, van der Poel HG, Horenblas S. Penile sparing surgery for penile cancer—does it affect survival? J Urol. 2014;192(1):120–5.
43. Kranz J, Parnham A, Albersen M, Sahdev V, Ziada M, Nigam R, et al. Zentralisierung der Harnröhre und Pseudoglansbildung nach partieller Penektomie. Urologe. 2017;56(10):1293–7.
44. Korets R, Koppie TM, Snyder ME, Russo P. Partial penectomy for patients with squamous cell carcinoma of the penis: the Memorial Sloan-Kettering experience. Ann Surg Oncol. 2007;14(12):3614–9.
45. Gonzalgo M, Parekh D. Hinman's Atlas of Urologic Surgery E-Book. Elsevier Health Sciences. Partial penectomy. 2012;113–8.
46. De Vries HM, Chipollini J, Slongo J, Boyd F, Korkes F, Albersen M, et al. Outcomes of perineal urethrostomy for penile cancer: a 20-year international multicenter experience. Urol Oncol. 2021;39(8):500.e9–500.e13.
47. Netter FH. Atlante di anatomia umana. Milano: Masson; 2007.
48. Koch MO, Smith JA Jr. Local recurrence of squamous cell carcinoma of the penis. Urol Clin North Am. 1994;21(4):739–43.
49. Ornellas AA, Kinchin EW, Nóbrega BL, Wisnescky A, Koifman N, Quirino R. Surgical treatment of invasive squamous cell carcinoma of the penis: Brazilian National Cancer Institute long-term experience. J Surg Oncol. 2008;97(6):487–95.
50. Meijer RP, Boon TA, van Venrooij GE, Wijburg CJ. Long-term follow-up after laser therapy for penile carcinoma. Urology. 2007;69(4):759–62.

51. Rothenberger KH, Hofstetter A. Laser therapy of penile carcinoma. Urologe A. 1994;33(4):291–4.
52. Yao HH, Sengupta S, Chee J. Penile sparing therapy for penile cancer. Transl Androl Urol. 2020;9(6):3195–209.
53. Saisorn I, Lawrentschuk N, Leewansangtong S, Bolton DM. Fine-needle aspiration cytology predicts inguinal lymph node metastasis without antibiotic pretreatment in penile carcinoma. BJU Int. 2006;97(6):1225–8.
54. Rosevear HM, et al. Utility of (1)(8)F-FDG PET/CT in identifying penile squamous cell carcinoma metastatic lymph nodes. Urol Oncol. 2012;30(5):723–6.
55. Hegarty PK, Dinney CP, Pettaway CA. Controversies in ilioinguinal lymphadenectomy. Urol Clin North Am. 2010;37(3):421–34.
56. Stuiver MM, Djajadiningrat RS, Graafland NM, Vincent AD, Lucas C, Horenblas S. Early wound complications after inguinal lymphadenectomy in penile cancer: a historical cohort study and risk-factor analysis. Eur Urol. 2013;64(3):486–92.
57. Yao K, Tu H, Li YH, Qin ZK, Liu ZW, Zhou FJ, et al. Modified technique of radical inguinal lymphadenectomy for penile carcinoma: morbidity and outcome. J Urol. 2010;184(2):546–52.
58. Koifman L, Hampl D, Koifman N, Vides AJ, Ornellas AA. Radical open inguinal lymphadenectomy for penile carcinoma: surgical technique, early complications and late outcomes. J Urol. 2013;190(6):2086–92.
59. La-Touche S, Ayres B, Lam W, Alnajjar HM, Perry M, Watkin N. Trial of ligation versus coagulation of lymphatics in dynamic inguinal sentinel lymph node biopsy for staging of squamous cell carcinoma of the penis. Ann R Coll Surg Engl. 2012;94(5):344–6.
60. Graafland NM, van Boven HH, van Werkhoven E, Moonen LM, Horenblas S. Prognostic significance of extranodal extension in patients with pathological node positive penile carcinoma. J Urol. 2010;184(4):1347–53.
61. Lughezzani G, Catanzaro M, Torelli T, Piva L, Biasoni D, Stagni S, et al. The relationship between characteristics of inguinal lymph nodes and pelvic lymph node involvement in penile squamous cell carcinoma: a single institution experience. J Urol. 2014;191(4):977–82.
62. Pizzocaro G, Piva L. Adjuvant and neoadjuvant vincristine, bleomycin, and methotrexate for inguinal metastases from squamous cell carcinoma of the penis. Acta Oncol. 1988;27(6b):823–4.
63. Leijte JA, Kerst JM, Bais E, Antonini N, Horenblas S. Neoadjuvant chemotherapy in advanced penile carcinoma. Eur Urol. 2007;52(2):488–94.
64. Bermejo C, Busby JE, Spiess PE, Heller L, Pagliaro LC, Pettaway CA. Neoadjuvant chemotherapy followed by aggressive surgical consolidation for metastatic penile squamous cell carcinoma. J Urol. 2007;177(4):1335–8.
65. Dickstein RJ, Munsell MF, Pagliaro LC, Pettaway CA. Prognostic factors influencing survival from regionally advanced squamous cell carcinoma of the penis after preoperative chemotherapy. BJU Int. 2016;117(1):118–25.
66. Pagliaro LC, Williams DL, Daliani D, Williams MB, Osai W, Kincaid M, et al. Neoadjuvant paclitaxel, ifosfamide, and cisplatin chemotherapy for metastatic penile cancer: a phase II study. J Clin Oncol. 2010;28(24):3851–7.
67. Lucky MA, Rogers B, Parr NJ. Referrals into a dedicated British penile cancer centre and sources of possible delay. Sex Transm Infect. 2009;85(7):527–30.
68. Nicolai N, Sangalli LM, Necchi A, Giannatempo P, Paganoni AM, Colecchia M, et al. A combination of cisplatin and 5-fluorouracil with a taxane in patients who underwent lymph node dissection for nodal metastases from squamous cell carcinoma of the penis: treatment outcome and survival analyses in neoadjuvant and adjuvant settings. Clin Genitourin Cancer. 2016;14(4):323–30.
69. Necchi A, Lo Vullo S, Nicolai N, Raggi D, Giannatempo P, Colecchia M, et al. Prognostic factors of adjuvant taxane, cisplatin, and 5-fluorouracil chemotherapy for patients with penile squamous cell carcinoma after regional lymphadenectomy. Clin Genitourin Cancer. 2016;14(6):518–23.

70. Sharma P, Djajadiningrat R, Zargar-Shoshtari K, Catanzaro M, Zhu Y, Nicolai N, et al. Adjuvant chemotherapy is associated with improved overall survival in pelvic node-positive penile cancer after lymph node dissection: a multi-institutional study. Urol Oncol. 2015;33(11):496.e17–23.

71. Pizzocaro G, Nicolai N, Milani A. Taxanes in combination with cisplatin and fluorouracil for advanced penile cancer: preliminary results. Eur Urol. 2009;55(3):546–51.

72. Bullen K, Matthews S, Edwards S, Marke V. Exploring men's experiences of penile cancer surgery to improve rehabilitation. Nurs Times. 2009;105(12):20–4.

73. Afonso LA, Cordeiro TI, Carestiato FN, Ornellas AA, Alves G, Cavalcanti SM. High risk human papillomavirus infection of the foreskin in asymptomatic men and patients with phimosis. J Urol. 2016;195(6):1784–9.

74. Muneer A, Horenblas S. Textbook of penile cancer. Cham: Springer International Publishing; 2016.

75. Kayes O, Minhas S, Allen C, Hare C, Freeman A, Ralph D. The role of magnetic resonance imaging in the local staging of penile cancer. Eur Urol. 2007;51(5):1313–8; discussion 8–9

76. Chu QD, Vezeridis MP, Libbey NP, Wanebo HJ. Giant condyloma acuminatum (Buschke-Lowenstein tumor) of the anorectal and perianal regions. Analysis of 42 cases. Dis Colon Rectum. 1994;37(9):950–7.

77. Guimaraes GC, Cunha IW, Soares FA, Lopes A, Torres J, Chaux A, et al. Penile squamous cell carcinoma clinicopathological features, nodal metastasis and outcome in 333 cases. J Urol. 2009;182(2):528–34; discussion 34

78. Cubilla AL, Reuter V, Velazquez E, Piris A, Saito S, Young RH. Histologic classification of penile carcinoma and its relation to outcome in 61 patients with primary resection. Int J Surg Pathol. 2001;9(2):111–20.

79. Barreto JE, Velazquez EF, Ayala E, Torres J, Cubilla AL. Carcinoma cuniculatum: a distinctive variant of penile squamous cell carcinoma: report of 7 cases. Am J Surg Pathol. 2007;31(1):71–5.

80. Crook J. Radiotherapy approaches for locally advanced penile cancer: neoadjuvant and adjuvant. Curr Opin Urol. 2017;27(1):62–7.

81. Crook J. Contemporary role of radiotherapy in the management of primary penile tumors and metastatic disease. Urol Clin North Am. 2016;43(4):435–48.

82. Korzeniowski MA, Crook JM. Contemporary role of radiotherapy in the management of penile cancer. Transl Androl Urol. 2017;6(5):855–67.

83. Alnajjar HM, MacAskill F, Christodoulidou M, Mosahebi A, Akers C, Nigam R, et al. Long-term outcomes for penile cancer patients presenting with advanced N3 disease requiring a myocutaneous flap reconstruction or primary closure-a retrospective single centre study. Transl Androl Urol. 2019;8(Suppl 1):S13–21.

84. Necchi A, Pond GR, Raggi D, Ottenhof SR, Djajadiningrat RS, Horenblas S, et al. Clinical outcomes of perioperative chemotherapy in patients with locally advanced penile squamous-cell carcinoma: results of a multicenter analysis. Clin Genitourin Cancer. 2017;15(5):548–55. e3

85. Nicholson S, Hall E, Harland SJ, Chester JD, Pickering L, Barber J, et al. Phase II trial of docetaxel, cisplatin and 5FU chemotherapy in locally advanced and metastatic penis cancer (CRUK/09/001). Br J Cancer. 2013;109(10):2554–9.

86. Djajadiningrat RS, Bergman AM, van Werkhoven E, Vegt E, Horenblas S. Neoadjuvant taxane-based combination chemotherapy in patients with advanced penile cancer. Clin Genitourin Cancer. 2015;13(1):44–9.

87. Chipollini J, Necchi A, Spiess PE. Outcomes for patients with node-positive penile cancer: impact of perioperative systemic therapies and the importance of surgical intervention. Eur Urol. 2018;74(2):241–2.

88. Azizi M, Aydin AM, Hajiran A, Lai A, Kumar A, Peyton CC, et al. Systematic review and meta-analysis-is there a benefit in using neoadjuvant systemic chemotherapy for locally advanced penile squamous cell carcinoma? J Urol. 2020;203(6):1147–55.

89. Robinson R, Marconi L, MacPepple E, Hakenberg OW, Watkin N, Yuan Y, et al. Risks and benefits of adjuvant radiotherapy after inguinal lymphadenectomy in node-positive penile cancer: a systematic review by the European Association of Urology Penile Cancer Guidelines Panel. Eur Urol. 2018;74(1):76–83.

90. Rippentrop JM, Joslyn SA, Konety BR. Squamous cell carcinoma of the penis: evaluation of data from the surveillance, epidemiology, and end results program. Cancer. 2004;101(6):1357–63.

91. Dorfinger K, Maier U, Base W. Parathyroid hormone related protein and carcinoma of the penis: paraneoplastic hypercalcemia. J Urol. 1999;161(5):1570.

92. Akashi T, Fuse H, Muraishi Y, Mizuno I, Nagakawa O, Furuya Y. Parathyroid hormone related protein producing penile cancer. J Urol. 2002;167(1):249.

93. Nicholson S, Tovey H, Elliott T, Burnett SM, Cruickshank C, Bahl A, et al. VinCaP: a phase II trial of vinflunine in locally advanced and metastatic squamous carcinoma of the penis. Br J Cancer. 2022;126(1):34–41.

94. Drager DL, Milerski S, Sievert KD, Hakenberg OW. Psychosocial effects in patients with penile cancer: a systematic review. Urologe A. 2018;57(4):444–52.

95. Maddineni SB, Lau MM, Sangar VK. Identifying the needs of penile cancer sufferers: a systematic review of the quality of life, psychosexual and psychosocial literature in penile cancer. BMC Urol. 2009;9:8.

96. Akers C, Plant H, Riley V, Alnajjar HM, Muneer A. Exploring penile cancer survivors' motivations and experiences of attending a support group: eUROGEN study. Int J Urol Nurs. 2021;15(1):20–6.

97. Hoffman MA, Renshaw AA, Loughlin KR. Squamous cell carcinoma of the penis and microscopic pathologic margins: how much margin is needed for local cure? Cancer. 1999;85(7):1565–8.

98. Agrawal A, Pai D, Ananthakrishnan N, Smile SR, Ratnakar C. The histological extent of the local spread of carcinoma of the penis and its therapeutic implications. BJU Int. 2000;85(3):299–301.

99. Djajadiningrat RS, van Werkhoven E, Meinhardt W, van Rhijn BW, Bex A, van der Poel HG, et al. Penile sparing surgery for penile cancer-does it affect survival? J Urol. 2014;192(1):120–5.

100. Opjordsmoen S, Waehre H, Aass N, Fossa SD. Sexuality in patients treated for penile cancer: patients' experience and doctors' judgement. Br J Urol. 1994;73(5):554–60.

101. Romero FR, Romero KR, Mattos MA, Garcia CR, Fernandes Rde C, Perez MD. Sexual function after partial penectomy for penile cancer. Urology. 2005;66(6):1292–5.

102. Wever L, de Vries HM, Dell'Oglio P, van der Poel HG, Donswijk ML, Sikorska K, et al. Incidence and risk factor analysis of complications after sentinel node biopsy for penile cancer. BJU Int. 2022; https://doi.org/10.1111/bju.15725.

103. Nabavizadeh R, Petrinec B, Nabavizadeh B, Singh A, Rawal S, Master V. Inguinal lymph node dissection in the era of minimally invasive surgical technology. Urol Oncol. 2020; https://doi.org/10.1016/j.urolonc.2020.07.026.

104. Patel KN, Salunke A, Bakshi G, Jayaprakash D, Pandya SJ. Robotic-Assisted Video-Endoscopic Inguinal Lymphadenectomy (RAVEIL) and Video-Endoscopic Inguinal Lymphadenectomy (VEIL) versus Open Inguinal Lymph-Node Dissection (OILND) in carcinoma of penis: comparison of perioperative outcomes, complications and oncological outcomes. A systematic review and meta-analysis. Urol Oncol. 2022;40(3):112.e11–22.

Association of Sexual Dysfunction and Neurological Disorders

19

Fatma Gokcem Yildiz

Abstract

Sexual dysfunction (SD) is common in neurological disorders due to the combination of lesions affecting neural control, neuropsycogenic consequences of the disease and pharmacological agents. SD significantly affects quality of life in not only neurological patients, but also their partners. Sexual function including arousal, desire, orgasm, erection and ejaculation is under the control of coordinated function of somatic and autonomic systems. The other brain network systems are also take part in functioning the sexual organs set in a complex neural hierarchy. This relation and interaction is increasingly being demonstrated over years with high quality neurophysiological and neuroimaging studies. SD is an underreported, underrecognised symptom for the neurology patients which impacts patients mental and physical health related quality of life. The major reason for this, is the lack of knowledge. Specialized neurologists dealing with the potential chronic neurological patients that can often be observed SD, urologists and andrologists should be aware of their patients for the management and diagnosis.

Sexual dysfunction (SD) is common in neurological disorders due to the combination of lesions affecting neural control, neuropsycogenic consequences of the disease and pharmacological agents. SD significantly affects quality of life in not only neurological patients, but also their partners. Thus, detailed investigations and the management of this patients should be undertaken in specialized centers. The treatment and evaluation of the patients should preferentially require collaboration of

F. G. Yildiz (✉)
Faculty of Medicine, Department of Neurology, Hacettepe University, Ankara, Turkey

© The Author(s), under exclusive license to Springer Nature
Switzerland AG 2022
S. Sarikaya et al. (eds.), *Andrology and Sexual Medicine*, Management of Urology,
https://doi.org/10.1007/978-3-031-12049-7_19

both neurology and urology departments. Regardless of the etiology; the damage of any neural features described above can cause SD.

Neural Control of Sexual Function

Sexual function including arousal, desire, orgasm, erection and ejaculation is under the control of coordinated function of somatic and autonomic systems. The other brain network systems are also take part in functioning the sexual organs set in a complex neural hierarchy. This relation and interaction is increasingly being demonstrated over years with high quality neurophysiological and neuroimaging studies. The cortical areas insula, temporal lobes, anterior cingulate cortex, periaqueductal grey matter and hypothalamus take part in central coordinating the sexual behavior via autonomic nervous system [1–4]. The facilitator and the inhibitory pathways through the spinal cord modulate the thoracolumbar sympathetic and sacral parasympathetic spinal levels. The control of sexual events for women and men genitals appear similarly; example lubrication of vagina, clitoris erection or the erection, ejaculation in male. Apart from the neuroanatomical structures; additional psychosocial pathologies, vascular or hormonal dysfunction also alter the sexuality. Although such a complex neural system provides normal sexual responses; the neurological lesions may lead SD at different anatomical levels. Normal erection function is arising after psychogenic and physical stimulation and under control of parasympathogenic fibers from sacral S2 to S4. These fibers travel though pelvic nerve, pelvic plexus and enters to corpus cavernosum. They start a process after releasing nitric oxide and acetylcholine both which causes smooth muscle relaxation and a blood influx to the tissue. The endothelium also releases more nitric oxide to sustain the erection. Intracavernosal pressure and phosphodiesterase 5 also contribute the maintaining the erection. Besides, ejaculation reflex is coordinated by sympathogenic fibers arise from thoracolumbar T10 to L2 and somatic fibers from S2–4 segments [4].

Dysfunction in Neurological Diseases

Regardless of the etiology; the damage of any neural features described above can cause SD (Fig. 19.1). The SD is more common than the other population in the patients with neurological diseases due to not only the lesions or neural damage, but also the therapies. The data about this information is related from the limited observational studies. In general SD appears as the loss of function or rarely hypersexuality. The main categories include loss of desire, failure of arousal, orgasmic dysfunction and sexual pain disorders in SD.

The medical history, screening tools like questionaries' and neurological examination takes part for the diagnosis of SD in neurologic patients. Neurological examination should include muscle stretch tests, deep tendon reflexes, detecting Babinski sign, sensation of touch and pinprick including perianal region, tonus of external

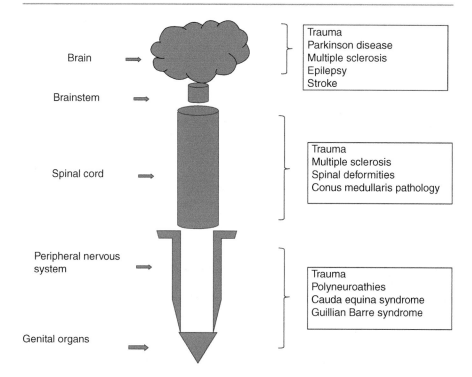

Fig. 19.1 Simplified illustration of neural control of sexual function and possible neurological disorders

anal sphincter, bulbocavernosus and anal reflexes. SD may appear not only with the patients with known neurological diseases; but also, it rarely be initial manifestation before the neurological diagnosis without finding a urological cause. Polyneuropathies, diseases related autonomic system dysfunction such as Parkinson plus syndromes multi system atrophy (MSA); structural that cause conus/cauda syndromes may be the early etiologies for the SD before the neurological diagnosis [5]. In such patients peripheral electromyography, electrodiagnostic test for needle EMG of anal sphincter, bulbocavernosus reflex testing and neuroimaging investigations are appropriate for detecting the main etiology.

Neurological Diseases

Trauma

Both head and the pelvic trauma may cause the SD by damaging the neural fibers directly. Pelvic floor nerves which are necessary for ejaculation and erection travel close to many of the pelvic organ anatomic neighborhood. Prostatectomies, cystectomies, rectal surgery, periaortic surgeries including aneurysm and bypass, retroperitoneal lymph node dissections in testicular cancers are the common surgical types which may damage the superior hypogastric plexus, postganglionic sympathomimetic nerves [6–9]. In general patients with head trauma has high rates of SD varies 36% to 54% [10]. The sexual disability may become after global injury or injury of focal regions. Although global injuries may result hypo sexuality, the focal prefrontal lobe regions may result hypo sexuality or hyper sexuality. Bilateral temporal lobe injuries also produce the Kluver-Bucy syndrome of hyper sexuality and hyper orality after head trauma [11]. Hypothalamic and pituitary damage associated with traumatic brain injuries may lead to change hormonal factors such as oxytocin, growth hormone, gonadotropins, prolactin hypothalamic peptidergic neurons of Orexin-A [12, 13].

Spinal Cord Injury and Abnormalities

Spinal cord injury impairs sexual dysfunction in men and women. Sensorimotor disability, bladder dysfunction are the major issues in patients that effect quality of life. Vaginal lubrication, and orgasm are generally affected in women, erection and ejaculation affected in women. The impaired sexual responses depend on the completeness and the level of the injury. Both genders become difficult to be aroused and its reported that the women are more effected that men [14].

The physical sensations including tingling and spasm are the most reported in men and women. Erection and ejaculatory capacity is most effected in men via the psychogenic and reflex pathways. The psychogenic pathway is mediated by the T12-L2 thoracolumbar sympathetic outflow. After a high lesion psychogenic erections are lost but reflex erections remain intact. Lower lesion levels generally reduce erectile capacity. Neural tube defects including lumbar vertebrae are the disorders of the spinal cord which may result any kind of SD [15, 16]. Tethered cord syndrome and its surgery are also included in the etiology of SD.

Multiple Sclerosis

Multiple Sclerosis (MS) is a demyelinating disease of central nervous system often causes disabling neurological symptoms in young adults. Sexual dysfunction is reported more common in MS patients than the general population with a rate of 50–90% in men and 60–80% in women [17, 18]. Several factors may contribute to SD in patients with MS. Primary SD may appear as a result of the demyelinating neural lesions and axonal damages' itself in which the pathways taking part of sexual function. Brainstem lesions, total lesion amount of the patients, limbic and paralimbic brain regions are more related with SD. Spinal cord lesions are also a major factor, especially in male erectile dysfunction [19].

Secondary MS related symptoms including spasticity, tremor, fatigue, bladder dysfunctions, immobility, cognitive and sensory dysfunction may effect SD. Emotional and psychosocial changes, depression and anxiety may also correlate with the SD. Some additional several medications may worsen the sexual function; patients should be warned about serotonin reuptake inhibitors. Although erectile dysfunction, ejaculatory dysfunction, anorgasmia and reduced libido are most frequent complaints in men; reduced libido, vaginal lubrication failure and anorgasmia are the most common SD presentations in women [20]. Some questions of symptomatology onset, duration and self-reported questionnaires like the MS Intimacy and Sexuality Questionnaire-19 (MSISQ-19) may help to detect the SD in patients.

Movement Disorders

Parkinson disease is a progressive neurodegenerative disorder with an autonomic, limbic and somatomotor systems involvement. Although SD is one of the disabling clinic aspect, it is poorly investigated. The prevalence is reported 35–65% of the Parkinson patients [21]. It is reported that men effected more than the women. This may be the complexity of the diseases itself. Motor control, cognitive, psychological, pharmacological components and interactions are crucial to discriminate the origin of sexual behaviors. Dopamine replacement therapy is the most common treatment of the symptoms. Dopamine promotes the sexual motivation and recognized as a pro-sexual neurotransmitter. Hyper sexuality may appear not only under L-dopa treatment, but also it may be a sign of frontal lobe disinhibition [22]. Apo morphine, D2 agonist, subcutaneous injections may result penis erection [22, 23]. In a previous study, treatment with deep brain stimulation of the subthalamic nucleus in men showed a slightly improvement over the satisfaction of sexual life [24]. Especially in medial optic area dopamine is releasing which causes sexual facilitation in men. Additionally, paraventricular nucleus which has oxytogenergic neurons, nucleus accumbens, mesolimbic areas, hippocampus, medulla oblongata has important role for the sexual behavior. The multifactor including aging, disability of movement disorder, autonomic dysfunction, neuropsychiatric status and pharmacotherapy may contribute the SD. Antidepressants, in particular selective serotonin reuptake inhibitors are associative in male and female. Increased sexual desire, vaginismus, decreased arousal, erectly dysfunction, premature ejaculation, decreased orgasm are the most self-reported categories. Erectly dysfunction is seen twice frequent than the healthy people. Autonomic dysfunction is important to discriminate the parkinsonian plus syndromes like multisystem atrophy (MSA) [25]. MSA patients are more likely to be affected because of the autonomic failure. The erectly dysfunction may be the appearance of the disease in men which should be questioned to the patients with other autonomic symptoms. Genital hyposensitivity was reported 56% of the women with MSA [26].

SD also discussed in patients with Huntington Disease which is an also neurodegenerative movement disorder disease. The most common symptoms are hypo sexual disorders (53–83%), hyperactive sexual disorder (6–30%), erectile (48–74%), ejaculatory dysfunctions (30–65%), lubrication problems (53–83%), and orgasmic dysfunction (35–78%) [27].

Epilepsy

The presence of SD in epilepsy is related multiple combination of factors including disease related, drug related and psychosocial factors. It discussed that all the factors alter the hypotalamo- pituitary releasing mechanisms or the epileptic discharges propagates the hormonal responses of gonadotropins and dopamine. And preferably right temporal epilepsy is also discussed to be a reason for SD in animal models. The prevalence of SD in epileptic women is variable with a rate of 10–75% [28].

This variable result may because of the small size of studies, the heterogeneity of epileptic syndromes and the variety of medical drugs. The patients with uncontrolled seizures, under polytherapy, higher seizure frequency are reported more SD. Hypo sexuality and sexual desire are more frequent SD domains in women with epilepsy [29]. Variable prevalence studies are reported in men, because of the heterogeneity of the patients as similar to women SD [30].

Erectile dysfunction and premature ejaculation are mainly affected and more common in men with epilepsy. Anti-epileptic drugs are also suspected of SD in previous studies. Decreased libido reported with pyrimidone, phenobarbital, carbamazepine and phenytoin [31, 32]. Carbamazepine is shown to be associated with low testosterone and high levels of sex hormone binding globulin. Oxcarbamezapine can cause similar hormonal responses like carbamazepine [33]. Valproic acid may cause impotence 10% of patients [34]. Topiramate may cause sexual disorders in 7.4% to 12.5% patients, likely causes orgasmic problems in women and erectly dysfunction in male [35]. A previous study indicates patients on lamotrigine therapy have improvement on sexual functions. It is suggested that the other newer antiepileptic drugs zonisamide, levetirasetam, gabapentine, pregabaline, locasamide can cause hyposexuality, anorgasmia and erectly dysfunction. It is not fully understood and likely be effected multifactorial. The changes of frequency after epilepsy surgery is not also clear; but its discussed that improvement may be present after surgery because of the reduction of antiepileptic drugs or reducing the frequency of seizures [36].

Epilepsy has also high association with psychosocial comorbidities and psychiatric disorders. Contribution of depression, anxiety, psychosis can play important role in management of patients. The prevalence of SD is increased with the comorbidities and antidepressant and antipsychotic treatment.

Stroke

Stroke is a disabling and mortal disease in which approximately 50% of the people experiences SD [37, 38]. It may occur in cerebral hemispheres, brainstem, midbrain or spinal cord which may cause varying SD depending the location. This condition often results because of multifactorial reasons. Direct result of stroke and comorbidities (diabetes, cardiac, hypertension…), the sensorimotor disabilities (hemiplegia, spasticity, bladder dysfunction, pain…), psychosomatic and cognitive issues are the related causes of SD in post stroke survivors. Erectly dysfunction, decline of libido, anorgasmia, ejaculation problems are frequent symptoms that seen 17% to 48% of the patients. Right hemispheric stroke patients are the more affected than the left hemispheric ones.

Peripheral Nerve Impairment

Different types of peripheral nerves (motor, somatic or autonomic) dysfunction may cause SD. The etiology of the axonal damage may be due to the direct nerve injury of the peripheral nerve or the small vascular impairment. Sensory stimuli of the genitals are important for sexual excitement. Penis and the clitoris has free nerve endings in glans superficial mucosa which of these are responding deep pressure, vigorous movement and pain. The mechanoreceptors are adapting by the afferent C and A-d fibers [39].

Pudendal nerve neuropathy, sacral plexus injuries, cauda equine syndrome are the focal nerve involvements. Diabetes mellitus, Vitamin B1–B12 deficits, uremia, Guillian Barres Syndrome, chronic demyelinating polyneuropathy, porphyria, pandysautonomia, alcoholism, Charcot–Marie–Tooth disease, Transthyretin amyloid polyneuropathy, hereditary sensory autonomic neuropathies, HIV-associated polyneuropathy, paraneoplastic autonomic neuropathy are the causes of polyneuropathies that cause SD [40–42].

Conclusion

SD is an underreported, underrecognised symptom for the neurology patients which impacts patients mental and physical health related quality of life. The major reason for this, is the lack of knowledge. Specialized neurologists dealing with the potential chronic neurological patients that can often be observed SD, urologists and andrologists should be aware of their patients for the management and diagnosis. Coordinating and counselling may provide to establish multidisciplinary approach for the healthcare of the patients. It is important to examine the patients individually to reach a successful therapy.

References

1. Holstege G, Georgiadis JR, Paans AM, Meiners LC, van der Graaf FH, Reinders AA. Brain activation during human male ejaculation. J Neurosci. 2003;23(27):9185–93.
2. Park K, Seo JJ, Kang HK, Ryu SB, Kim HJ, Jeong GW. A new potential of blood oxygenation level dependent (BOLD) functional MRI for evaluating cerebral centers of penile erection. Int J Impot Res. 2001;13(2):73–81. https://doi.org/10.1038/sj.ijir.3900649.
3. Karama S, Lecours AR, Leroux JM, Bourgouin P, Beaudoin G, Joubert S, et al. Areas of brain activation in males and females during viewing of erotic film excerpts. Hum Brain Mapp. 2002;16(1):1–13.
4. Baird AD, Wilson SJ, Bladin PF, Saling MM, Reutens DC. Neurological control of human sexual behaviour: insights from lesion studies. J Neurol Neurosurg Psychiatry. 2007;78(10):1042–9. https://doi.org/10.1136/jnnp.2006.107193.

5. Podnar S, Oblak C, Vodusek DB. Sexual function in men with cauda equina lesions: a clinical and electromyographic study. J Neurol Neurosurg Psychiatry. 2002;73(6):715–20. https://doi.org/10.1136/jnnp.73.6.715.

6. Jensen PT, Groenvold M, Klee MC, Thranov I, Petersen MA, Machin D. Early-stage cervical carcinoma, radical hysterectomy, and sexual function. A longitudinal study. Cancer. 2004;100(1):97–106. https://doi.org/10.1002/cncr.11877.

7. Carson CC 3rd, Hubbard JS, Wallen E. Erectile dysfunction and treatment of carcinoma of the prostate. Curr Urol Rep. 2005;6(6):461–9. https://doi.org/10.1007/s11934-005-0042-1.

8. Zippe CD, Raina R, Massanyi EZ, Agarwal A, Jones JS, Ulchaker J, et al. Sexual function after male radical cystectomy in a sexually active population. Urology. 2004;64(4):682–5.; ; discussion 5–6. https://doi.org/10.1016/j.urology.2004.05.056.

9. Hendren SK, O'Connor BI, Liu M, Asano T, Cohen Z, Swallow CJ, et al. Prevalence of male and female sexual dysfunction is high following surgery for rectal cancer. Ann Surg. 2005;242(2):212–23. https://doi.org/10.1097/01.sla.0000171299.43954.ce.

10. Sandel ME, Williams KS, Dellapietra L, Derogatis LR. Sexual functioning following traumatic brain injury. Brain Inj. 1996;10(10):719–28. https://doi.org/10.1080/026990596123981.

11. Lilly R, Cummings JL, Benson DF, Frankel M. The human Kluver-Bucy syndrome. Neurology. 1983;33(9):1141–5. https://doi.org/10.1212/wnl.33.9.1141.

12. Bondanelli M, De Marinis L, Ambrosio MR, Monesi M, Valle D, Zatelli MC, et al. Occurrence of pituitary dysfunction following traumatic brain injury. J Neurotrauma. 2004;21(6):685–96. https://doi.org/10.1089/0897715041269713.

13. Lieberman SA, Oberoi AL, Gilkison CR, Masel BE, Urban RJ. Prevalence of neuroendocrine dysfunction in patients recovering from traumatic brain injury. J Clin Endocrinol Metab. 2001;86(6):2752–6. https://doi.org/10.1210/jcem.86.6.7592.

14. Stoffel JT, Van der Aa F, Wittmann D, Yande S, Elliott S. Fertility and sexuality in the spinal cord injury patient. World J Urol. 2018;36(10):1577–85. https://doi.org/10.1007/s00345-018-2347-y.

15. Boemers TM, van Gool JD, de Jong TP. Tethered spinal cord: the effect of neurosurgery on the lower urinary tract and male sexual function. Br J Urol. 1995;76(6):747–51. https://doi.org/10.1111/j.1464-410x.1995.tb00767.x.

16. Decter RM, Furness PD 3rd, Nguyen TA, McGowan M, Laudermilch C, Telenko A. Reproductive understanding, sexual functioning and testosterone levels in men with spina bifida. J Urol. 1997;157(4):1466–8.

17. Mattson D, Petrie M, Srivastava DK, McDermott M. Multiple sclerosis. Sexual dysfunction and its response to medications. Arch Neurol. 1995;52(9):862–8. https://doi.org/10.1001/archneur.1995.00540330040012.

18. Lew-Starowicz M, Rola R. Prevalence of sexual dysfunctions among women with multiple sclerosis. Sex Disabil. 2013;31(2):141–53. https://doi.org/10.1007/s11195-013-9293-9.

19. Li V, Haslam C, Pakzad M, Brownlee WJ, Panicker JN. A practical approach to assessing and managing sexual dysfunction in multiple sclerosis. Pract Neurol. 2020;20(2):122–31. https://doi.org/10.1136/practneurol-2019-002321.

20. Orasanu B, Frasure H, Wyman A, Mahajan ST. Sexual dysfunction in patients with multiple sclerosis. Mult Scler Relat Disord. 2013;2(2):117–23. https://doi.org/10.1016/j.msard.2012.10.005.

21. Jacobs H, Vieregge A, Vieregge P. Sexuality in young patients with Parkinson's disease: a population based comparison with healthy controls. J Neurol Neurosurg Psychiatry. 2000;69(4):550–2. https://doi.org/10.1136/jnnp.69.4.550.

22. Uitti RJ, Tanner CM, Rajput AH, Goetz CG, Klawans HL, Thiessen B. Hypersexuality with antiparkinsonian therapy. Clin Neuropharmacol. 1989;12(5):375–83. https://doi.org/10.1097/00002826-198910000-00002.

23. Montorsi F, Perani D, Anchisi D, Salonia A, Scifo P, Rigiroli P, et al. Apomorphine-induced brain modulation during sexual stimulation: a new look at central phenomena related to erectile dysfunction. Int J Impot Res. 2003;15(3):203–9. https://doi.org/10.1038/sj.ijir.3900999.

24. Farmer SF. Sexual wellbeing in Parkinson's disease. J Neurol Neurosurg Psychiatry. 2004;75(9):1232. https://doi.org/10.1136/jnnp.2004.043927.
25. Kirchhof K, Apostolidis AN, Mathias CJ, Fowler CJ. Erectile and urinary dysfunction may be the presenting features in patients with multiple system atrophy: a retrospective study. Int J Impot Res. 2003;15(4):293–8. https://doi.org/10.1038/sj.ijir.3901014.
26. Raccagni C, Indelicato E, Sidoroff V, Daniaux M, Bader A, Toth B, et al. Female sexual dysfunction in multiple system atrophy: a prospective cohort study. Clin Auton Res. 2021;31(6):713–7. https://doi.org/10.1007/s10286-021-00825-2.
27. Szymus K, Bystrzynski A, Kwasniak-Butowska M, Konkel A, Lesnicka A, Nowacka M, et al. Sexual dysfunction in Huntington's disease—a systematic review. Neurol Neurochir Pol. 2020;54(4):305–11. https://doi.org/10.5603/JNNS.a2020.0025.
28. Demerdash A, Shaalan M, Midani A, Kamel F, Bahri M. Sexual behavior of a sample of females with epilepsy. Epilepsia. 1991;32(1):82–5. https://doi.org/10.1111/j.1528-1157.1991.tb05616.x.
29. Rathore C, Henning OJ, Luef G, Radhakrishnan K. Sexual dysfunction in people with epilepsy. Epilepsy Behav. 2019;100(Pt A):106495. https://doi.org/10.1016/j.yebeh.2019.106495.
30. Laumann EO, Nicolosi A, Glasser DB, Paik A, Gingell C, Moreira E, et al. Sexual problems among women and men aged 40-80 y: prevalence and correlates identified in the Global Study of Sexual Attitudes and Behaviors. Int J Impot Res. 2005;17(1):39–57. https://doi.org/10.1038/sj.ijir.3901250.
31. Herzog AG, Drislane FW, Schomer DL, Pennell PB, Bromfield EB, Dworetzky BA, et al. Differential effects of antiepileptic drugs on sexual function and hormones in men with epilepsy. Neurology. 2005;65(7):1016–20. https://doi.org/10.1212/01.wnl.0000178988.78039.40.
32. Rattya J, Turkka J, Pakarinen AJ, Knip M, Kotila MA, Lukkarinen O, et al. Reproductive effects of valproate, carbamazepine, and oxcarbazepine in men with epilepsy. Neurology. 2001;56(1):31–6. https://doi.org/10.1212/wnl.56.1.31.
33. Svalheim S, Tauboll E, Luef G, Lossius A, Rauchenzauner M, Sandvand F, et al. Differential effects of levetiracetam, carbamazepine, and lamotrigine on reproductive endocrine function in adults. Epilepsy Behav. 2009;16(2):281–7. https://doi.org/10.1016/j.yebeh.2009.07.033.
34. Mattson RH, Cramer JA, Collins JF. A comparison of valproate with carbamazepine for the treatment of complex partial seizures and secondarily generalized tonic-clonic seizures in adults. The Department of Veterans Affairs Epilepsy Cooperative Study No. 264 Group. N Engl J Med. 1992;327(11):765–71. https://doi.org/10.1056/NEJM199209103271104.
35. Chen LW, Chen MY, Chen KY, Lin HS, Chien CC, Yin HL. Topiramate-associated sexual dysfunction: a systematic review. Epilepsy Behav. 2017;73:10–7. https://doi.org/10.1016/j.yebeh.2017.05.014.
36. Baird AD, Wilson SJ, Bladin PF, Saling MM, Reutens DC. Sexual outcome after epilepsy surgery. Epilepsy Behav. 2003;4(3):268–78. https://doi.org/10.1016/s1525-5050(03)00085-4.
37. Korpelainen JT, Kauhanen ML, Kemola H, Malinen U, Myllyla VV. Sexual dysfunction in stroke patients. Acta Neurol Scand. 1998;98(6):400–5. https://doi.org/10.1111/j.1600-0404.1998.tb07321.x.
38. Giaquinto S, Buzzelli S, Di Francesco L, Nolfe G. Evaluation of sexual changes after stroke. J Clin Psychiatry. 2003;64(3):302–7. https://doi.org/10.4088/jcp.v64n0312.
39. Podnar S, Vodusek DB. Sexual dysfunction in patients with peripheral nervous system lesions. Handb Clin Neurol. 2015;130:179–202. https://doi.org/10.1016/B978-0-444-63247-0.00011-0.
40. Alves M, Conceicao I, Luis ML. Neurophysiological evaluation of sexual dysfunction in familial amyloidotic polyneuropathy—Portuguese type. Acta Neurol Scand. 1997;96(3):163–6. https://doi.org/10.1111/j.1600-0404.1997.tb00260.x.
41. Ferriere G, Guzzetta F, Kulakowski S, Evrard P. Nonprogressive type II hereditary sensory autonomic neuropathy: a homogeneous clinicopathologic entity. J Child Neurol. 1992;7(4):364–70. https://doi.org/10.1177/088307389200700406.
42. Burk K, Weiss A. Impotence after recovery from Guillain-Barre syndrome. N J Med. 1998;95(11):31–4.

Testosterone Replacement Therapy

20

Cem Haymana and Alper Sonmez

Abstract

The aim of testosterone replacement therapy (TRT) is to provide the development of and maintain the secondary sex characteristics and to improve the symptoms and signs due to testosterone deficiency in patients with androgen deficiency. Testosterone replacement should be applied in patients with hypogonadism who have symptoms and signs of androgen deficiency associated with low testosterone levels. TRT has positive effects on secondary sex characteristics, sexual functions, muscle strength, physical functions, mood and bone density. Several testosterone preparations such as oral preparations, parenteral testosterone esters, transdermal testosterone patch, testosterone gels and transdermal testosterone tablets are available for the treatment of male hypogonadism. The adequacy of testosterone therapy is assessed according to the clinical response and serum testosterone levels. The biochemical goal in treatment is to keep testosterone levels at mid-normal range. After starting TRT, serum testosterone, hematocrit and PSA levels should be measured periodically, and digital rectal examination should be performed in the follow-up. TRT is contraindicated in patients with metastatic prostate and breast cancers. Before starting TRT, men with a history of prostate cancer or are at high risk for developing prostate cancer should be identified. Testosterone therapy is also not recommended in patients with increased hematocrit values, patients with obstructive sleep apnea, uncontrolled heart failure and lower urinary tract symptoms.

C. Haymana · A. Sonmez (✉)
Department of Endocrinology and Metabolism, University of Health Sciences Gulhane
Faculty of Medicine, Ankara, Turkey
e-mail: yusufalper.sonmez@sbu.edu.tr

© The Author(s), under exclusive license to Springer Nature
Switzerland AG 2022
S. Sarikaya et al. (eds.), *Andrology and Sexual Medicine*, Management of Urology,
https://doi.org/10.1007/978-3-031-12049-7_20

The overall aim of the testosterone replacement therapy (TRT) is to induce and maintain the secondary sex characteristics and improve the symptoms of androgen deficiency. Testosterone replacement should be administered to patients with hypogonadism who have symptoms and signs of androgen deficiency associated with low testosterone levels. Testosterone replacement is not effective in patients with symptoms of androgen deficiency but with normal testosterone levels. Also, the off-label usage for antiaging purposes or to increase muscle mass or sexual desire should be discouraged because of potential adverse effects. The specific symptoms and signs for androgen deficiency are decreased libido and morning erections, loss of body hair, gynecomastia, small testicles, and low bone mineral density.

The main goal in testosterone replacement is to keep testosterone levels within normal ranges. The normal range for testosterone in adults is quite broad and is based on morning blood samples of a healthy young male. Testosterone levels decrease gradually and progressively with age. However, the physiologic significance of this decline is unclear.

Effects of TRT

The dose-related effects of TRT may vary in different tissues and in different clinical situations. The effects of testosterone therapy on libido continue to increase until testosterone levels reach normal levels. No additional increase in libido is seen at supraphysiologic testosterone levels. However, the effect of TRT on muscle strength increases in proportion to serum testosterone levels, and muscle strength continues to increase at supraphysiologic levels.

In patients with severe and long-standing androgen deficiency, TRT may cause sexual, behavioral and physical complications in the patient. To alleviate these problems, it is important to inform the patients and their partners about the side effects and complications of the treatment. Starting with a lower beginning dose of TRT for a few months and then increasing to a full replacement dosage may result in a more gradual transition from hypogonadism to eugonadism, leading to less severe problems [1].

Secondary Sexual Characteristics

Testosterone replacement to patients who have not completed pubertal development, provides the development of secondary sex characteristics such as deepening of the voice, facial and body hair growth, penile enlargement and pigmentation of scrotum, and increase the muscle and bone mass [2].

Sexual Functions

Testosterone replacement improves libido, erectile functions, and sexual activity in hypogonadal patients with low libido and sexual dysfunction. However, testosterone treatment had no effect on libido and sexual activity in hypogonadal patients with testosterone levels in the normal range [3, 4]. There is no effect of TRT on the ejaculatory function of patients with hypogonadism.

Body Composition, Muscle Strength, and Physical Function

Testosterone replacement increases the muscle strength and fat-free mas in hypogonadal men [5, 6]. TRT also reduces the whole body, intraabdominal, and intermuscular fat. These effects are related to the administered testosterone dose.

Well-Being, Depressive Symptoms and Cognition

Testosterone treatment also has important effects on the mood. In this regard, TRT improves the positive aspects of mood and reduces the negative aspects. However, this effect is less significant in older hypogonadal men. TRT has not been shown to have a positive effect on depressive symptoms in men with clinical depression [7]. The effect of TRT on fatigue is inconsistent. Similarly, TRT had no effect on cognitional function in older hypogonadal men.

Bone Mineral Density

Bone density and vertebral and femoral bone strength improves after TRT in hypogonadal men [8, 9]. However, the effect of TRT on the fracture risk is unknown. So far, testosterone replacement is not an approved modality for the treatment of osteoporosis or for reducing the risk of fractures. If the risk of fracture is high in hypogonadal patients receiving TRT, osteoporosis should be treated with a pharmacological agent. In hypogonadal men with osteoporosis who are not at high risk for bone fracture, osteoporosis treatment can be delayed until the response to TRT will be seen.

TRT in the Late Onset Hypogonadism

Late onset hypogonadism (LOH) is characterized by the signs and symptoms due to androgen deficiency with no reason of low testosterone levels other than aging. Older men have mildly reduced levels of total serum testosterone with a much significant reduction of free testosterone due to a rise in SHBG with age. Although LOH negatively affects the quality of life in elderly patients, the use of TRT in this patient group is still controversial. Some short term trials showed that testosterone replacement may improve the sexual function, mood and bone density in these patients [10], long-term studies with higher number of patients are needed to clarify the criteria for treatment. Also, the risks and benefits associated with testosterone replacement in this population should be carefully assessed. Many position statements and clinical guidelines recommend the administration of TRT in individually selected cases in patients with LOH [11–14]. TRT should only be administered in elderly men with clinically significant symptoms of androgen deficiency and low serum testosterone levels confirmed by at least two separate measurements, especially after the potential benefits and risk of treatment have been discussed with the patient.

Testosterone Formulations

Several testosterone preparations are available for the treatment of male hypogonadism. These include oral testosterone preparations, parenteral testosterone esters, transdermal testosterone patch, testosterone gels and transdermal testosterone tablets (Table 20.1).

Oral Formulations

Testosterone is well absorbed from the small intestine and is rapidly metabolized in the liver. Therefore, it is very difficult to maintain normal testosterone levels with the use of oral testosterone preparations. Adding an alkyl group in the 17-alpha position of the testosterone molecule slows its catabolism by the liver. These preparations have low bioavailability and have the serious hepatic side effects. For these reasons, the 17-alpha alkylated androgens should generally not be used to treat testosterone deficiency.

Another bioavailable oral testosterone preparation, testosterone undecanoate, has been introduced in recent years. This lipophilic preparation is absorbed from the intestinal lymphatic system and bypasses the first-pass hepatic effect. However, it has some serious adverse effects such as cardiovascular events and increase in blood pressure. Serum testosterone concentrations reach the peak level approximately 5 h after the application and the effect continues for 8–12 h. It is administered relatively in high doses, at doses of 40–80 mg, b.i.d. or t.i.d. This frequent application requirement also reduces the compliance of the patient. Testosterone levels decline rapidly following discontinuation of the drug, which may become a desirable feature, especially in elderly patients with prostate disease or comorbidities.

Parenteral Testosterone Formulations

Parenteral testosterone has been used in the treatment of hypogonadism since 1950s. In current formulations, the 17β-hydroxyl group of testosterone is esterified. This esterification increases the oil solubility of testosterone, resulting in a slower release, and prolonged half-life. The intramuscular formulations approved for the treatment are T cypionate (TC), T enanthate (TE), T propionate (TP) and T undecanoate (TU).

Table 20.1 Testosterone formulations in the treatment of male hypogonadism

Formulation	Typical starting dose	Advantages	Disadvantages
Testosterone enanthate or cypionate	150–200 mg IM every 2 wk or 75–100 mg/wk	• Extensive clinical use • Inexpensive with self-injection • Dose flexibility	• Discomfort due to IM injection, • Fluctation in testosterone levels, • More frequent erythrocytosis than transdermal testosterone
Injectable long-acting T undecanote	1000 mg IM initially and at 6 wk., then 1000 mg IM every 10–14 wk	• Less frequent injection, • Longer maintenance of normal T levels, • No apparent fluctuations in T levels or symptoms	• Discomfort due to IM injection, • Large-volume injection (4 mL), • No possible self-injection, • Rarely, cough immediately after injection
Transdermal testosterone gels 1%, 1.62%, or 2%	50–100 mg of 1% transdermal gel; 20.25–81 mg of 1.62% gel or 40–70 mg of 2% transdermal gel Applied to skin; shoulders or trunk	• Dose flexibility, • Easy application, • Little skin irritation, • Less frequent erythrocytosis than injectable testosterone	• Risk of contact transfer of testosterone to partner or child, • Daily application, • Expensive, • Moderately high dihydrotestosterone levels
Testosterone axillary solutions	60 mg of testosterone solution	• Good skin tolerability	• Risk of contact transfer of testosterone to partner or child, • Daily application, • Expensive, • Moderately high dihydrotestosterone levels

(continued)

Table 20.1 (continued)

Formulation	Typical starting dose	Advantages	Disadvantages
Transdermal testosterone patch	2.5 or 5 mg (one patch) or 7.5 mg or 10 mg (one 2.5-mg plus 5.0-mg patch or two 5-mg patches) applied daily over non-pressure areas	• Easy application,	• In some patients, two patches may be needed daily,
		• Mimics normal circadian variation when applied nightly,	• Frequent skin irritation,
		• Less frequent erythrocytosis than injectable formulations	• Expensive
Transbuccal testosterone	30 mg tablet applied between cheek and gum bid	• Convenience,	• Twice-daily application,
		• No injections,	• Gum related adverse events,
		• Physiologic T levels	• Altered or bitter taste,
			• No dose flexibility,
			• Expensive
Testosterone pellets	Pellets containing 600–1200 mg T implanted SC	• Requires infrequent administration,	• Requires surgical incision,
		• Longer maintenance of normal T levels	• Risk of local hematoma and infection,
			• Large number of pellets,
			• Not easily removed,
			• Spontaneous extruding
Nasal testosterone gel	11 mg two or three times daily	• Rapid absorption, Avoidance of first pass metabolism	• Multiple daily application,
			• Local nasal side effects,
			• Not appropriate for patients with nasal disorders
Oral testosterone undecanoate	40–80 mg oral, two or three times daily with meals	• Convenience of	• Variable bioavailability due to fat content of meals
		• oral administration	

These are effective, safe and inexpensive preparations for the treatment of hypogonadism. Among these preparations, TU has the longest duration of action. TE and TC have similar pharmacokinetic profiles and are considered clinically equivalent [15, 16]. However, maintaining physiological testosterone levels by these parenteral formulations is more limited when compared to transdermal gel formulations.

The usual starting dose of TE and TC is 150–200 mg IM every 2 weeks. After injection, testosterone levels reach supraphysiologic levels for a short period and decrease gradually over 2 weeks to the lower end of normal levels or below. These extreme rises and falls in testosterone concentrations lead to fluctuations in the patient's energy levels, mood, and libido. Shortening the dosing intervals and applying at lower doses may provide a decrease in fluctuations.

Testosterone ester combinations have been widely used for the treatment of male hypogonadism. The aim of this application is to reduce fluctuations in testosterone levels by combining short-acting and long-acting testosterones (e.g., TP + TE). However, this administration increases the initial testosterone peaks resulting in wider fluctuation.

The long-acting testosterone preparation TU is administered as an IM injection into the gluteus muscle at a dose of 1000 mg. The second dose is administered 6 weeks after the first application, and then the application is continued at intervals of 10–14 weeks. The pharmacokinetic profile of TU does not demonstrate the supraphysiologic testosterone peaks. TU provides the testosterone concentration within the normal ranges. After the TU injection, coughing may occur in some patients. Although the exact cause is not known, it is hypothesized to be related to fat droplet microembolism due to large volume of castor oil administration [17].

Transdermal Testosterone Formulations

Testosterone gels and solutions are available for the treatment of male hypogonadism. Different formulations are available in 1%, 1.62% and 2% solutions and gels of testosterone. 1% concentration forms as unit dose packets include 25 mg/2.5 g or 50 mg/5 g of testosterone and there is a multi-dose metered pump that provides 12.5 mg of testosterone per actuation. Also, 2% gel and solution forms is available in a metered-dose pump. For gels forms, a starting dose of once daily 50 mg in the morning is generally recommended. Based on the serum testosterone concentration, the dose can be increased to 100 mg in 25 mg increments. The common application areas of gel forms are shoulders, upper arm or abdomen. Patients should be advised to wash their hands and avoid contact with other people after applying the gel forms.

Another transdermal formulation is the administration of testosterone as patch. The patches include 2 or 4 mg testosterone. The recommended starting dose is 4 mg every night to the back, abdomen, upper arm or thighs. The administration sides should be rotated and should not be used again in 7 days. Testosterone should be measured 2 weeks after the initiation of treatment. The effectiveness of the transdermal patch is limited by lack of adherence or discontinuation, often due to skin reactions. Easy, non-invasive application and rapid reversal after removal and maintaining normal circadian rhythm of testosterone are the advantages of the patch application. However, the effectiveness of the patch application is often limited by lack of adherence or discontinuation due to skin reactions.

Transdermal formulations provide more physiologic testosterone concentration compared to parenteral formulations. The patch application maintains a normal circadian rhythm of testosterone and the gel formulations provide steady-state serum testosterone concentration.

Other Formulations

A transbuccal tablet which contains 30 mg testosterone is available for the treatment of male hypogonadism. With this application, testosterone is released from the buccal mucosa into the systemic circulation at a controlled and constant rate.

Another formulation is subcutaneous testosterone pellet. Testosterone pellets are implanted with a trocar into the subcutaneous fat tissue of the buttocks, lower abdominal wall or thigh under sterile conditions using a local anesthetic. Pellet extrusion, infection, and fibrosis are the main adverse events due to this formulation [18].

There is also a nasal testosterone gel application. The gel is applied to the nostrils using a metered dose pump applicator. The minimal transfer risk of gel to a partner is the advantage of the application. However, the administration of t.i.d. is inconvenient and the allergies and nasal or sinus pathologies may cause the trouble.

Monitoring

The adequacy of testosterone therapy is assessed by the clinical response and serum testosterone levels. Symptoms and signs of androgen deficiency should be assessed at 2 or 3 months after initiation of treatment or dose change. When the dose is stable, controls at 6–12 month intervals will be sufficient. The goal in testosterone treatment is to keep testosterone levels at mid-normal range [14].

Measurement time of serum testosterone may vary depending on the preparation used. In patients using TE or TC, serum testosterone concentration should be measured midway between the two injections. In patients using transdermal testosterone preparations, serum testosterone concentration can be measured at any time. However, it should not be forgotten that testosterone reaches its peak level in 6–8 h in patch applications and measurements should be made 8–10 h after patch application. Testosterone concentrations in gel applications can vary significantly. For this reason, it is useful to adjust the dose by measuring testosterone concentration at least twice [19]. In patients using buccal tablet, serum testosterone concentration can be measured at any time, preferably in the morning.

Testosterone and hematocrit levels should be measured at 3–6 and 12 months and annually after starting TRT. Serum prostate specific antigen (PSA) measurement and digital rectal examination should be performed 3–12 months after starting TRT.

Contraindications of TRT

Prostate Cancer

Testosterone therapy may stimulate the growth of androgen dependent malignancies. Therefore, TRT is contraindicated in patients with metastatic prostate cancer. Digital rectal examination and a serum PSA measurement should be performed in a patient older than 50 years of age (or has a history of prostate cancer in a first-degree relative) before the initiation of TRT. If a prostate nodule or an elevated PSA value (>4 or >3 ng/mL in a man of high risk) is detected, a urologic evaluation should be done.

Breast Cancer

Testosterone is aromatized to estradiol and may stimulate the growth of ER-positive breast cancer. Therefore, men who have breast cancer should not be treated with TRT. Before the initiation of TRT, a careful breast examination should be performed for suspicious masses.

Severe Lower Urinary Tract Symptoms

Lower urinary tract symptoms (LUTS) should be assessed by the International Prostate Symptom Score (IPSS) before the initiation of TRT. Severe LUST (IPSS score > 19) due to benign prostatic hyperplasia should be treated before the TRT.

Erythrocytosis

Testosterone therapy stimulates the erythropoiesis because of increased erythropoietin, bone marrow stimulation, and suppression of hepcidin. Therefore, hematocrit levels should be measured before the treatment. If the patient has high hematocrit levels (>54%), the etiology should be sought and treated before starting treatment.

Obstructive Sleep Apnea

In patients with severe and untreated sleep apnea, TRT may worsen the sleep-disordered breathing.

Uncontrolled Heart Failure

Testosterone therapy can cause fluid retention and therefore worsen the clinical situation in patients with uncontrolled heart failure.

Adverse Effects Associated with TRT

Prostate Cancer

Although TRT increases the prostate volume and the PSA levels, there is no evidence that testosterone treatment causes prostate carcinoma. However, the potential for testosterone stimulation of occult prostate carcinoma exists. On the other hand, TRT may stimulate the growth of androgen dependent cancers such as metastatic prostate cancer and breast cancer. Therefore, patients with these cancers should not be given testosterone. However, there is no clear evidence that testosterone therapy can stimulate the growth and progression of subclinical prostate cancer.

Before starting TRT, men with a history of prostate cancer or are at high risk for developing prostate cancer should be identified. Therefore, in men over age 50 years or 40 years with high risk for prostate cancer, serum PSA levels should be measured, and digital rectal examination should be performed before the initiation of treatment and 3 months and 1 year after the initiation of therapy. If a prostate nodule is detected, or if PSA levels increase by more than 1.4 ng/mL or exceed 4 ng/dL in 1-year period, the patient should be referred to the urology department.

Lower Urinary Tract Symptoms (LUTS)

TRT does not increase the risk of LUTS. However, it is not known that testosterone therapy worsens the LUTS in men who have severe LUTS at baseline [20, 21].

Erythrocytosis

A testosterone-induced increase in hematocrit can occur, although clinically significant polycythemia is rare, unless the drug is being abused. This increase is more frequent in older men than in young men [22]. In hematocrit values exceeding 54%, testosterone therapy should be discontinued, the dose should be reduced or a different formulation should be used. Testosterone therapy can be restarted at lower doses when hematocrit levels return to normal ranges. In some cases, phlebotomy can also be used to lower hematocrit levels

Cardiovascular Effects

The data about the effect of TRT on the major adverse cardiovascular events (MACE) are inconsistent. Several randomized controlled studies and meta-analyses showed a relationship between TRT and MACE [23–29]. However, there are several methodological problems such as heterogeneity of eligibility criteria, dosing, formulations and duration of testosterone therapy and the inability to prespecify and judge cardiovascular outcomes in these studies. As a result, studies fail to show a causal relationship between testosterone therapy and cardiovascular events.

Venous Thromboembolism

The relationship between testosterone therapy and venous thromboembolism are also not clear. There very few venous thromboembolism cases in the RCTs to show this relationship [19, 30]. Some case reports have suggested that the risk of VTE may be increased within the first 6 months after starting TRT, particularly in the presence of thrombophilia [31, 32].

Reversible Infertility

Reversible infertility is a common adverse effect due to negative feedback resulting in a low FSH and a lack of stimulation of spermatogenesis. It may last 12 months to regain.

baseline sperm concentration after discontinuing TRT. Therefore, it may not be appropriate to start testosterone therapy, especially in patients with hypogonadotropic hypogonadism who have a fertility plan within 6–12 months. Men who desire fertility should be treated with human chorionic gonadotropin which acts like LH to stimulate endogenous testosterone production but not suppressing spermatogenesis.

Acne and Skin Irritation

Acne may occur during the testosterone replacement. However, topical, or systemic acne medications are not needed in general. Skin irritation is quite common with the testosterone patch and is one of its major disadvantages.

References

1. Matsumoto AM. Hormonal therapy of male hypogonadism. Endocrinol Metab Clin N Am. 1994;23:857–75.
2. Giagulli VA, Triggiani V, Carbone MD, Corona G, Tafaro E, Licchelli B, Guastamacchia E. The role of long-acting parenteral testosterone undecanoate compound in the induction of secondary sexual characteristics in males with hypogonadotropic hypo-gonadism. J Sex Med. 2011;8(12):3471–8.
3. Brock G, Heiselman D, Maggi M, Kim SW, Rodríguez Vallejo JM, Behre HM, McGettigan J, Dowsett SA, Hayes RP, Knorr J, Ni X, Kinchen K. Effect of testosterone solution 2% on testosterone concentration, sex drive and energy in hypogonadal men: results of a placebo controlled study. J Urol. 2016;195(3):699–705.
4. Cunningham GR, Stephens-Shields AJ, Rosen RC, Wang C, Bhasin S, Matsumoto AM, Parsons JK, Gill TM, Molitch ME, Farrar JT, Cella D, Barrett-Connor E, Cauley JA, Cifelli

D, Crandall JP, Ensrud KE, Gallagher L, Zeldow B, Lewis CE, Pahor M, Swerdloff RS, Hou X, Anton S, Basaria S, Diem SJ, Tabatabaie V, Ellenberg SS, Snyder PJ. Testosterone treatment and sexual function in older men with low testosterone levels. J Clin Endocrinol Metab. 2016;101(8):3096–104.

5. Bhasin S, Storer TW, Berman N, Yarasheski KE, Clevenger B, Phillips J, Lee WP, Bunnell TJ, Casaburi R. Testosterone replacement increases fat-free mass and muscle size in hypogonadal men. J Clin Endocrinol Metab. 1997;82(2):407–13.

6. Woodhouse LJ, Gupta N, Bhasin M, Singh AB, Ross R, Phillips J, Bhasin S. Dose-dependent effects of testosterone on regional adipose tissue distribution in healthy young men. J Clin Endocrinol Metab. 2004;89(2):718–26.

7. Pope HG Jr, Amiaz R, Brennan BP, Orr G, Weiser M, Kelly JF, Kanayama G, Siegel A, Hudson JI, Seidman SN. Parallel-group placebo-controlled trial of testosterone gel in men with major depressive disorder displaying an incomplete response to standard antidepressant treatment. J Clin Psychopharmacol. 2010;30(2):126–34.

8. Snyder PJ, Kopperdahl DL, Stephens-Shields AJ, Ellenberg SS, Cauley JA, Ensrud KE, Lewis CE, Barrett-Connor E, Schwartz AV, Lee DC, Bhasin S, Cunningham GR, Gill TM, Matsumoto AM, Swerdloff RS, Basaria S, Diem SJ, Wang C, Hou X, Cifelli D, Dougar D, Zeldow B, Bauer DC, Keaveny TM. Effect of testosterone treatment on volumetric bone density and strength in older men with low testosterone: a controlled clinical trial. JAMA Intern Med. 2017;177(4):471–9.

9. Aminorroaya A, Kelleher S, Conway AJ, Ly LP, Handelsman DJ. Adequacy of androgen replacement influences bone density re- sponse to testosterone in androgen-deficient men. Eur J Endocrinol. 2005;152(6):881–6.

10. Snyder PJ, Bhasin S, Cunningham GR, Matsumoto AM, Stephens-Shields AJ, Cauley JA, Gill TM, Barrett-Connor E, Swerdloff RS, Wang C, Ensrud KE, Lewis CE, Farrar JT, Cella D, Rosen RC, Pahor M, Crandall JP, Molitch ME, Cifelli D, Dougar D, Fluharty L, Resnick SM, Storer TW, Anton S, Basaria S, Diem SJ, Hou X, Mohler ER 3rd, Parsons JK, Wenger NK, Zeldow B, Landis JR, Ellenberg SS, Testosterone Trials Investigators. Effects of testosterone treatment in older men. N Engl J Med. 2016;374(7):611–24.

11. Wang C, Nieschlag E, Swerdloff R, Behre HM, Hellstrom WJ, Gooren LJ, et al. Investigation, treatment and monitoring of late-onset hypogonadism in males: ISA, ISSAM, EAU, EAA and ASA recommendations. Eur J Endocrinol. 2008;159:507–14.

12. Isidori AM, Balercia G, Calogero AE, Corona G, Ferlin A, Francavilla S, et al. Outcomes of androgen replacement therapy in adult male hypogonadism: recommendations from the Italian society of endocrinology. J Endocrinol Investig. 2015;38:103–12.

13. Dimopoulou C, Ceausu I, Depypere H, Lambrinoudaki I, Mueck A, Pérez-López FR, et al. EMAS position statement: testosterone replacement therapy in the aging male. Maturitas. 2016;84:94–9.

14. Bhasin S, Brito JP, Cunningham GR, Hayes FJ, Hodis HN, Matsumoto AM, Snyder PJ, Swerdloff RS, Wu FC, Yialamas MA. Testosterone therapy in men with hypogonadism: an endocrine society clinical practice guideline. J Clin Endocrinol Metab. 2018;103(5):1715–44.

15. Schulte-Beerbuhl M, Nieschlag E. Comparison of testosterone, dihydrotestosterone, luteinizing hormone, and follicle-stimulating hormone in serum after injection of testosterone enanthate of testosterone cypionate. Fertil Steril. 1980;33:201–3.

16. Schurmeyer T, Nieschlag E. Comparative pharmacokinetics of testosterone enanthate and testosterone cyclohexanecarboxylate as assessed by serum and salivary testosterone levels in normal men. Int J Androl. 1984;7:181–7.

17. Alexander WP, Yiqun H, Jeffrey DF. Occurrence of pulmonary oil microembolism after testosterone undecanoate injection: a postmarketing safety analysis. Sex Med. 2020;8(2):237–42.

18. Seftel A. Testosterone replacement therapy for male hypogonadism: part III. Pharmacologic and clinical profiles, monitoring, safety issues, and potential future agents. Int J Impot Res. 2007;19(1):2.

19. Swerdloff RS, Pak Y, Wang C, Liu PY, Bhasin S, Gill TM, Matsumoto AM, Pahor M, Surampudi P, Snyder PJ. Serum testosterone (T) level variability in T gel-treated older hypogonadal men: treatment monitoring implications. J Clin Endocrinol Metab. 2015;100(9):3280–7.

20. Debruyne FMJ, Behre HM, Roehrborn CG, Maggi M, Wu FCW, Schröder FH, Jones TH, Porst H, Hackett G, Wheaton OA, Martin Morales A, Meuleman E, Cunningham GR, Divan HA, Rosen RC, RHYME Investigators. Testosterone treatment is not associated with increased risk of prostate cancer or worsening of lower urinary tract symptoms: prostate health outcomes in the Registry of Hypogonadism in Men. BJU Int. 2017;119(2):216–24.

21. Kathrins M, Doersch K, Nimeh T, Canto A, Niederberger C, Seftel A. The relationship between testosterone-replacement therapy and lower urinary tract symptoms: a systematic review. Urology. 2016;88:22–32.

22. Coviello AD, Kaplan B, Lakshman KM, Chen T, Singh AB, Bhasin S. Effects of graded doses of testosterone on erythropoiesis in healthy young and older men. J Clin Endocrinol Metab. 2008;93(3):914–9.

23. Haddad RM, Kennedy CC, Caples SM, Tracz MJ, Boloña ER, Sideras K, Uraga MV, Erwin PJ, Montori VM. Testosterone and cardiovascular risk in men: a systematic review and meta-analysis of randomized placebo-controlled trials. Mayo Clin Proc. 2007;82(1):29–39.

24. Srinivas-Shankar U, Roberts SA, Connolly MJ, O'Connell MDL, Adams JE, Oldham JA, Wu FCW. Effects of testosterone on muscle strength, physical function, body composition, and quality of life in intermediate-frail and frail elderly men: a randomized, double-blind, placebo-controlled study. J Clin Endocrinol Metab. 2010;95(2):639–50.

25. Basaria S, Coviello AD, Travison TG, Storer TW, Farwell WR, Jette AM, Eder R, Tennstedt S, Ulloor J, Zhang A, Choong K, Lakshman KM, Mazer NA, Miciek R, Krasnoff J, Elmi A, Knapp PE, Brooks B, Appleman E, Aggarwal S, Bhasin G, Hede-Brierley L, Bhatia A, Collins L, LeBrasseur N, Fiore LD, Bhasin S. Adverse events associated with testosterone administration. N Engl J Med. 2010;363(2):109–22.

26. Nair KS, Rizza RA, O'Brien P, Dhatariya K, Short KR, Nehra A, Vittone JL, Klee GG, Basu A, Basu R, Cobelli C, Toffolo G, Dalla Man C, Tindall DJ, Melton LJ III, Smith GE, Khosla S, Jensen MD. DHEA in elderly women and DHEA or testosterone in elderly men. N Engl J Med. 2006;355(16):1647–59.

27. Emmelot-Vonk MH, Verhaar HJJ, Nakhai Pour HR, Aleman A, Lock TMTW, Bosch JLHR, Grobbee DE, van der Schouw YT. Effect of testosterone supplementation on functional mobility, cognition, and other parameters in older men: a randomized controlledtrial. JAMA. 2008;299(1):39–52.

28. Borst SE, Shuster JJ, Zou B, Ye F, Jia H, Wokhlu A, Yarrow JF. Cardiovascular risks and elevation of serum DHT vary by route of testosterone administration: a systematic review and meta-analysis. BMC Med. 2014;12(1):211–5.

29. Alexander GC, Iyer G, Lucas E, Lin D, Singh S. Cardiovascular risks of exogenous testosterone use among men: a systematic review and meta-analysis. Am J Med. 2017;130(3):293–305.

30. Baillargeon J, Urban RJ, Morgentaler A, Glueck CJ, Baillargeon G, Sharma G, Kuo Y-F. Risk of venous thromboembolism in men receiving testosterone therapy. Mayo Clin Proc. 2015;90(8):1038–45.

31. Martinez C, Suissa S, Rietbrock S, Katholing A, Freedman B, Cohen AT, Handelsman DJ. Testosterone treatment and risk of venous thromboembolism: population based case-control study. BMJ. 2016;355:i5968.

32. Glueck CJ, Prince M, Pate N, Pate J, Shah P, Mehta N, Wang P. Thrombophilia in 67 patients with thrombotic events after starting testosterone therapy. Clin Appl Thromb Hemost. 2016;22(6):548–53.

Biochemical Analysis and Laboratory Tests in Andrology and Sexual Medicine

21

Ege Mert Ozgurtas and Taner Ozgurtas

Abstract

Andrology is the field of medicine that deals with matter affecting the male reproductive system. Laboratory tests are an essential part of andrology and are commonly resorted to by physicians as they yield important data for the patients' evaluation process. There are cases where laboratory tests are significant for therapy and monitoring.

The most called-upon test in an andrology laboratory is semen analysis. With infertility affecting up to 13–15% of couples worldwide, it is not surprising that semen analysis is such a common test. In most infertility cases, the medical approach is to rule out the female-factor infertility with a detailed history and clinical examination. Once that is ruled out a semen analysis is in order for both the future management and treatment process.

The testes are responsible for producing the spermatozoa within the seminiferous tubules and sexual hormones in the interstitial cells. Any process that affects sperm production and quality is potentially harmful to male fertility. Therefore a semen analysis, which provides data from which a prognosis of fertility or the diagnosis of infertility can be extrapolated, is the primary laboratory test.

Hormonal evaluation is also a very important part of any andrology laboratory as hormones - testosterone in particular - regulate many aspects of male reproduction. Measuring serum total testosterone levels may be very helpful for the diagnosis of conditions related to male reproduction such as delayed puberty and hypogonadism, which has many clinical manifestations like sexual dysfunctions,

E. M. Ozgurtas
Third Medical Student, Baskent University Faculty of Medicine, Ankara, Turkey
e-mail: taner.ozgurtas@sbu.edu.tr

T. Ozgurtas (✉)
Biochemistry Department, Gulhane School of Medicine, University of Health Science, Ankara, Turkey

S. Sarikaya et al. (eds.), *Andrology and Sexual Medicine*, Management of Urology, https://doi.org/10.1007/978-3-031-12049-7_21

reduced libido, gynecomastia and such. Many hypogonadism patients with low serum total testosterone levels are treated with testosterone therapy but in some cases there might be need for further evaluation of different hormones.

Andrology is the field of medicine that deals with matter affecting the male reproductive system. The earliest use of this term appeared in 1891 in the Journal of American Medical Association when it reported on the formation of American Andrological Association [1].

In general, the female partner is evaluated by a gynecologist who orders a semen analysis for the male. If the semen analysis results are abnormal, then male infertility is suspected [2].

Male infertility is directly or indirectly responsible for 60% of cases involving reproductive-age couples with fertility-related issues. Nevertheless, the evaluation of male infertility is often underestimated or postponed [2]. In recent years, a decline in semen quality across Africa, Europe, North America, and Asia has been reported [3, 4]. This seems to suggest that male infertility is a growing global problem. This diagnostic procedure may not always identify the cause of male infertility as 25% of infertility cases worldwide are considered as unexplained [5].

Semen analysis is a basic test for evaluating male fertility potential, as it plays an essential role in driving the future management and treatment of infertility in couples. Manual semen analysis includes the evaluation of both macroscopic and microscopic parameters [6].

Manual Semen Analysis

The patient should be provided with clear instructions for collecting the semen sample [7, 8]. The initial fraction of the ejaculate contains the highest concentration of sperm, and so if any fraction is lost, this must be duly recorded. After 2–7 days of abstinence, the entire semen sample is collected in a sterile cup. After collection, the sample is placed in an incubator at 37 °C for 30–60 min to allow liquefaction before being analyzed [6].

Qualitative and Quantitative Test of Semen

A semen examination should be performed immediately after liquefaction and no longer than 60 min after ejaculation [7]. A manual semen analysis includes macroscopic and microscopic evaluation. It is important to mix the sample well using a vortex mixer before any examination, to resuspend the cellular fraction.

1. Macroscopic examination
   The ejaculate consists of secretions from seminal vesicle (70%), prostate (25%), epididymis, vas deferens, bulbourethral, and urethral glands (~5% in

total) and sperm (~5%). The macroscopic evaluation includes liquefaction, viscosity, appearance of the ejaculate, volume, and pH [5, 9].
2. Microscopic examination

The sample is examined under a phase-contrast microscope. Microscopic evaluation allows the calculation of sperm concentration, total sperm count and sperm motility. The presence of round cells, white blood cells, and sperm agglutination are also examined during microscopic evaluation [5, 9].

Significance of Quality Control in an Andrology Laboratory

The importance of QC in semen analysis was introduced for the first time in the fourth edition of the WHO manual [10]. Quality indicators are the measures of QC to monitor the accuracy and precision of a particular test or procedure and to identify any out-of-range values. Quality indicators in the pre-analytical phase are:

- specimen identification,
- test order accuracy,
- time to analysis,
- patient's waiting time for the appointment,
- waiting times in the laboratory.

QC in the analytical phase includes instrument function checks, instrument calibration and maintenance checks. Competency and proficiency of testing personnel is an important component of the analytical QC [6].

To ensure quality in the post-analytical phase, the laboratory personnel should double check that all results on the worksheet are correctly reported both manually and in the electronic medical records.

There are two equally important ways of doing a quality check in the laboratory:

1. Internal quality control (IQC): Implementing IQC at all stages requires checking all the critical points during the work routine such as temperature control, equipment maintenance and the technical performance by individual technologists.
2. External quality control (EQC): it is defined as a method to check the laboratory performance by an external agency, as a tool to assess the accuracy and detect systematic variations [7] QC samples are used to monitor technicians and trainees, and to validate new equipment, supplies and procedures.

Endocrine Evaluation

Endocrine evaluation is suggested when the following scenarios are present [11]:

- a sperm concentration, <10 million/mL;
- erectile dysfunction;

- hypospermia (volume <1 mL) or
- signs and symptoms of endocrinopathies or hypogonadism.

A Sperm Concentration < 10 Million/mL

Azoospermia (a-, without + − zoo– » Greek zôion, animal + − spermia– » Greek sperma, sperm/seed) is defined by the absence of sperm in the ejaculate. According to global estimates, 1 out of 100 men at reproductive age and up to 10% of men with infertility are azoospermic [12, 13]. The differential diagnosis between obstructive (OA) and nonobstructive azoospermia (NOA) is the first step in the clinical management of azoospermic patients with infertility. It affects patient management and treatment outcomes [13].

Each having very different etiologies and treatments. NOA (which includes primary testicular failure and secondary testicular failure) is differentiated from OA by clinical assessment (testis consistency/volume), laboratory testing (FSH), and genetic testing (karyotype, Y chromosome microdeletion, or specific genetic testing for hypogonadotropic hypogonadism) [14].

The severe spermatogenic deficiency observed in NOA patients is often a consequence of primary testicular failure affecting mainly spermatogenic cells (spermatogenic failure (STF)) or related to a dysfunction of the hypothalamus-pituitary-gonadal axis (hypogonadotropic hypogonadism (HH)). The differential diagnosis between STF and HH is also essential because the former is linked with severe and untreatable conditions, whereas the latter can be effectively treated with gonadotropin therapy [9, 15].

OA is typically accompanied by preservation of normal exocrine and endocrine function, and normal spermatogenesis in the testis [16]. OA is the consequence of physical blockage to the male excurrent ductal system. NOA includes nonobstructive causes of azoospermia, including toxic exposures or abnormal testicular development [17]. NOA results from either primary testicular failure (elevated LH, FSH, small testes affecting up to 10% of men presenting with infertility), secondary testicular failure (congenital hypogonadotropic hypogonadism with decreased LH and FSH, small testes) [18].

OA Laboratory values, most significantly FSH, is normal in OA and usually elevated in NOA due to lack of normal negative feedback on the hypothalamus and pituitary by inhibin B and testosterone [14].

NOA includes primary testicular failure (elevated LH, FSH, small testes affecting up to 10% of men presenting with infertility), secondary testicular failure (congenital hypogonadotropic hypogonadism with decreased LH and FSH, small testes), and those with an incomplete or ambiguous picture of testicular failure [14].

Erectile Dysfunction

In men, erectile dysfunction (ED) and ejaculatory dysfunction are the most reported sexual dysfunction. Hormones can regulate many aspects of male reproduction. Endocrine disorders, including hypogonadism, thyroid diseases and hyperprolactinaemia, has been implicated in the pathogenesis of ED [19]. Testosterone is the major hormonal regulator of penile development and physiology, and affects both the central and peripheral levels of the ejaculatory process [20].

Aromatase is responsible for the conversion of testosterone to estrogen and localized abundantly in the male reproductive system. Levels of estradiol have been demonstrated to be correlated with the incidence and severity of ED [21].

Although high estradiol milieu may adversely affect male sexual function, a moderate estradiol value is beneficial. Men with decreased estradiol levels reported low libido and sexual activity, which could be improved by estrogen administration [22]. Estrogen can influence mood, mental state, cognition, and emotion through an interaction with serotonin receptors [23]. In men with aromatase deficiency, estrogen treatment enhances libido, sexual activity, and erotic fantasies [24]. In addition, sympathetic excitation might be modulated by estrogen, whereas parasympathetic sexual excitation might be dominated by testosterone [25].

Signs and Symptoms of Endocrinopathies or Hypogonadism

The 2010 Endocrine Society guideline suggests using a repeated measurement of morning Total Testosterone (TT) to confirm the diagnosis of hypogonadism in symptomatic men. In men with borderline TT levels and expected alterations in sex hormone binding globülin (SHBG) levels (such as in older men, obesity, or thyroid disorders), measuring Free Testosterone (FT) concentrations [26]. Currently, directly measuring FT remains technically challenging and expensive [26, 27]. Instead of equilibrium dialysis, calculated FT (cFT) is commonly used, with the most commonly used calculation (the Vermeulen formula) being based on the law of mass action [26, 28].

Hormonal Evaluation

The minimal evaluation includes the assessment of serum follicle-stimulating hormone (FSH) and total testosterone (TT) levels, which reflect germ cell epithelium and Leydig cell status, respectively. Follicle-stimulating hormone (FSH) and testosterone are the essential hormones driving spermatogenesis [15, 29]. Testosterone is produced by the Leydig cells under luteinizing hormone (LH) stimulation. Adequate levels of intratesticular testosterone are critical for sperm maturation [30]. By contrast, FSH is mainly responsible for increasing sperm production, and it collaborates with intratesticular testosterone to promote cell proliferation [31]. In general, there is an inverse relationship between FSH levels and spermatogonia quantity [32, 33]. When spermatogonia number is absent or remarkably reduced, FSH levels increase; when spermatogonia number is normal, FSH levels are within normal ranges [34].

The initial test for diagnosing androgen deficiency is serum total testosterone [35]. These signs and symptoms can be categorized as specific (reduced libido, decreased spontaneous erections, gynecomastia, loss of body hair, testicular atrophy, infertility, and hot flushes), or nonspecific (decreased energy, decreased motivation, depressed mood, sleepiness, reduced muscle bulk, increased body fat, increased body mass index, and diminished physical performance) [26].

TT assays are used in males with the primary aim of confirming the clinical diagnosis of hypogonadism or delayed puberty, and in women to confirm the diagnosis and cause of hyperandrogenism. In both sexes, testosterone circulates in plasma largely bound to proteins, only 1–2% being unbound (free testosterone), 25–50% being specifically bound with high affinity to the sex hormone binding globulin (SHBG) and 50–75% being albumin-bound. Most of the weakly albumin-bound testosterone dissociates (half-dissociation time 51 s) [36] whereas the SHBG—testosterone complex (half-dissociation time 420 s) remains intact [37]. It is generally referred to as bioavailable testosterone, is biologically active (bioavailable testosterone = free testosterone + albumin-bound testosterone) via interaction with the androgen receptor [38, 39].

Recommendations: Routine Measurement of TT

1. Men presenting with the following conditions should be screened for low TT:
    (a) Sexual symptoms including decreased libido, ED, and decreased frequency of morning erections [LoE = 1, Grade = B].
    (b) Clinical conditions associated with insulin resistance (obesity, type 2 diabetes, and MetS) should be screened for TD because it is often comorbid [LoE = 2, Grade = B].
    (c) Infertility [LoE = 2, Grade = B] (this is discussed in more detail in subsequent section).
    (d) Osteoporosis and height loss or low trauma fractures likely indicate TD because asymptomatic low T can be a negative contributor and can be corrected with TTh [LoE = 1, Grade = B].
    (e) HIV-associated weight loss [LoE = 2, Grade = B].
    (f) Long-acting opioid use [LoE = 2, Grade = B].
    (g) High-dose glucocorticoid use [LoE = 1, Grade = B] [40]

Measuring Serum TT Levels

It has been recommended that blood samples for diagnosing TD should be obtained in the morning, usually from 08:00 to 11:00 AM, because of the diurnal rhythm of serum TT in which values are highest in the early morning [26]. A single low TT value should always be confirmed by a second measurement because a substantial number of men have normal values on repeat testing [41]. Although measurement of serum TT is the first step in the diagnosis of androgen deficiency, TT concentrations may not be reliable in patients with conditions that result in alterations in serum SHBG levels. The low SHBG levels lead to low serum TT levels in the absence of hypothalamic, pituitary, or testicular disease. The next step in this patient's evaluation is measurement of FT. In these cases, measurement of FT is helpful.

It is important to note that men presenting with low serum TT levels (T < 150 ng/dL) and increased prolactin levels or suppressed luteinizing hormone (LH) and follicle-stimulating hormone levels should undergo pituitary magnetic resonance imaging rule out a pituitary adenoma [26].

Methods to Measure Serum TT

Total Testosterone (TT)
The main screening test for hypogonadism is the measurement of serum TT. The immunoassays—performed by most laboratories in the everyday clinical setting— are relatively inexpensive and readily available.

Free Testosterone (FT)
TT circulates in the blood mainly bound to proteins, especially to SHBG. Because unbound T readily crosses the cell membrane and bound T does not, many experts consider FT and bioavailable T to be more accurate indicators of androgen status than TT [42]. The commercial radioimmunoassays are capable of distinguishing eugonadal from hypogonadal males, at very low levels, as observed in women and children, methods lack accuracy and precision. Reliable methods involving LC–MSMS for the direct measurement of free testosterone [43].

Testosterone deficiency (TD), also known as hypogonadism. TD varies from various defects in virilization to an almost complete female phenotype. Sexual dysfunctions are a prominent symptom of TD and often the presenting symptom [44–46]. Low sexual desire and decreased nocturnal and morning erections are clearly associated with TD. Several studies have demonstrated that the T threshold at 320 ng/dL (11 nmol/L) for the decrease of morning erections and 245 ng/dL (8.5 nmol/L) for erectile dysfunction (ED) [44]. TT levels below 200 ng/dL (7 nmol/L) are in most cases associated with impairment of sexual function and nocturnal erections, and the effect of TT seems to reach its maximum benefit from levels of at least 350 to 400 ng/dL (12–16 nmol/L) [47]. There seems to be a gray zone, from 200 to 400 ng/dL [41].

Recommendations: Laboratory Diagnosis of TD

The following investigations are recommended in patients with suspected TD:

1. Steps for diagnosis of TD
   Step 1. Morning determination of TT [LoE = 2, Grade = A].
   Step 2. In case of a low level (defined as TT < 12 nmol/L or 350 ng/dL), we recommend: Repeating the TT measurement [LoE ¼ 3, Grade ¼ A]. Measuring with serum LH and prolactin measurements [LoE = 1, Grade = B].
2. In individuals with clinically suspected TD, SHBG levels should be assessed if TT is low to normal or borderline, especially in obese or older men [LoE = 2, Grade = C] [40].

TT levels below the normal range are common in men, especially after 50 years of age. However, low TT levels are not associated with symptoms of TD in every case.

Osteoporosis low TT can be found in up to 20% of men with symptomatic vertebral fractures and 50% of elderly men with hip fractures [48]. TT effects on men's bone are mostly linked to its aromatization into estradiol (E2) [49]. In a cohort study of men at least 65 years old, the major predictor of non-vertebral fracture risk was a low bioavailable E2 followed by the association of low bioavailable TT with high SHBG levels [40].

Late-onset hypogonadism could be clinically defined by the presence of the three preceding sexual symptoms associated with a TT level lower than 320 ng/dL (11 nmol/L) and an FT level lower than 6.4 ng/dL (6.4 pg/mL, 220 pmol/L).

Opioids according to a recent meta-analysis of 17 studies, TT levels are suppressed in men with regular opioid use, regardless of opioid type, including methadone and tramadol [49]. Acute administration of dexamethasone has been shown to significantly decrease T in serum and at the muscle level [40].

TD can result from:

- Decreased testicular synthesis of T owing to impaired Leydig cell function (hypergonadotropic hypogonadism; primary hypogonadism)
- Decreased testicular synthesis of T owing to inadequate gonadotropic stimulation of Leydig cells (hypogonadotropic hypogonadism; secondary hypogonadism)

In addition, TD symptoms, in the presence of a TT level within the reference range, can result from (i) impaired androgen receptor function, (ii) androgen receptor blockade, and (iii) increased SHBG, resulting in a decrease in free T (FT) [40].

TD: Medical Approach and Monitoring

1. The laboratory diagnosis of hypogonadism should include two morning TT levels. In individuals with moderately low or borderline TT, SHBG levels should be assessed (especially in obese or older men)
2. Symptomatic men with TT lower than 12 nmol/L or 350 ng/dL should be treated with TTh.
3. There is no compelling evidence that T treatment causes PCa or PCa progression.
4. TTh should not be used in men who are trying to produce a pregnancy.
5. Current commercially available preparations of T (with the exception of the 17a-alkylated ones) are safe and effective.
6. Selective estrogen receptor modulators (SERMs) and hCG can be safely used to increase endogenous T levels in hypogonadal men [40].

There are two primary widely considered indications for Testosterone therapy (TTh) in adult men with low TT circulating levels;

- After hypophysectomy
- Signs or symptoms of TD associated with low circulating TT values [40].

TTh and Male Fertility

TTh can lead to impaired spermatogenesis because T is a natural contraceptive. T inhibits gonadotropin-releasing hormone and gonadotropin secretion and thus can cause lead to hypospermatogenesis [50]. Complete inhibition of intratesticular T can result in azoospermia [51, 52]. Success rates of recovering spermatogenesis after TTh have been shown with human chorionic gonadotropin (hCG) alone or in combination with human menopausal gonadotropin [53].

Alternatives to TTH

A more appropriate approach in many young men with the diagnosis of hypogonadism is to increase their own endogenous T production.

Selective Estrogen Receptor Modulators (SERMs)

SERMs inhibit estrogen feedback to the hypothalamus, which in turn results in an increase in the gonadotropins follicle-stimulating hormone and LH. Clomiphene citrate is a SERM that is commonly used off-label in men to increase endogenous T levels.

Aromatase Inhibitors Aromatase inhibitors inhibit the conversion from T to E2. Examples of aromatase inhibitors include anastrozole, testolactone, and letrozole.

Human Chorionic Gonadotropin hCG injections have been shown to increase endogenous serum T levels [40].

Adverse Events and Monitoring with TTH

Adverse effects appear to be particularly significant in elderly patients and are often dependent on the method of TTh. Reported adverse effects include [40]:

- Erythrocytosis
- Gynecomastia
- Hepatotoxicity (primarily with oral methylated formulations)
- Acne or oily skin
- Impaired sperm production and fertility
- Edema

Follow-Up and Monitoring

Patients should be evaluated at 3 months after initiation of TTh and then every 6–12 months thereafter to assess serum T levels, symptomatic improvement, PSA and digital rectal exam changes, and changes in hematocrit [40].

Most of the reported side effects of TTh had occurred in subjects with high baseline serum TT. This has led to an FDA warning allowing the use of T only in cases of confirmed low T levels and only in "men with disorders of the testicles, pituitary gland or brain that cause hypogonadism", as to avoid "attempts to relieve symptoms in men who have low T for no apparent reason other than aging" [54].

Other Hormones

Symptoms of hypogonadism are often reported by subjects with normal serum testosterone (T) levels. T is irreversibly converted to dihydro-T (DHT) by the microsomal enzyme 5α-reductase, which exists in three isoforms present in multiple tissues of the male body. DHT can be associated with symptoms of hypogonadism in biochemically eugonadal men.

Serum DHT measurement might be helpful once the diagnosis of hypogonadism has been ruled out but should not be routinely included in the primary diagnostic process [55].

Compared to DHT, T has a twofold lower affinity to the androgen receptor (AR) and a fivefold faster dissociation rate [56], which is largely compensated by significantly higher serum concentrations.

If the testosterone level is low, a second collection is recommended along with free testosterone, LH and prolactin measurements. While T is secreted under the direct stimulus of pituitary LH, in turn secreted following hypothalamic GnRH stimulus. Highly elevated FSH and LH levels, when associated with low-normal or below normal testosterone levels, suggest diffuse testicular failure and may have either a congenital (e.g., Klinefelter syndrome) or acquired cause. Concomitant low levels of FSH and LH may implicate hypogonadotropic hypogonadism (HH). This condition may be congenital or secondary to a prolactin-producing pituitary tumor [2]. Low FSH levels (e.g., < 1.5 mIU/mL), combined with low LH (e.g., < 1.5 mIU/mL), and low testosterone levels (e.g., < 300 ng/dL) indicate primary or secondary HH [15, 29]. Typically, patients with NOA-STF present with elevated FSH (>7.6 mIU/mL) and low testosterone (<300 ng/dL) levels, whereas those with OA show normal FSH and testosterone levels. Other hormones can also be assessed, including inhibin B, prolactin, estradiol, 17-hydroxyprogesterone, and sex hormone-binding globulin (SHBG) [29]. Inhibin-B levels reflect Sertoli cell integrity and spermatogenesis status [57].

Serum estradiol levels should be determined in patients presenting with gynecomastia. Infertile patients with a testosterone to estradiol ratio less than 10 can harbor significant but reversible seminal alterations [58].

Serum prolactin (PRL) levels should be determined in infertile men with a complaint of concomitant sexual dysfunction or when there is clinical or laboratory evidence of pituitary disease; however, hyperprolactinemia is rarely a cause of infertility in healthy men [59].

PRL has been primarily shown to regulate lactation but, subsequently, it was demonstrated to play a role in over 300 biological functions [60]. On the other hand, dopamine is the major supervisor of sexual function, playing a prevalently stimulatory role on desire, arousal, and orgasm [61, 62]. PRL may potentially represent a peripheral marker of orgasm. Chronic hyperprolactinemia acting on both motivational and instinctive levels as well as an inhibitory effect on gonadal function either in male or females [63, 64]. Certainly, sexual dysfunction, mainly characterized by decreased libido and/or erectile dysfunction (ED) represents the most common initial clinical presentation of men with hyperprolactinemia [65].

This review highlights the fundamental role of andrology laboratory for both diagnostic and therapeutic purposes.

References

1. The Chicago Medical Record, between 1891 and 1927, a crucial period in the development of the city's medical community.
2. Esteves SC, Miyaoka R, Agarwal A. An update on the clinical assessment of the infertile male. Clinics (Sao Paulo). 2011;66(4):691–700.
3. Dissanayake DMIH, Keerthirathna WLR, Peiris LDC. Male infertility problem: a contemporary review on present status and future perspective. Gend Genome. 2019;3:247028971986824.
4. Agarwal A, Mulgund A, Hamada A, Chyatte MR. A unique view on male infertility around the globe. Reprod Biol Endocrinol. 2015;13:37.
5. Khatun A, Rahman MS, Pang MG. Clinical assessment of the male fertility. Obstet Gynecol Sci. 2018;61:179–91.
6. Agarwal A, Sharma R, Gupta S, Finelli R, Parekh N, MKP S, Pompeu CP, Madani S, Belo A, Darbandi M, Singh N, Darbandi S, Covarrubias S, Sadeghi R, Arafa M, Majzoub A, Caraballo M, Giroski A, McNulty K, Durairajanayagam D, Henkel R. Standardized laboratory procedures, quality control and quality assurance are key requirements for accurate semen analysis in the evaluation of infertile male. World J Mens Health. 2022;40(1):52–65.
7. World Health Organisation. WHO laboratory manual for the examination and processing of human semen. 5th ed. Geneva: WHO; 2010.
8. Baskaran S, Finelli R, Agarwal A, Henkel R. Diagnostic value of routine semen analysis in clinical andrology. Andrologia. 2021;53:e13614.
9. World Health Organisation. WHO laboratory manual for the examination of human semen and sperm-cervical mucus interaction. 4th ed. Cambridge: Cambridge University Press; 1999.
10. Sokol RZ, Swerdloff RS. Endocrine evaluation. In: Lipshultz LI, Howards SS, editors. Infertility in the male. 3rd ed. New York: Churchill Livingstone; 1997. p. 210–8.
11. Cocuzza M, Alvarenga C, Pagani R. The epidemiology and etiology of azoospermia. Clinics. 2013;68(Suppl. 1):15–26.
12. Olesen IA, Andersson AM, Aksglaede L, Skakkebaek NE, Rajpert-de Meyts E, Joergensen N, Juul A. Clinical, genetic, biochemical, and testicular biopsy findings among 1213 men evaluated for infertility. Fertil Steril. 2017;107(1):74–82.
13. Wosnitzer M, Goldstein M, Hardy MP. Review of azoospermia. Spermatogenesis. 2014;4:e28218.
14. Esteves SC. Clinical management of infertile men with nonobstructive azoospermia. Asian J Androl. 2015;17:459–70.
15. Fraietta R, Zylbersteijn DS, Esteves SC. Hypogonadotropic hypogonadism revisited. Clinics. 2013;68(Suppl. 1):81–8.
16. Practice Committee of American Society for Reproductive Medicine in Collaboration with Society for Male Reproduction and Urology. The management of infertility due to obstructive azoospermia. Fertil Steril. 2008;90(Suppl):S121–4.
17. Jarow JP, Espeland MA, Lipshultz LI. Evaluation of the azoospermic patient. J Urol. 1989;142:62–5.
18. Fuchs EF, Burt RA. Vasectomy reversal performed 15 years or more after vasectomy: correlation of pregnancy outcome with partner age and with pregnancy results of in vitro fertilization with intracytoplasmic sperm injection. Fertil Steril. 2002;77:516–9.

19. O'connor DB, et al. The relationships between sex hormones and sexual function in middle-aged and older European men. J Clin Endocrinol Metab. 2011;96:E1577–87.
20. Corona G, Jannini EA, Vignozzi L, Rastrelli G, Maggi M. The hormonal control of ejaculation. Nat Rev Urol. 2012;9:508.
21. Schulster M, Bernie AM, Ramasamy R. The role of estradiol in male reproductive function. Asian J Androl. 2016;18:435.
22. Finkelstein JS, et al. Gonadal steroids and body composition, strength, and sexual function in men. N Engl J Med. 2013;369:1011–22.
23. Cooke PS, Nanjappa MK, Ko C, Prins GS, Hess RA. Estrogens in male physiology. Physiol Rev. 2017;97:995.
24. Vignozzi L, et al. Estrogen mediates metabolic syndrome-induced erectile dysfunction: a study in the rabbit. J Sex Med. 2014;11:2890–902.
25. Motofei I. The etiology of premature ejaculation starting from a bihormonal model of normal sexual stimulation. Int J Impot Res. 2001;13:49.
26. Bhasin S, Cunningham GR, Hayes FJ, et al. Testosterone therapy in men with androgen deficiency syndromes: an Endocrine Society clinical practice guideline. J Clin Endocrinol Metab. 2010;95:2536–59.
27. Rosner W, Auchus RJ, Azziz R, Sluss PM, Raff H. Position statement: utility, limitations, and pitfalls in measuring testosterone: an Endocrine Society position statement. J Clin Endocrinol Metab. 2007;92:405–13.
28. Vermeulen A, Stoica T, Verdonck L. The apparent free testosterone concentration, an index of androgenicity. J Clin Endocrinol Metab. 1971;33:759–67.
29. Esteves SC, Miyaoka R, Agarwal A. An update on the clinical assessment of the infertile male. Clinics. 2011;66:691–700.
30. Oduwole OO, Peltoketo H, Huhtaniemi IT. Role of follicle-stimulating hormone in spermatogenesis. Front Endocrinol. 2018;9:763.
31. Ishikawa T, Fujioka H, Fujisawa M. Clinical and hormonal findings in testicular maturation arrest. BJU Int. 2004;94:1314–6.
32. Martin-du-Pan RC, Bischof P. Increased follicle stimulating hormone in infertile men. Is increased plasma FSH always due to damaged germinal epithelium? Hum Reprod. 1995;10:1940–5.
33. Andrade DL, Viana MC, Esteves SC. Differential diagnosis of azoospermia in men with infertility. J Clin Med. 2021;10:3144.
34. Basaria S. Male hypogonadism. Lancet. 2014;383(9924):1250–63.
35. Manni A, Partridge WM, Cefalu W, et al. Bioavailability of albumin-bound testosterone. J Clin Endocrinol Metab. 1985;62:705–10.
36. Mendel CM. Rates of dissociation of sex-steroid hormone-binding globulin: a reassessment. J Steroid Biochem Mol Biol. 1990;37:251–3.
37. Vermeulen A, Ando S. Metabolic clearance rate and interconversions of androgens and the influence of the free androgen fraction. J Clin Endocrinol Metab. 1979;48:320–6.
38. Saez JM, Forest MG, Morera AM, Bertrand J. Metabolic clearance rate and blood production rate of testosterone and dihydrotestosterone in normal subjects, during pregnancy and in hyperthyroidism. J Clin Invest. 1972;51:1226–34.
39. Khera M, Adaikan G, Buvat J, Carrier S, El-Meliegy A, Hatzimouratidis K, McCullough A, Morgentaler A, Torres LO, Salonia A. Diagnosis and treatment of testosterone deficiency: recommendations from the Fourth International Consultation for Sexual Medicine (ICSM 2015). J Sex Med. 2016;13(12):1787–804.
40. Brambilla DJ, O'Donnell AB, Matsumoto AM, McKinlay JB. Intraindividual variation in levels of serum testosterone and other reproductive and adrenal hormones in men. Clin Endocrinol. 2007;67(6):853–62.
41. Winters SJ, Kelley DE, Goodpaster B. The analog free testosterone assay: are the results clinically useful? Clin Chem. 1998;44:2176–82.

42. Wang C, Catlin DH, Demers ML, Starcevic B, Swerdloff RS. Measurement of total serum testosterone in adult men: comparison of current laboratory methods versus liquid chromatography-tandem mass spectrometry. J Clin Endocrinol Metab. 2004;89:534–43.

43. Wu FC, Tajar A, Beynon JM, et al. Identification of late-onset hypogonadism in middle-aged and elderly men. N Engl J Med. 2010;363:123–35.

44. Buvat J, Maggi M, Guay A, et al. Testosterone deficiency in men: systematic review and standard operating procedures for diagnosis and treatment. J Sex Med. 2013;10:245–84.

45. Maggi M, Buvat J. Standard operating procedures: pubertas tarda/delayed puberty—male. J Sex Med. 2013;10:285–93.

46. Buvat J, Bou JG. Significance of hypogonadism in erectile dysfunction. World J Urol. 2006;24:657–67.

47. Tuck SP, Francis RM. Testosterone, bone and osteoporosis. Front Horm Res. 2009;37:123–32.

48. Irwig MS. Male hypogonadism and skeletal health. Curr Opin Endocrinol Diabetes Obes. 2013;20:517–22.

49. Bawor M, Bami H, Dennis BB, et al. Testosterone suppression in opioid users: a systematic review and meta-analysis. Drug Alcohol Depend. 2015;149:1–9.

50. Sun YT, Irby DC, Robertson DM, et al. The effects of exogenously administered testosterone on spermatogenesis in intact and hypophysectomized rats. Endocrinology. 1989;125:1000–10.

51. McLachlan RI, O'Donnell L, Meachem SJ, et al. Hormonal regulation of spermatogenesis in primates and man: insights for development of the male hormonal contraceptive. J Androl. 2002;23:149–62.

52. Weinbauer GF, Nieschlag E. Gonadotrophin-releasing hormone analogue-induced manipulation of testicular function in the monkey. Hum Reprod. 1993;8(Suppl 2):45–50.

53. Burris AS, Clark RV, Vantman DJ, et al. A low sperm concentration does not preclude fertility in men with isolated hypogonadotropic hypogonadism after gonadotropin therapy. Fertil Steril. 1988;50:343–7.

54. Corona G, Goulis DG, Huhtaniemi I, et al. European Academy of Andrology (EAA) guidelines on investigation, treatment and monitoring of functional hypogonadism in males: endorsing organization: European Society of Endocrinology. Andrology. 2020;8:970–87.

55. Sansone A, Kliesch S, Dugas M, Sandhowe-Klaverkamp R, Isidori AM, Schlatt S, Zitzmann M. Serum concentrations of dihydrotestosterone are associated with symptoms of hypogonadism in biochemically eugonadal men. J Endocrinol Investig. 2021;44:2465–74.

56. McEwan IJ, Brinkmann AO, et al. Androgen physiology: receptor and metabolic disorders. In: Feingold KR, Anawalt B, Boyce A, et al., editors. Endotext. South Dartmouth, MA: MDText.com, Inc.; 2000–2001.

57. Adamopoulos DA, Koukkou EG. Value of FSH and inhibin-B measurements in the diagnosis of azoospermia—a clinician's overview. Int J Androl. 2010;33:e109–13.

58. Raman JD, Schlegel PN. Aromatase inhibitors for male infertility. J Urol. 2002;167:624–9.

59. Sigman M, Jarow JP. Endocrine evaluation of infertile men. Urology. 1997;50:659–64.

60. Goffin V, Binart N, Touraine P, Kelly PA. Prolactin: the new biology of an old hormone. Annu Rev Physiol. 2002;64:47–67.

61. Bancroft J. The endocrinology of sexual arousal. J Endocrinol. 2005;186:411–27.

62. Genazzani AR, Gastaldi M, Bidzinska B, et al. The brain as a target organ of gonadal steroids. Psichoneuroendocrinology. 1992;17:385–90.

63. Doherty PC, Wu DE, Matt KS. Hyperprolactinemia preferentially inhibits erectile function in adrenalectomized male rats. Life Sci. 1990;47:141–8.

64. Aoki H, Fujioka T, Matsuzaka J, Kubo T, Nakamura K, Yasuda N. Sup pression by prolactin of the electrically induced erectile response through its direct effect on the corpus cavernosum penis in the dog. J Urol. 1995;154:595–600.

65. Buvat J. Influence of primary hyperprolactinemia on human sexual behavior. Nouv Press Med. 1982;11:3561–3.

Printed by Printforce, United Kingdom